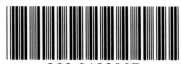

369 0123367

D1428929

Oxford Medical Publications

Oxford Textbook of
Public Health

VOLUME 1

Oxford Textbook of
Public Health

FIFTH EDITION

The scope of public health

Roger Detels

Distinguished Professor of Epidemiology and Infectious Diseases, Schools of
Public Health and Medicine, University of California, Los Angeles, Los Angeles,
California, USA

Robert Beaglehole

Professor Emeritus, University of Auckland, Auckland, New Zealand

Mary Ann Lansang

Professor of Medicine and Clinical Epidemiology, College of Medicine,
University of the Philippines, Manila, The Philippines

Martin Gulliford

Professor of Public Health, Department of Public Health Sciences,
King's College London, London, United Kingdom

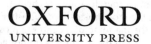

OXFORD
UNIVERSITY PRESS

OXFORD
UNIVERSITY PRESS

Great Clarendon Street, Oxford ox2 6DP

Oxford University Press is a department of the University of Oxford.
It furthers the University's objective of excellence in research, scholarship,
and education by publishing worldwide in

Oxford New York

Auckland Cape Town Dar es Salaam Hong Kong Karachi
Kuala Lumpur Madrid Melbourne Mexico City Nairobi
New Delhi Shanghai Taipei Toronto

With offices in

Argentina Austria Brazil Chile Czech Republic France Greece
Guatemala Hungary Italy Japan Poland Portugal Singapore
South Korea Switzerland Thailand Turkey Ukraine Vietnam

Oxford is a registered trademark of Oxford University Press
in the United Kingdom and in certain other countries.

Published in the United States
by Oxford University Press Inc., New York

© Oxford University Press 2009

The moral rights of the author have been asserted
Database right Oxford University Press (maker)

First edition 1984
Second edition 1991
Third edition 1997
Fourth edition 2002 (reprinted in paperback 2004, 2005 twice)
Fifth edition 2009

British Library Cataloguing in Publication Data
Data available

Library of Congress Cataloguing in Publication Data
Data available

Typeset by Cepha Imaging Pvt. Ltd., Bangalore, India
Printed by L.E.G.O.S.p.A.

ISBN 978–0–19–921870–7 (Set)
ISBN 978–0–19–957943–3 (Vol. 1)
ISBN 978–0–19–957944–0 (Vol. 2)
ISBN 978–0–19–957945–7 (Vol. 3)

1 3 5 7 9 10 8 6 4 2

Available as a set only

Oxford University Press makes no representation, express or implied, that the drug
dosages in this book are correct. Readers must therefore always check the product
information and clinical procedures with the most up-to-date published product
information and data sheets provided by the manufacturers and the most recent codes of
conduct and safety regulations. The authors and the publishers do not accept responsibility
or legal liability for any errors in the text or for the misuse or misapplication of material in
this work. Except where otherwise stated, drug dosages and recommendations are for the
non-pregnant adult who is not breastfeeding.

Preface to the fifth edition

Much has happened in the world and in the field of public health since the publication of the 4th edition of the *Oxford Textbook of Public Health*. Sudden acute respiratory syndrome (SARS) has come and gone, H5N1, H1N1 and the probability of new variant influenzas are the emerging infectious diseases of greatest concern, the health gap between rich and poor countries and within many countries has widened, HIV continues to be a major problem despite the development of effective treatments and strategies to prevent mother-to-child transmission, wars continue to be waged causing massive loss and disruption of human life and displacement of people, violence and terrorism have increased, and the epidemics of obesity and asthma have intensified. Our inability to effectively meet disasters has been demonstrated with the tsunami devastating northern Indonesia, Sri Lanka, and southern Thailand (2004), although the rapid, effective response by the Chinese to the Sichuan earthquake (2008) gives evidence that our ability to respond to natural disasters is improving.

On the positive side, the World Health Organization and member states are in the process of developing international reporting systems for emerging diseases, we have made strides in preventing chronic diseases such as cancer and heart disease (although these diseases are already a major cause of morbidity and mortality in low- and middle-income countries), polio has been eliminated in much of the world through effective new immunization strategies, and environmental pollution and global warming are now recognized as major problems and have attracted political concern—a major step in implementing effective solutions. Further, the burgeoning field of genomics holds promise of transforming both medicine and public health, but we must be concerned that it is applied to the improvement of the health of individuals and society and not used to discriminate against genetically vulnerable persons. Although private organizations have long contributed to public health, there has been a recent surge in private support of public health, particularly in the field of HIV/AIDS. While these contributions have had very positive effects on the health of people, particularly in low- and middle-income countries, they have also had unexpected impacts.

Public health continues to be a dynamic, exciting field which challenges creative thinking and demands implementation of innovative strategies. For the 5th edition of the Textbook, we have outlined these continuing and new public health problems and have recruited authors who are leaders in recognizing and addressing them. Although we have continued dividing the basic structure of the Textbook into three major topic areas, the scope of public health, the methods of public health, and the practice of public health, we have added chapters to reflect the growth and changes in the field since 2002 and the emergence of new public health strategies. Thus, we have added new chapters on management of public health disasters, collective violence including war, applications of genomics to the field of public health, gene–environment interactions, clinical epidemiology, private support of public health, and the global health agenda for the twenty-first century, among others. All other chapters have been updated, most of them by new leaders in their respective fields. Further, we have recruited public health professionals from all the major regions of the world, reflecting the global scope of public health and the textbook.

We hope that this 5th edition will contribute to the advancement of the field of public health through its presentation of the scope, concerns, strategies, and applications of the field. The Textbook is intended for public health researchers, practitioners, students of the field, and other health professionals who wish to understand the field and their opportunities for contributing to the health and well-being of the people of the world.

Roger Detels
Robert Beaglehole
Mary Ann Lansang
Martin Gulliford

Introduction to Volume 1: The scope of public health

The scope of public health is vast and ever widening. Volume 1 of the *Oxford Textbook of Public Health* provides a conceptual framework encompassing the scope of public health as it strives to cope with the enormous challenges of the twenty-first century.

Despite remarkable health gains achieved in the world over the past century, the increasing complexity of human interactions has considerably expanded public health concerns. Traditional public health approaches to epidemics have had to be redefined in the face of new global threats like severe acute respiratory syndrome (SARS) and avian influenza, as well as older microbial diseases with new biosecurity implications. The growing burden of noncommunicable diseases, the severe consequences of global warming, the repercussions of globalization, and the serious social dislocations resulting from rapid urbanization and armed conflicts have escalated the challenges to public health.

The persistence of HIV/AIDS, malaria, and tuberculosis, particularly among low- and middle-income countries, has spurred public health practitioners to utilize innovations in the fields of vaccinology, genomics, and proteomics to implement realistic solutions through sound health policies and systems strengthening, community engagement, and intersectoral partnerships. A major concern of public health is the growing recognition of the social determinants of health and the wide health disparities among nations, income groups, genders, and social classes. This concern for social justice and equity requires that public health professionals incorporate strategies from the social sciences, ethics, and human rights in the collective and organized pursuit of 'health for all'.

Volume 1 maps the breadth of public health through four updated sections: the history and development of public health, determinants of health and disease, public health policies, and public health law and ethics. Chapter 1.1 provides an overarching framework for public health and defines an expanded list of 13 functions covering the range of technology, social sciences, and politics. The next three chapters (Chapters 1.2–1.4) describe how public health has evolved in the context of rich and poor countries as well as those in economic transition, and the unique roles of the public and private sectors in addressing inequities in these different settings.

Critical to the development of interventions for public health problems is a thorough understanding of the structural and intermediary determinants of social inequities, coupled with a participative approach to address these determinants through intersectoral

policies (Chapter 2.2). Globalization can potentially aggravate health inequities; hence, the economic, social, and political processes associated with these transnational interactions must be recognized and effectively managed (Chapter 2.1). The behavioural determinants, once viewed as the dominant factors for health and disease, are discussed within an ecological frame, thus providing a more integrated view of the complex interplay of behaviour with biologic, economic, political, and environmental factors (Chapter 2.3). In Chapters 2.4–2.7, important biologic determinants are elaborated. Genetic risks, which are increasingly being understood through the Human Genome Project, as well as genome-based technologies, have a growing potential to yield important public health interventions in the future, but there are also complex behavioural, economic, and ethical concerns that must be considered (Chapter 2.4). Almost taken for granted by the developed world, but still critically inadequate in many parts of the globe, are safe water, basic sanitation, food security, and good nutrition. Chapters 2.5 and 2.6 discuss the health risks and challenges associated with their absence, shortage, or—in the case of obesity—oversupply. Chapter 2.7 reviews the major infectious diseases, which remain significant causes of ill health globally and which present new threats with the emergence of new microbial pathogens and increasing antimicrobial resistance. The risks to human health and survival posed by a variety of environmental exposures, greenhouse gas accumulation, and ozone depletion, among others, are described in Chapter 2.8 and require urgent collaborative action.

There is ample evidence to demonstrate the value of providing essential packages through quality health services in reducing risks and improving health (Chapter 2.9). By assessing the burden of disease and underlying risk factors (Chapter 2.10), it is possible to prioritize the essential health care packages and interventions that will be most cost-effective and equitable in a given population.

An understanding of health determinants must translate into effective policies and strategies for action. Many countries have responded by addressing these root causes systemically and developing mechanisms to reduce health inequities (Chapter 3.1). With few exceptions, many high-income countries have used knowledge generated from biomedical and public health research to protect and improve public health (Chapter 3.2). In contrast, multiple factors such as poor governance, inadequate financing of health care, the distortion of national health priorities vis-à-vis global health initiatives, and an inadequate evidence base for decision-making are common features of the policy environment in low- and middle-income countries (Chapter 3.3). Of paramount importance to effective policy-making is strong public health leadership at all levels, characterized by strategic thinking in addressing public health problems and the ability to engage and mobilize multiple stakeholders in the process (Chapter 3.4).

In the last section of Volume 1, Chapter 4.1 affirms the commitment of public health to achieve the 'highest attainable standard of health' and offers a rights-based approach to health (Chapter 4.1). This human right is elaborated in the context of public health legislation (Chapter 4.2) and international public health instruments (Chapter 4.3). Finally, the evolution of principles and guidelines of public health and research ethics are discussed in Chapter 4.4, with particular attention given to the principle of social justice as it relates to public health practice and research.

The extensive responsibilities and dynamic scope of public health described in this volume dictate that public health professionals employ a wide range of disciplines, seek and build intersectoral partnerships and international coalitions, and, most importantly, engage communities to achieve the goals of improving population health and promoting equity for all.

Brief Contents

Contents

List of contributors

Quarraisha Abdool Karim Columbia University (Department of Epidemiology), University of KwaZulu Natal (School of Family Medicine and Public Health) and CAPRISA (Centre for the AIDS Programme of Research in South Africa), South Africa.
Chapter 9.13 Acquired immunodeficiency syndrome

Salim S. Abdool Karim, Pro Vice Chancellor (Research), University of KwaZulu-Natal; Director, Centre for the AIDS Programme of Research in South Africa (CAPRISA); Professor in Clinical Epidemiology, Columbia University Adjunct; Professor in Medicine, Cornell University, South Africa.
Chapter 9.13 Acquired immunodeficiency syndrome

Maia Ambegaokar London School of Hygiene and Tropical Medicine, London, UK.
Chapter 3.4 Leadership in public health

Ian Anderson Professor for Indigenous Health, Centre for Health and Society & Onemda VicHealth Koori Health Unit, School of Population Health, University of Melbourne, Melbourne, Australia.
Chapter 11.5 Ethnic minorities and indigenous peoples

Roy M. Anderson Rector, Imperial College London, London, UK.
Chapter 6.16 Mathematical models of transmission and control

Samira Asma Associate Director, Global Tobacco Control, Centers for Disease Control and Prevention, USA.
Chapter 10.1 Tobacco

Gunilla Backman Senior Researcher, Human Rights Centre, University of Essex, UK.
Chapter 4.1 The right to the highest attainable standard of health

Rajiv Bahl Medical Officer, Department of Child and Adolescent Health and Development, World Health Organization, Geneva, Switzerland.
Chapter 11.3 Child health

Dean Baker Professor and Director, Center for Occupational and Environmental Health, University of California, Irvine, CA, USA.
Chapter 8.5 Occupational health

Hilary J. Bambrick Senior Lecturer, School of Medicine, University of Western Sydney, Campbelltown NSW Australia; Visiting Fellow, National Centre for Epidemiology and Population Health, The Australian National University, Canberra ACT, Australia.
Chapter 2.8 The global environment

Catherine R. Bateman School of Public Health and Community Medicine, University of New South Wales, Sydney, Australia.
Chapter 11.8 Forced migrants and other displaced populations

Robert Beaglehole Professor Emeritus, University of Auckland, Auckland, New Zealand.
Chapter 12.5 Prevention and control of chronic, non-communicable diseases

Ruth L. Berkelman Department of Epidemiology, Rollins School of Public Health, Emory University, Atlanta, GA, USA.
Chapter 6.17 Public health surveillance

Douglas Bettcher Director, Tobacco Free Initiative, World Health Organization, Geneva, Switzerland.
Chapter 4.3 International public health instruments
Chapter 10.1 Tobacco

Zulfiqar Ahmed Bhutta Husein Lalji Dewraj Professor of Pediatrics, and Chairman, Department of Pediatrics & Child Health, The Aga Khan University, Karachi, Pakistan.
Chapter 2.7 Infectious diseases

Stella Bialous President, Tobacco Policy International, San Francisco, USA.
Chapter 10.1 Tobacco

Fred Binka Dean School of Public Health, College of Health Sciences, University of Ghana, Legon, Ghana.
Chapter 5.2 Information systems and community diagnosis in low- and middle-income countries

Jennifer Bishop Department of Food Safety, Zoonoses and Foodborne Diseases, World Health Organization, Geneva, Switzerland.
Chapter 4.3 International public health instruments

Marike Boezen Unit Chronic Airway Diseases (head), Department of Epidemiology, University Medical Center Groningen, University of Groningen, Groningen, The Netherlands.
Chapter 9.4 Chronic obstructive pulmonary disease and asthma

Paolo Boffetta International Agency for Research on Cancer, Lyon, France.
Chapter 9.3 Neoplasms

Diana Bonta Vice President, Public Affairs, Kaiser Foundation Health Plans and Hospitals, Southern California Region, USA.
Chapter 7.5 Governance and management of public health programmes

Cynthia Boschi-Pinto Medical Officer, Department of Child and Adolescent Health and Development, World Health Organization, Geneva, Switzerland.
Chapter 11.3 Child health

James Bowen Center at Evergreen, Kirkland, WA, USA.
Chapter 9.10 Neurologic diseases, epidemiology, and public health

James W. Buehler Department of Epidemiology, Rollins School of Public Health, Emory University, Atlanta, GA, USA.
Chapter 6.17 Public health surveillance

Wylie Burke Professor and Chair, Department of Medical History and Ethics, University of Washington, Seattle, WA, USA.
Chapter 2.4 Genomics and public health

Jason W. Busse Assistant Professor, Department of Clinical Epidemiology & Biostatistics, McMaster University, Hamilton, Ontario, Canada; Scientist, Institute for Work & Health, Toronto, Ontario, Canada.
Chapter 6.11 Clinical epidemiology

Julie E. Byles Director, Research Centre for Gender, Health and Ageing Faculty of Health, University of Newcastle, NSW, Australia.
Chapter 11.7 Health of older people

Meredith Cagle Cagle Consulting Services.
Chapter 7.5 Governance and management of public health programmes

Simon Carroll Associate Director, Centre for Community Health Promotion Research, University of Victoria, Canada.
Chapter 7.3 Health promotion, health education, and the public's health

Margaret Chan Director General, World Health Organization, Geneva, Switzerland.
Chapter 12.14 Global health agenda for the twenty-first century

Venkatraman Chandra-Mouli Head, Adolescent Health and Development, Department of Child and Adolescent Health and Development (CAH), World Health Organization, Geneva, Switzerland.
Chapter 11.4 Adolescent health

Leda Chatzi Department of Social Medicine, Medical School, University of Crete, Heraklion, Greece.
Chapter 6.3 Cross-sectional studies

Chien-Jen Chen Academician and Distinguished Research Fellow, Genomics Research Center, Academic Sinica, National Taiwan University School of Medicine, Taipei, Taiwan.
Chapter 8.1 Environmental health issues in public health

Virasakdi Chongsuvivatwong Professor of Community Medicine, Epidemiology Unit, Faculty of Medicine, Prince of Songkla University, Hatyai, Thailand.
Chapter 12.5 Prevention and control of chronic, non-communicable diseases

Aileen Clarke Associate Clinical Professor in Public Health & Health Services Research, Health Sciences Research Institute, Warwick Medical School, University of Warwick, Coventry, UK.
Chapter 12.2 Needs assessment: A practical approach

Thomas Clasen Department of Infectious and Tropical Diseases, London School of Hygiene and Tropical Medicine, London, UK.
Chapter 2.5 Water and sanitation

Myles Cockburn Associate Professor, Department of Preventive Medicine, Keck School of Medicine; Department of Geography, College of Letters, Arts and Sciences, University of Southern California, USA.
Chapter 8.2 Radiation and public health

Bernadette Daelmans Department of Child and Adolescent Health and Development, World Health Organization, Geneva, Switzerland.
Chapter 11.3 Child health

Peter Davis Department of Sociology, University of Auckland, New Zealand.
Chapter 7.6 Public health sciences and policy in high-income countries

Manuel M. Dayrit Director, Human Resources for Health, World Health Organization, Geneva, Switzerland.
Chapter 3.4 Leadership in public health

Judith Bueno de Mesquita Senior Researcher, Human Rights Centre, University of Essex, UK.
Chapter 4.1 The right to the highest attainable standard of health

Katherine DeLand Senior Technical Officer, Tobacco Free Initiative, World Health Organization, Geneva, Switzerland.
Chapter 4.3 International public health instruments
Chapter 10.1 Tobacco

Rodolfo Dennis Head, Departments of Medicine and Research, Fundacion Cardioinfantil; Professor of Medicine, Pontificia Universidad Javeriana, Bogota, Colombia.
Chapter 6.11 Clinical epidemiology

Roger Detels Distinguished Professor of Epidemiology and Infectious Diseases, Schools of Public Health and Medicine, University of California, Los Angeles, Los Angeles, CA, USA.
Chapter 1.1 The scope and concerns of public health
Chapter 6.1 Epidemiology: The foundation of public health
Chapter 9.13 Acquired immunodeficiency syndrome
Chapter 12.13 Private support of public health

Ana V. Diez-Roux Department of Epidemiology, University of Michigan School of Public Health, Ann Arbor, MI, USA.
Chapter 6.2 Ecologic variables, ecologic studies, and multilevel studies in public health research

Allan Donner Department of Epidemiology and Biostatistics, Schulich School of Medicine and Dentistry, University of Western Ontario London, Ontario, Canada.
Chapter 6.8 Methodological issues in the design and analysis of community intervention trials

Manjit Dosanjh Advisor to the Director General, Life Sciences and International Organisations, CERN, Geneva.
Chapter 8.2 Radiation and public health

John M. Douglas, Jr Director, DSTDP, NCHHSTP, CDC, Atlanta, GA, USA.
Chapter 9.12 Sexually transmitted infections

Jeroen Douwes Associate Director, Centre for Public Health Research, Massey University Wellington Campus, Wellington, New Zealand.
Chapter 9.4 Chronic obstructive pulmonary disease and asthma

Lesley Doyal Professor of Gender and Health, School for Policy Studies, University of Bristol, Bristol, UK; Visiting Professor, University of Cape Town, South Africa.
Chapter 11.2 Women, men, and health

Shah Ebrahim Professor of Public Health, Department of Epidemiology & Population Health, London School of Hygiene and Tropical Medicine, London, UK.
Chapter 11.7 Health of older people

Matthias Egger Professor of Epidemiology and Public Health, Institute of Social & Preventive Medicine (ISPM), University of Bern, Switzerland.
Chapter 6.14 Systematic reviews and meta-analysis

Marcos Espinal Executive Secretary, Stop TB Partnership, Geneva, Switzerland.
Chapter 9.14 Tuberculosis

Daniel Ferrante World Health Organization, Geneva, Switzerland.
Chapter 10.1 Tobacco

Josep Figueras Director, European Observatory on Health Systems and Policies, Head, WHO Centre for Health Policy, Brussels.
Chapter 12.10 Strategies for health services

J. Peter Figueroa Chief, Epidemiology & AIDS, Ministry of Health, Kingston, Jamaica.
Chapter 7.7 Public health sciences and policy in low- and middle-income countries

Louise Finer Senior Researcher, Human Rights Centre, University of Essex, UK.
Chapter 4.1 The right to the highest attainable standard of health

Baruch Fischhoff Howard Heinz University Professor, Department of Social and Decision Sciences, Department of Engineering and Public Policy; Department of Social and Decision Sciences, Carnegie Mellon University, Pittsburgh, PA, USA.
Chapter 8.8 Risk perception and communication

Olivier Fontaine Department of Child and Adolescent Health and Development, World Health Organization, Geneva, Switzerland.
Chapter 11.3 Child health

Sven Francque Division of Gastroenterology and Hepatology, University Hospital Antwerp, Belgium.
Chapter 9.16 Chronic hepatitis and other liver disease

Melvyn Freeman Extraordinary Professor, University of Stellenbosch, South Africa.
Chapter 9.7 Public mental health

Julio Frenk Dean, Harvard School of Public Health, Boston, USA.
Chapter 3.3 Health policy in developing countries

Lawrence M. Friedman Independent Consultant, Rockville, MD, USA.
Chapter 6.7 Methodology of intervention trials in individuals

Fu Paul Fu, Jr. Associate Professor of Pediatrics and Public Health, David Geffen School of Medicine at UCLA, and UCLA School of Public Health, CA, USA.
Chapter 5.1 Information systems in support of public health in high-income countries

Michelle Funk Michelle Funk, Coordinator, Mental Health Policy and Service Development (MHP), Department of Mental Health and Substance Abuse, World Health Organization, Geneva, Switzerland.
Chapter 9.7 Public mental health

Gary Giovino Senior Research Scientist and Director, Tobacco Control Program, Roswell Park Cancer Institute, Buffalo, USA.
Chapter 10.1 Tobacco

Lynn R. Goldman Professor, Environmental Health Sciences, Johns Hopkins University, Bloomberg School of Public Health, Baltimore, MD, USA.
Chapter 12.8 Environmental health practice

Bernard D. Goldstein Professor, Department of Environmental and Occupational Health, University of Pittsburgh Graduate School of Public Health, Pittsburgh, PA, USA.
Chapter 8.7 Toxicology and risk assessment in the analysis and management of environmental risk

Octavio Gómez-Dantés Researcher, National Institute of Public Health, Mexico.
Chapter 3.3 Health policy in developing countries

Miguel Angel González-Block Executive Director of the Center for Health Systems Research, INSP—National Public Health Institute, Mexico.
Chapter 3.3 Health policy in developing countries

Fernando González-Martín International Health Regulations Secretariat, World Health Organization, Geneva, Switzerland.
Chapter 4.3 International public health instruments

Sherwood L. Gorbach Professor of Public Health, Medicine, and Molecular Biology/Microbiology, Tufts University School of Medicine, Boston, MA, USA.
Chapter 2.7 Infectious diseases

Lawrence W. Green Adjunct Professor, Department of Epidemiology and Biostatistics, School of Medicine, University of California at San Francisco, CA, USA.
Chapter 2.3 Behavioural determinants of health and disease

Manfred S. Green Center for the Study of Bioterrorism, Tel Aviv University, Israel Center for Disease Control, Ministry of Health, Israel.
Chapter 10.8 Public health aspects of bioterrorism

Sander Greenland Professor, Department of Epidemiology and Department of Statistics University of California, Los Angeles, CA, USA.
Chapter 6.12 Validity and bias in epidemiological research
Chapter 6.13 Causation and causal inference

Emily Grundy Centre for Population Studies, London School of Hygiene and Tropical Medicine, London, UK.
Chapter 7.2 Demography and public health

Martin Gulliford Department of Public Health Sciences, King's College London, London, UK.
Chapter 2.9 Health services as determinants of population health
Chapter 11.5 Ethnic minorities and indigenous peoples

Davidson R. Gwatkin The World Bank, Washington, DC, USA.
Chapter 12.4 Reducing health inequalities in developing countries

Davidson H. Hamer Associate Professor of International Health and Medicine, Department of International Health, Boston University School of Public Health, Department of Medicine, Boston University School of Medicine; Adjunct Associate Professor of Nutrition, Tufts University Friedman School of Nutrition Science and Policy, Boston, MA, USA.
Chapter 2.7 Infectious diseases

Christopher Hamlin Professor, Department of History, and in the Program of History and Philosophy of Science, University of Notre Dame, Notre Dame, IN, USA; Honorary Professor, Department of Public Health and Policy, London School of Hygiene and Tropical Medicine, London, UK.
Chapter 1.2 The history and development of public health in developed countries

Summer Hammide Student researcher, UCLA School of Public Health.
Chapter 4.3 International public health instruments

Marian T. Hannan Associate Professor of Medicine, Harvard Medical School, Co-Director of Musculoskeletal Research, Institute for Aging Research, Hebrew SeniorLife, Boston, MA, USA.
Chapter 9.9 Musculoskeletal diseases

Piya Hanvoravongchai Lecturer in Health Policy, Department of Public Health and Policy, London School of Hygiene and Tropical Medicine, London, UK.
Chapter 12.11 Public health workers

David Heymann Assistant Director General, Health Security and Environment, and Polio Eradication, World Health Organization, Geneva, Switzerland.
Chapter 9.17 Emerging and re-emerging infections

Robert A. Hiatt Co-Chair, Department of Epidemiology and Biostatistics, School of Medicine, University of California at San Francisco, CA, USA.
Chapter 2.3 Behavioural determinants of health and disease

Marcia Hills Professor, School of Nursing, Director, Centre for Community Health Promotion Research President, Canadian Consortium for Health Promotion Research University of Victoria, Canada.
Chapter 7.3 Health promotion, health education, and the public's health

Katherine J. Hoggatt Assistant Professor, Department of Epidemiology, University of Michigan, Ann Arbor, MI, USA.
Chapter 6.13 Causation and causal inference

Walter W. Holland Emeritus Professor of Public Health Medicine, Visiting Professor, LSE Health and Social Care, London School of Economics and Political Science, London, UK.
Chapter 3.1 Overview of policies and strategies
Chapter 12.7 Population screening and public health

T. Déirdre Hollingsworth Department of Infectious Disease Epidemiology, Faculty of Medicine, Imperial College London, London, UK.
Chapter 6.16 Mathematical models of transmission and control

Robert L. Hubbard Director, National Development and Research Institutes, Raleigh, NC, USA.
Chapter 10.2 Drug abuse

Paul Hunt UN Special Rapporteur on the right to the highest attainable standard of health (2002–2008); Professor, Human Rights Centre, University of Essex (England); Adjunct Professor, University of Waikato, New Zealand.
Chapter 4.1 The right to the highest attainable standard of health

Adnan A. Hyder Johns Hopkins University, Bloomberg School of Public Health, Department of International Health; Center for Injury Research & Policy, Baltimore, MD, USA.
Chapter 10.4 Injury prevention and control: The public health approach

Sopon Iamsirithaworn International Field Epidemiology Training Program, Bureau of Epidemiology, Department of Disease Control, Ministry of Public Health, Thailand.
Chapter 6.4 Principles of outbreak investigation

Alec Irwin Associate Director, François-Xavier Bagnoud Center for Health and Human Rights, Harvard School of Public Health, Boston, USA.
Chapter 2.2 Overview and framework

Philip James London School of Hygiene and Tropical Medicine, London, UK; International Obesity TaskForce, IASO, London, UK.
Chapter 9.5 Obesity

Dean T. Jamison Professor, Department of Global Health, University of Washington, Seattle, WA, USA.
Chapter 7.4 Cost-effectiveness analysis: Concepts and applications

Stephen Jan Senior Health Economist, The George Institute for International Health; Associate Professor, Faculty of Medicine, University of Sydney, NSW, Australia.
Chapter 12.1 Need: What is it and how do we measure it?

Don C. Des Jarlais Director of Research, Baron Edmond de Rothschild Chemical Dependency Institute, Beth Israel Medical Center, New York, NY, USA; Professor of Epidemiology and Population Health, Albert Einstein College of Medicine, Bronx, NY, USA.
Chapter 10.2 Drug abuse

Mary L. Kamb International Coordinator, Division of STD Prevention, Centers for Disease Control & Prevention (CDC), USA.
Chapter 9.12 Sexually transmitted infections

Nancy Kass Phoebe R. Berman Professor of Bioethics and Public Health, Berman Institute of Bioethics, Johns Hopkins Bloomberg School of Public Health, Baltimore, USA.
Chapter 4.4 Ethical principles and ethical issues in public health

Jennifer L. Kelsey Professor Emeritus, Stanford University School of Medicine, Department of Health Research and Policy, Stanford, CA, USA; Professor (part-time), University of Massachusetts Medical School, Departments of Medicine and of Family Medicine and Community Health, Worcester, MA, USA.
Chapter 9.9 Musculoskeletal diseases

Leeka Kheifets Professor, UCLA School of Public Health, Department of Epidemiology, Los Angeles, CA, USA.
Chapter 8.2 Radiation and public health

Rajat Khosla Senior Researcher, Human Rights Centre, University of Essex, UK.
Chapter 4.1 The right to the highest attainable standard of health

Muin J. Khoury Director, National Office of Public Health Genomics, Centers for Disease Control and Prevention, Atlanta, GA, USA.
Chapter 2.4 Genomics and public health

Robert J. Kim-Farley Professor, Departments of Epidemiology and Community Health Sciences, UCLA School of Public Health, Los Angeles, USA.
Chapter 12.6 Principles of infectious disease control

Mary Kindhauser Office of the Director General, World Health Organization, Geneva, Switzerland.
Chapter 12.14 Global health agenda for the twenty-first century

Richard S.G. Knight Professor of Clinical Neurology, National CJD Surveillance Unit, University of Edinburgh, Western General Hospital, Edinburgh, UK.
Chapter 9.11 The transmissible spongiform encephalopathies

Manolis Kogevinas Professor and co-Director, Centre for Research in Environmental Epidemiology (CREAL) Municipal Institute of Medical Research (IMIM), Barcelona, Spain.
Chapter 6.3 Cross-sectional studies

David Koh Head, Department of Community, Occupational and Family Medicine; Yong Loo Lin School of Medicine, National University of Singapore, Singapore.
Chapter 8.5 Occupational health

Dragana Korljan Human Rights Officer, Office of the High Commissioner for Human Rights.
Chapter 4.1 The right to the highest attainable standard of health

Walter A. Kukull Professor, Epidemiology, Director, Nat'l Alzheimer's Coord Ctr (NACC), Department of Epidemiology, University of Washington, Seattle, WA, USA.
Chapter 9.10 Neurologic diseases, epidemiology, and public health

Vipat Kuruchittham Lecturer, College of Public Health Sciences, Chulalongkorn University, Bangkok, Thailand.
Chapter 5.2 Information systems and community diagnosis in low- and middle-income countries

Kamakshi Lakshminarayan Assistant Professor, Department of Neurology, School of Medicine, University of Minnesota, Minneapolis, USA.
Chapter 9.2 Cardiovascular and cerebrovascular diseases

Mary Ann Lansang Professor of Medicine and Clinical Epidemiology, College of Medicine, University of the Philippines, Manila.
Chapter 7.7 Public health sciences and policy in low- and middle-income countries
Chapter 12.2 Needs assessment: A practical approach

Kelley Lee Head, Public and Environmental Health Research Unit, London School of Hygiene and Tropical Medicine, London, UK.
Chapter 2.1 Globalization

June Leung Intern, Hospital Authority, Hong Kong Special Administrative Region, People's Republic of China.
Chapter 10.1 Tobacco

Barry S. Levy Adjunct Professor of Public Health, Tufts University School of Medicine, Sherborn, MA, USA.
Chapter 10.6 Collective violence: War

Khanchit Limpakarnjanarat Communicable Disease Surveillance and Response (CSR), Department of Communicable Diseases (CDS), WHO SEARO.
Chapter 12.12 Planning for and responding to public health needs in emergencies and disasters

Annette Lin A candidate for a JD (juris doctorate) and MPH (masters of public health) joint degree at the University of California in Los Angeles, CA, USA.
Chapter 4.3 International public health instruments

Paul J. Lioy Professor and Vice Chair, Department of Environmental and Occupational Medicine, RWJMS, Deputy Director of Government Relations and Director of the Exposure Science Division of the Environmental and Occupational Health Sciences Institute (EOHSI), Robert Wood Johnson Medical School (RWJMS), UMDNJ and Rutgers University, Piscataway, NJ, USA.
Chapter 8.4 The science of human exposures to contaminants in the environment

Alexander Lo Dak Wai Solicitor, Hong Kong; Solicitor, England and Wales (non-practising); Chinese Medical Practitioner, Hong Kong; Professional Consultant, School of Law, The Chinese University of Hong Kong.
Chapter 4.2 Comparative national public health legislation

Donald Lollar Senior Research Scientist, National Center on Birth Defects and Developmental Disabilities, Centers for Disease Control and Prevention, United States Department of Health and Human Services, Atlanta, GA, USA.
Chapter 11.6 People with disabilities

A.D. Lopez School of Population Health, University of Queensland, Brisbane, Australia.
Chapter 2.10 Assessing health needs: The global burden of disease approach

Adetokunbo Lucas Adjunct Professor, Harvard University, Cambridge, MA, USA.
Chapter 3.3 Health policy in developing countries

Jeff Luck Department of Health Services, UCLA School of Public Health, CA, USA.
Chapter 5.1 Information systems in support of public health in high-income countries

Russell V. Luepker Mayo Professor, Division of Epidemiology and Community Health School of Public Health University of Minnesota, Minneapolis, USA.
Chapter 9.2 Cardiovascular and cerebrovascular diseases

Johan P. Mackenbach Department of Public Health, Erasmus MC, University Medical Centre Rotterdam, Rotterdam, The Netherlands.
Chapter 12.3 Socioeconomic inequalities in health in high-income countries: The facts and the options

Dermot Maher Senior Clinical Epidemiologist, Medical Research Council/Uganda Virus Research Institute, Entebbe, Uganda.
Chapter 9.14 Tuberculosis

Lindiwe Makubalo Chief Director, Health Information, Epidemiology, Evaluation & Research, Department of Health, South Africa.
Chapter 7.7 Public health sciences and policy in low- and middle-income countries

Zoe Marshman Clinical Lecturer in Dental Public Health School of Clinical Dentistry, Claremont Crescent, Sheffield, UK.
Chapter 9.8 Dental public health

Robyn Martin Professor of Public Health Law, Centre for Research in Primary and Community Care, University of Hertfordshire, Hatfield, UK; Visiting Professor, The Chinese University of Hong Kong; Honorary Professor, London School of Hygiene and Tropical Medicine, London, UK; Director, European Public Health Law Network.
Chapter 4.2 Comparative national public health legislation

Jose Martines Department of Child and Adolescent Health and Development, World Health Organization, Geneva, Switzerland.
Chapter 11.3 Child health

Elizabeth Mason Director Department of Child and Adolescent Health and Development (CAH), World Health Organization, Geneva, Switzerland.
Chapter 11.3 Child health

Colin Douglas Mathers Coordinator, Mortality and Burden of Disease, Department of Health Statistics and Informatics, World Health Organization, Geneva, Switzerland.
Chapter 2.10 Assessing health needs: The global burden of disease approach

Di McIntyre Professor and South African Research Chair in 'Health and Wealth', Health Economics Unit, School of Public Health and Family Medicine, University of Cape Town.
Chapter 12.1 Need: What is it and how do we measure it?

Martin McKee European Centre on Health of Societies in Transition, London School of Hygiene and Tropical Medicine, London, UK.
Chapter 12.10 Strategies for health services

Anthony J. McMichael NHMRC Australia Fellow, National Centre for Epidemiology and Population Health, The Australian National University, Canberra ACT Australia.
Chapter 2.8 The global environment

Pierre-André Michaud, Médecin chef, Unité multidisciplinaire de santé des adolescents, Lausanne, Switzerland.
Chapter 11.4 Adolescent health

Peter Michielsen, Division of Gastroenterology and Hepatology, University Hospital Antwerp, Belgium.
Chapter 9.16 Chronic hepatitis and other liver disease

Edward Mills Canada Research Chair, Global Health, Faculty of Health Sciences, University of Ottawa, Ottawa, Ontario, Canada.
Chapter 6.11 Clinical epidemiology

Mark R. Montgomery Professor of Economics, Stony Brook University; and Senior Associate, Population Council, NY, USA.
Chapter 10.7 Urban health in low- and middle-income countries

Gavin Mooney Professor of Health Economics, Department of Public Health, University of Sydney, Australia and Health Economics Unit, University of Cape Town, South Africa.
Chapter 12.1 Need: What is it and how do we measure it?

Myfanwy Morgan Professor of Sociology and Health, Department of Public Health Sciences, King's College London, London, UK.
Chapter 7.1 Sociology and psychology in public health
Chapter 11.5 Ethnic minorities and indigenous peoples

Richard Morrow Professor of International Health, Johns Hopkins Bloomberg School of Public Health, Baltimore, MD, USA.
Chapter 9.15 Malaria

William Moss Associate Professor of Epidemiology, Johns Hopkins Bloomberg School of Public Health, Baltimore, MD, USA.
Chapter 9.15 Malaria

Alvaro Muñoz Professor of Epidemiology, Johns Hopkins Bloomberg School of Public Health, Baltimore, MD, USA.
Chapter 6.6 Cohort studies

C.J.L. Murray Institute for Health Metrics and Evaluation, University of Washington, Seattle, USA.
Chapter 2.10 Assessing health needs: The global burden of disease approach

F. Javier Nieto Professor and Chair, Department of Population Health Sciences, University of Wisconsin School of Medicine and Public Health, Madison, WI, USA.
Chapter 6.6 Cohort studies

D. James Nokes KEMRI-Wellcome Trust Programme, Kilifi, Kenya; Reader, Department of Biological Sciences, University of Warwick, Coventry, UK.
Chapter 6.16 Mathematical models of transmission and control

Ellen Nolte Senior Lecturer, European Centre on Health of Societies in Transition, London School of Hygiene and Tropical Medicine, London, UK.
Chapter 12.10 Strategies for health services

Don Nutbeam Provost and Deputy Vice Chancellor, University of Sydney, NSW, Australia.
Chapter 12.9 Structures and strategies for public health intervention

Roderico H. Ofrin Technical Officer, Emergency and Humanitarian Action, WHO SEARO.
Chapter 12.12 Planning for and responding to public health needs in emergencies and disasters

Jane Ogden Professor of Health Psychology, Department of Psychology, University of Surrey, Guildford, UK.
Chapter 7.1 Sociology and psychology in public health

Lisa Oldring Special Advisor to Mary Robinson, GAVI Fund Board of Directors.
Chapter 4.1 The right to the highest attainable standard of health

Jørn Olsen Professor and Chair, Department of Epidemiology, School of Public Health, UCLA, CA, USA.
Chapter 12.5 Prevention and control of chronic, non-communicable diseases

Adrian Ong Office of the Director General, World Health Organization, Geneva, Switzerland.
Chapter 12.14 Global health agenda for the twenty-first century

Krishna M. Palipudi Senior Survey Statistician, Office on Smoking and Health, Centers for Disease Control and Prevention (CDC), Atlanta, Georgia, USA.
Chapter 10.1 Tobacco

George C. Patton VicHealth Professor of Adolescent Health, Centre for Adolescent Health, Murdoch Children's Research Institute, Melbourne, Australia.
Chapter 11.4 Adolescent health

Sarah Payne Reader in Social Policy, School for Policy Studies, University of Bristol, Bristol, UK.
Chapter 11.2 Women, men, and health

Neil Pearce Director, Centre for Public Health Research, Massey University Wellington Campus, Wellington, New Zealand.
Chapter 9.4 Chronic obstructive pulmonary disease and asthma

Corinne Peek-Asa Professor, University of Iowa, Occupational and Environmental Health, Injury Prevention Research Center, Iowa City, IA, USA.
Chapter 10.4 Injury prevention and control: The public health approach

John Powell Associate Clinical Professor of Epidemiology and Public Health, Health Sciences Research Institute, Warwick Medical School, University of Warwick, Coventry, UK.
Chapter 12.2 Needs assessment: A practical approach

John Powles Senior Lecturer in Public Health Medicine, Department of Public Health and Primary Care, Institute of Public Health, Robinson Way, Cambridge, UK.
Chapter 3.2 Public health policy in developed countries

Deborah Prothrow-Stith Professor, Harvard University School of Public Health, Boston, Mass, USA.
Chapter 10.5 Interpersonal violence prevention: A recent public health mandate

Denis J. Protti Professor, Health Information Science, Human & Social Development Building, University of Victoria, Victoria, Canada; Visiting Professor, Health Informatics, City University, London, UK.
Chapter 5.1 Information systems in support of public health in high-income countries

Laura Punnett Professor, Department of Work Environment; Director, Center to Promote Health in the New England Workplace (CPH-NEW); Senior Associate, Center for Women and Work (CWW), University of Massachusetts Lowell, MA, USA.
Chapter 8.6 Ergonomics and public health

Pekka Puska Director General, National Public Health Institute (KTL), Helsinki, Finland.
Chapter 6.9 Community-based intervention studies in high-income countries

Mario Raviglione Director, Stop TB Department, World Health Organization, Geneva, Switzerland.
Chapter 9.14 Tuberculosis

K. Srinath Reddy President, Public Health Foundation of India, New Delhi, India.
Chapter 1.4 The development of the discipline of public health in countries in economic transition: India, Brazil, China

Margaret Reid Professor of Women's Health, Public Health and Health Policy, Community Based Sciences, University of Glasgow, Glasgow, UK.
Chapter 7.1 Sociology and psychology in public health

Peter G. Robinson School of Clinical Dentistry, University of Sheffield, UK.
Chapter 9.8 Dental public health

Robin Room Professor, School of Population Health, University of Melbourne; and Director, AER Centre for Alcohol Policy Research, Turning Point Alcohol & Drug Centre, Fitzroy, Victoria, Australia.
Chapter 10.3 Alcohol

Julia Royall Chief, Office of International Programs, US National Library of Medicine, USA.
Chapter 5.3 Web-based public health information dissemination and evaluation

Jonathan Samet Professor, University of Southern California, Los Angeles, California, USA.
Chapter 10.1 Tobacco

Rodolfo Saracci Director of Research in Epidemiology, IFC-National Research Council, Pisa Italy.
Chapter 9.1 Gene–environment interactions and public health

Benedetto Saraceno Director, Department of Mental Health and Substance Abuse, Acting Director, Department of Chronic Diseases and Health Promotion, World Health Organization, Geneva, Switzerland.
Chapter 9.7 Public mental health

Jorgen Schlundt Director, Department of Food Safety, Zoonoses and Foodborne Diseases, World Health Organization, Geneva, Switzerland.
Chapter 4.3 International public health instruments

Eleanor B. Schron Program Director, National Heart, Lung, and Blood Institute, National Institutes of Health ,Bethesda, MD, USA.
Chapter 6.7 Methodology of intervention trials in individuals

John C. Scott President, Center for Public Service Communications, Arlington, Virginia, USA.
Chapter 5.3 Web-based public health information dissemination and evaluation

Than Sein Director, Noncommunicable Diseases and Mental Health, World Health Organization, Regional Office for Southeast Asia, New Delhi, India.
Chapter 1.3 The history and development of public health in low- and middle-income countries

Shira Shafir Department of Epidemiology, School of Public Health, UCLA, CA, USA.
Chapter 8.3 Control of microbial threats: Population surveillance, vaccine studies, and the microbiological laboratory

Prakash S. Shetty Professor of Public Health Nutrition, Institute of Human Nutrition, School of Medicine, University of Southampton, Southampton, UK.
Chapter 2.6 Food and nutrition

Daniel Shouval Liver Unit, Hadassah-Hebrew University Hospital, Jerusalem, Israel.
Chapter 9.16 Chronic hepatitis and other liver disease

Victor W. Sidel Distinguished University Professor of Social Medicine, Montefiore Medical Center and the Albert Einstein College of Medicine, Bronx, NY, USA; Adjunct Professor of Public Health at Weill Medical College of Cornell University in New York City, NY, USA.
Chapter 10.6 Collective violence: War

Elliot R. Siegel Associate Director for Health Information Programs Development, US National Library of Medicine, US National Institutes of Health, US Department of Health and Human Services, Bethesda, MD, USA.
Chapter 5.3 Web-based public health information dissemination and evaluation

Chitr Sitthi-Amorn Professor and Senior Consultant, College of Public Health Sciences, Chulalongkorn University, Bangkok, Thailand.
Chapter 5.2 Information systems and community diagnosis in low- and middle-income countries

George Davey Smith Professor of Clinical Epidemiology, Department of Social Medicine, University of Bristol, UK.
Chapter 6.14 Systematic reviews and meta-analysis

Ian Smith Office of the Director General, World Health Organization, Geneva, Switzerland.
Chapter 12.14 Global health agenda for the twenty-first century

Orielle Solar Ministry of Health, Chile; and World Health Organization, Geneva, Switzerland.
Chapter 2.2 Overview and framework

Frank Sorvillo Department of Epidemiology, School of Public Health, UCLA, CA, USA.
Chapter 8.3 Control of microbial threats: Population surveillance, vaccine studies, and the microbiological laboratory

Jonathan Sterne Professor of Medical Statistics and Epidemiology, Department of Social Medicine, University of Bristol, UK.
Chapter 6.14 Systematic reviews and meta-analysis

Alison Stewart Principal Associate, Foundation for Genomics and Population Health, Cambridge, UK.
Chapter 2.4 Genomics and public health

Allison Streetly Programme Director, NHS Sickle Cell and Thalassaemia Screening Programme, Department of Public Health Sciences, King's College London, London, UK.
Chapter 12.7 Population screening and public health

Steven Sugden The Hygiene Centre, Department of Infectious and Tropical Diseases, London School of Hygiene and Tropical Medicine, London, UK.
Chapter 2.5 Water and sanitation

Patrick S. Sullivan Department of Epidemiology, Rollins School of Public Health, Emory University, Atlanta, GA, USA.
Chapter 6.17 Public health surveillance

Sheena G. Sullivan National Center for AIDS/STD Control and Prevention, Chinese Center for Disease Control and Prevention, Beijing China; Edith Cowan University, Perth, Australia.
Chapter 6.10 Community-based intervention trials in low- and middle-income countries
Chapter 12.13 Private support of public health

Julien O. Teitler Associate Professor of Social Work and Sociology, Columbia University, New York, NY, USA.
Chapter 11.1 The changing family

Tim Tenbensel School of Population Health, University of Auckland, New Zealand.
Chapter 7.6 Public health sciences and policy in high-income countries

Puja Thakker Research Associate, Public Health Foundation of India, New Delhi, India.
Chapter 1.4 The development of the discipline of public health in countries in economic transition: India, Brazil, China

Elma B. Torres Director, Health Safety and Environmental Management Consultancy Services, Inc., Philippines.
Chapter 12.8 Environmental health practice

Peter Tugwell Canada Research Chair in Health Equity; Director, Centre for Global health, Institute of Population Health, University of Ottawa, Canada.
Chapter 6.11 Clinical epidemiology

Kumnuan Ungchusak Director, Bureau of Epidemiology and International Health Regulation (IHR) Focal point Department of Diseases Control, Ministry of Public Health, Thailand.
Chapter 6.4 Principles of outbreak investigation

Nigel Unwin Professor of Epidemiology, Institute of Health and Society, Newcastle University, UK.
Chapter 9.6 The epidemiology and prevention of diabetes mellitus

Pierre van Damme Centre for the Evaluation of Vaccination, Vaccine & Infectious Disease Institute, University of Antwerp, Belgium.
Chapter 9.16 Chronic hepatitis and other liver disease

Koen Van Herck Centre for the Evaluation of Vaccination, Vaccine & Infectious Disease Institute, University of Antwerp, Belgium.
Chapter 9.16 Chronic hepatitis and other liver disease

Erkki Vartiainen Director, Department of Health Promotion and Chronic Disease Prevention, Helsinki, Finland.
Chapter 6.9 Community-based intervention studies in high-income countries

Carlo La Vecchia Head, Laboratory of General Epidemiology, Istituto di Ricerche Farmacologiche 'Mario Negri', Milano, Italy.
Chapter 9.3 Neoplasms

Jeanette Vega Vice Minister of Health, Chile.
Chapter 2.2 Overview and framework

Gemma Vestal World Health Organization, Geneva, Switzerland.
Chapter 10.1 Tobacco

Paolo Vineis Chair in Environmental Epidemiology, Imperial College London, UK.
Chapter 9.1 Gene–environment interactions and public health

Hester J.T. Ward Consultant in Epidemiology and Public Health, National CJD Surveillance Unit, University of Edinburgh, Western General Hospital, Edinburgh, UK.
Chapter 9.11 The transmissible spongiform encephalopathies

Noel S. Weiss School of Public Health and Community Medicine, University of Washington, WA, USA.
Chapter 6.5 Case–control studies

Vivian Welch Institute of Population Health, University of Ottawa, Ottawa, Canada.
Chapter 6.11 Clinical epidemiology

Suwit Wibulpolprasert Senior Advisor on Disease Control, Ministry of Public Health, Thailand.
Chapter 12.11 Public health workers

Gail Williams School of Population Health, Faculty of Health Sciences, University of Queensland, Australia.
Chapter 6.15 Statistical methods

Marilyn Wise School of Public Health, University of Sydney, NSW, Australia.
Chapter 12.9 Structures and strategies for public health intervention

Fred B. Wood Office of Health Information Programs Development, US National Library of Medicine, US National Institutes of Health, Bethesda, MD, USA.
Chapter 5.3 Web-based public health information dissemination and evaluation

Zunyou Wu Director, National Center for AIDS/STD Control and Prevention, Chinese Center for Disease Control and Prevention, Beijing, China.
Chapter 6.10 Community-based intervention trials in low- and middle-income countries

Derek Yach Vice-President, Global Health Policy, PepsiCo Foundation, USA.
Chapter 10.1 Tobacco

Gonghuan Yang Deputy Director, China Center for Disease Prevention and Control, Beijing, China.
Chapter 10.1 Tobacco

Ron Zimmern Executive Director, Foundation for Genomics and Population Health, Cambridge, UK.
Chapter 2.4 Genomics and public health

Paul Zimmet Director Emeritus and Director of International Research, Baker IDI Heart and Diabetes Institute, Melbourne Australia.
Chapter 9.6 The epidemiology and prevention of diabetes mellitus

Anthony B. Zwi School of Public Health and Community Medicine, University of New South Wales, Sydney, Australia.
Chapter 11.8 Forced migrants and other displaced populations

SECTION 1

The development of the discipline of public health

1.1

The scope and concerns of public health

Roger Detels

Abstract

Public health is the art and science of preventing disease, prolonging life, and promoting health through the organized efforts of society. The goal of public health is the biologic, physical, and mental well-being of all members of society. Thus, unlike medicine, which focuses on the health of the individual patient, public health focuses on the health of the public in the aggregate. To achieve this broad, challenging goal, public health professionals engage in a wide range of functions involving technology, social sciences, and politics. Public health professionals utilize these functions to anticipate and prevent future problems, identify current problems, identify appropriate strategies to resolve these problems, implement these strategies, and finally, evaluate their effectiveness.

In this chapter, we introduce the reader to the scope and current major concerns of public health as we enter the twenty-first century, giving examples of each. It is the goal of the chapter to assist the readers in understanding the conceptual framework of the field, which will help them in placing the subsequent more detailed chapters in the context of the entire field of public health.

Introduction

There have been many definitions and explanations of public health. The definition offered by the Acheson Report (Acheson 1988) has been widely accepted:

Public health is the science and art of preventing disease, prolonging life, and promoting health through the organized efforts of society.

This definition underscores the broad scope of public health and the fact that public health is the result of society's efforts as a whole, rather than that of single individuals.

In 2003, Detels defined the goal of public health as:

The biologic, physical, and mental well-being of all members of society regardless of gender, wealth, ethnicity, sexual orientation, country, or political views.

This definition or goal emphasizes equity and the range of public health interests as encompassing not just the physical and biologic, but also the mental well-being of society. Both the World Health Organization (WHO) and Detels' goals or definitions depict public health as being concerned with more than merely the elimination of disease.

To achieve the WHO goal of 'health for all', it is essential to bring to bear many diverse disciplines to the attainment of optimal health, including the physical, biologic, and social sciences. The field of public health has adapted and applied these disciplines for the elimination and control of disease, and the promotion of health.

Functions of public health

To accomplish its task of ensuring the well-being of the population, public health must perform a wide range of functions, which are listed in Table 1.1.1. The primary functions are to prevent disease and injuries and to promote healthy lifestyles and good health habits; but in order to succeed in these two objectives, public health must perform additional functions.

Public health *identifies*, *measures*, and *monitors* community health needs through surveillance of disease and risk factors (e.g. smoking) trends. Analysis of these trends and the existence of a functioning health information system provides the essential information for predicting or anticipating future community health needs.

In order to ensure the health of the population, it is necessary to *formulate*, *promote*, and *enforce* sound health policies to prevent and control disease and to reduce the prevalence of factors impairing the health of the community. These include policies requiring reporting of highly transmissible diseases and health threats to the community and control of environmental threats through the regulation of environmental hazards (e.g. water and air quality standards and smoking). It is important to recognize that influencing politics, particularly in a democracy, is an essential function of public health.

There are limited resources that can be devoted to public health and the assurance of high-quality health services. Thus, an essential function of public health is to effectively *plan*, *manage*, and *administer cost-effective health services*, and to ensure their availability to all segments of society.

In every society, there are *health inequalities* that limit the ability of some members to achieve their maximum ability to function.

Table 1.1.1 Functions of public health

1.	Prevent disease and injuries.
2.	Promote healthy lifestyles and good health habits.
3.	Identify, measure, monitor, and anticipate community health needs.
4.	Formulate, promote, and enforce essential health policies.
5.	Organize and ensure high-quality, cost-effective public health and health-care services.
6.	Reduce health disparities and ensure access to health care for all.
7.	Promote and protect a healthy environment.
8.	Disseminate health information and mobilize communities to take appropriate action.
9.	Plan and prepare for natural and man-made disasters.
10.	Reduce interpersonal violence and aggressive war.
11.	Conduct research and evaluate health-promoting/disease-preventing strategies.
12.	Develop new methodologies for research and evaluation.
13.	Train and ensure a competent public health workforce.

Source: Adapted from Office of the Director, National Public Health Performance Standards Program. *10 essential public health services*. [Online]. Centers for Disease Control; 1994. (Available from: http://www.cdc.gov/od/ocphp/nphpsp/EssentialPHServices.htm) and Pan American Health Organization. *Essential public health services*. [Online]. 2002. (Available from: http://www.sopha.cpha.ca/english/ephf_e.html)

Although these disparities primarily affect the poor, minority, rural, and remote populations and the vulnerable, they also impact on society as a whole, particularly in regard to infectious and/or transmissible diseases. Thus, there is not only an ethical imperative to reduce health disparities, but also a pragmatic rationale.

Technological advances and increasing commerce have done much to improve the quality of life, but these advances have come at a high cost to the environment. In many cities of both the developed and developing world, the poor quality of air—contaminated by industry and commerce—has affected the respiratory health of the population, and has threatened to change the climate, with disastrous consequences. We have only one world. If we do not take care of it, we will ultimately have difficulty living in it. Through education of the public, formulation of sound regulations, and influencing policy, public health must restore and monitor the environment to *ensure that the population can live in a healthy environment.*

To ensure that each individual in the population functions to his or her maximum capacity, public health needs to *educate the public and stimulate the community* to take appropriate actions towards the optimal conditions for the health of the public. Ultimately, public health cannot succeed without the support and active involvement of the community.

We cannot predict, and rarely can we prevent, the occurrence of natural and man-made disasters, but we can prepare for them to ensure that the resulting damage is minimized. Thus, *disaster preparedness* is an essential component of public health, whether the disaster is an epidemic such as influenza or the occurrence of typhoons.

Unfortunately, in the modern world, interpersonal *violence and war* have become common. In some segments of society (particularly among adolescent and young adult minority males), violence

has become the leading cause of death and productive years of life lost. Public health cannot ignore that violence and wars are major factors dramatically reducing the quality of life for millions.

Many of the advances in public health have become possible through *research*. Research will continue to be essential for identifying health problems and the optimal strategies for confronting public health problems. Strategies that seem very logical may, in fact, not succeed for a variety of unforeseen reasons. Therefore, public health systems and programmes cannot be assumed to function cost-effectively without continuous monitoring and evaluation. Thus, it is essential that new public health strategies undergo rigorous evaluation before being scaled up, and once scaled up, periodically reviewed to ensure their continuing effectiveness.

Over the last century, the quality of research has been enhanced by the *development of new methodologies*, particularly in the fields of epidemiology, biostatistics, and laboratory sciences. The development of the computer has increased our ability to analyse massive amounts of data, and to use multiple strategies to aid in the interpretation of data. As new technologies continue to be developed, it is essential that public health continues to use these new technologies to develop more sophisticated research strategies in order to address public health issues.

The quality of public health is dependent on the competence and vision of the public health *workforce*. Thus, it is an essential function of public health to *ensure the continuing availability of a well-trained, competent workforce* at all levels, including leaders with the vision essential to ensure the continued well-being of society and the implementation of innovative, effective public health measures.

Contemporary health issues

Underlying almost all the pubic health problems of the world is the issue of poverty. More than half of the world's population lives below the internationally defined poverty line. Although the majority of the world's poor live in developing countries, there are many poor living in the wealthiest countries of the world—underscoring the disparity of wealth between developed and developing countries as well as between the poor and the rich in all countries. Unfortunately, the disparity between the rich and the poor is increasing, not only within countries, but also between rich and poor countries. It is incumbent on public health to reduce these disparities to ensure that all members of the global society share in a healthy quality of life.

The twentieth century witnessed the transition of major disease burdens, defined by death, from infectious and/or communicable diseases to chronic diseases (Table 1.1.2). In 1900, the leading cause of death in the United States and other developed countries was reported to be pneumonia and influenza. By the end of the century, diseases of the heart were the leading cause of death, and pneumonia and influenza dropped to the seventh place, primarily affecting the elderly. Commensurately, the average lifespan increased significantly, compounding the problems introduced by population growth. The reduction in communicable diseases was not primarily due to the development of better treatments, although vaccines played an important role in the second half of the twentieth century, but through public efforts to reduce crowding and improve housing, improve nutrition, and provide clean water and safe disposal of wastes.

By 1980, many leading public health figures felt that infectious diseases had been eliminated as a primary concern for public

Table 1.1.2 Leading causes of death in the United States (1900, 1950, 1990, 1997, 2001)

	1900	1950	1990	1997	2001
Diseases of the heart	167	307	152	131	248
Malignant neoplasms	81	125	135	126	196
Cerebrovascular disease	134	89	28	26	58
Chronic obstructive lung diseases	—	4	20	13	44
Motor vehicle injuries	—	23	19	16	15
Diabetes mellitus	13	14	12	13	25
Pneumonia and influenza	210	26	14	13	22
HIV infection	—	—	10	6	5
Suicide	11	11	12	11	10
Homicide and legal intervention	1	5	10	8	7

Values expressed as rates per 100 000, age-adjusted.
Source: Updated from McGinnis JM, Foege WH. Actual causes of death in the United States. *Journal of the American Medical Association* 1993; **270**:2007–12 and Department of Health and Human Services, National Center for Health Statistics *Health, United States, 1999*. Washington (DC): US Government Printing Office; 1999.

health; however, the discovery and expanding pandemic of acquired immunodeficiency syndrome (AIDS) caused by the human immunodeficiency virus (HIV) in the early 1980s, and subsequently, sudden acute respiratory syndrome (SARS) outbreaks in the late 1990s demonstrated the fallacy of their thinking. Although infectious and/or communicable diseases persist as a major public health concern, globally, even in poor, developing countries, chronic

diseases have become a major health problem. In fact, 74 per cent of the deaths due to non-communicable or chronic diseases at the beginning of the twenty-first century occurred in developing countries. This, of course, reflects that the majority of the world's population lives in developing countries with limited resources and incomes. Communicable diseases, however, still accounted for 30 per cent of the deaths worldwide in 2005 (Fig. 1.1.1). This statistic is particularly disturbing, as the majority of the communicable diseases are now preventable through vaccines, improved sanitation, behavioural interventions, and better standards of living.

An essential step in defining health is to identify appropriate methods for measuring it. Traditionally, public health has defined disease in terms of mortality rates because they are relatively easy to obtain and death is indisputable. The use of mortality rates, however, places the greatest emphasis on diseases that end life, and tends to ignore those which compromise function and quality of life without causing death. Thus, the problems of mental illnesses, accidents, and disabling conditions are seriously underestimated if one uses only mortality to define health.

Two other strategies to measure health that evolved in the last half of the twentieth century have been 'years of productive life lost' (YPLL) (Lopez *et al.* 2006) and 'disability-adjusted life years' (DALYs) (Murray & Lopez 1995). The former emphasizes those diseases that reduce the productive lifespan (currently arbitrarily defined as 75 years), whereas the latter emphasizes those diseases that compromise function but also includes a measure of premature mortality. Using either of these alternatives to define health results in very different orderings of diseases and/or health problems as public health priorities (Fig. 1.1.1).

Using death to identify disease priorities, the leading cause is chronic diseases, which account for 61 per cent of the diseases worldwide (Fig. 1.1.1). Among the chronic diseases, cardiovascular diseases account for almost half (49 per cent) of the deaths.

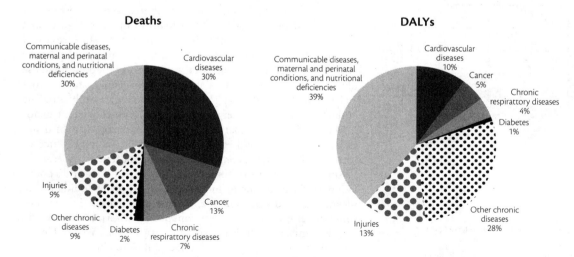

Fig. 1.1.1 Main causes of death and global burden of disease (DALYs) in the world for all ages, projections for 2005.
Source: World Health Organization. *Preventing chronic diseases: A vital investment*. [Online]. 2005. Available from: http://whqlibdoc.who.int/publications/2005/9241563001_eng.pdf.

The proportion, however, varies markedly by regions of the world and level of affluence of the countries. Communicable diseases remain the major cause of death only in Africa, although they account for a significant proportion of deaths in Southeast Asia and the eastern Mediterranean (Figs 1.1.2 A and B). The major victims of these communicable diseases are infants and children under five. The persistence of communicable diseases in these areas represents a major public health challenge.

DALYs and YPLL may be considered as better measures of the quality of life and functioning capacity of a country than mortality. Using DALYs to establish global disease priorities emphasizes communicable diseases and injuries, which tend to disproportionately affect the young, and reduces the relative importance of cardiovascular diseases and other chronic diseases that primarily affect the elderly (Fig. 1.1.1). The WHO has projected that the ranking of total DALYs for neuropsychiatric disorders, injuries, and noncommunicable and/or chronic diseases will increase by 2020,

whereas the ranking for communicable diseases other than HIV/AIDS will decline (Figs 1.1.3A–D) (Mathers & Loncar 2006). Communicable diseases, which currently account for 40 per cent of the DALYS, are expected to decline to 30 per cent by 2030 (Mathers & Loncar 2006).

On the other hand, according to projections by the WHO, HIV, tuberculosis, and malaria (currently major communicable disease problems globally) will account for an even greater number of YPLL per 1000 population by 2030, whereas other communicable diseases will yield to intervention efforts and account for progressively fewer YPLL (Fig. 1.1.4). The YPLL per 1000 population due to chronic diseases that tend to affect older people, however, is projected to remain constant, perhaps reflecting the optimism regarding the development of strategies for earlier diagnosis and better drugs to sustain life with these conditions.

Communicable diseases

The WHO's regional offices working with individual countries have conducted intensive immunization programmes against the major preventable infectious diseases of childhood, but there are significant barriers to complete coverage, including poverty, geographic obstacles, low levels of education, civil unrest and wars, and mistrust of governments. Poverty, weak governments, and misuse of funds have also prevented the control of disease vectors, provision of clean water, and safe disposal of sanitation, all essential for the control of communicable diseases. Another major factor in the rapid spread of communicable diseases has been the rapid growth in transportation. It is now possible for an individual with a communicable disease to circumnavigate the globe while still infectious and asymptomatic. Thus, cases of SARS were reported throughout Southeast Asia and as far as Canada within weeks of the recognition of the first cases in Hong Kong (Lee 2003).

Another source of communicable diseases is the continuing emergence of new infectious agents, many of them adapting to humans from animal sources. Figure 1.1.5 identifies new disease outbreaks from 1981 to 2003, including newly drug-resistant variants of new diseases occurring worldwide. Changes in food production, crowding of animals, mixing of live animal species in 'wet markets' in Asia and elsewhere, and the introduction of hormones and antibiotics into feed have all contributed to the emergence of these new diseases. Table 1.1.3 lists many of the new diseases that have been recognized since 1980. In addition to the diseases listed in this table, antibiotic-resistant strains of known agents have emerged rapidly due, in part, to the widespread inappropriate use of antibiotics. Thus, resistant strains of gonorrhoea, staphylococcus, tuberculosis, and malaria have become major problems. The latter two have now emerged as two of the three current major infectious disease problems globally. The development of drug-resistant malaria has been compounded by the emergence of vectors resistant to the commonly used chemical insecticides.

Approximately one billion people, one sixth of the world's population, suffer from one or more tropical disease, including Buruli ulcer, Chagas' disease, cholera, dengue, dracunculiasis, trypanosomiasis, leishmaniasis, leprosy, lymphatic filariasis, onchocerciasis, schistosomiasis, helminthiasis, and trachoma (World Health Organization 2006). The functional ability of those who suffer from one or more of these diseases is severely compromised, in turn affecting the ability of the poorest countries, which suffer the greatest burden of these tropical diseases, to compete in the

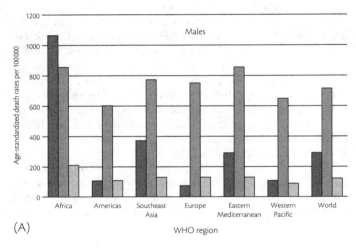

(A)

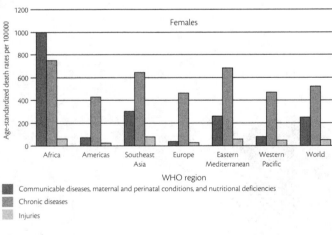

(B)

Fig. 1.1.2 Projected main caused of death by WHO region for all ages, 2005: (A) males and (B) females.
Source: World Health Organization. Main causes of death and global burden of disease (DALYs), world, all ages, projections for 2005. [Online]. Available from: http://www.who.int/chp/chronic_disease_report/contents/part2.pdf [accessed 2007 May].

Income group	Rank	Disease or injury	Per cent of total deaths
Worldwide	1	Ischaemic heart disease	13.4
	2	Cerebrovascular disease	10.6
	3	HIV/AIDS	8.9
	4	COPD	7.8
	5	Lower respiratory infections	3.5
	6	Trachea, bronchus, lung cancers	3.1
	7	Diabetes mettitus	3.0
	8	Road traffic accidents	2.9
	9	Perinatal conditions	2.2
	10	Stomach cancer	1.9
High-income countries	1	Ischaemic heart disease	15.8
	2	Cerebrovascular disease	9.0
	3	Trachea, bronchus, lung cancers	5.1
	4	Diabetes mellitus	4.8
	5	COPD	4.1
	6	Lower respiratory infections	3.6
	7	Alzheimer's and other dementias	3.6
	8	Colon and rectum cancers	3.3
	9	Stomach cancer	1.9
	10	Prostate cancer	1.8
Middle-income countries	1	Cerebrovascular disease	14.4
	2	Ischaemic heart disease	12.7
	3	COPD	12.0
	4	HIV/AIDS	6.2
	5	Trachea, bronchus, lung cancers	4.3
	6	Diabetes mellitus	3.7
	7	Stomach cancer	3.4
	8	Hypertensive heart disease	2.7
	9	Road traffic accidents	2.5
	10	Liver cancers	2.2
Low-income countries	1	Ischaemic heart disease	13.4
	2	HIV/AIDS	13.2
	3	Cerebrovascular disease	8.2
	4	COPD	5.5
	5	Lower respiratory infections	5.1
	6	Perinatal conditions	3.9
	7	Road traffic accidents	3.7
	8	Diarrhoeal diseases	2.3
	9	Diabetes mellitus	2.2
	10	Malaria	1.8

Fig. 1.1.3A Ten leading causes of death by income group (baseline scenario), 2030.
Source: Mathers CD, Loncar D. Projections of global mortality and burden of disease from 2002 to 2030. *PLoS Medicine* 2006;**3**(11):e442. Available from: http://medicine.plosjournals.org/perlserv/?request=slideshow&type=table&doi=10.1371/journal.pmed.0030442&id=9665 [accessed 2007 May].

world marketplace. However, major strides have been achieved in reducing the burden of diseases such as leprosy, guinea worm disease, and lymphatic filariasis. Continuing efforts are needed to further reduce the burden of these and other tropical diseases.

We now recognize that we will continue to see new human pathogens emerging in the future, and need to be prepared to contain them. Table 1.1.4 lists the factors that contribute to the emergence of these new agents and disease threats. Unless the world faces the consequences of changing the environment in which we live, newly emerging diseases will continue to plague us.

Chronic diseases

With the increasing control of communicable diseases and the increasing lifespan, chronic diseases have emerged as the major global health problem in both developed and developing countries. Even in developing countries, chronic diseases have assumed greater importance. The prevalence of type 2 diabetes in rural India is 13.2 per cent (Chow & Raju 2006). Cardiovascular diseases have become a major cause of death in China. Eighty-seven per cent of stroke deaths occur in low- and/or middle-income countries (Lopez *et al.* 2007).

The causes of chronic diseases are many and complex (Fig. 1.1.6). Although the immediate causes are factors such as increasing blood pressure, increasing blood glucose, abnormal lipids and fat deposition, and diabetes, the underlying causes are behavioural and social. These behavioural factors include unhealthy diets that substitute pre-packaged and fast foods high in fats for a balanced diet, physical inactivity, and tobacco use; these in turn are the products of social change, including globalization, urbanization, and aging. Some chronic diseases have been associated with infectious disease agents. For example, *Chlamydia pneumoniae* has been implicated in the development of atherosclerosis (Kuo & Campbell 2000), and hepatitis C as a leading cause of hepatocellular (liver) cancer.

Another aspect of chronic diseases is the increasing survival of compromised individuals who would not otherwise have survived, many of whom are handicapped. These individuals require modified environments to experience a reasonable quality of life and to realize their full potential in order to contribute to society.

Most chronic diseases can be reduced by a combination of healthy behaviours, including not smoking, moderate alcohol use, and exercise (Breslow & Breslow 1993). Many developed countries have been promoting healthy lifestyles, but there is need for greater

Group	Cause	Average annual change (per cent) in age-standardized death rate	
		Males	Females
All causes		−0.8	−1.1
Group I		−1.4	−1.9
	Tuberculosis	−5.4	−5.3
	HIV/AIDS	3.0	2.1
	Malaria	−1.3	−1.5
	Other infectious diseases	−3.4	−3.3
	Respiratory infections	−2.7	−3.4
	Perinatal conditions[a]	−1.7	−1.9
	Other Group I	−3.0	−3.6
Group II		0.0	−0.8
	Cancer	−0.2	−0.4
	Lung cancer	0.1	0.3
	Diabetes mellitus	1.1	1.3
	Cardiovascular diseases	−1.1	−1.2
	Respiratory diseases	0.3	−0.1
	Digestive diseases	−1.3	−1.7
	Other Group II	−0.7	−1.1
Group III		0.0	−0.2
	Unintentional injuries	−0.2	−0.2
	Road traffic accidents	1.1	1.1
	Intentional injuries	0.2	−0.2
	Self-inflicted injuries	−0.3	−0.4
	Violence	0.4	0.2

[a]Causes arising in the perinatal period as defined in the ICD, principally prematurity and birth asphyxiz, and does not include all deaths occurring in the neonatal period (under 1 mo).
DOI: 10.1371/journal.pmed.0030442.t001

Fig. 1.1.3B Projected global tobacco-caused deaths (baseline scenario), by cause, 2015.
Source: Mathers C.D., Loncar D. Projections of global mortality and burden of disease from 2002 to 2030. *PLoS Medicine* 2006;**3**(11):e442. Available from: http://medicine.plosjournals.org/perlserv/?request=slideshow&type=table&doi=10.1371/journal.pmed.0030442&id=9667 [accessed May 2007].

Category	Disease or injury	2002 rank	2030 ranks	Change in rank
Within top 15	Perinatal conditions	1	5	−4
	Lower respiratory infections	2	8	−6
	HIV/AIDS	3	1	+2
	Unipolar depressive disorders	4	2	+2
	Diarrhoeal diseases	5	12	−7
	Ischaemic heart disease	6	3	+3
	Cerebrovascular disease	7	6	+1
	Road traffic accidents	8	4	+4
	Malaria	9	15	−6
	Tuberculosis	10	25	−15
	COPD	11	7	+4
	Congenital anomalies	12	20	−8
	Hearing loss, adult onset	13	9	+4
	Cataracts	14	10	+4
	Violence	15	13	+2
Outside top 15	Self-inflected injuries	17	14	+3
	Diabetes mellitus	20	11	+9

Fig. 1.1.3C Changes in rankings for 15 leading causes of DALYs (baseline scenario), 2002 and 2030.
Source: Mathers C.D., Loncar D. Projections of global mortality and burden of disease from 2002 to 2030. *PLoS Medicine* 2006;**3**(11):e442. Available from: http://medicine.plosjournals.org/perlserv/?request=slideshow&type=table&doi=10.1371/journal.pmed.0030442&id=9669.

emphasis and development of these programmes in developing countries, where the major global burden of chronic diseases occurs.

Mental illness

Public health professionals have only relatively recently recognized the need to address the mental health needs of society on a global scale, partly due to the difficulties in defining it. It is now estimated that 10 per cent of the world's population suffers from mental illness at any given time, and that mental illness represents 12 per cent of the global burden of disease. Mortality rates seriously underestimate the burden of mental health on society. Mental illness accounts for 31 per cent of DALYs, a better measure of its impact on society (Murray & Lopez 1995). However, the true extent of mental illness is probably greater—only 73 per cent of the countries have a formal mental health reporting system, and only 57 per cent have done epidemiologic studies or have data collection systems for documenting mental illness (World Health Organization 2001).

Income group	Rank	Disease or injury	Per cent of total DALYs
Worldwide	1	HIV/AIDS	12.1
	2	Unipolar depressive disorders	5.7
	3	Ischaemic heart disease	4.7
	4	Road traffic accidents	4.2
	5	Perinatal conditions	4.0
	6	Cerebrovascular disease	3.9
	7	COPD	3.1
	8	Lower respiratory infections	3.0
	9	Hearing loss, adult onset	2.5
	10	Cataracts	2.5
High-income countries	1	Unipolar depressive disorders	9.8
	2	Ischaemic heart disease	5.9
	3	Alzheimer and other dementias	5.8
	4	Alcohol use disorders	4.7
	5	Diabetes mellitus	4.5
	6	Cerebrovascular disease	4.5
	7	Hearing loss, adult onset	4.1
	8	Trachea, bronchus, lung cancers	3.0
	9	Osteoarthritis	2.9
	10	COPD	2.5
Middle-income countries	1	HIV/AIDS	9.8
	2	Unipolar depressive disorders	6.7
	3	Cerebrovascular disease	6.0
	4	Ischaemic heart disease	4.7
	5	COPD	4.7
	6	Road traffic accidents	4.0
	7	Violence	2.9
	8	Vision disorders, age-related	2.9
	9	Hearing loss, adult onset	2.9
	10	Diabetes mellitus	2.6
Low-income countries	1	HIV/AIDS	14.6
	2	Perinatal conditions	5.8
	3	Unipolar depressive disorders	4.7
	4	Road traffic accidents	4.6
	5	Ischaemic heart disease	4.5
	6	Lower respiratory infections	4.4
	7	Diarrhoeal diseases	2.8
	8	Cerebrovascular disease	2.8
	9	Diabetes mellitus	2.8
	10	Malaria	2.5

Fig. 1.1.3D Ten leading causes of DALYs by income group and sex (baseline scenario), 2030.
Source: Mathers C.D., Loncar D. Projections of global mortality and burden of disease from 2002 to 2030. *PLoS Medicine* 2006;**3**(11):e442. Available from: http://medicine.plosjournals.org/perlserv/?request=slideshow&type=table&doi=10.1371/journal.pmed.0030442&id=9671 [accessed 2007 May].

Global provisions for treatment of mental illness are still significantly below what is necessary to adequately address the problem. Although 87 per cent of the world's governments offer some mental health services at the primary-care level, 30 per cent of them have no relevant programme and 28 per cent have no budget specifically identified for mental health. Mental illness robs society of a significant number of potentially productive persons. With the diminishing proportion of productive people of working age and the increasing proportion of elderly dependants, it is important to assist those who are not productive because of mental illness to become healthy, productive members of society.

Population changes

Although the rate of growth of the world's population has slowed in the latter half of the twentieth century, the world's population, currently over 6.5 billion people, is estimated to grow to 9 billion by 2050 (Fig. 1.1.7) (United States Census Bureau 2006). The growth in the population will be mostly among the elderly and the old elderly (those over 80 years of age). By 2050, at least 30 per cent of the population in most developed countries and in China will be over 65 years of age (Fig. 1.1.8). In the United States, the number of elderly is expected to double over the next 30 years. Because women survive longer, the majority of the elderly will be women. The gender ratio (M:F) for the world's population was 101.4 in 2007, but is estimated to be 101.3 by 2010. However, among those 80 years and over, the ratio was 56.3 in 2007 and is estimated to be 57.3 by 2010.

Currently, one of the major problems facing the world is the deterioration of the environment caused by the increasing numbers of people and the accumulation of wastes produced by them, their vehicles, and the industries they support. Thus, the quality of the air that we breathe has declined, especially in developing countries, where increased economic output has come at the expense of the environment. The most polluted cities of the world are concentrated in developing countries, which have the least capacity and political will to reduce pollutants. Pollution of the world's oceans, which receive massive amounts of biological and chemical wastes annually, affects not only the quality of the water but also the ability of the ocean to sustain marine life, an important source of food.

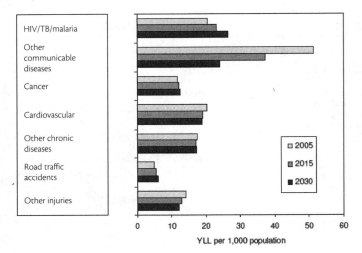

Fig. 1.1.4 Trends in global years of life lost (YLL) per 1000 population, by broad cause group and income group, 2002–2030 (2005).
Source: Mathers C.D., Loncar D. *Updated projections of global mortality and burden of disease, 2002–2030: data sources, methods and results.* Geneva: World Health Organization; 2005. Available from: http://www.who.int/healthinfo/statistics/bodprojections2030/en/index.html [accessed 2007 May].

As the population grows, there is increasing pressure to provide food, water, and other necessities to maintain a high quality of life. Fertile farmlands are increasingly being converted to residential areas. Thus, more people need to be supported on less land. Will agricultural efficiency grow at a rate commensurate with population growth? Will we be able to find alternative fuel sources when oil and other natural resources are depleted? Will we be able to provide sufficient water to sustain populations and agriculture, currently a major global problem?

The well-being of society is dependent on the ratio of those who produce to those who are dependent. The fact that the majority of the population growth in the coming decades will be among the old and old elderly, not through increasing birth rates, will result in a diminishing proportion of producers and an increasing proportion of dependants. In 2000, the proportion of the world's population who were 60 years and over was 10 per cent; by 2050, it will be 50 per cent. This will be further exacerbated because the majority of the oldest elderly will be single women who traditionally have more limited resources and lower levels of education, particularly in developing countries. Thus, the productivity and efficiency of those who produce must increase if we are to sustain or improve the quality of life for all. Improved technology and strategies will be required to increase worker productivity.

The occurrence of disease in old age is directly correlated with unhealthy behaviours developed in early life. Unfortunately, concurrent with population growth, there has been a worldwide epidemic of obesity and decreased physical activity, which has increased the proportion of elderly who suffer from chronic debilitating diseases in both the developed and developing world. Thus, unless efforts to promote health lifestyles are successful, not only will there be an increase in the proportion of elderly, but also an increasing proportion of them will require supportive care, placing a further economic burden on society.

Other public health issues

Oral health

Good dental health is essential for maintaining adequate nutrition and a healthy quality of life. However, it was estimated that in 2004 there was an average of 1.6 decayed, missing, or filled teeth (DMFT) among children 12 years old globally (WHO Oral Health Program 2004). The number of DMFT ranged from a low of 0.3 in Togo and Rwanda to 6.3 per 12-year-old in Martinique. The percentage of

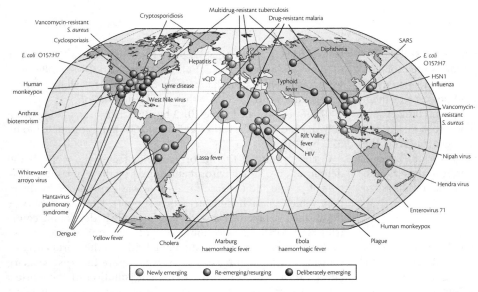

Fig. 1.1.5 Emerging and re-emerging disease worldwide, 1981–2003.
Source: Morens D.M., Folkers G.K., Fauci A.S. *Nature* 2004; **430**:242–9. Updated and reproduced with permission of A. Fauci [2007 June].

Table 1.1.3 Newly identified infectious diseases and pathogens

Year	Disease/pathogen
2004	Avian influenza (human cases)
2003	SARS
1999	Nipah virus
1997	H5N1 (avian influenza A virus)
1996	New variant Creutzfelt-Jacob disease; Australian bat lyssavirus
1995	Human herpes virus 8 (Kaposi's sarcoma virus)
1994	Savia virus; Hendra virus
1993	Hanta virus pulmonary syndrome (Sin Nombre virus)
1992	*Vibrio cholerae* O139
1991	Guanarito virus
1989	Hepatitis C
1988	Hepatitis E; human herpes virus 6
1983	HIV
1982	*Escherichia coli* O157:H7; Lyme borreliosis; human T-lymphotropic virus type 2
1980	Human T-lymphotropic virus

Source: World Health Organization. Workshop presentation by David Heymann. Geneva: World Health Organization; 1999.

adults in the United Kingdom with total tooth loss in 1998 was 13 per cent, and increased with decreasing social class (Table 1.1.5) and education (Fig. 1.1.9). These high rates of DMFT and tooth loss reflect poor dental hygiene and preventive care (Pine & Harris 2007). Unfortunately, many people believe that dental care is an expendable luxury, and that visits to dentists are only necessary when there is a problem. Poor dental hygiene is probably a major reason for the 119 730 cases of oral cancer worldwide in 2000, and why the five-year prevalence of oral cancer is estimated to be 6.8 per cent globally (WHO Oral Health Program 2004). Even in Western Europe, the five-year prevalence of oral cancer was estimated at almost 50 000 cases (WHO Oral Health Program 2004). Clearly the public health message regarding the importance of good dental hygiene, regular tooth brushing, and regular dental check ups is not reaching the majority of the people.

Injuries

Injuries and violence caused 9 per cent of all deaths and 12 per cent of the global burden of diseases in 2002, accounting for 5.2 million deaths (World Health Organization 2004). Deaths due to injuries are almost three times greater in developing than in developed countries. However, most of the injuries do not cause death, but may result in disability. Furthermore, they occur more commonly among younger persons and children.

Injuries can be broadly categorized in the following groups: motor vehicle accidents, suicide, homicide, and other unintentional injuries, including occupational injuries and falls. Motor vehicle accidents account for the largest proportion of deaths due to injury (Fig. 1.1.10); globally, they were the sixth leading cause of death in

2001, and the third leading cause of YPLL lost in the United States in 2000. The WHO projects that motor vehicle accidents will become the third highest cause of DALYs globally by 2020. Falls, particularly among the elderly, are a major cause of DALYs, and ranked thirteenth globally in 1999 according to the WHO.

Occupational injuries are another major cause of death and DALYs. Globally, over 350 000 deaths and 270 million injuries are currently attributable to occupation-related factors annually. The burden is greater in developing countries, where the drive to produce goods cheaply has been given greater importance than providing a safe work environment.

Homicide, violence, and suicide

Homicide, violence, and suicide represent a growing problem, particularly among the young. Homicide and suicide are among the top ten leading causes of death in the United States. In some minority groups in the United States, homicide and violence are the leading cause of death of youth, followed by suicide. In China, suicide remains the leading cause of death among women in rural areas. Globally, the WHO predicts that homicide and suicide will account for an increasing proportion of deaths. Unfortunately, the WHO predicts that by 2020, war will become the sixth leading cause of DALYs, violence the twelfth, and self-inflicted injuries the fourteenth.

Unintentional injuries are largely preventable through community and governmental intervention. Thus, improved roads, separation of different modes of transportation, enactment, and enforcement of seat belt and helmet laws, and improved designs of ladders and other equipment and tools have all been shown to significantly reduce injuries and deaths due to accidents. Stronger emphasis on a safer work environment, especially in developing countries, will significantly reduce both injuries and the severity of injuries that occur in the workplace.

Vulnerable populations

Public health has always been concerned with the health and well-being of vulnerable groups who require special attention. The definition of a vulnerable population and who constitute a vulnerable population varies by time, situation, and culture, but the common characteristic across all vulnerable groups is their susceptibility to adverse health and poor quality of life. Often, they live at the margins of society and have difficulty accomplishing the basic functions of living and accessing healthcare. Thus, they require assistance. In many societies, particularly in developing countries, the family acts as the safety net for these groups; but if the family itself is vulnerable, this safety net is absent. Societies with resources have developed social support programmes that assist the vulnerable, but these programmes seldom cover the full range of vulnerable groups, and may not adequately support those whom they target. Universal healthcare is one component of assisting the vulnerable, but presently, even in rich, developed countries such as the United States, healthcare is not available to all, and strategies to fund universal healthcare are difficult to implement.

The list of vulnerable groups includes the poor, minorities, women, children, the elderly, the handicapped, the illiterate, orphans and street children, immigrants, refugees and displaced people, the homeless, and the mentally ill. In certain situations, other groups may be considered vulnerable. For example, in the face of epidemics such as HIV/AIDS, one could also consider adolescents to be a vulnerable group.

Table 1.1.4 Factors contributing to the emergence or re-emergence of infectious diseases

1.	Human 'demographic change' by which persons begin to live in previously uninhabited remote areas of the world and are exposed to new environmental sources of infectious agents, insects, and animals.
2.	Breakdowns of sanitary and other public health measures in overcrowded cities and in situations of civil unrest and war.
3.	Economic development and changes in the use of land, including deforestation, reforestation, and urbanization.
4.	Climate changes cause changes in geography of agents and vectors.
5.	Changing human behaviours, such as increased use of child-care facilities, sexual and drug-use behaviours, and patterns of outdoor recreation.
6.	Social inequality.
7.	International travel and commerce that quickly transport people and goods vast distances.
8.	Changes in food processing and handling, including foods prepared from many different animals and transported great distances.
9.	Evolution of pathogenic infectious agents by which they may infect new hosts, produce toxins, or adapt by responding to changes in the host immunity (e.g. influenza, HIV).
10.	Development of resistance of infectious agents such as *Mycobacterium tuberculosis* and *Neisseria gonorrhoeae* to chemoprophylactic or chemotherapeutic medicines.
11.	Resistance of the vectors of vector-borne infectious diseases to pesticides.
12.	Immunosuppression of persons due to medical treatments or new diseases that result in infectious diseases caused by agents not usually pathogenic in healthy hosts (e.g. leukaemia patients).
13.	Deterioration in surveillance systems for infectious diseases, including laboratory support, to detect new or emerging disease problems at an early stage.
14.	Illiteracy limits knowledge of prevention strategies.
15.	Lack of political will—corruption, other priorities.
16.	Biowarfare/bioterrorism—an unfortunate potential source of new or emerging disease threats (e.g. anthrax and letters).
17.	War, civil unrest—creates refugees, food and housing shortages, increased density of living, etc.
18.	Famine.

In almost every country, developed or developing, there are homeless people, many of whom suffer from multiple problems, including mental illness. Complicating the ability of many vulnerable groups, including the homeless, mentally ill, alcoholics, and drug addicts, to achieve good health and to function adequately are poverty, prejudice, and stigmatization by society. Thus, we not only need programmes to assist the vulnerable, but also to encourage society to take action to assist them in realizing their maximum potential.

Complicating the issue of vulnerable groups is the fact that the specific problems and needs of each of these groups are different, and thus require differing specific public health action. For some of these groups, such as mothers and children and the handicapped,

there are well-established programmes, although coverage is far from complete and the quality of these programmes varies widely. For others, such as the illiterate and migrants, there are fewer established programmes. If we are to meet the public health goal of 'Health for All', we need to identify and assist the vulnerable groups within societies to achieve their maximum possible health and function.

The environment

Environmental health comprises those aspects of human health, including quality of life, that are determined by physical, chemical, biological, social, and psychosocial processes in the environment. (WHO)

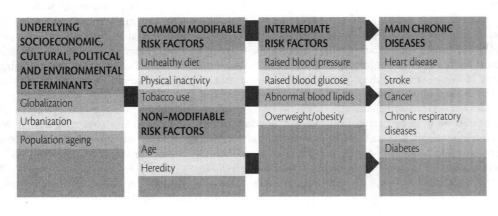

Fig. 1.1.6 Causes of chronic diseases. *Source*: World Health Organization. Main causes of death and global burden of disease (DALYs), world, all ages, projections for 2005. [Online]. Available from: http://www.who.int/chp/chronic_disease_report/contents/part2.pdf [accessed 2007 May].

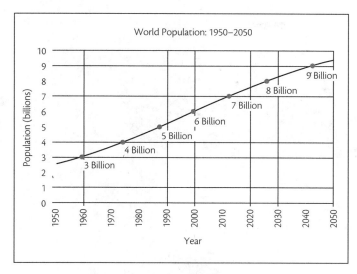

Fig. 1.1.7 World population, 1950–2050.
Source: United States Census Bureau. *International database.* [Online]. 2006 Aug. Available from: http://www.census.gov/ipc/www/idbnew.html [accessed 2007 May].

The number of known chemicals globally exceeds 14 million, of which over 60 000 are commonly used. All of these ultimately end up in the environment. They are the result of the huge proliferation of industry, technology, and automobiles in the twentieth century. Murray and Lopez (1996) have estimated that 1 379 238 DALYs are caused annually by environmental exposures. As we enter the twenty-first century, the number of pollutants will continue to increase.

Problems of the environment occur at the personal level (at home and the workplace), the community level (air and water pollution), and globally (global warming, hazardous and radioactive waste). Although these problems may be viewed separately, they are in fact all global issues affecting both local and remote populations. Thus, air pollution caused by slash-and-burn cultures in Sumatra severely affects the health of residents of Singapore and Malaysia. Industrial pollutants released in the industrial states of Northeastern United States cause acid rain, which adversely affects crops and people in the Midwestern United States and southern Canada. Pollution of rivers upstream can adversely affect communities and countries downstream, as happened in 2005 when nitrobenzene was released into the Songhua River in Heilongjiang, China, contaminating drinking water downriver in both China and Siberia, Russia.

Air pollution

The rapid increase in automobiles and industry has caused widespread air pollution in most urban areas of the world, the worst occurring in the developing countries, which have rapidly industrialized at the expense of their environment. Now, in the early part of the twenty-first century, many of these countries are realizing the need to protect the environment. Unfortunately, reversal of decades of pollution is far more difficult and costly than prevention.

The harmful effects of air pollution extend beyond the environment. Many members of society, including asthmatics and persons with chronic respiratory disease, are vulnerable to even relatively low levels of pollutants. Studies of the urban air in Southern

California have demonstrated that children chronically exposed to high levels of both primary pollutants and photochemical oxidants have decreased lung function (Detels *et al.* 1979). Recent studies have demonstrated that children living near freeways in Southern California also suffer long-term lung damage (Gauderman *et al.* 2007). Levels of pollutants observed in many developing countries, especially in China and India, are considerably higher than in developed countries, but few studies have documented the cost of these high levels of pollutants to the health of children, as well as adults, in these countries. Thus, the true cost of uncontrolled industrialization in these countries is not known.

Water pollution

Those who live in developed countries take the provision of safe drinking water for granted, but 40 per cent of the world's population does not have access to clean drinking water, a basic necessity of life. As the world population expands, the production of waste increases, and the problem of protecting water supplies also increases. Approximately 60 per cent of the world does not have adequate facilities for waste disposal. Even in leading cities in developed countries, pollution of the water supply occurs, as happened in Milwaukee, Wisconsin, when cryptosporidia contaminated the water supply, causing severe illness and death, especially in vulnerable populations compromised by immune deficiency disorders (MacKenzie *et al.* 1994). The increased rate of upper respiratory infections and gastrointestinal disorders among surfers and others using the ocean for recreational purposes has been well documented. Beaches in most urban areas are frequently closed when the sewage disposal systems become overwhelmed. Acid rain from industrialization has caused acidification of lakes, making them inhospitable for fish and other marine life, thus compromising the food supply. Recently there has been discussion about whether the benefits of omega-3 fatty acids found in fish outweigh the risk of mercury poisoning among those who eat large quantities of fish. Ensuring a safe, adequate water supply for people in both developed and developing countries must become a public health priority.

Other pollutants

As the population of the world rapidly increases and technology produces new substances and processes, not only the amount of pollutants, but also the varieties of pollutants increases. As new substances are developed, their use should not be permitted until plans and provisions have been developed and implemented for their safe disposal. This seldom happens!

Biodegradable pollutants have a limited lifespan in the environment, but we are increasingly producing non-biodegradable substances such as plastics, which are now ubiquitous, and hazardous materials such as radioactive wastes that persist for generations. It is likely that the amount of these hazardous substances will increase as natural energy sources are exhausted by the burgeoning and increasingly affluent population. The problem of discarding these waste products safely has become a major public health issue. Developed countries are now paying developing countries to accept their hazardous waste products. This strategy does not solve the problem, but shifts it to those countries that have fewer resources with which to deal with the problem, thus solving a local problem but creating a global problem! A major public health issue of the twenty-first century will be global warming due to the release of carbon dioxide and other 'greenhouse gases'.

2000

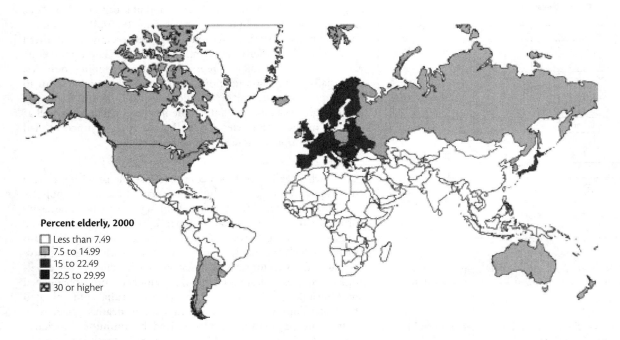

Percent elderly, 2000
☐ Less than 7.49
▨ 7.5 to 14.99
■ 15 to 22.49
■ 22.5 to 29.99
▨ 30 or higher

2050

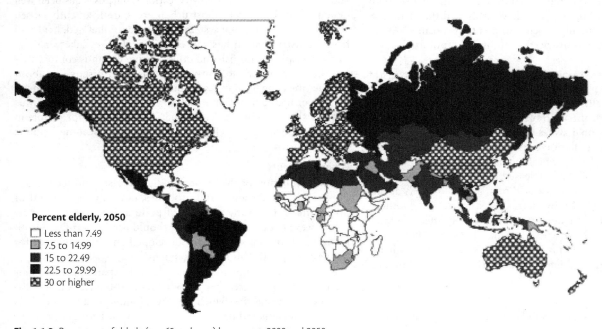

Percent elderly, 2050
☐ Less than 7.49
▨ 7.5 to 14.99
■ 15 to 22.49
■ 22.5 to 29.99
▨ 30 or higher

Fig. 1.1.8 Percentage of elderly (age 65 and over) by country, 2000 and 2050.
Source: Kaneda T. Percentage of elderly (ages 65 and over) by country, 2000 and 2050. [Online]. Population Reference Bureau.
Available from: http://www.prb.org/Articles/2006/iticalWindowforPolicymakingonPopulationAginginDevelopingCountries.
aspx [accessed 2007 May].
United Nations Population Division, *World Population Prospects: The 2004 Revision* (New York: United Nations, 2005).

Rescuing the environment

The key to rescuing the environment is to induce the political will of the countries of the world to take steps towards reversing and preventing further degradation of the environment. Global warming represents an example of these problems. The United States is the major producer of carbon dioxide and other greenhouse gases responsible for global warming, yet it is one of the few countries unwilling to sign the treaty on global warming! In order to induce the political will to protect the environment and public health globally, political leaders will need to collaborate with other countries

Table 1.1.5 Percentages of adults with total tooth loss in the United Kingdom for different age, gender, and social class groups in 1978, 1988, and 1998

	1978	1988	1998
Age (years)			
25–34	4	1	0
35–44	13	4	1
45–54	32	17	6
55–64	50	37	20
65 and over	79	67	45
All ages	30	21	13
Gender			
Male	25	16	10
Female	33	25	15
Both	30	21	13
Social class of head of household			
I, II, III NM (skilled non-manual)	22	15	8
III M (skilled manual)	29	24	15
IV, V (unskilled)	38	32	22
All	30	21	13

Source: Walker and Cooper (eds), 2000; Todd and Lader, 1991
Petersen PE. Inequalities in oral health: the social context for oral health. In: *Community oral health*. 2nd ed. London: Quintessence Publishing; 2007. p. 38.

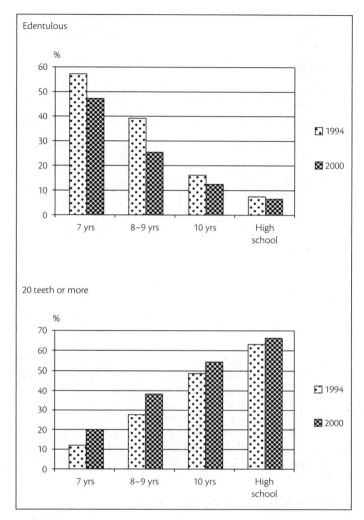

Fig. 1.1.9 Percentages of interviewed elderly (65 years or more) who reported being edentulous or having at least 20 teeth present in relation to number of years having attended school and year of study.
Source: Petersen PE. Inequalities in oral health: the social context for oral health. In: *Community oral health*. 2nd ed. London: Quintessence Publishing; 2007. p. 39.

to confront cultural norms, strong economic interests (e.g. industry), and current attitudes of much of the world's population. Regulations will need to be promulgated and implemented, which, out of necessity, will compromise the current lifestyle of much of the world's population. It is unlikely that risk from environmental pollution and hazardous waste can be reduced to zero. Thus, the concept of 'acceptable risk' will be a part of the process. Determining the level of acceptable risk might not be a scientific process, but a political one in which public health must play a strong role.

Occupational health

Occupational diseases are different from other diseases, not biologically, but socially. (Henry Sigerist 1958)

In 1999, Dr. Jukke Takala, Chief of the International Labour Organization's Health and Safety Programme, estimated that there were 1.1 million work-related deaths, 250 million work-related injuries, and 160 million cases of occupational disease annually worldwide (International Labour Organization 1999). Twelve million of these serious injuries occurred among young workers. This is more people than those who have myocardial infarcts (heart attacks), strokes, or newly diagnosed malignancies annually. A significant proportion of these deaths and injuries are preventable by improving safety in the workplace. However, safeguarding the worker is often given less priority than the need to produce cheap goods, especially in developing countries.

The nature of the workplace is constantly changing, with increasing proportions of workers being involved in communications and services rather than production of goods. Increasingly, the production of goods is moving from developed countries to developing countries, where labour costs are cheaper and safety regulations are fewer. Increasingly, women are entering the workforce and must juggle work and family. Because the costs of healthcare are rising more rapidly than the cost of living, industry is seeking relief from providing healthcare benefits, and healthcare is increasingly not provided as part of the employment package. Shifting from a formal full-time workforce to an informal part-time workforce is one strategy for reducing labour costs. Thus, the informal part-time workforce, not usually able to receive work-related benefits, now represents 50 per cent or more of the workforce globally. This segment of the workforce is particularly vulnerable to injury and limited access to healthcare.

As noted earlier, the population is aging, and the proportion of the population that produces is diminishing. In response to this

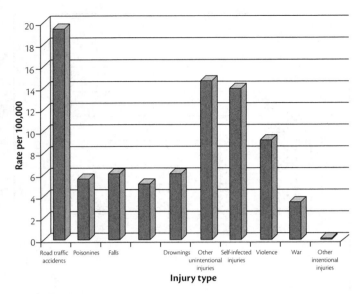

Fig. 1.1.10 Global injury DALY rates per 1 000 000 population, 2001. *Source*: Merson M.H., Black R.E., Mills J.E., editors. *International public health*. 2nd ed. Sudsbury [MA]: Jones & Bartlett; 2006. p. 326.

change, the age of eligibility for social security benefits in the United States is increasing, and mandatory retirement is being phased out. It is now projected that the proportion of workers over the age of 60 will increase to 20 per cent in Japan and 10 per cent in the United States by 2030 (Population Projections 2000). The needs of older workers are different from those of younger workers. Thus, the changing nature of the workforce will require changes in work safety regulations and health benefits to ensure a healthy, productive workforce.

Provision of and access to healthcare

Access to preventive and curative care is a requirement for health in every society, whether rich or poor. Access to healthcare has long been a problem for the poor and for rural residents, especially in developing countries. However, in the United States, access to healthcare is even a problem for the middle class. Health insurance is prohibitively expensive and beyond the reach of many in the middle class, unless it is subsidized by the employers. Increasingly, employers are attempting to free themselves from the cost of health insurance for their employees through a variety of strategies. Thus, the proportion of those without healthcare is likely to increase. The elderly also have problems with healthcare; because healthcare costs increase with age, insurance companies are less willing to cover the elderly, and many governments, even in developed countries, do not provide adequate support for the elderly. In developing countries, the rural poor are particularly at risk. Few health professionals are willing to work in rural areas, and the cost of providing care in less populated areas is greater than in urban areas. Innovative strategies are needed to ensure that the rural poor and elderly have access to reasonable healthcare.

Bioterrorism and war

Bioterrorism has been used as a weapon for hundreds of years. In the middle ages, corpses of plague victims were catapulted into castles under siege. Recently, anthrax was used to contaminate the

US postal system, resulting in several deaths. There has been a sharp increase in terrorist activities in this century. The WHO and public health agencies of individual countries have developed plans to quickly diagnose and control bioterrorist incidents. These threats to the health of the public will continue until we address the underlying causes of terrorism and bioterrorism.

Few actions can have the magnitude of negative impact on the health of the public that war has. Men, women, and children are killed, homes are destroyed, major segments of the population become displaced refugees, and the social and/or economic fabric of the countries involved is destroyed. Recovery usually takes years to decades. The outside world, particularly those countries adjacent to warring nations, must cope with the huge influx of displaced persons, and action needs to be implemented to help those still in the country suffering from the impact of the war. In many cases, the so-called rationale for the aggressive action is spurious. One suspects that had the billions of dollars that were spent on the wars in Iraq, Vietnam, and Afghanistan been put into humanitarian and public health support, it would probably have achieved a greater goal and more goodwill, not only on the part of the nations involved, but globally. The world must find a better way to resolve international conflicts.

Ethics in public health

Although ethics is implicit in the delivery of public health, it was only after the Second World War and the recognition that 'scientific experiments' in Nazi Germany violated human rights that an emphasis was placed on recognizing the ethics of public health actions, particularly research. The Declaration of Helsinki (World Medical Association 2002), the Belmont Report (US National Commission for the Protection of Human Subjects of Biomedical and Behavioral Research 1978), and the Council for International Organizations of Medical Science (CIOMS 2002) have promulgated ethical guidelines for research and the establishment of institutional review boards worldwide to ensure that medical and/or public health research is conducted ethically and does not violate human rights. However, there are inherent ethical conflicts in many public health actions. For example, the human rights of 'typhoid Mary', a typhoid carrier who insisted on working as a cook, were violated when she was incarcerated to prevent her from preparing food that initiated epidemics. Protecting the human rights of a man to refuse testing for HIV may result in his unknowingly infecting his wife, yet-to-be-born children, and other sexual contacts. By protecting his human rights, the human rights of his wife or partner and future family will be violated.

Implementing public health programmes and research often results in ethical conflicts and the need to balance the good of society against potential harm to the individual. It is usually necessary to inform society, particularly those who will be involved in the public programme or research, about the nature of the ethical conflicts inherent in action. For example, a trial evaluating the effectiveness of prophylactic treatment to prevent HIV infection in sex workers in Cambodia was stopped by the prime minister, who felt that the prevention trial exploited Cambodian sex workers. A more intense effort on the part of the researchers to inform the public and politicians about the nature of the study and the potential benefit to sex workers, not only in Cambodia but everywhere, might have averted this unfortunate outcome.

Public health interventions

One important task of public health professionals is to raise the level of anxiety of the public about public health problems to the level at which they will be willing to take an appropriate action. Raising the level of anxiety efficiently will result in inadequate or no action. On the other hand, raising the level too high will promote a fatalistic attitude and, as in the case of the recent HIV/AIDS epidemic, may promote stigmatization and isolation of affected individuals, seriously complicating the task of intervention. The difficulty for the public health professional is creating the level of anxiety that results in the required action.

Public health interventions can be divided into four categories: social/biologic/environmental, behavioural, political, and structural. The public health professional must use strategies in all four categories to achieve the maximum health of the public.

Social, biologic, and/or environmental interventions

The strategy that has had the greatest impact on improving the health of the public has been an improved standard of living, including provision of clean water and safe disposal of wastes. Unfortunately, these interventions have not reached much of the world where crowding, unsafe and insufficient water, and accumulation of wastes, and a lack of economic development persist.

The most cost-effective biologic intervention strategy is immunization, in part because it requires minimal behavioural change and usually only a single action. The WHO has taken the lead in promoting vaccine coverage worldwide through its Expanded Programme on Immunization. The appropriate use of vaccines has virtually eliminated the majority of childhood infections from the developed countries and significantly reduced them in most developing countries. Smallpox, a major infectious disease problem until the latter half of the twentieth century, has now been eliminated. We are well on our way to eliminating polio, but more challenges, such as hepatitis and tuberculosis, remain. Next may be measles. However, it is important to realize that development and production of a vaccine is only the first step. An effective vaccine against smallpox was available for over 150 years before smallpox was eliminated. The key was the strategy of vaccine coverage, 'search and contain', that permitted global elimination of the disease. Thus, the strategy for utilizing the vaccine is perhaps equally important as the efficacy of the vaccine itself.

Another biologic strategy is to eliminate the vectors of disease, the major approach currently in use for the control of dengue, arboviral diseases, and many of the parasitic diseases. However, overzealous use of pesticides can also create problems. For example, dichloro-diphenyl-trichloroethane (DDT), used widely in the twentieth century as an insecticide, still contaminates the food supply, creating other health problems, including the risk of malignancy.

Treatment can also be considered a biologic intervention strategy. To confront tuberculosis, one of the major infectious diseases of the twenty-first century, directly observed treatment short course (DOTS) has been successfully implemented in countries where the disease persists. Treatment of sexually transmitted infections and contacts is a major strategy for control of transmission, but has yet to prove effective in stopping the current epidemic.

Behavioural interventions

Most public health interventions depend ultimately on behaviour, whether it is personal or community behaviour. At the personal or individual level, promotion of good health habits and avoidance of smoking, excess alcohol use, and other dependency disorders are important interventions that have a major impact on health. At the community level, attitudes towards acceptable sexual behaviour and persons with dependency disorders and stigmatizing diseases are key to establishing community 'norms' that promote a healthy lifestyle and include all segments of society. However, modifying individual behaviour and community norms is difficult; it is even more difficult to ensure persistence of the modified behaviour. Yet, the majority of the public health interventions will not be successful unless they are embraced and sustained by the community at the local, national, and international levels. The success of the antismoking campaigns in the United States and Britain and population control in China (the one-child policy) affirm that it is possible to change community norms.

Many theories identifying strategies to modify behaviour have been proposed. One of the most interesting is the Popular Opinion Leader model proposed by Jeffrey Kelly (2004), which utilizes the natural leaders found in any social group as agents of change. In the United States, this strategy has been demonstrated to change behaviour in groups of men who have sex with men, and is now being evaluated in other populations worldwide.

Political interventions

Public health *is* politics. Any process that involves obtaining the support of the public will involve politics and differing points of view. For example, the campaign to stop smoking was strongly opposed by the tobacco industry, which spent millions of dollars trying to counter the many reports on the adverse health effects of smoking. Countering the efforts of the tobacco industry required obtaining the political support of the public in order to pass laws and regulations limiting smoking, placing health warnings on cigarette packages, and raising taxes on cigarettes.

If we are to succeed in safeguarding the oceans, inland waters, and the air we breathe, it will be through the political process. This process has already begun in many of the developed countries, which have passed strong laws regulating the emissions from automobiles and factories. Now this process must be expanded to the developing countries, where the worst pollution is currently occurring.

One of the most urgent issues before the public today is the battle over emission of 'greenhouse gases', which are causing a rise in temperatures globally. This temperature rise will adversely affect the quality of life of our children, grandchildren, and their grandchildren. Unfortunately, we have not yet achieved the political will to take the necessary steps to reverse this detrimental warming trend. The United States, the richest, most politically powerful nation in the world, even refuses to sign an international treaty signed by many other nations to address this problem.

It is important that the political process to improve the health of the public be based on sound scientific evidence. Pushing agendas not based on sound scientific evidence will undermine the credibility of public health professionals and our ability to accomplish our legitimate goals. Obtaining this evidence is not always easy. For example, accumulating evidence on the long-term (induction period of years to decades) impact of adverse exposures is not easily established, and often requires extrapolation from data on the impact of acute high-dose exposures to lower doses. This often requires relying on models, which are difficult for the public to understand, and are often subject to debate within the scientific community.

Structural interventions

The end result of the political process is the passage of laws and regulations. This action, if implemented, can have a very significant impact on the improvement of the health of the public. For example, the law reducing the maximum speed in California from 65 to 55 miles per hour had a significant impact on lowering the automobile fatality rate; unfortunately, this lower speed limit has been reversed. The passage and enforcement of helmet laws for motorcycles in Indonesia has reduced the incidence of associated brain injuries and deaths. The incidence of lung cancer and heart disease among men in California has been significantly reduced, probably due to the laws regulating smoking and the high taxes imposed on cigarettes. Many of the current public health problems of the world, particularly those involving protection of the environment, can be addressed through structural changes requiring passage and implementation of laws and regulations. To accomplish this will require changing the attitudes and behaviour of the public.

Private support of public health

Private support has played an important role in the development of public health, especially in the twentieth century. The Rockefeller Foundation supported the first school of public health in the United States at Johns Hopkins University; set up the International Health Commission in 1913; established the China Medical Board in 1914, which established the first public health university in China, the Peking Union Medical College, in 1921; and has continued to contribute to global health since its founding in 1913 (Berman 1983; Brown 1979). Other foundations, including the Ford Foundation, the Carnegie Foundation, and the Robert Wood Johnson Foundation, have made similar significant contributions to public health.

Private support of public health has been implemented through three strategies: establishment of charitable foundations by industry; development of international, national, and local non-governmental organizations (NGOs); and direct contributions by industry. Each makes and can continue to make a significant contribution to the health of the public.

Foundations have contributed enormously to the advancement of public health, but most often identify their own priorities for funding. Usually they provide support for important public health needs, but foundations and public health leaders do not always agree on what the most important priorities are. Thus, massive infusions of money into public health by organizations such as the Gates Foundation, which makes contributions to fight HIV, malaria, and tuberculosis, can have a significant positive impact, but they also tend to influence public health priorities. Some argue that developing strong public health infrastructures in developing countries will have a much greater impact on improving health than focusing funds on specific health issues (Garrett 2007).

NGOs tend to focus on specific health problems (e.g. American Cancer Society), specific health issues such as refugee health or medical care for the underserved (e.g. Doctors without Borders),

and specific populations (e.g. drug users and sex workers). Often they can be more effective in reaching vulnerable populations and specific health problems and issues because they are closer to the problem than health professionals who must confront a broad range of concerns. Public health programmes can increase their cost-effectiveness by cooperating with NGOs in addressing specific issues, health problems, and populations.

Industry is often viewed as part of the problem. Certainly, industry is frequently the source of public health problems (e.g. air and water pollution). On the other hand, economic development can lead to an improved economic situation that reduces poverty and benefits all of society. However, industry, particularly the advertising industry, has clearly demonstrated that they are better at creating demand and influencing lifestyles than public health. Thus, it would behoove public health to learn from industry and to work with industry to develop and implement healthy economic growth, while safeguarding the environment and benefiting the public.

Private support has greatly benefited public health in the twentieth century. The challenge for the twenty-first century is for public health and private support to agree on the most effective use of private funds for achieving public health goals.

The future of public health

Public health does not lack challenges requiring solutions: emerging infections will continue to present new problems. Public health professionals recognize the threat that H5N1 influenza may mutate to cause human-to-human transmission, but given a virus as labile as influenza, other pandemics are also likely to occur. Early recognition of new strains by genetic monitoring of circulating influenza viruses will help.

An increasing proportion of the world's population will live to be old. We have been successful at adding 'years to life', but chronic diseases such as Alzheimer's have reduced the quality of life of the years of life added. We must now concentrate on adding 'life to years', helping older people to continue to be productive.

We cannot afford to continue to ignore the quality of the environment. Continuing contamination of the air and water will not only cause and/or exacerbate chronic and infectious diseases, but will rob us of important sources of food. Addressing these problems will require eliciting the political will and commitment of the public and changes in lifestyle. Unchecked population growth will further exacerbate the problem of protecting the environment.

Despite the economic and health advances of the past century, disparities between the rich and the poor are widening. This gap must be narrowed if not eliminated, not at the expense of those who are better-off, but by improving the economic situation and health of the poor and disadvantaged.

Injuries and violence are robbing an increasing number of people of their ability to function and to enjoy a reasonable quality of life. Injuries can be easily prevented through a variety of preventive strategies, including better design of the workplace and tools such as ladders, but also include implementing behavioural and structural strategies. Violence and war represent greater challenges, and will most likely require new strategies not hitherto widely used in public health.

We in public health know what needs to be done to significantly reduce chronic diseases such as cardiovascular diseases, stroke, and cancer, but we need to develop more effective ways to change behaviour and promote healthy lifestyles.

We have made tremendous strides to improve the health of the public, but the challenge to do better remains. In subsequent chapters, public health experts discuss the challenges and potential solutions in detail.

References

Acheson E.D. On the state of the public health [the fourth Duncan lecture]. *Public Health* 1988;**102**(5):431–437.

Berman E.H. *The ideology of philanthropy: the influence of the Carnegie, Ford, and Rockefeller foundations on American foreign policy.* New York (NY): University of New York Press; 1983.

Breslow L., Breslow N. Health practices and disability: some evidence from Alameda County. *Preventive Medicine* 1993;**22**:86–95.

Brown E.R. *Rockefeller medicine men: medicine and capitalism in America.* Berkeley (CA): University of California Press; 1979.

Chow C.K, Raju R. The prevalence and management of type 2 diabetes in India. *Diabetes Care* 2006;**29**:1717–1718.

Council for International Organization of Medical Sciences (CIOMS). *International ethical guidelines for biomedical research involving human subjects.* Geneva: World Health Organization; 2002.

Department of Health and Human Services, National Center for Health Statistics, *Health, United States, 1999.* Washington (DC): US Government Printing Office; 1999.

Detels R., Rokaw S.N., Coulson A.H. et al. The UCLA population studies of chronic obstructive respiratory disease: I. Methodology and comparison of lung function in areas of high and low pollution. *American Journal of Epidemiology* 1979;**109**(1):33–58.

Garrett L. The challenge of public health. *Foreign Affairs;* 2007 Jan/Feb.

Gauderman W.J., Vora H., McConnell K. et al. Effect of exposure to traffic on lung development from 10 to 18 years of age: a cohort study. *Lancet* 2007;**369**:571–577.

Sigerist H.E. *A History of Medicine.* Oxford and New York: Oxford University Press, 1958–1961.

International Labour Organization. Report of the 15th World Congress on Occupational Safety and Health. [Online]. 1999. Available from: http://www.ilo.org/public/english/bureau/inf/pr/1999/9.htm [accessed 2007 May].

Kaneda T. Percentage of elderly (ages 65 and over) by country, 2000 and 2050. [Online]. Population Reference Bureau. Available from: http://www.prb.org/Articles/2006/ACriticalWindowforPolicymakingonPopulationAginginDevelopingCountries.aspx [accessed 2007 May].

Kelly J.A. Popular opinion leaders and HIV prevention peer education: resolving discrepant findings, and implications for the development of effective community programmes. *AIDS Care* 2004;**16**(2):139–50.

Kuo C.C, Campbell L.A. Detection of Chlamydia pneumoniae in arterial tissues. *Journal of Infectious Diseases* 2000;**181**:S432–S436.

Lopez A., Mathers C., Ezzati M., Jamison D., Murray C. Global and regional burden of disease and risk factors, 2001: a systematic analysis of population health data. *Lancet* 367(9524):1747–1757, 2007.

Lee S.H. The SARS epidemic in Hong Kong. *Journal of Epidemiology and Community Health* 2003;**57**(9):652–4.

Lopez A.D, Mathers C.D, Ezzati M. et al. Global burden of disease and risk factors. In: *Disease control priorities project.* Oxford: Oxford University Press; 2006.

MacKenzie W.R., Hoxie N.J., Proctor M.E. et al. A massive outbreak in Milwaukee of cryptosporidium infection transmitted through the public water supply. *New England Journal of Medicine* 1994;**331**:161–7.

Mathers C.D., Loncar D. Projections of global mortality and burden of disease from 2002 to 2030. [Online]. *PLoS Medicine* 2006;**3**(11):e442.

McGinnis J.M., Foege W.H. Actual causes of death in the United States. *Journal of the American Medical Association* 1993;**270**:2007–2012.

Merson M.H., Black R.E., Mills J.E., eds. *International public health.* 2nd edn. Sudsbury (MA): Jones & Bartlett; 2006. p. 326.

Murray C.J.L., Lopez A.D. A comprehensive assessment of mortality and disability from diseases, injuries, and risk factors in 1990, and projected to 2020. In: *The global burden of disease.* Cambridge (MA): Harvard University Press; 1995. vol 1.

Murray C.J.L., Lopez A.D. (eds). The global burden of disease. In: *The global burden of disease.* Cambridge (MA): Harvard University Press; 1996. (Global burden of disease and injury series; vol 1).

Office of the Director, National Public Health Performance Standards Program. *10 essential public health services.* [Online]. Centers for Disease Control; 1994. Available from: http://www.cdc.gov/od/ocphp/nphpsp/EssentialPHServices.htm

Pan American Health Organization. *Essential public health services.* [Online]. 2002. Available from: http://www.sopha.cpha.ca/english/ephf_e.html

Petersen P.E. Inequalities in oral health: the social context for oral health. In: *Community oral health.* 2nd edn. London: Quintessence Publishing; 2007. p. 38–39.

Pine C., Harris R. *Community oral health.* London: Quintessence Books; 2007.

Population Projections. *Health Affairs;* 2000 May/June.

United States Census Bureau. *International database.* [Online]. 2006. Available from: http://www.census.gov/ipc/www/idbnew.html [accessed 2007 May].

US National Commission for the Protection of Human Subjects of Biomedical and Behavioral Research. *The Belmont report.* Washington (DC): US National Commission for the Protection of Human Subjects of Biomedical and Behavioral Research; 1978.

WHO Oral Health Program. [Online]. Sweden: Malmo University; 2004. Available from: http://www.whocollab.od.mah.se/index.html [accessed 2007 May].

World Health Organization. *Atlas mental health resources in the world, 2001.* [Online]. 2001. Available from: http://whqlibdoc.who.int/whr/2001/WHR_2001.pdf [accessed 2007 May].

World Health Organization. Causes of chronic diseases. [Online]. 2005. Available from: http://www.who.int/chp/chronic_disease_report/contents/part2.pdf [accessed 2007 May].

World Health Organization. Indicators for Policy and Decision Making in Environmental Health. Geneva, Switzerland: WHO; 1997.

World Health Organization. *Injury Report.* [Online]. 2004. Available from: http://www.wpro.who.int/internet/templates/HLT_Topic.aspx?NRMODE=Published&NRORIGINALURL=%2Fhealth_topics%2Finjuries_and_violence_prevention%2F&NRNODEGUID=%7BF17BB93C-267E-49F1-B089-F4C4710AED39%7D&NRCACHEHINT=NoModify Guest [accessed 2007 May].

World Health Organization. Main causes of death and global burden of disease (DALYs), world, all ages, projections for 2005. [Online]. Available from: http://www.who.int/chp/chronic_disease_report/contents/part2.pdf [accessed 2007 May].

World Health Organization. Neglected tropical diseases—hidden successes, emerging opportunities. [Online]. 2006. Available from: http://whqlibdoc.who.int/hq/2006/WHO_CDS_NTD_2006.2_eng.pdf [accessed 2007 May].

World Health Organization. Trends in global years of life lost (YLL) per 1,000 population, by broad cause group and income group, 2002–2030. [Online]. 2005. Available from: http://www.who.int/healthinfo/statistics/bodprojectionspaper.pdf [accessed 2007 May].

World Health Organization. *World Health Report, 2001.* Geneva: World Health Organization; 2001.

World Medical Association. *Declaration of Helsinki.* 5th revision. Washington (DC): World Medical Association; 2002.

The history and development of public health in developed countries

Christopher Hamlin

Abstract

This chapter explores the problem of defining the proper domain of public health as a science and department of public action. It examines three elements of public health, which have been important in its past in the developed world: The response to epidemics, the policing of towns (and states) in ordinary times, and efforts to produce a systematic betterment of population health. The chapter also argues that a 'golden age' from 1880 to 1970, when public health rationales were relatively unquestioned, has given way to a new era of complexity: The agenda of public health is less clear and there has been renewed fundamental debate on such ancient issues as how to understand cause as well as on what kinds of changes are possible and warranted.

Introduction

Much more than is usually realized, public health is both a central and a problematic element of the history of the developed world—here conceived as Europe and the 'Neo Europes'; that is, the set of nations in broad latitude bands of the northern and southern hemispheres in which European institutions and biota have been particularly successful (Crosby 1986).

Over the last three centuries, health status has changed profoundly in these regions; arguably, it is in terms of health that our lives differ most strikingly from those of our ancestors. We live longer. Rarely do parents experience the death of their young children; rarely do young adults experience the gradual 'consumption' of pulmonary tuberculosis. Affluence and transportation mean most of us are no longer subject to periodic famines, and much less subject to epidemics of deadly infectious diseases, although we are less confident about that than we were two decades ago. Nor are most of us wracked with chronic pain, with abscesses, or with induced deformities. Most of us do not see life as a continuously painful experience and death as a merciful release, a view that is rather commonly found in books of theology from three centuries ago (Browne 1964).

Our health is adversely affected by aspects of the world we have built and the ways we choose to live individually and communally.

A good deal is known about how to prevent those effects even if we do not always do so. Nonetheless, an expectation of health and a preoccupation with it are hallmarks of modernity. The freedom of action that ideally characterizes the lives of individuals in the developed world is predicated on health; so much of the agenda of development concerns health, that this transformation has some claim to be seen as one of the monumental changes in human history. It might be argued that economic and political progress are subordinate to securing health—they are means; health, which surely translates into life, liberty, and the pursuit of happiness, is the end.

Surprisingly, the history of public health is under-studied. Few general texts give it much attention (but see McNeill 1976); there remain vast gaps in empirical knowledge, and relatively little comparative work (but see Baldwin 1999; Porter 1999; Kunitz 2007). Compared with the grand dramas of history, public health has sometimes seemed to historians a marginal and uncontroversial function of modern society. After all, we provide medicine, collect and evaluate demographic data, test water, and keep cities clean in roughly similar ways, according to the conventions of science, technology, and public administration that developed mainly in the nineteenth century. This view partly reflects a distortion of the history of public health by the modern professions and institutions of public health, which have often found it prudent to reduce the significance of the fact that they are necessarily political, even if their business is politics by medical means.

Public health is treated more broadly in this chapter. It is concerned with the general questions of how, why, and in what manners states came to take an interest in the peoples' health. The questions of what 'health' is, of what we mean by 'public', and of what we understand to be the proper domain of 'public health' are, and have always been, contested matters. To define public health as that part of health that is the responsibility of the state does not help: What constitutes the state, and what are presumed to be state responsibilities vary in time and place. However broadly or narrowly we define 'health', it will be clear that many public actions affect the public's health, yet will not necessarily be seen to belong to the domain of 'public health' or its predecessors.

An examination of actions taken in the name of the public to protect or improve the health of the public will illuminate the enigmatic relationship between that universal goal, the health of the public, and public health as an institution—as a profession, science, component of public administration, and theme of moral and political philosophy (Porter 1999; Fee 1993; Rosen 1958). Within that framework, there will be more diversity, contingency, complexity, and controversy in its history than is usually apparent. Ultimately, however, there can be no single narrative. A history of public health is necessarily part of an ongoing conversation about a programme of social change that is both rational and moral. The story we tell about it will depend on what we think public health should be, just as our notions of it will themselves reflect the evolution of the professions and institutions we have inherited, and of the myths, memories, and sensibilities that sustain them.

Themes and problems in the history of public health

It will help at the outset to recognize several of the most troublesome issues that face any historian of public health. Among these are the following:

I. The units of public health: States and publics

- *The public and the state:* 'State' and 'public' are not always interchangeable terms. The state, concerned with population, may arrive at different health-related policies from a public sphere of groups of citizens, carrying out a rational and critical dialogue among equals (Sturdy 2002).

- *The diversity of states:* Even when widely accepted reasons of the state and agendas of state responsibility arose, not every state was in the position to act on them. The focus of public health was quite often at the level of local states, whose responsibility and jurisdiction were often unclear or overlapping. But the state itself was an artificial unit for addressing problems, like many epidemic diseases, which were global in nature.

- *Goals of the state:* Although health is now thought of in terms of the biological autonomy of individuals, this has rarely, and only recently, been the goal of programmes of public health. Health sometimes has meant a good supply of labour or of soldiers, control of excess population, protection of élites, enhancement of the genetic stock of a population, or environmental stability.

II. The condition that is truly health

- *The definition of health:* The combating of epidemic infectious diseases has often seemed to be the core of public health. When we go beyond these diseases, questions arise of what level and kind of physical and mental well-being the state should guarantee or require of its citizens, and of the status of health as a source of imperatives vis-à-vis other sources of imperatives such as the market, the environment, or individual liberty. What sort of normality will a society demand?

- *The problem of causation of disease:* In a broad sense, diseases have many causes—personal, social, cultural, political, and economic, as well as biological. Among the multiple antecedents that converge in the production of an epidemic or endemic disease, there are numerous opportunities to intervene (MacMahon & Pugh 1970: Chapter 2). Notions of rights that must be respected, or of political or technical practicality,

narrow that list. Discussion of cause has often included notions of responsibility or preventability—of where in a social system there is flexibility, of who or what must change to prevent disease.

- *Equality and rights—race, class, gender:* The idea of 'health for all' disguises the fact that the interests of the so-called public have not always been the interests of all of its members. Public health actions have often reflected, and sometimes exacerbated, a view of the world in which some groups were seen primarily as a threat to others. Often, views of the standards of health that were properly matters for the state varied with respect to different groups: Key divisions were by sex, by age (infants, working adults, and the aged all had a different status), by wealth, and by race, religion, or historical heritage (indigenous people had a different status from colonial rulers). Whether the public's response to disease was to advise, aid, or condemn, or to imprison, banish, or kill, reflected the allocation of rights and the distribution of power more than the status of the biological threat.

III. The health that is truly public

- *Health and public health:* Most modern states have in principle distinguished aspects of health that are the business of the public from those that are for the individual to pursue in the medical marketplace, although the borders have been drawn in many different ways.

- *Medical and non-medical public health:* Although public health has evolved into an ancillary medical science, with occasional involvement of relevant areas of engineering and the social sciences, the fact that health has been improved by many non-medical factors—prosperity, town planning, architecture, religious and humanitarian charity, the power of organized labour, and even the enlargement of political or economic rights—suggests that any comprehensive account of improved health must include these factors.

- *Health as authority:* Given the amorphous nature of the concept of health and its status as the supreme good of human existence, it has been attractive as an imperative for political action. If other 'reasons of state' carry more immediacy, public health has better claim to the moral high ground because it is seen to be universal and apolitical, exactly the qualities that make it attractive to act politically in the name of health.

These issues are too many to address fully, but they inform what follows. The history of public health in the developed world can be conceived in terms of three relatively distinct missions: Public health as a reaction to epidemics, as a form of police, and as a means of human betterment. Public health was initially reactive; faced with epidemic disease, early modern European states closed borders and ports, instituted fumigation, shut down dangerous (smelly) trades, and isolated victims. Second, public health acted as a form of police. It is probably the case that wherever humans live in communities, customs arise for the regulation of behaviour and the maintenance of the communal environment. Gradually, much of the enforcement of community standards became medical. The control of food adulteration or prostitution, of the indigent and the transient, or concern over dung or smoke overlapped with the control of epidemics, but went well beyond it, and occurred in normal as well as in epidemic times.

Finally, public health became a proactive political vision for improvement of the health of all. Well into the nineteenth century, the view remained common that high urban or infant death rates were inevitable. A proactive public health involved the determination that normal conditions of health, if they could be improved, were not acceptable conditions of health. This shift was partly due to technical achievements—such as smallpox inoculation, and later, vaccination—and to better demographic information, but it rested on changed conceptions of human rights coupled with greater technical and economic optimism. Such visions sustained the building of comprehensive urban water and sewerage systems before there was wide acceptance that these needed to be universal features of cities; such visions have periodically led public health to venture beyond traditional medical bounds, to recognize, for example, nuclear warfare or gun violence as public health problems.

The public health of epidemic crisis: Reaction

Regardless of their virulence and pervasiveness, epidemic and, even more so, endemic diseases do not necessarily warrant comment or action—they may simply be acknowledged as part of life. For the public to decide to fight an epidemic, it must believe it can do something to mitigate the problem, and it must be just sufficiently concerned. It is true that a belief in *the possibility of effective action* is a prerequisite for public health; one of the most intriguing problems in its history is the emergence of this belief. It does not coincide with the replacement of the supernatural by naturalistic explanations of disease causation. 'Will-of-God' explanations of disease have sometimes incited public action, but on other occasions implied abject resignation.

Similarly, naturalistic explanations—attributing epidemics to a mysterious element in the atmosphere or, as in the case of classical conceptions of smallpox, to a normal process of fermentation in the growing body—have on some occasions been taken as proof that we can do nothing beyond giving supportive care and on other occasions have sanctioned preventive public action. In each case, assessments of technical and political practicality are mixed with assessments of propriety: Is taking such action part of our cultural destiny?

These issues are already evident in the first European account of a widely fatal epidemic, the unidentified plague that struck Athens in 430 BC. Athenians both recognized contagion and acknowledged a duty to aid the afflicted, as Thucydides informs us, but these recognitions did not translate into expectations of prevention, mitigation, or escape (Carmichael 1993; Longrig 1992; Nutton 2000; Thucydides 1950). Few fled; on the contrary, the epidemic was exacerbated by an influx from the countryside. Although it was appreciated that those who survived the disease were unlikely to be affected again, and some hoped it would bring permanent immunity from all afflictions, the main response was to accept one's fate. The disease was attributed to the seasons, as well as to the gods, and was said to have be prophesied. Such resignation would be central to the moral philosophies of the Roman world, Stoicism and Epicureanism, both of which taught one to accept what was fated or necessary (Veyne 1987). Later writers in the Christian world attributed the failure of Islam to take active steps against plague to such an outlook. Although classical Islamic doctors developed a science of hygiene to a remarkable degree (Gori 2002), it did not follow that one should apply this knowledge in an epidemic: If plague came, that was Allah's will. To fight it would be futile and impious; one's duty was to trust (Conrad 1992; Dols 1977).

In contrast, the response to epidemic disease in the medieval Christian Latin countries was activism. One could prevent disease from taking hold in a community, or extinguish it if it did, or at least avoid it personally. This activism had many avenues, indicative of the syncretism of Medieval Latin culture. In the Old and New Testaments alone, disease had a multiplicity of significations. It represented the dispensation of God to an individual, perhaps as punishment or a test. To act against disease by intervening to help others stricken by a dangerous epidemic was an act of devotion. If one died in such a situation, it was a sign of grace; if one did not die, and helped to save others, this was equally a sign of grace. The laws of hygiene in the Pentateuch permitted a naturalistic interpretation of disease. Unclean acts or other transgressions, such as failing to isolate lepers from society, generated the retribution of disease, perhaps through God's appointed secondary or natural causes. Disease might even be naturally communicable; in such a case, communal decisions to maintain the Levitical laws were means not only of acting against potential epidemics but also of policing the community, and perhaps, of augmenting its welfare (Amundsen & Ferngren 1986; Dorff 1986; Douglas 1966; Lieber 2000; Winslow 1980). Such views would become widespread among nineteenth-century sanitarians.

The two diseases that did spur medieval Europeans to comment and react were leprosy and the plague. Although it is difficult to assess the number of lepers in medieval Europe, the common view is that there was a vast overreaction, in terms of both investment in institutions to house victims of the disease—there were said to be several thousand leprosaria—and the detection and isolation of cases to prevent transmission. In keeping with the prominence of leprosy in the Bible, the professionals who diagnosed it were churchmen, not medical men. The diagnosis was a loose one; it might be based on skin blemishes alone.

Often it involved an accusation. It led to the expulsion of the victim from ecclesiastical and civil society, symbolized in a ceremony resembling a funeral. Subsequently, no one was to touch or come near the leper or to touch what the leper touched. The theory of contagion provided the rationale for such action, but Skisnes (1973) has argued that the clinical characteristics of the disease itself—for example, its slow development, the visible disfigurement it produced—triggered such a reaction (Brody 1974; Carmichael 1997; Richards 1977; Touati 2000). Even if leprosy precautions did embody empirical knowledge of contagion, it, like most other diseases, belonged to the sphere of providence. While leprosy was sometimes seen as a punishment of sin, it might also reflect grace: God's singling out of an individual to bear a particular burden of suffering.

The prototypical institutional responses to epidemic disease, however, were those that arose in response to plague. The first wave of plague, the Black Death, spread across Europe from 1347 to 1353, and thereafter the disease returned to most areas about once every two decades for the next three centuries. This was a catastrophic disease, with case-fatality rates ranging from 30 to nearly 100 per cent depending on the strain of 'plague' (the identity of the microbe has recently been questioned; for a review, see Carmichael 2003), the means of transmission, and the immunological state of the population. Plague and accompanying diseases reduced the

European population by roughly a third or more in the fourteenth century and were responsible for only a very slow population growth during the following two centuries. As in the case of leprosy, the aetiology of plague and the associated means of prevention and mitigation of the disease were conceived in terms of divine will and natural processes, although even more clearly than with leprosy the distinction is misleading: Nature, whether in the courses of the stars, in meteorological phenomena, or in the process of contagion, was God's instrument (Nohl 1926; Ziegler 1969).

It is clear that in many communities the coming of plague was unacceptable. It could not be reconciled with the usual course of events, but indicated some fundamental violation of the cosmos, of an order which included human society. Boccaccio (1955), whose *Decameron* is a document on the Black Death, testifies to one form of activism—a discarding of social convention and religious duty, a devil-may-care indulgence in the present founded on the recognition that life was short and the future uncertain. Those with the means often fled plague-ridden places. Others, taking the view that the plague reflected God's just anger with hopelessly corrupt civil and ecclesiastical authority, saw a clear need to take charge of matters temporal and spiritual, to cleanse themselves, the state, and the church. Righteousness would end the plague.

Thus, the plague precipitated a social crisis, as would epidemics of other diseases in subsequent centuries. Beyond the massive disruption caused by high mortality and morbidity and an interruption of commerce and industry, the loss of faith in the conventions and institutions of society was a critical blow. Why respect property, family, or communal obligations, pay taxes, invest money, or tolerate rivals and others? Latent tensions within society had an excuse to become active.

When people acted precipitately and independently, civil and ecclesiastical institutions were threatened, and it is in their responses that we clearly see the emergence of public health as a form of public authority. For a state, to act in a crisis was to keep the state going; one maintained authority by acting authoritatively. If some state actions were rational in terms of the naturalistic aspects of theories of the plague, the viability of civic authority itself was probably more crucial than any lives they might save.

All these issues are evident in the manifold responses to plague from the mid-fourteenth to the early eighteenth century. Particularly in Germany, the response to the Black Death was to challenge civil and ecclesiastical authority. In 1349, lay flagellant groups paraded from town to town, giving public penitential performances to end the plague. Although they were usually well received, and their practices were unorthodox, the movement did draw attention to what the Church had failed to do, and Pope Clement VI condemned it.

However, the state response to such actions could not have been uniform, for medieval and early states were not monoliths but fragile alliances of multiple levels and kinds of authority, existing in continual tension with one another. In Basel, the majority Christian population blamed the plague on Jews—either it came by direct divine action because Jews had been allowed to live in the town, or through a natural agent with which the Jews had presumably poisoned the town's water. The town's Jews were rounded up, sequestered on an island, and burned. Here it was a local state, the town council, which took the action. Its credibility was at stake; it needed to be seen to act boldly in order to secure an end to the epidemic, its action built on pre-existing anti-Semitism. To the central state,

the Holy Roman Empire, such actions against one group of its subjects verged on anarchy. Emperor Charles IV condemned the persecution and asserted on the basis of medical and religious authority that the Jews were not responsible for the plague (Ziegler 1969).

In contrast, the approaches to plague prevention and control developed in the next two centuries in the Italian city-states were humane, focused mainly on naturalistic intervention, and probably relatively successful. Plague control measures emerged out of a tradition of close municipal management, and in a cosmopolitan intellectual environment. Italy, after all, was the main European centre for receiving Galenic and Islamic medical knowledge; included were concepts of hygiene, disease causation, and the purification of enclosed spaces. The preventive measures taken in Italian city-states were eclectic. They included the development of the forty-day hold on ships or other traffic coming from potentially infected places (the quarantine), the isolation of victims (and families of victims), and numerous means of purifying the air and/or destroying contamination: Bonfires, burning sulphur, burning clothes and bedding, washing surfaces with lime or vinegar, and killing or removing urban animals. Such actions were predicated on an understanding that the disease moved from place to place through some medium or media, possibly involving, although probably not limited to, person-to-person contact.

Although the eclecticism of this response is certainly indicative of uncertainty about how plague spread, the actions do show a responsive civil authority (Carmichael 1986; Cipolla 1979, 1992). Indeed, in some ways plague prevention initiatives were themselves a means of state growth. Plague control required officials to oversee quarantine or isolation procedures. It required a staff to disinfect, and a structure to gather information on health conditions at remote ends of the state. An embassy, which in the high Middle Ages signified an official visit by one state to another, became the permanent presence of one state in the territory of another in the Italian city-states. Its initial purpose was to monitor the public health in the host country and to send word home if plague broke out (Cipolla 1981; Slack 1985).

Plague set the template for responses to epidemics of other diseases (often generically called plague)—flight, exacerbation of social tensions leading to scapegoating, a heightening of religious seriousness (often combined with a collapse of normal customs and obligations), and a mix of pragmatic efforts to disinfect people, places, goods, or the environment, and to isolate victims or potentially contagious strangers, and somehow to control the poor (Carmichael 1986; Briggs 1961). The particular mix of these actions reflected the current state of debate between proponents of atmospheric theories, including miasmatic theories, which located the origins of the epidemic in some unusual state of air, and of contagionist theories, which emphasized various forms of interpersonal transmission, and presumed that epidemics could spread only as far as infected humans (or human products) carried them. Only rarely were contagionist and environmental explanations mutually exclusive, as a wide range of factors were implicated in disease (Kinzelbach 2006; Pelling 2001).

Thus, in the nineteenth century, the series of cholera pandemics which arrived in Europe in the early 1830s brought forth accusations by the poor that the rich were poisoning them (particularly the doctors who wanted their bodies for teaching and research), and by the rich that the poor wantonly persisted in living in disease-nurturing squalor. It also engendered calls for public fasts, pure living, and declamations against sinful society, and a variety of attempts to disinfect, quarantine, and isolate (Briggs 1961; Delaporte 1986; Durey 1979; Evans 1990; McGrew 1965; Richardson 1988; Rosenberg 1962; Snowden 1995). In nineteenth-century America, the response to yellow fever and malaria was regular flight and the abandonment of cities during the summer by those who could afford to do so (Ellis 1992; Humphreys 1992). The summer home, in cooler, cleaner, and higher ground, became a mark of upper-middle-class life.

Significant alterations of that pattern came through efforts to control three other diseases: Venereal diseases (particularly syphilis), smallpox, and a mix of diseases including typhus, typhoid, relapsing fever, and a mix of ill-defined conditions known as continued fever (or just 'fever').

Whether syphilis came to Europe from America or Africa, or had been present in Europe in a milder form (perhaps labelled as leprosy), has been much debated. What is clear is that a virulent epidemic often known as the French disease or pox began to spread quickly in the last years of the fifteenth century, and can be traced to the intercourse between Italian prostitutes and French and Spanish soldiers during the siege of Naples in 1494. The connection between the disease and sex was made quickly, partly because of the initial symptoms on the external genitalia—the more expressive German term *lustseuche* had been adopted by 1510. As had not been the case with plague or leprosy, syphilis represented a serious epidemic disease that constituted a state problem (surely, plague was a state problem?), particularly because it affected military strength, but which was not susceptible to large-scale public action. It was further complicated by having variable symptoms and effects, having a long course during parts of which it was not clearly manifest, and varying in contagiousness and virulence.

If syphilis was to be controlled, states must prevail on individuals to avoid behaviours that spread the disease. One might expect the moral opprobrium related to contracting a disease usually acquired through illicit sexual contact to have had some role in discouraging such practices, but it did not. For an adventurous young man, a case of pox was a cost of doing business, even a badge of achievement. The disease was deemed curable, chiefly through mercurial treatments. Although there are suggestions that by the eighteenth century syphilis had become something to hide (though not necessarily for moral reasons), such was not the case during the sixteenth century, when the disease was spreading rapidly (Arrizabalaga 1993; Arrizabalaga *et al.* 1997).

State attention shifted from cure to prevention only in the eighteenth century, partly because syphilis was becoming more clearly distinguished from other venereal conditions and as the varied phenomena of tertiary syphilis were becoming more evident. Whereas the European states varied significantly in the priority they put on syphilis as a public problem, their approaches did not vary greatly: The disease was to be controlled by regulating prostitutes, who were regarded as the reservoir that maintained the contagion. Such approaches may well have had a significant effect in controlling the disease, but they exposed tensions between state and individual rights that have since become common in public health.

Such conflicts developed first in the United Kingdom following the first Contagious Diseases Act of 1862, even though its programme against venereal disease was much smaller than that of France, where regulation of prostitution was a central feature of public hygiene (Baldwin 1999). The British Act allowed the police in designated garrison towns to arrest and inspect women presumed to be prostitutes and to confine infected women in hospital. It led to a sustained campaign for repeal, which was ultimately successful in 1885. The repealers represented a broad coalition: Some objected that the legislation was morally indefensible because it acquiesced in the immoral industry of prostitution, others that it singled out women as responsible for a problem that was as much the responsibility of the men who used the services of prostitutes, while still others objected that the practice of arresting women was arbitrary (except with respect to class) and stigmatized working-class women who were not prostitutes (McHugh 1982; Walkowitz 1980).

The problem that the British parliament faced stemmed from liberal principles of human rights. Ironically, the Contagious Diseases Act had been touted as respecting rights—the rights of men: The state would inspect women because male soldiers and sailors would not put up with genital inspection. Nor should they be expected to in a state in which the male franchise was broadening and the public was becoming increasingly uneasy with declarations that part of its population existed as cannon fodder. But recognizing the rights of men simply made it all the more clear that they were not accorded to women.

The issues that arose in combating venereal diseases arose in a more general way with regard to smallpox. While the ninth-century doctor Al-Razi had viewed smallpox as a normal childhood condition, a particularly dangerous stage of growth, it had become more virulent in fifteenth- and sixteenth-century Europe (Clendening 1942)—why the change? By the eighteenth century, it had accounted for 10–15 per cent of the deaths. It was then widely recognized as a contagious disease of childhood. Many parents intentionally exposed their young children to it: Sooner or later, one would be exposed, and the older child who died from it was a multi-year investment lost; the younger one who survived was subsequently immune.

Small pox induction had arisen in many parts of the world. Independently of medical statistics, it was recognized that some means of inducing the disease made it significantly less virulent. Mortality rates of 25 per cent or more might drop to a few per cent. Notwithstanding assertions that such practice defied providence, and its inherently counter-intuitive character, such logic and experience had much to do with the relatively rapid acceptance of inoculation after 1721, when it was introduced into Western Europe by Lady Mary Wortley Montagu, a well-connected aristocrat who had observed the process in Turkey. It was first taken up in the British Isles; its subsequent spread depended on the patronage of royalty and nobility, on increases in the safety of the procedure, especially when carried out by the most highly skilled practitioners, and the acquiescence of at least a segment of the medical profession (Hopkins 2002; Miller 1957; Razzell 1977).

In 1798, the English practitioner Edward Jenner made immunization significantly safer by introducing the practice of vaccination with cowpox. Increasingly, smallpox prevention, hitherto a personal matter, became a state concern. Presumably, the institutions that orchestrated quarantines could also ensure universal vaccination. But here too there was ambiguity: In whose interests were vaccination programmes to be undertaken? England began offering free vaccination in 1840, made it compulsory in 1853, and instituted fines for non-compliance in 1873. The initial assumption that all would take advantage of this free medical service proved unfounded; as the authorities sought to give the vaccination laws more teeth, they encountered growing opposition and decreasing rates of compliance.

In 1898, anti-vaccinationists gained permission for conscientious objectors to forgo having their children vaccinated. The opposition was able to show that the dangerous procedure was not carried out everywhere with sufficient skill or care, and a real decline in smallpox meant decreasing risk to the unvaccinated. But mandatory vaccination also exposed underlying tension between the state and the public: In an atmosphere of distrust of the state, the more insistent the state became, the more convinced the public became that the state's actions were not in their interests (Baldwin 1999; Brunton, in press; Durbach 2005; Porter & Porter 1988). Yet anti-vaccination movements were sporadic and often isolated: Certainly, lack of opposition did not necessarily signify trust in the state?

It is important to emphasize that for most of the history of the West, efforts to combat epidemic disease had not reflected any sense of obligation to the health of individuals. At stake was the military, commercial, and cultural welfare of the state, and often, the protection of élites: The welfare of individual subjects (a better term than 'citizens' for much of the period) was incidental. Although states devoted substantial resources to enforcing quarantines and other health regulations (and absorbed considerable costs in lost commerce), it would be misleading to think of them acting in some quasi-contractual way as agents for groups of individuals who had recognized that public actions were necessary to secure their own health. Although many places had town or parish doctors, and there was often an expectation that the state take steps to protect the welfare of its subjects (such as making food affordable in times of dearth), early modern political theorists recognized no obligation of the state to protect the health of individuals. What was at risk in an epidemic was the state itself: The collection of taxes, the maintenance of defence, the continuance of commerce, and even the orderly transfer of property at a time of high mortality.

Perhaps, nowhere was the tension between individual and state so great as in the combating of what was called 'continued fever'. Typhus, typhoid, relapsing fever, and yellow fever were among the several epidemic diseases that appeared or became increasingly prominent in the aftermath of the Black Death. This continued fever (malaria was generally distinguished as 'remittent' or 'intermittent' fever) was endemic as well as epidemic, and amidst vast disagreement about classification and cause, there was general agreement about its frequent association with social catastrophe and squalor—with war, jails, pestilence, famine, and overcrowded slums (Geary 1995; Hamlin 1998, 2006; Smith 1981; Wilson 1978). Although it was often associated with class, it did not limit itself to the poor. Many theorists believed the fever could spread from poor to rich, whether by person-to-person contact or by diffusion through some environmental medium from hovels and slums to mansions. But, as would later be the case with tuberculous diseases, it was not clear whether one could disentangle any single factor from the many conditions of poverty, nor did medical men necessarily think it made sense to try.

The public action that might have been taken was the comprehensive improvement of living conditions—the prevention of overcrowded dwellings; the insurance of sufficient food, fuel, and clothing; the provision of personal and environmental cleanliness, a safe work place, and a non-exhausting work day—in short, all the physical and social changes that would produce a sound human being.

Yet, such far-reaching actions to defend the state also threatened to transform it, and in essential ways—in its social distinctions, its institutions of property, even in the political rights it recognized. When the young Prussian radical doctors Rudolph Virchow and Sebastian Neumann investigated a typhus outbreak in Silesia in 1848, they argued that liberal political and economic reforms were the antidote to the squalor which caused the epidemic (Rosen 1947). Irish physicians made similar diagnoses in the pre-famine years—perhaps a little more on the Irish contribution because it is not as well-known as Virchow *et al.*

The public health of communal life: Police

Beyond the response to epidemic outbreaks of specific diseases, Western societies had from early times taken steps to regulate their communities for the common good or the public peace. By the eighteenth century, the term generally used for such efforts was 'police', but the control of crime was only a small part of it. It generally referred to matters of internal public order; that is, to all aspects of government other than military and diplomatic affairs, the raising of funds, import and export duties, matters of land tenure, and civil litigation. Common police functions included:

- The enforcement of basic rules of public behaviour
- The enforcement of standards of building construction and use, with regard to noxious trades and basic sanitation
- The care for the poor, the disabled, and for abandoned children or orphans
- The regulation of hours and modes of work
- The conduct of markets and the quality of the commodities sold in them
- The regulation of marriage and midwifery
- The supply of water to people and the treatment of cattle and other animals
- The inspection and regulation of transients and prostitutes
- The appropriate disposal of the dead, both human and animal
- The prevention of fire and injury
- The investigation of accidental deaths and other forensic matters
- The maintenance of population statistics
- The regulation of medical practice

Sometimes, town or public doctors were involved in this enforcement, and some of these matters—such forensic diagnosis—were overtly medical, at least as often doctors were part of the domain to be regulated.

The issues under the heading of police constituted problems at various levels: For individuals as town dwellers, or adjoining property owners within a neighbourhood, for towns as corporate entities, and for regional or national states. Public health, in the sense of a recognized obligation to protect the health of the people through public regulation, was only rarely the rationale for police, although improvement in the public's health was likely often a consequence of police action. Some matters of police represented public means for the resolution of disputes between individuals as property owners, such as those that arose when the drainage, smoke, or dung of one person's premises encroached on another's.

At a municipal level, a widespread concern with the policing of commerce and manufacture reflected the town's dependence on its markets. The privileges of trade and industry within a town were rarely free; the concern with the quality of foods and drugs was less a matter of consumers' health than of fair competition, consumer satisfaction, and maintenance of the market's good reputation. And it was in the interest of guilds, such as the medical guilds, to keep out outsiders—the regulation of medical practice was in the self-interest of established practitioners, even if done under the auspices of maintaining the quality of public medical care. Finally, at the state level, concern with midwifery, nutrition, or demographic statistics did not necessarily reflect concern with individuals' health. Early modern statecraft equated state strength with population. In the crudest forms of that equation that population was understood as cannon fodder.

The character of institutions of police varied considerably, although most medieval (and ancient) European towns had some kind of institution(s) to carry out the tasks listed earlier (Hope & Marshall 2000). Typically, these mirrored the political structure of the state. In medieval Islamic towns, a *muhtasib*, an appointee of the caliph (or in early modern Spain, a *mutasaf*) oversaw public morals and commerce, but also regulated medical and veterinary practice, refuse disposal, water supply, the cleansing of the public baths, and the licensing of prostitutes (Karmi 1981; López-Piñero 1981; Palmer 1981). In England, where the state was weak and towns strong, police institutions were more community-based; this bottom-up character of dispute resolution would evolve into common law. Among medieval English institutions of local government were the *leet* juries (groups of citizens who biannually perambulated through the town and 'presented' the nuisances they found to the magistrates, who would order abatement), and the courts of sewers, which acted similarly in trying to resolve conflicts about drainage. Whenever a landowner altered drainage patterns, others were affected, often deleteriously. The sewers court was a means of minimizing those adverse effects and compensating for the damage when they were unavoidable. In a similar way, London's Assize of Nuisances managed disputes between neighbours about the location and cleansing of privies (Chew & Kellaway 1973; Leongard 1989; Novak 1996; Redlich & Hirst 1970; Webb & Webb 1922).

The concept of 'nuisance', if not the term, underlay much of the work of public police. In the Anglo-French tradition, a 'nuisance' was an accusation, subsequently backed by a legal determination, that actions on one person's property or in the public domain annoyed and/or interfered with the enjoyment of another's rights (Novak 1996; Blackstone 1892; Hamlin 2002). Common forms of 'nuisance' included conditions offensive to health and sensibility, such as concentrations of pig manure or butchers' waste, as well as antisocial forms of behaviour.

It is clear that the business of the public police did affect health in many ways and also that it covered much of what would later belong to the domain of public health. The priority, however, was usually with amenity, morality, and conflict resolution. However, although the motives and contexts of police initiatives were broader than public health matters, there were overlaps in both practice and theory. The police institutions in late medieval Italian city-states evolved from means of plague response (Carmichael 1986), and almost always, a poorly administered town was looked upon as ripe for an epidemic. Moreover, within Hippocratic and Galenic frameworks, amenity was not clearly distinct from health: To feel well

was to be well; unpleasant sights or smells, noises or incidents, even if they led to nothing we would recognize as disease, constituted both a form of trespass and an assault on health (Carlin 2005). Concepts of specific diseases and vectors were far in the future. Notwithstanding the occasional speculation, such as that of the sixteenth-century Italian doctor Girolamo Fracastoro that each disease might be the product of an invisible living seed, most medical men were not thinking about individual diseases in a way that would encourage them to look for discrete distinguishing causes. Because amenity, order, and health were so closely linked, a medical rationale could provide a basis for social action on behalf of a community.

Too little is known about the operation of these police institutions. What is known suggests that their performance varied enormously. It also suggests that the popular image of the pre-modern town as filthy and ungoverned is misleading. There may well have been filth on the streets, but clearly in some cases it was put there at prescribed hours prior to the rounds of the municipal street sweepers, who would collect it for manure or otherwise dispose of it. Many urban cottage industries—dyeing, soap making, the treating of leather or textiles—did use unpleasant animal products; complaints about them often reflect the struggle between classes for control of the urban environment, with wealthy merchants or professionals appealing to supposedly universal standards of sensibility and health to enhance their status over those who worked in what Guillerme calls the fermentation industries (Guillerme 1988; Kearns 1988).

Two examples of the ongoing legacy of such institutions of police can be seen in the regulation of the food supply and the evolution of the concept of 'nuisances' in Anglo-American public health. The fight for pure food and drugs that developed in the later nineteenth century is often seen as an early manifestation of consumerism, and equally, the product of advances in chemistry, microscopy, and bacteriology as applied to foods. Currently, regulation of the food supply is one of the most common duties of public health departments—efficient inspection of meat- and milk-processing plants and institutional kitchens is seen as an essential component of a civilized society. There were changes in the late nineteenth century in the recognition of a wider range of food contaminants, and due to the need to grapple with a more ingenious group of food adulterers, whose doings were better hidden by an increasingly complicated system of food production and distribution.

But, the concerns of consumers with food safety and their view that food inspection was a duty of government was old and widely shared. The concern of many medieval food inspection officers was with honest weights and measures, but quality was always implicit—the just measure did not satisfy if the ale was diluted. Although there might not have always been objective ways of determining food quality, consumers knew and enforced a moral economy on transgressing vendors: The records of civil discord are packed with the trashing of shops and the thrashing of vendors (Thompson 1971).

Traditions of market regulation affected public health more broadly. Concern about water quality in metropolitan London, for example, reflected consumer outrage at high prices and poor quality and quantity of the water well before there was any epidemiological evidence of it causing cholera. Equally, public willingness to accept that epidemiological evidence was tied to anger at paying too much for an irregular and visibly dirty water supply

(Hamlin 1990; Taylor & Trentmann 2005). It is also likely, although difficult to show, that the ready acceptance of the new scientific forms of food inspection in the late nineteenth century reflected consumer expectations that the service was necessary and appropriate for government to undertake (Waddington 2006).

In the case of environmental nuisances too, institutions of public health took over from long-standing institutions for settling civil disputes. Whereas in earlier centuries the concept had been very broad—including excessive noise, disturbances of the peace, the blocking of customary light—by the mid-nineteenth century, the quintessential nuisance had become urban dung, human and animal, and action against nuisances acquired a basis in statute law that supplemented its status in civil law. Beginning with the first English Nuisances Removal Act of 1847, passed in an expectation of the return of cholera, doctors, and later a new functionary called an inspector of nuisances (later a sanitary inspector), were charged with identifying nuisances and taking steps to have them removed (Hamlin 2005; Wilson 1881). The change from civil to criminal law reflects a recognition that a legal tradition built upon the power of property was ill-suited to a situation in which most property was not occupied by its owners, and which depended upon an outrage to sensibility was ill-suited to a situation in which most peoples' sensibilities were insufficiently attuned to the particular states of environment presumed to be associated with cholera.

Although this change was an emergency response, its effects were more far reaching. It represented the investing of community standards for health in a permanent institution with enforcement powers, rather than leaving them to be worked out incident-by-incident, through common law.

The inspectors of nuisances did not restrict themselves to documented causes of disease, but continued to respond to community complaints, which sometimes were primarily aesthetic. They became the defenders of the ever-rising standards of middle-class life, and however far their activities might stray from any direct relation to disease control, they carried with them the authority of public health imperative (Hamlin 1988, 2005; Kearns 1991).

Towards the end of the nineteenth century, some epidemiologists, recognizing that the tracing of cases and contacts informed by the new science of bacteriology provided a more exact means of disease control, suggested that concern with general environmental quality was an unjustified expense that deflected the attention of public health departments from what really mattered (Cassedy 1962; Rosenkrantz 1974). In some cases, they were effective in severing sanitation and public works from public health, but often they found that the public, who tended to support clean streets and pleasant neighbourhoods, continued (and continues) to appeal to public health as justification for their concern. More common than the wholesale replacement of sanitation by bacteriology was the emergence of what has been called a 'sanitary–bacteriological synthesis' (Barnes 2006). Here too, scientific medicine, however distantly it might be linked to the environmental condition under scrutiny, gave public action a legitimacy that would otherwise have been difficult to create.

The medicalization of public police that these examples suggest was clearly underway by the mid-eighteenth century. The concept of medical police first arose in Germany and Austria, later in Scotland, Scandinavia, Italy, and Spain; in France the rough equivalent was *hygiene publique*. In America and in England, the term and concept never really caught on (Carroll 2002). Medicine's rise to prominence reflected an alliance between medical practitioners who sought state patronage and the 'enlightened despots'—rulers who, such as Austria's Joseph II, sought a science of good government that would significantly strengthen their states. Increasingly, rulers like Joseph felt obliged to test their policies against some tenets of rationality; health seemed to offer a well-defined arena of rational government, a set of means to improve the state and to measure the progress of that improvement (Rosen 1974a,b). How much the regulation of personal behaviour could improve the health of soldiers and sailors was becoming recognized; why not practice the same techniques on the rest of society? The effect of this medicalization was to move matters of police further from the realm of local social relations and towards an all-encompassing scientific rationality.

The classic text of eighteenth-century medical police is Johann Peter Frank's six volume *System einer Vollständingen Medicinischen Polizey*, or *A System of Complete Medical Police*, which appeared between 1779 and 1819 (Frank 1976). Frank (1745–1821) had a distinguished career as a medical professor and a public health and hospital administrator, mainly in Vienna. He began his giant work with a discussion of reproductive health (two volumes), including suggestions for the regulation (and encouragement) of marriage, prenatal care, obstetrical matters, and infant feeding and care. He turned then to diet, personal habits, public amusements, and healthy buildings. The fourth volume covered public safety, which involved everything from accident prevention to the injuries supposedly inflicted by witches, the fifth volume dealt with safe means of interment, and the sixth with the regulation of the medical profession. In Frank's cameralist view, anything that adversely affected health was a matter for public policy and an appropriate subject for regulation—rights, traditions, property, and freedom had no status if they interfered with the welfare of the population.

In its most far-reaching definitions, modern public health approaches the domain of a comprehensive police. It also recognizes that a wide range of factors are implicated in health conditions—current public health concerns include the effects of violent entertainment, the prevention of gun violence, and the conditions of the work place. But in modern liberal democracies, much of what Frank saw as the obvious business of the state is deeply problematic. For, in the nineteenth century, public health shifted radically in mission and constituency. It became less a means of maintaining the state, and more a means by which the state served its sovereign citizens with an (increasing) standard of health that they (increasingly) took as a right of citizenship.

The public health of human potential

We often think that health is a service that governments owe their citizens, that what separates past from present is not intent but simply sufficient knowledge of the means to provide that service—this is not so. A public health that is not merely reactive or regulative but which takes as its goal the reduction of rates of preventable mortality and morbidity, and sees this as its duty to its populace, is a product of the eighteenth century. It is also one of the most remarkable changes of sensibility in human history. Its causes are complex but poorly understood; it clearly did require the development both of knowledge of the problem and of the means to solve it. The concepts of preventable mortality and excess morbidity required being able to show that both death and illness existed at much higher rates in some places than in others.

Although there were a few attempts in seventeenth and eighteenth century Europe to determine local bills of mortality, they were too few to provide a basis for comparison. In contrast, by the late nineteenth century, annual mortality rates were an important focus of competition among English towns. The central government's public health officials, notably John Simon, chief medical officer of the Privy Council from 1857 to 1874, badgered towns with poor showings. Simon and his successors urged them to analyse the reasons for their excess mortality and to take appropriate action (Brand 1965; Eyler 1979; Lambert 1965; Wohl 1983). By the end of the century, and during the twentieth century, reliable morbidity statistics were available to provide a better understanding of the remediable causes of disease. The gathering of such data, and after about 1920 their analysis by means of statistical inference, has become a central part of modern public health (Desrosières 1998; Magnello 2002).

The mission of prevention was also tied to a very real growth in knowledge of the means of prevention. The widespread adoption of inoculation, and after 1800, of vaccination for smallpox was the first clearly effective means to intervene decisively to prevent a deadly disease. Initially through the development of the numerical method and the cultivation of pathological anatomy in the Parisian hospitals in the first decades of the nineteenth century, and subsequently through bacteriological and later serological methods, infectious diseases were distinguished and their discrete causes and vectors identified (Ackerknecht 1967; Bynum 1994). Such recognition ultimately led not only to the 'magic bullet' thinking of vaccine development, but also underwrote campaigns to improve water quality and provide other means of sanitation, and sometimes, as with tuberculosis and typhoid, programmes to identify, monitor, and regulate carriers.

Yet these factors alone cannot account for the widespread conviction that human health could, and must be, significantly improved—they are means, not ends. Whatever the symbolic significance of effective action against smallpox in boosting confidence, vaccination successes did not imply that all infectious diseases were amenable to a similar strategy. In most cases, the new medical knowledge did not precede the determination to improve the health of all but was developed in the process of achieving that goal. A great deal of success was achieved despite quite erroneous conceptions of the nature of the diseases and their causes. The great sanitary campaign against urban filth (based on a vague and flexible concept of pathogenic miasms) is the best-known example (Barnes 2006).

Recognition of differential mortality was not new in the early 1800s, but it did not necessarily convey a need for action. That there was a mortality penalty associated with poverty, infancy, and urban living was clear; but some regarded the town as a necessary corrective to the overfecundity of the countryside, and characterized the poor peasant as occupying a fixed station in life, one whose chief attributes were higher mortality than the virtuous middle classes (though not necessarily than the profligate aristocracy) as well as compensating benefits, such as lowered anxiety (Sadler 1830; Weyland 1968). And even humane and optimistic writers saw infant mortality rates of 25 per cent or more as providential (Roberton 1827). To the influential eighteenth-century Lutheran clergyman Christoph Christian Sturm, God's providence was evident in the symmetry of the curve of mortality by age: Mortality rates were high among the very young and very old, and low in between (Strum 1832).

This is in contrast with the modern sensibility which admits no justifiable reason (beyond, perhaps, the climatic factors that determine the range of some disease vectors) for differential mortality or morbidity. These changes in sensibilities towards state provision can be divided into three periods: An age of liberalism from 1790 to 1880; a golden age of public health to 1970; and a more confusing post-modern period in the last four decades, which may, at least in its most positive aspects, be seen as a return to liberalism.

The age of liberalism: Health in the name of the people, 1790–1880

The social and intellectual movement known as liberalism, which began to prevail in the second half of the eighteenth century, included a wide range of philosophical, political, economic, and religious ideas, but at its heart were notions of individual freedom and responsibility, and usually, of equality in some form. In 1890, when John Simon, England's first chief medical officer and a pioneer of state medicine, surveyed progress in public health during the past two centuries in his *English Sanitary Institutions*, he included a lengthy chapter on the 'New Humanity'. In it, he covered the antislavery movement, the rise of Methodism, growing concern about cruelty to criminals and animals, legislation promoting religious freedom, the replacement of patronage by principle as the motor of parliamentary democracy, the introduction of free markets, the rationalization of criminal and civil law, and efforts towards international peace. Simon saw little need to explain how this concerned public health; he was sketching a fundamental change in 'feeling' that underlay changes in public health policy.

> Society had become readier than before to hear individual voices which told of pain or asked for redress of wrong; abler . . . to admit that justice does not weight her balances in relation to the ranks, creeds, colours, or nationalities of men.

No longer were humans so much cannon fodder; the best policies were those which maximized 'human worth and welfare' (Simon 1890; compare with Pettenkofer 1941; Coleman 1974; Haskell 1985).

What Simon recognized was that with the granting of equal political and economic rights and responsibilities, it had become impossible to see health status as appropriately constrained by class, race, or sex. Nineteenth-century French and English liberals recognized that some—particularly women, children, and the poor—still suffered ill health disproportionately, but they saw such consequences as incidental, accidental, and increasingly, as unnecessary and objectionable: In principle, all had an equal claim to whatever version of human and health rights a society was prepared to recognize. As Simon also recognized, this change in feeling was both the cause and effect of the widening distribution of political power.

And yet liberalism was no clear and compact doctrine, and its implications for public health were, and still are, by no means clear. Few of the pioneers of liberal political theory bothered to translate human rights into terms of health. They wrote mainly with middle-class men in mind, and saw the threats to life, liberty, and property as political rather than biosocial. The expansion (or translation) of political rights into rights to health was gradual, piecemeal (it has never been the rallying cry of revolution), complicated, and even fundamentally conflictual—it was, and is, not always the case that the choices free individuals make will protect the public's health, or even their own. Concern with public health arose accidentally, and in different ways and at different times in the developed nations. At the beginning of the twenty-first century, an obligation to maintain and/or improve the health of all citizens exists only in varying degrees.

Many early liberals found health rights hard to recognize because so much of public health had been closely associated with the medical police functions of an overbearing state. In revolutionary France, the first instinct was to free the market in medical practice by abolishing medical licensing, a policy quickly recognized as disastrous for maintaining the armies of citizen–soldiers who were protecting the nation (Foucault 1975; Riley 1987; Weiner 1993; Brockliss & Jones 1997). Even after new, meritocratic, and science-based medical institutions had been established, the cadre of public health researchers that it fostered—at the time, the world's leaders in epidemiology is this France?—found it difficult to conceive how their findings of the preventable causes of disease could be translated into proposals for preventive legislation. Poverty, and to some degree, working and living conditions were dictated by the market; government mandates would induce dependence or simply shift the problem elsewhere. Thus, France was the scientific leader in public health for the first half of the nineteenth century without finding a viable political formula for translating that knowledge into prevention (LaBerge 1992; Coleman 1982).

In early-nineteenth-century Britain, the ideas of T.R. Malthus led a broad range of learned public opinion, both liberal and conservative, to similar conclusions. Disease was among the natural checks that kept population within the margins of survival. Successful prevention of disease would be temporary only; it would postpone an inevitable equilibration of the food–population balance that would occur through some other form of human catastrophe (Hamlin 1998; Dean 1991). Malthusian sentiment blocked attempts to establish foundling hospitals. Notwithstanding the fact that such institutions were notoriously deadly to their inmates, it was felt that their existence encouraged irresponsible procreation—faced with full economic responsibility for their actions, men (or women, depending on how one viewed the prevailing legal arrangements for child support) would stifle their urges (McClure 1981). Malthusian views were prominent in British policy with regard to Ireland, Scotland, and India.

By 1850, in both France and England, it was no longer possible to maintain what for many was a complacent and convenient faith in the welfare-maximizing actions of a completely free society. A number of factors shattered this faith. First, no government ever adopted the programme of the early nineteenth-century liberals in full. In Central, Eastern, and Southern Europe, the old concerns of state security continued to govern their public health. In Sweden and later France, concern about a state was weakened by depopulation-fostered attention to the health and welfare of individuals.

Second, working-class parties, although often generally sympathetic with political liberalism, saw no advantage in economic liberalism. Often, they demanded adherence to the moral economy of the old order, in which governments damped fluctuations in grain prices and enforced the working conditions that craft guilds had established. Most important is that many liberals themselves arrived at what is properly called a biosocial vision, a concept of society which recognized that it was impractical, inhumane, and injudicious to impose economic and political responsibilities on people who were biologically incapable of meeting those responsibilities: Liberty had biological prerequisites.

These considerations were central to debates in France and Britain in the 1830s and 1840s. Governments in both countries were apprehensive of revolution and wary of an alienated underclass, urban and rural, of people who could not be trusted with political rights and seemed immune to the incentives of the market. Such people represented a reservoir of disease, both literal physical disease and metaphorical social disease, that could infect those clinging precariously to the lower rungs of respectability. Reformers proposed to somehow transform these dangerous classes, usually with Bibles, schools, or experimental colonies. Such was the political background against which Edwin Chadwick (1800–1884), secretary of the English bureau charged with overseeing the administration of local poor relief, developed 'the sanitary idea' in the late 1830s (Finer 1952; Hamlin 1998; Lewis 1952; Richards 1980; Chadwick 1965).

Chadwick justified public investment in comprehensive systems of water and sewerage on the grounds that saving lives—particularly of male breadwinners—would be recompensed in lowered costs for the support of widows and orphans. But he also suggested that sanitation would remoralize the underclass, and for many supporters, this was its most important feature. Politically, sanitation was a brilliant idea, as every other general reform was deeply controversial: Proposals for religion and education were plagued by sectarianism, calls to improve welfare by allowing free trade in grain (leading to lower food prices) ran afoul of powerful agricultural interests, proposals for regulating working conditions were unacceptable to powerful industrial interests. Notwithstanding complaints that towns should be allowed to reform in their own ways and their own good time rather than being forced to adopt Chadwick's technologies and deadlines, sanitation achieved remarkable popularity in nineteenth-century Britain. It was the locus of hope not just for improved health, but in general, for a prettier, happier, and better world.

In treating insanitation as the universal cause of disease, Chadwick hoped to establish a public health that was truly liberal. He sought to deflect attention from other causes of disease, such as malnutrition and overwork, for these were areas of great potential conflict between public health and liberal policy. For many, the liberty of the free (or more properly in the case of women, the unmarried) adult to bargain in the market for labour without state intervention to limit hours or kinds of work was axiomatic. And the need for food was to be the spur for work and self-improvement. Interventions by what has recently been called a 'nanny state' seemed to imply an obligation to the state and to affirm the desirability of dependence and subjugation. There were grounds for such concern: The relations of political status to health were fraught with ambiguity. Frank had written passionately of misery as a cause of disease amongst the serfs of Austrian Italy, but had not advocated the elimination of serfdom. Virchow argued, in 1848, that liberal political rights were the answer to typhus in Silesia, and in Scotland, WP Alison argued on the contrary that too rigorous a liberal regime was the cause of poverty-induced typhus (Frank 1941; Rosen 1947; Weindling 1984; Hamlin 2006).

For about a generation, from 1850 to 1880, sanitation was unchallenged in Britain (and in much of its empire) as the keystone of improved health. Chadwick's campaigns led to a series of legislative acts—beginning with the Public Health Act of 1848 and culminating with a comprehensive act in 1875—that established state standards for urban sanitation and a bureau of state medicine, staffed by medical officers in central and local units of government and charged with detecting, responding to, and preventing outbreaks of disease (Wohl 1983).

Outside Britain, although the ideals of sanitation might have had similar appeal, they did not warrant the same conclusions about state responsibility or sanitary technology. The English paradigm of a water-centred sanitary system was adopted only in the twentieth century (Simson 1978; Göckjan 1985; Goubert 1989; Labisch 1992; Münch 1993; Ramsey 1994; Melosi 2000; Hennock 2000). Often, the heritage of medical police was more prominent than that of sanitary engineering. Networks of local medical officers to control contagious disease transmission through the regulation of travel and prostitution were important.

Through the 1880s, the United States remained an exceptional case, coming closest to following a policy that an individual's health was a private matter alone. The national government maintained a system of marine hospitals along the coasts and navigable rivers, less for controlling the spread of epidemics than for relieving ports of the burden of caring for sick seamen. In the early 1880s, it established a National Board of Health to advance knowledge on public health issues of common import, but despite a superb research performance, the Board was scrapped within a few years on the grounds that public health was the business of individual states and cities (Duffy 1990).

Often dominated by rural interests, many state legislatures had little enthusiasm for public health. Louisiana, which established a state board of health to combat yellow fever, was an exception (Ellis 1992). Towns and cities were more active, but often only sporadically, taking steps when faced with epidemics. States that did establish boards of health usually focused on specific problems rather than on public health in general: In Massachusetts, the allotment of pure water resources was a key issue; elsewhere, it was food quality, care for the insane, vital statistics, or the threat of immigrants (Rosenkrantz 1972; Shattuck 1972; Kraut 1994). In Michigan, concern about kerosene quality (it was being adulterated with volatile and explosive petroleum fractions) and arsenical wallpaper dyes spurred the establishment of a state board of health in 1873 (Duffy 1990).

1880–1970: The golden age of public health?

By the 1880s, the classic liberalism of the first half of the nineteenth century was giving way to a resurgent statism. The European nations, the United States, and later, Japan competed for colonies and international influence. If the newly liberated or the newly enfranchised had some claim to a right to health, they also had a duty to the state to be healthy. In most of the industrialized nations, there was renewed interest in monitoring social conditions.

Although the emerging techniques of empirical social research gave this inquiry the aura of quantitative precision, the surveys disclosed little that was distinctly new about the lives or health of the mysterious poor, the usual targets of public health and social reform. Much of it seemed new, however, because it now registered as problematic (Turner 2001). For example, the enormous contribution of infant deaths to total mortality had long been clear, but only towards the end of the century did infant mortality, persistently high even in relatively well-sanitized Britain, become a

problem in itself as distinct from an indicator of sanitary conditions in general. The health conditions of women too, and of workers, began to command attention in a way that they had not done previously (Sellars 1997).

Although these newly recognized public health problems partly reflected the changing distribution of political power, they also reflected anxiety about the nation's vulnerability, and even the decadence of its population. Worried about the strengths of their armies, states such as Britain discovered in the 1890s that too few of those they would call up were competent to be mobilized, and they attributed the problem to a vast range of causes: Poor nutrition (coupled with lack of sunlight in smoky cities), bad sanitation, bad mothering, and bad heredity (Soloway 1982; Pick 1989; Porter 1991a, 1999; Stradling & Thorsheim 1999). Epidemics of smallpox following the Franco-Prussian War of 1870 and again in the 1890s disclosed the gaps in vaccination programmes (Baldwin 1999; Brunton in press). The usual response was to redouble the state's efforts to take responsibility for the immune status of its population. The persistence of syphilis registered at a new level of unacceptability (Brandt 1985; Baldwin 1999).

This led to an expanded public health, one highly successful in terms of reduced mortality and morbidity. It was undertaken jointly in the name of the state and the people, but it involved the regulation of an individual's life—home, work, family relations, recreation, sex—that went beyond the medical police of the previous century. From a later standpoint, such intimate regulation of the individual by the state may seem overbearing, but, with some notable exceptions, the populations of developed countries accepted it as an appropriate and even desirable role for the state.

New diseases, or old diseases that were (or seemed) more prevalent or virulent, new institutions for the practice of public health medicine, and advances in medical and social science contributed to this new relation between states and people. During the 1860s, a long-standing analogy of disease with fermentation matured into the germ theory of disease as the research of Louis Pasteur and John Tyndall made clear the dependence of fermentation on some microscopic living ferment (Pelling 1978; Worboys 2000).

During the 1880s, primarily through the work of emerging German and French schools of determinative bacteriologists, it became possible to distinguish many microbe species from one another, to ascertain the presence of particular species with some degree of confidence, and therefore, to link individual species with particular diseases (Bulloch 1938). Through serological tests developed in the succeeding decades, the presence of a prior infection could be determined, regardless of whether anyone had noticed symptoms.

Notwithstanding the increasing recognition of the many ways by which microbial agents of disease were transmitted from person to person, the effect of the rise of the germ theory was to focus attention on the body that housed and reproduced the germ—for example, the well-digger working through a mild case of typhoid—even when there were alternative strategies (water filtration or, by the second decade of the twentieth century, chlorination) that protected the public reasonably well most of the time (Hamlin 1990; Melosi 2000). The general interest in the human as germ-bearer and culture medium brought with it an emphasis on the labour-intensive business of case-tracing, of keeping track not only of those who showed symptoms of the disease but also those with whom they had contact.

In the key diseases of typhoid fever, syphilis, and tuberculosis, concern with the inspection and regulation of people was exacerbated by the recognition that not all who were infected were symptomatic. The case of 'Typhoid Mary' Mallon, the asymptomatic typhoid carrier who lived for 26 years as an island-bound 'guest' of the City of New York, is notorious, but it was also important in the working out of both legal limits and cultural sensibilities with regard to the trade-off between civil rights and public health (Leavitt 1996). Newly virulent forms of diphtheria and scarlet fever, deadly childhood diseases transmitted person to person or by common domestic media, also gave immediacy to decisive public health intervention.

Such monitoring could not have occurred without a large rank and file of local public health officers. It was during the late nineteenth century that public health was identified as a distinct division of medicine and when most of the developed countries solidified a reasonably complete network of municipal and regional public health officers: In Germany, the *Kreisartz*; in France, the *Officier de Santé*; and in Britain, the Medical Officer of Health, assisted by the sanitary inspector. Increasingly, these officers worked as part of hierarchical national health establishments to which they reported local health conditions and from which they received expert guidance.

Whereas preceding generations of public doctors had often been drawn from the ranks of undercapitalized young doctors, beginning in the mid-1870s, many were specially trained and certified for public health work (Novak 1973; Watkin 1984; Acheson 1991; Porter 1991b). A commitment to public health was increasingly incompatible with ordinary medical practice, not wholly because of its specialized knowledge, but because it was built upon a quite different ethic. There had long been economic tension between public and private medicine in areas of practice such as vaccination, in which public authorities either took over entirely or inadequately compensated private practitioners for services that had traditionally been part of the ordinary medical marketplace (Brunton, in press; White 1991).

But monitoring healthy carriers and those who might be susceptible to disease introduced a new regime of medicine—one which responded to an ethic of public good, even if there were no client-defined complaints. Effectively, bacteriology, epidemiology, and associated measures of immunological status redefined disease away from the patient complaint. The healthy carrier might see no need to seek medical care, but to the public health doctor that person was a social problem. On occasion, private doctors were appealed to for a diagnosis (bronchitis, pneumonia) that would protect one from the health officer's diagnosis of tuberculosis, which would bring loss of employment and social stigma (Smith 1988).

Rivalling the germ theory as the major motif of public health thinking from the 1890s to the 1950s was the application of the emerging science of heredity to the improvement of human populations—the science and practice of eugenics (Paul 1995; Kevles 1995). Whether or not eugenic concerns were the source of the greatest anxiety about the public's health is debatable, but they were the locus of the greatest hope for health progress, the home of a residue of utopianism that had coloured the medical police and sanitary literature. Even more than other forms of public health, eugenics exposed a class, and sometimes a racial, division that had long been a part of public health: Much public health practice was predicated on a distinction between those, usually the poor, who

were seen as the objects of public health efforts and those, often the well-to-do, who authorized intervention, whether to improve the lot of the poor, to protect 'society', or perhaps even to block the physical or moral contagia that might infect their own class (Kraut 1994; Anderson 1995; Bashford & Hooker 2001; Carlin 2005). Eugenics appealed mainly to those with wealth and power: Those others who were to be improved rarely identified heredity as the source of their problems.

Such an attitude is reflected in the most infamous application of the eugenic viewpoint, the attempt by Nazi Germany to exterminate Jews and other 'races' regarded as inferior and unfit not only to intermarry with so-called 'true Aryans', but even to exist. Although historians' views of the origins of the Holocaust differ, some of the immediate precedents for a state policy of negative eugenics—the prevention of the reproduction of those regarded as unfit—came from the sterilization laws that American states had begun to pass in the first decade of the century. The American laws focused on persistent immorality or criminality, and on what was called 'feeble-mindedness'.

In Germany, the acceptance of sterilization translated rather easily into the acceptance of euthanasia of the permanently institutionalized, and on to the extreme measures of the death camps, which were conceived of as facilities of state medicine. Even during the Holocaust, the prevailing rationality remained that of public health: The trade-off between individual rights and the welfare of the state was a part of the working moral world of the public health officer. Just as an excision of corrupt or cancerous matter might be necessarily to maintain the body of the individual, so too an excision of a part of society might be necessary to maintain the health of the nation (Lifton 1986).

The horrors of the extreme version of eugenics practised in Nazi Germany have discredited eugenics to such a degree that it is difficult to recapture how central it seemed to reformers of the left as well as of the far right. It appealed for a number of reasons. First, it explained the failure of prior reforms, particularly sanitation, which was to have effected the thorough physical and moral renewal of the lower classes.

Second, it seemed to be implied by Darwin's discoveries, which were themselves founded on deep familiarity with the remarkable transformations achieved by scientific agriculturalists in animal breeding. Those discoveries seemed particularly applicable within the utilitarian framework of the new statism: The task of governments was to reverse the trend towards decadence and produce uniform, reliable humans. Such concerns became powerful especially for nations that perceived themselves to be in demographic crisis, such as Sweden, which was experiencing depopulation and persistent tuberculosis, and the United States, where successive groups of immigrants found reasons to deplore the effects on the nation of the next immigrant group (Johannisson 1994; Kraut 1994; Broberg & Roll-Hansen 1996).

Finally, it flattered those who held power and prominence by assuring them that this was no accident. It offered a simple explanation, one resistant to empirical falsification, of all that was wrong, and a simple remedy for improvement based on an attractive sociological formula: More sex for those who should breed (sometimes with new partners) and less for those regarded as inferior.

Eugenics sanctioned an enormous range of practices. Although eugenists focused attention on the human genotype and urged the inadequacy of public health programmes that ignored heredity, they were by no means uniformly dismissive of social and environmental reforms. These were needed to allow the better stock to fulfil its potential and because many believed that nurture *could* affect nature: Heredity might be a limiting factor, but significant reforms were needed to fulfil hereditary potential. In almost every country in which eugenics was prominent—the United States, Britain, Japan, Germany, Russia, Brazil, and Argentina—it fitted into a comprehensive concept of social hygiene, albeit one that translated rather easily into racial hygiene (Schneider 1990; Stepan 1991; Porter 1991a; Gallagher 1999).

A third element of this phase of the development of public health was the rise of nutritional science. Although the effects of food on health had broadly been central to Western medicine throughout its history, and it was no mystery that poor food led to poor health, with the exception of the linkage between scurvy and a lack of fresh vegetables, matters of malnutrition and famine had remained outside public health. Remarkably, a science of nutrition that discriminated the particular effects of particular foods only began to take shape in the second half of the nineteenth century, chiefly in the new institutes of agricultural science where animal diets were being studied (Carpenter 1994). Most important was the link of several clinically distinct conditions with a deficit in trace substances in the diet. Particularly remarkable were Goldberger's association of pellagra in the American south with a too heavy reliance on maize, and the recognition of the roles of vitamin D and sunlight in the emergence of rickets. By the 1930s, public health included attention to a varied diet which ensured adequate vitamins (Etheridge 1972; Apple 1996; Marks 2003; Kunitz 2007). Diet, like genes, loomed in the public imagination as the cause of all troubles, and a universal source of hope.

Thus, during this golden age of public health, people in the developed world learned to fear three malign entities: The invisible germs of disease, which might come through the most casual contact; the mysterious genes in their gonads; and the peculiar set of trace nutrients that their food might not contain. Their health and survival depended on all these, yet governments could control them only partially; successful control depended on their behaviour. Hence, a significant role of public health was to educate, advise, and admonish. The citizen, particularly the female citizen, was now being asked to uphold a new standard of cleanliness and to clean things that were not visibly dirty with new kinds of disinfectants. It became important to exercise new prudence in choosing a mate and controlling sexuality. A doctor was required to see whether the baby was being properly fed (Apple 1987; Hoy 1995; Tomes 1998).

Ignorance heightened these hygienic demands. It was clear from tuberculin tests, for example, that exposure to tuberculosis was widespread, in some places nearly universal, but far from clear what was required for exposure to evolve into pulmonary consumption: Whether it was a matter of concentrated exposure, the victim's own constitution, or the diet and environment. All seemed plausible; the advice of public health authorities (who were concerned with infected cases and with their potential for infecting others) involved every aspect of life. It was not simply a matter of not spitting, but of disinfecting eating utensils, clothes, and bedclothes; transforming relations with a spouse, family, and co-workers; and changing diet, leisure activities, and the climate of dwellings (Newsholme 1935; Dubos & Dubos 1987; Smith 1988; Barnes 1995).

Some modern historians have been surprised that these long lists of seemingly exhausting and impossible hygienic expectations,

each with no guarantee of health, did not trigger widespread resentment, victim-blaming, and excessive violations of rights (Armstrong 1983). Four factors are important: First, this was an age stunned by scientific and technical achievement and lacking for the most part a critical vocabulary for mediating expert advice. Second, it was an age of mass aspiration to middle-class standards of living, which were manifested in health, behaviour, and cleanliness. Third, all this was taking place against the backdrop of falling mortality and morbidity, and increasing domestic comfort. Fourth, these efforts were redolent with the ethos of progressive development of the community and the state (Lewis 1986).

The return of liberalism, 1970 to the present day: Lifestyle, environment, and welfare

The decades following the Second World War brought a marked shift in the focus of public health and the expectations of the public. In the developed world, the infectious diseases that had so long been the chief focus of public health receded, with polio being the last of the shock epidemics to fall victim to immunizations, antibiotics, or epidemiological or environmental control (Rogers 1990). With the conquest of fascism and the subsequent decline of communism, liberalism re-emerged. This was symbolized in the mission statement of the World Health Organization (WHO) that health and welfare were the birthright of all (WHO 1968). It was the obligation of states to deliver that right to their populations, who now, at least in the developed world, were made up of those who saw themselves as individual free agents, diverse perhaps in culture but equal in rights. In such a situation, the conflict between the imperatives of public health and civil rights re-emerged. It remains the most formidable issue that public health faces.

The retreat of infectious disease made clearer the failure of the developed nations to grapple with chronic diseases, some of which were the price of longer lifespans (Fox 1993). Some of these were clearly conditions that could be prevented by changes in behaviour: Epidemiological studies in the 1950s and 1960s showed the deadly effects of good living—of smoking and a rich diet (Susser 1985; Marks 1997; Porter 1999). A new set of personal disciplines emerged to control lifestyle diseases and prevent accidents—as well as not smoking, avoiding fats, recreational drugs, and alcohol, exercising one's heart and shedding weight, and using condoms (not to mention flossing and straightening one's teeth), one was to use seat belts and child harnesses, cope with childproof caps on medicine bottles, and accept a fluoridated water supply. All these measures met with objections in terms of their intrusion into personal liberty or on culture, or because they were found to be irksome or unpleasant.

Another feature of post-war public health concern was the shift from individual hygiene back to the environment (Hays 1987; Gottlieb 1993). To many, these heart diseases and cancers, along with other diseases and pathological conditions that seemed even more serious—for example, other forms of cancer, birth defects, lowered sperm counts—had broader structural causes and could be prevented only by comprehensive changes in the physical and social environment (Epstein 1979; McNeill 2000). Thus, part of the liberal resistance to public health imposition was the argument that a focus on disciplining lifestyles came at the cost of attention to grander and more serious political issues (Tesh 1987; Turshen 1987; Levins & Lopez 1999).

Although this new environmentalism had links with the nineteenth-century view of public health as environmental improvement, there were greater differences. The fear of insidious invisible radiation or the toxic chemicals that might lurk in numerous consumer products reflects the terror of germs or of the invisible odourless miasmas which germs replaced; however, the blame was quite differently directed. The new problems of environmental public health were those in which individuals were victimized by corporate oligopolies and by the governments they influence.

Although Chadwick and his associates had warned of vested interests, such as those that perpetuated slum housing, nineteenth-century environmental health problems had a communal character that was missing from the twentieth. Everyone in a nineteenth-century town produced excrement, smoke, ash, and rubbish; the great problem was to find within the community the will and means to act collectively (Wohl 1977; Kearns 1988). Few in a twentieth-century community produced radiation or toxic chemical waste, and the reasons why nothing was done about these seemed all too clear. Public health had failed in its police function; an institution that had evolved to stop the selling of spoiled food by the individual grocer or restaurateur could not cope with the conglomerate or the vast industry that sold goods whose harmful effects were less obvious and slower to appear but which might be much more widely distributed.

The result was an increasingly adversarial relationship between the people and the public health institutions that were supposedly safeguarding their health. To the degree that governments were seen as colluding with the proliferation of these dangerous materials, institutions of public health, as departments of government, were implicated too (Steneck 1984; Brown & Mikkelsen 1990; Edelstein 2004). An epidemiology that spoke the language of 'risk factors' could seem a way to dodge the blame (Rothstein 2003). Even the establishment of new departments of environmental protection, although it might be a means to apply new kinds of expertise to problems of environmental health, did not fundamentally alter the climate of distrust. Public health again became a matter for grassroots political agitation with the emergence of neopopulist Green parties, whose platforms gave prominent attention to health as part of environmental good, and who put their marginality to established governments at the centre of their appeal to the electorate. Public participation became an increasingly important concern (Jasanoff 2005). Nor could victims be confident that the government's epidemiologists would even recognize their disease unless a community of sufferers took it upon themselves to agitate for attention (Packard et al. 2004).

Such a focus on bad environmental policy even informed the response to AIDS and to other new infectious diseases, such as Ebola fever, that appeared in the 1980s and 1990s. Although it became clear that these diseases could be largely controlled through the traditional means of changes in personal behaviour and isolation or restriction of the activities of victims, these recognitions were not fully reassuring. They did little to deflect demand for a vaccine, or the investment of hope in curative medicine. They too could be seen as environmental diseases, caused by environmental changes that had allowed animal viruses to acquire secondary human hosts for whom they were highly virulent. Chief among these changes was the unwise exploitation of tropical forests by a globalizing oligopoly that put profit ahead of prudence (Garrett 1995).

Even those diseases most closely linked to lifestyle choice could be attributed to the broader social environment. People smoked, drank, used drugs, ate too much or vastly too little, practised unsafe sex, spent hours immobilized before televisions absorbing images of violence, hit their spouses and children, or shot their co-workers or themselves because they could no longer cope. To expect disciplined personal behaviour from alienated people living in a stressful world was unrealistic, and the institutions of public health should recognize this.

But the critics were ambivalent as to what such an analysis implied. For some, the obvious response was to remake a society whose support structures were more consistent with the health behaviours it wished to promote. How absurd, for example, for a state to subsidize the production of tobacco and the addiction to it of people in other nations, while blaming its own citizens for smoking (Brandt 2006). For others, such a response sounded like an even more invidiously intrusive state, bent on removing not only the means by which we satisfied unhealthful temptations, but also the temptations themselves. In this 'critical public health' view, the lifestyle agenda was suspicious. It was the public health agenda of an untrustworthy state, not that its people would have chosen. It was not clear that the personal benefits of delayed or denied gratification were worth it: Perhaps one should just enjoy life and rely on the miracles of modern medicine for redemption (Petersen & Lupton 1996).

This view, together with the emergence of widespread cancers and other chronic illnesses for which there was no clear preventive strategy, including the debilitating conditions of ageing, raised the question of why supportive and curative medical care did not form a part or priority in public health. It also raised the question of how far-reaching were the health obligations of the liberal state to its citizens. This issue had vexed public health practitioners throughout the liberal era, although it had often been suppressed because it was seen as too politically volatile.

In socialist or social democratic politics, or where the legacy of medical police remained strong (even when adopted, as in Sweden, by a democratic polity), there was often no clear boundary between public health and the public medical care most people demanded and received (Porter 1999). But elsewhere, the recognition that public health was bound up in the larger issue of human welfare, which in turn included the rest of medical care, was problematic. Many of the newly prominent diseases were not infectious; they could be experienced privately without disturbing community or state, hence the reactive and police rationales for public health did not apply. But they did disrupt the fulfilment of human potential, exacted great costs on productivity, and hence could justly take their place among the demands citizens could make of their governments.

In France, Germany, and Russia, public health services had emerged from, and had remained closely linked to, medical services for the poor (Labisch 1992; Solomon 1994; Ramsey 1994). In mid-nineteenth-century England, Edwin Chadwick, notwithstanding his own post as chief administrator of relief to the poor and the existence of a comprehensive national network of poor law medical officers, had deliberately severed public health (which he equated with sanitary engineering and saw as exclusively preventive) from medical care for the poor. Such medical care was second-rate, grudgingly made available because it was seen as a constitutional right. Expectations of effectiveness were low, however: It was hoped that the poor quality of public medical relief would spur the poor to pay for something better. While moderating the focus on sanitary engineering, Chadwick's English successors retained a distinction between public health medicine and social welfare, which seemed to them only marginally medical and to have more to do with the moral chastisement of the feckless or the warehousing of the incompetent or neglected (Hamlin 1998).

In Ireland, by contrast, an integrated system of public health, welfare, and medical care did emerge during the late nineteenth century, but more by accident than design (Cassell 1997). At the end of the nineteenth century, the Fabian socialists presented British parliament with a clear choice. The Fabians (mainly Beatrice Webb) proposed a much expanded scheme of prevention, although one which made even greater demands on personal and social behaviour as the price the citizen must pay for greater guarantees from the state. The liberals, whose view prevailed, would not discipline personal hygiene, but offered instead an insurance plan to pay for the medical care needed by stricken working men (Fox 1986; Eyler 1997). It was a policy acceptable to the rank and file of the medical profession and that retained and reinforced the split between public health and medicine.

Subsequent efforts to expand state responsibility for health into matters of care and cure have generally worked when medical professions have seen them as advantageous, yet the relationship between even this expanded public medicine and the broader questions of social welfare remain problematic (Starr 1982; Fox 1986; Levins & Lopez 1999; Epstein 2003). The kinds of objections that were made to Webb's scheme still arise: However laudable prevention as a goal, ironically, as we have seen with the concerns about lifestyles and the environment, the strategies and priorities of the preventive public health of the last two centuries have not always been those most desired by the masses of people. To many it has seemed that if the state was going to discipline behaviour for its own purposes, those who suffered that imposition deserved compensation for their trouble when things still went wrong.

Such logic was clearest in compensating veterans of wars. It underwrote the post-war establishment of Britain's National Health Service, which would provide 'health for heroes' and sustains the Veterans Administration medical system in the United States as it lurches from scandal to reform. Thus, what some have complained of as an unrealistic demand for risk-free living, in which people demand a political right to complete freedom of action without accepting responsibility for the consequences (as if one could somehow live free of one's biological self), may be better understood as a complaint about the fairness of the basic social contract of modern societies.

This problem of the relationship between the institutions of public health and the citizenry on whose behalf they claim to act is the greatest challenge currently facing public health in the developed world. That the problems that confront both public health and regular medical practice often stem from a wide range of social causes is plain. That it is so difficult to develop political will to respond to these problems is not chiefly a matter of epidemiological uncertainty. Such pathological phenomena are clearly the product of many causes on many levels, and accordingly, there are numerous points of access where defensible preventive measures might be taken. But almost all of them are likely to intrude on what are claimed as personal or cultural rights, and almost always attempts to act will be met with the response that it is fairer to act elsewhere.

In such cases, epidemiology necessarily requires a large supplement, not from ethics so much as from a moral and political philosophy, that must be acceptable to an increasingly diverse community. Without such a foundation, public health is forced to take refuge in science that is frequently challenged; but simultaneously, it is not clear whether the professional and educational institutions of public health, or the legal, political, and administrative structures that create and maintain it, will be able to initiate and implement a satisfactory enquiry about how these conflicting rights are to be adjudicated.

Key points

◆ Economic and political progress are subordinate to securing health—they are the means; health is the end.

◆ Most modern states have distinguished aspects of health that are the business of the public from those that are for the individual to pursue.

◆ Public health, in the sense of a recognized obligation to protect the health of the people, was only rarely the rationale for policy.

◆ In the nineteenth century, public health shifted radically in mission and constituency. It became less a means of maintaining the state and more a means by which the state served its citizens.

◆ A new set of personal disciplines emerged to control lifestyle diseases and prevent accidents.

◆ Efforts to expand state responsibility for health into matters of care and cure have generally worked when medical professions have seen them as advantageous.

References

Acheson R. The British diploma in public health: birth and adolescence. In: Fee E, Acheson R, editors. *A history of education in public health: health that mocks the doctors rules.* Oxford University Press; 1991. pp. 44–82.

Ackerknecht E. *Medicine at the Paris hospital, 1794–1848.* Baltimore: Johns Hopkins University Press; 1967.

Bynum W.F. *Science and the practice of medicine in the nineteenth century.* Cambridge University Press; 1994.

Amundsen D., Ferngren G. The early Christian tradition. In: Numbers R., Amundusen D., editors. *Caring and curing: health and medicine in the Western religious traditions.* New York (NY): Macmillan; 1986. pp. 40–64.

Anderson W. Excremental colonialism: public health and the poetics of pollution. *Critical Inquiry* 1995;**21**:640–69.

Apple R. *Mothers and medicine: a social history of infant feeding, 1890–1950.* Madison (WI): University of Wisconsin Press; 1987.

Apple R.D. *Vitamania: vitamins in American culture.* New Brunswick (NJ): Rutgers University Press; 1996.

Armstrong D. *The political economy of the body.* Cambridge University Press; 1983.

Arrizabalaga J., Henderson J., French R. *et al. The great pox: the French disease in Renaissance Europe.* New Haven (CT): Yale University Press;1997.

Arrizabalaga J. Syphilis. In: Kiple K, editor. *Cambridge world history of human disease.* Cambridge: Cambridge University Press; 1993. pp. 1025–33.

Baldwin P. *Contagion and the state in Europe, 1830–1930.* New York (NY): Cambridge University Press; 1999.

Barnes D. *The great stink of Paris and the nineteenth-century struggle against filth and germs.* Baltimore (MD): Johns Hopkins University Press; 2006.

Barnes D. *The making of a social disease: tuberculosis in nineteenth-century France.* Berkeley (CA): University of California Press; 1995.

Bashford, A., Hooker, C., editors, *Contagion: Historical and Cultural Studies.* London, New York: Routledge; 2001.

Blackstone W. *Commentaries on the laws of England.* New York (NY): Strouse; 1892.

Boccaccio, G. *The Decameron.* London: Dutton; 1955.

Brand J.L. *Doctors and the state: the British medical profession and government action in public health, 1870–1912.* Baltimore (MD): Johns Hopkins University Press; 1965.

Brandt A. *No magic bullet: a social history of venereal disease in the United States since 1880.* New York (NY): Oxford University Press; 1985.

Brandt A. *The cigarette century: the rise, fall and deadly persistence of the product that defined America.* New York (NY): Basic Books; 2006.

Briggs A. Cholera and society in the nineteenth century. *Past and Present* 1961;**19**:76–96.

Broberg G., Roll-Hansen N., editors. *Eugenics and the welfare state: sterilization policy in Denmark, Sweden, Norway and Finland.* East Lansing (MI): Michigan State University Press; 1996.

Brockliss L., Jones C. *The medical world of early modern France.* Oxford: Clarendon Press; 1997.

Brody S. *The disease of the soul; leprosy in medieval literature.* Ithaca (NY): Cornell University Press; 1974.

Brown P., Mikkelsen E. *No safe place: toxic waste, leukemia, and community action.* Berkeley (CA): University of California Press; 1990.

Browne T. Religio medici. In: *Religio medici and other works.* Oxford: Clarendon Press; 1964.

Brunton D. *Political medicine: the construction of vaccination policy across Britain, 1800–1871.* University of Rochester Press; in press.

Bulloch W. *The history of bacteriology.* New York (NY): Oxford University Press; 1938.

Carlin C., editor. *Imagining contagion in early modern Europe.* New York (NY): Macmillan Palgrave; 2005.

Carmichael A. Leprosy: larger than life. In: Kiple K, editor. *Plague, pox, and pestilence.* New York (NY): Barnes and Noble; 1997. pp. 50–7.

Carmichael A. Plague and more plagues. *Early Science and Medicine* 2003;**8**:253–66.

Carmichael A. *Plague and the poor in Renaissance Florence.* Cambridge: Cambridge University Press; 1986.

Carmichael A. Plague of Athens. In: Kiple K, editor. *Cambridge world history of human disease.* Cambridge: Cambridge University Press; 1993. pp. 934–7.

Carpenter K. Protein and energy: a study of changing ideas in nutrition. Cambridge University Press; 1994.

Carroll P. Medical police and the history of public health. *Medical History* 2002;**46**:461–94.

Cassedy J. *Charles V: Chapin and the public health movement.* Cambridge (MA): Harvard University Press; 1962.

Cassell R.D. *Medical charities, medical politics: the Irish dispensary system and the poor law, 1836–1872.* Woodbridge, Suffolk: Royal Historical Society/Boydell Press; 1997.

Chadwick E. Report on the sanitary condition of the labouring population of Great Britain. Edinburgh University Press; 1965.

Chew H., Kellaway W.E., editors. *London assize of nuisance, 1301–141: a calendar.* London: London Record Society; 1973.

Cipolla C. Faith, reason, and the plague in seventeenth century Tuscany. New York (NY): Norton; 1979.

Cipolla C. *Fighting the plague in seventeenth-century Italy.* Madison (WI): University of Wisconsin Press; 1981.

Cipolla C. *Miasmas and disease: public health and the environment in the pre-industrial age.* Potter E, translator. New Haven (CT): Yale University Press; 1992.

Clendening L. *Source book of medical history.* New York (NY): Dover Publications; 1942.

Coleman W. *Death is a social disease: public health and political economy in early industrial France.* Madison (WI): University of Wisconsin Press; 1982.

Coleman W. Health and hygiene in the *Encyclopedie*: A medical doctrine for the bourgeoisie. *Journal of the History of Medicine* 1974;**29**:399–421.

Coleman W. *Yellow fever in the North: the methods of early epidemiology.* Madison (WI); University of Wisconsin Press; 1987.

Conrad L. Epidemic disease in formal and popular thought in early Islamic society. In: Ranger T, Slack P, editors. *Epidemics and ideas: essays on the historical perception of pestilence.* Cambridge University Press; 1992. pp. 77–99.

Crosby A. *Ecological imperialism: the biological expansion of Europe, 900–1900.* Cambridge University Press; 1986.

Dean M. *The constitution of poverty: toward a genealogy of liberal governance.* London: Routledge; 1991.

Delaporte F. *Disease and civilization, the cholera in Paris, 1832.* Cambridge (MA): MIT Press; 1986.

Desrosières A. The politics of large numbers: A history of statistical reasoning. Naish C, translator. Cambridge (MA): Harvard University Press; 1998.

Dols M. *The Black Death in the Middle East.* Princeton (NJ): Princeton University Press; 1977.

Dorff E. The Jewish tradition. In: Numbers R, Amundusen D, editors. *Caring and curing: health and medicine in the Western religious traditions.* New York (NY): Macmillan; 1986. pp. 5–39.

Douglas M. Purity and danger: an analysis of the concepts of pollution and taboo. London: Routledge; 1966.

Dubos R., Dubos J. *The white plague: tuberculosis, man and society.* New Brunswick (NJ): Rutgers University Press; 1987.

Duffy J. *The sanitarians: a history of American public health.* Urbana (IL): University of Illinois Press; 1990.

Durbach N. *Bodily Matters: The Anti-vaccination Movement in England, 1853–1907.* Durham: Duke University Press; 2005.

Durey M. *The return of the plague: British society and cholera, 1831–32.* Dublin: Gill and MacMillan; 1979.

Edelstein M. *Contaminated communities: social and psychological impacts of residential toxic exposure.* 2nd ed. Boulder (CO): Westview; 2004.

Ellis J.H. *Yellow fever and public health in the New South.* Lexington (KY): University Press of Kentucky; 1992.

Epstein R. Let the shoemaker stick to his last: a defense of the 'old' public health. *Perspectives in Biology and Medicine* 2003;**46**:s138–s159.

Epstein S. *The politics of cancer.* Revised edition. New York (NY): Anchor; 1979.

Etheridge E. *The butterfly caste: a social history of pellagra in the South.* Westport (CT): Greenwood Press; 1972.

Evans R.J. *Death in Hamburg: society and politics in the cholera years, 1830–1910.* London: Penguin Books; 1990.

Eyler J. *Sir Arthur Newsholme and state medicine, 1885–1935.* Cambridge University Press; 1997.

Eyler J.M. *Victorian social medicine: the ideas and methods of William Farr.* Baltimore (MD): Johns Hopkins University Press; 1979.

Fee E. Public health, past and present: a shared social vision. In: Rosen G, editor. *A history of public health.* Expanded edition. Baltimore (MD): Johns Hopkins University Press; 1993. pp. ix–lxvii.

Finer S.E. *The life and times of Sir Edwin Chadwick.* London: Methuen; 1952.

Foucault M. *The birth of the clinic.* New York (NY): Vintage; 1975.

Fox D. *Health policies, health politics: British and American experience, 1911–1965.* Princeton (NJ): Princeton University Press; 1986.

Fox D. *Power and illness: the failure and future of American health policy.* Berkeley (CA): University of California Press; 1993.

Frank J.P. *A system of complete medical police; selections from Johann Peter Frank.* Baltimore (MD): Johns Hopkins University Press; 1976.

Frank J.P. Academic address on the people's misery. *Bulletin of the History of Medicine* 1941;**9**:88–100.

Gallagher N. *Breeding better Vermonters.* Hanover (NH): University Press of New England; 1999.

Garrett L. *The coming plague: newly emerging diseases in a our world of balance.* New York (NY): Penguin; 1995.

Geary L. Famine, fever, and the bloody flux. In: Poirteir C, editor. *The Great Irish Famine.* Dublin: Mercier Press; 1995. pp. 74–85.

Göckjan G. Kurieren und Staat Machen: Gesundheit und Medizin in der burgerlichen welt. Frankfurt am Main: Suhrkamp; 1985. pp. 19.

Gori L. Arabic treatises on environmental pollution upto the end of the thirteenth century. *Environment and History* 2002.**8**:475–88.

Gottlieb R. *Forcing the spring: the transformation of the American environmental movement.* Washington (DC): Island Press; 1993.

Goubert J.P. *The conquest of water.* Wilson A, translator. London: Polity Press; 1989.

Guillerme A. *The age of water: the urban environment in the north of France, AD 300–1800.* College Station (TX): Texas A & M University Press; 1988.

Hamlin C. *A science of impurity: water analysis in nineteenth century Britain.* Adam Hilger/University of California Press; 1990.

Hamlin C. Environmental sensibility in Edinburgh, 1839–1840: the 'fetid irrigation' controversy. *Journal of Urban History* 1994;**20**:311–39.

Hamlin C. Muddling in bumbledom: local governments and large sanitary improvements: the cases of four British towns, 1855–1885. *Victorian Studies* 1988;**32**:55–83.

Hamlin C. Predisposing causes and public health in the early nineteenth century public health movement. *Social History of Medicine* 1992;**5**: 43–70.

Hamlin C. *Public health and social justice in the age of Chadwick: Britain 1800–1854.* Cambridge University Press; 1998.

Hamlin C. Public sphere to public health: the transformation of 'nuisance'. In: Sturdy S, editor. *Medicine, health, and the public sphere in Britain, 1600–2000.* London: Routledge; 2002. pp. 190–204.

Hamlin C. Sanitary policing and the local state, 1873–74: a Statistical study of English and Welsh towns. *Social History of Medicine* 2005; **18**:39–61.

Hamlin C. William Pulteney Alison, the Scottish philosophy, and the making of a political medicine. *Journal of the History of Medicine and Allied Sciences* 2006:547–66.

Haskell T. Capitalism and the origins of the humanitarian sensibility. *American Historical Review* 1985;**90**:339–61.

Hays S. *Beauty, health, and permanence: environmental politics in the United States, 1955–1985.* Cambridge University Press; 1987.

Hennock E.P. The urban sanitary movement in England and Germany, 1838–1914: a comparison. *Continuity and Change* 2000;**15**:269–96.

Hope V., Marshall E., editors. *Death and disease in the ancient city.* London: Routledge; 2000.

Hopkins D. *Princes and peasants: smallpox in history.* New edition. Chicago (IL): University of Chicago Press; 2002.

Hoy S. *Chasing dirt: the American pursuit of cleanliness.* New York (NY): Oxford University Press; 1995.

Humphreys M. *Yellow fever and the South.* New Brunswick (NJ): Rutgers University Press; 1992.

Jasanoff S. *Designs on nature: science and democracy in Europe and the United States.* Princeton (NJ): Princeton University Press; 2005.

Johannisson K. The people's health: public health policies in Sweden. In: Porter D, editor. *The history of public health and the modern state.* Amsterdam: Rudopi; 1994. pp. 165–82.

Karmi G. State control of the physician in the Middle Ages: an Islamic model. In: Russell A, editor. *The town and state physician in Europe from the Middle Ages to the Enlightenment.* Wolfenbüttel, Germany: Herzog August Bibliothek; 1981. pp. 63–84.

Kearns G. Cholera, nuisances, environmental management in Islington, 1830–1855. In: Bynum WF, Porter R, editors. *Living and dying in London.* London: Wellcome Institute for the History of Medicine; 1991. pp. 94–125.

Kearns G. Private property and public health reform in England, 1830–1870. *Social Science and Medicine* 1988;**26**:187–99.

Kevles D. *In the name of eugenics: genetics and the uses of human heredity.* Cambridge (MA): Harvard University Press; 1995.

Kinzelbach A. Infection, contagion, and public health in late Medieval and early Modern German imperial towns. *Journal of the History of Medicine* 2006;**61**:369–89.

Kraut A. *Silent travelers: germs, genes, and the 'immigrant menace'.* New York (NY): Basic Books; 1994.

Kunitz S. *The Health of Populations: General Theories and Particular Realities.* New York: Oxford University Press; 2007.

LaBerge A. *Mission and method: the early-nineteenth-century French public health movement.* Cambridge University Press; 1992.

Labisch A. *Homo hygienicus: Gesundheit und Medizin in der Neuzeit.* New York (NY): Campus; 1992.

Lambert R. *Sir John Simon and English social administration.* London: McGibbon and Kee; 1965.

Leavitt J. *Typhoid Mary: captive to the public's health.* Boston (MA): Beacon Press; 1996.

Leongard J., editor. *London viewers and their certificates, 1508–1558: certificates of the sworn viewers of the City of London.* London: London Record Society; 1989.

Levins R., Lopez C. Toward an ecosocial view of health. *International Journal of Health Services* 1999;**29**:261–93.

Lewis J. *What price community medicine? The philosophy, practice, and politics of public health since 1919.* Brighton: Wheatsheaf Books; 1986.

Lewis R.A. *Edwin Chadwick and the public health movement, 1832–1854.* London: Longmans Green; 1952.

Lieber E. Old Testament 'leprosy', contagion and sin. In: Conrad LI, Wujastyk K, editors. *Contagion: perspectives from pre-Modern societies.* Aldershot, UK: Ashgate; 2000. pp. 99–136.

Lifton R. *The Nazi doctors: medical killing and the psychology of genocide.* New York (NY): Basic Books; 1986.

Longrig J. Epidemic, ideas and classical Athenian society. In: Ranger T, Slack P, editors. *Epidemics and ideas: essays on the historical perception of pestilence.* Cambridge University Press; 1992. pp. 21–44

López-Piñero J.M. The medical profession in sixteenth-century Spain. In: Russell A, editor. *The town and state physician in Europe from the Middle ages to the Enlightenment.* Wolfenbüttel, Germany: Herzog August Bibliothek; 1981. pp. 85–98.

MacMahon B., Pugh T. *Epidemiology: pinciples and methods.* Boston (MA): Little, Brown; 1970.

Magnello E. The introduction of mathematical statistics into medical research: the roles of Karl Pearson, Major Greenwood, and Austin Bradford Hill. In: Magnello E, Hardy A, editors. *The road to medical statistics.* Amsterdam: Rodopi; 2002. pp. 95–123.

Marks H. Epidemiologists explain pellagra: gender, race, and political economy in the work of Edgar Sydenstricker. *Journal of the History of Medicine and Allied Sciences* 2003;**58**:34–55.

Marks H. *The progress of experiment: science and therapeutic reforming the United States, 1900–1990.* Cambridge University Press; 1997.

McClure R. *Coram's children: the London Foundling Hospital in the eighteenth century.* New Haven (CT): Yale University Press; 1981.

McGrew R. *Russia and the cholera, 1823–1832.* Madison (WI): University of Wisconsin Press; 1965.

McHugh P. *Prostitution and Victorian social reform.* London: Croom Helm; 1982.

McNeill J.R. *An environmental history of the twentieth-century world.* New York (NY): Norton; 2000.

McNeill W. *Plagues and peoples.* New York (NY): Anchor Doubleday; 1976.

Melosi M. *The sanitary city: urban infrastructure in America from colonial times to the present.* Baltimore (MD): Johns Hopkins University Press; 2000.

Miller G. *The adoption of inoculation for smallpox in England and France.* Philadelphia (PA): University of Pennsylvania Press; 1957.

Münch P. *Stadthygiene im 19 und 20 jahrhundert*. Göttingen, Germany: Vandenhoeck und Ruprecht; 1993.

Newsholme A. *Fifty years in public health: a personal narrative with comments*. Vol 1: *The years preceding 1909*. London: George Allen and Unwin; 1935.

Nohl J. *The Black Death*. London: George Allen and Unwin; 1926.

Novak SJ. Professionalism and bureaucracy: English doctors and the Victorian public health administration. *Journal of Social History* 1973;**6**:440–62.

Novak WJ. *The people's welfare: law and regulation in nineteenth-century America*. Chapel Hill (NC): University of North Carolina Press; 1996.

Nutton V. Did the Greeks have a name for it? Contagion and contagion theory in classical antiquity. In: Conrad LI, Wujastyk K, editors. *Contagion: perspectives from pre-Modern societies*. Aldershot, UK: Ashgate; 2000. pp. 137–62.

Packard RM, Brown PJ, Berkelman RL *et al*., editors. Introduction: emerging illnesses as social process. In: *Emerging illnesses and society: negotiating the agenda of public health*. Baltimore (MD): Johns Hopkins University Press; 2004.

Palmer R. Physicians and the state in post-medieval Italy. In: Russell A, editor. *The town and state physician in Europe from the Middle Ages to the Enlightenment*. Wolfenbüttel, Germany: Herzog August Bibliothek; 1981. pp. 47–62.

Paul DB. *Controlling human heredity: 1865 to the present*. Atlantic Highlands (NJ): Humanities Press; 1995.

Pelling M. *Cholera, fever, and English medicine, 1825–1865*. Oxford University Press; 1978.

Pelling M. The meaning of contagion: reproduction, medicine and metaphor. In: Bashford A, Hooker C, editors. *Contagion: historical and cultural studies*. London: Routledge; 2001. pp. 15–38.

Petersen A., Lupton D. *The new public health: health and self in the age of risk*. London: Sage; 1996.

Pettenkofer M. *The value of health to a city* [translation, with an introduction by HE Sigerist]. Baltimore (MD): Johns Hopkins University Press; 1941.

Pick D. *Faces of degeneration: a European disorder, c. 1848–1918*. Cambridge University Press; 1989.

Pickstone JV. Dearth, dirt, and fever epidemics: rewriting the history of British 'public health', 1780–1850. In: Ranger T, Slack P, editors. *Epidemics and ideas: essays on the historical perception of pestilence*. Cambridge University Press; 1992. pp. 125–48.

Porter D., Porter R. The politics of prevention: anti-vaccinationism and public health in nineteenth century England. *Medical History* 1988;**32**:231–52.

Porter D. 'Enemies of the race': biologism, environmentalism, and public health in Edwardian England. *Victorian Studies* 1991a;**34**:159–78.

Porter D. *Health, civilization and the state*. London: Routledge; 1999.

Porter D. Stratification and its discontents: professionalization and conflict in the British public health service, 1848–1914. In: Fee E, Acheson R, editors. *A history of education in public health: health that mocks the doctor's rules*. Oxford University Press; 1991b. pp. 83–113.

Ramsey M. Public health in France. In: Porter D, editor. *The history of public health and the modern state*. Amsterdam: Rudopi; 1994. pp. 45–118.

Razzell P. *The conquest of smallpox: the impact of inoculation on smallpox mortality in eighteenth century England*. Firle, Sussex: Caliban; 1977.

Redlich J., Hirst F. *The history of local government in England* [reissue of Book I of *Local government in England*]. 2nd ed. New York (NY): Augustus Kelley; 1970.

Richards P. State formation and class struggle. In: Corrigan P, editor. *Capitalism, state formation, and Marxist theory*. London: Quartet; 1980. pp. 49–78.

Richards P. *The medieval leper and his northern heirs*. Totowa (NJ): Rowman and Littlefield; 1977.

Richardson R. *Death, dissection, and the destitute*. London: Penguin; 1988.

Riley JC. *The eighteenth century campaign to avoid disease*. London: Macmillan; 1987.

Roberton J. *Observations on the mortality and physical management of children*. London: Longman, Rees, Orme, Brown; 1827.

Rogers N. *Dirt and disease: polio before FDR*. New Brunswick (NJ): Rutgers University Press; 1990.

Rosen G, editor. Cameralism and the concept of medical police. In: *From medical police to social medicine: essays on the history of health care*. New York (NY): Science History; 1974a. pp. 120–41.

Rosen G, editor. The fate of the concept of medical police, 1780–1890. In: *From medical police to social medicine: essays on the history of health care*. New York (NY): Science History; 1974b. pp. 142–58.

Rosen G. *A history of public health*. New York (NY): MD Publications; 1958.

Rosen, G. What is social medicine: a genetic analysis of the concept. *Bulletin of the History of Medicine* 1947;**21**:674–733.

Rosenberg C: *The cholera years: the United States in 1832, 1849, and 1866*. Chicago (IL): University of Chicago Press; 1962.

Rosenkrantz B. *Public health and the state: changing views in Massachusetts, 1842–1936*. Cambridge (MA): Harvard University Press; 1972.

Rosenkrantz BG. Cart before horse: theory, practice and professional image in American public health, 1870–1920. *Journal of the History of Medicine* 1974;**29**:55–73.

Rothstein W. *Public health and the risk factor: a history of an uneven medical revolution*. Rochester (NY): University of Rochester Press; 2003.

Sadler M. *The law of population*. A treatise in six books, in disproof of the superfecundity of human beings, and developing the real principle of their increase. London: John Murray; 1830.

Schneider WH. *Quality and quantity: the quest for biological regeneration in 20th century France*. Cambridge University Press; 1990.

Sellars C. *Hazards of the job: from industrial disease to environmental health science*. Chapel Hill (NC): University of North Carolina Press; 1997.

Shattuck L. *Report of a general plan for the promotion of public and personal health, devised, prepared, and recommended by the commissioners … relating to a sanitary survey of the state*. New York: Arno; 1972.

Simon J. *English sanitary institutions, reviewed in their course of development, and in some of their political and social relations*. London: Cassell; 1890.

Simson JV. Die Flussverungsreinigungsfrage im Jahrhundert. *Vierteljahrschirft für sozial-und wirtschaftgeschichte* 1978;**65**:370–90.

Skisnes O. Notes from the history of leprosy. *International Journal of Leprosy* 1973;**41**:220–37.

Slack P. *The impact of the plague in Tudor and Stuart England*. London: Routledge and Kegan Paul; 1985.

Smith DC. Medical science, medical practice, and the emerging concept of typhus. In: Bynum WF, Nutton V, editors. *Theories of fever from Antiquity to the Enlightenment*. London: Wellcome Institute for the History of Medicine; 1981. pp. 121–34.

Smith FB. *The retreat of tuberculosis, 1850–1950*. London: Croom Helm 1988.

Snowden F. *Naples in the time of cholera 1884–1911*. Cambridge University Press; 1995.

Solomon SG. The expert and the state in Russian public health: continuities and changes across the revolutionary divide. In: Porter D, editor. *The history of public health and the modern state*. Amsterdam: Rudopi; 1994. pp. 183–223.

Soloway RA. *Birth control and the population question in England, 1877–1930*. Chapel Hill (NC): University of North Carolina Press; 1982.

Starr P. *The social transformation of American medicine*. New York (NY): Basic Books; 1982.

Steneck N. *The microwave debate*. Cambridge (MA): MIT Press; 1984.

Stepan N. *The hour of eugenics: race, gender, and nation in Latin America*. Ithaca (NY): Cornell University Press; 1991.

Stradling D., Thorsheim P. The smoke of great cities: British and American efforts to control air pollution, 1860–1914. *Environmental History* 1999;**4**:6–31.

Sturdy S., editor. Introduction: medicine, health, and the public sphere. *Medicine, health, and the public sphere in Britain, 1600–2000*. London: Routledge; 2002. pp. 190–204.

Sturm C.C. *Sturm's reflections on the works of God, and his providence throughout all nature*. Philadelphia (PA): Woodward; 1832.

Susser M. 'Epidemiology in the United States after World War II: the evolution of technique.'. *Epidemiologic Reviews* 1985;**7**:147–77.

Taylor V., Trentmann F. From users to consumers: water politics in nineteenth-century London. In: Trentmann F, editor. *The making of the consumer: knowledge, power and identity in the modern world*. Oxford: Berg; 2005.

Tesh S.N. *Hidden arguments: political ideology and disease prevention*. New Brunswick (NJ): Rutgers University Press; 1987.

Thompson E.P. The moral economy of the English crowd in the eighteenth century. *Past and Present* 1971;**50**:76–136.

Thucydides. *The history of the Peloponnesian War*. Crawley R, translator. New York (NY): EP Dutton; 1950.

Tomes N. *The gospel of germs: men, women, and the microbe in American life*. Cambridge (MA): Harvard University Press; 1998.

Touati F-O. Contagion and leprosy: myth, ideas and evolution in medieval minds and societies. In: Conrad LI, Wujastyk K, editors. *Contagion: perspectives from pre-Modern societies*. Aldershot, UK: Ashgate; 2000. pp. 179–201.

Turner S. What is the problem with experts?. *Social Studies of Science* 2001;**31**:123–49.

Turshen M. *The politics of public health*. New Brunswick (NJ): Rutgers University Press; 1987.

Veyne P., editor. The Roman empire. In: *A history of private life. Vol I: From pagan Rome to Byzantium*. Goldhammer A, translator. Cambridge (MA): Belknap Press of Harvard University Press; 1987. pp. 222–32.

Waddington K. *The bovine scourge: meat, tuberculosis and public health, 1850–1914*. Woodbridge, UK: Boydell; 2006.

Walkowitz J. *Prostitution and Victorian society: women, class and the state*. Cambridge University Press; 1980.

Watkin D. The English revolution in social medicine, 1889–1911. Unpublished PhD thesis. University of London; 1984.

Webb S., Webb B. *English local government from the Revolution to the Municipal Corporations Act: statutory authorities for special purposes*. London: Longmans Green; 1922.

Weindling P. Was social medicine revolutionary? Rudolph Virchow and the Revolution of 1848. *Bulletin of the Society for the Social History of Medicine* 1984;**34**:13–8.

Weiner D. *The citizen-patient in revolutionary and imperial Paris*. Baltimore (MD): Johns Hopkins University Press; 1993.

Weyland J. *The principles of population and production as they are affected by the progress of society with view to moral and political consequences* [original, 1816]. New York (NY): Augustus Kelley; 1968.

White K. *Healing the schism: epidemiology, medicine and the public's health*. New York (NY): Springer; 1991.

Wilson F.R. *A practical guide for inspectors of nuisances*. London: Knight; 1881.

Wilson L. Fevers and science in early nineteenth century medicine. *Journal of the History of Medicine* 1978;**33**:386–407.

Winslow C.A. *The conquest of epidemic disease: a chapter in the history of ideas* [original ed 1943]. Madison (WI): University of Wisconsin Press; 1980.

Wohl A. *The eternal slum: housing and social policy in Victorian London*. London: Edward Arnold; 1977.

Wohl A.S. *Endangered lives: public health in Victorian Britain*. Cambridge (MA): Harvard University Press; 1983.

Worboys M. *Spreading germs: disease theories and medical practice in Britain, 1865–1900*. Cambridge University Press; 2000.

World Health Organization. *Constitution of the World Health Organization in WHO Basic Documents*. 19th ed. Geneva: World Health Organization; 1968.

Ziegler P. *The Black Death*. New York (NY): Harper Torchbooks; 1969.

1.3

The history and development of public health in low- and middle-income countries

Than Sein

Introduction

Public health broadly deals with identification of health problems that affect the entire population with mechanisms to address these problems effectively. Historically, public health interventions are those that promote and protect people's health, and are chiefly undertaken by the governments. Ko Ko (1986) charted the progress of public health development over five eras—empirical health, basic science, clinical science, public health, and political science. Detels and Breslow (2000) described public health as a process of mobilizing local, state, national, and international resources to ensure the conditions in which people can be healthy. Beaglehole and Bonita (2004) referred to it as a collective action for sustained population-wide health improvement, emphasizing the hallmarks of sustained health actions and interventions addressing the health of the whole population. The notion of public within the term, public health, encompasses the interventions for health development by the people themselves individually and collectively, in addition to those carried out by the government or its agents. In general, public health is a comprehensive measure by the government and the people, covering promotive, preventive, curative, and rehabilitative aspects. Public health actions, for many centuries and even today, mainly focus on prevention and control of diseases or conditions that particularly affect a large number of people. Public health interventions not only deal with control and management of diseases, but also address the prevention or reduction of risks and root causes of these problems. Since fundamental characteristics of public health actions lie primarily on the social and other determinants of health, that are outside the domain of the health sector and also beyond the individual's action, these actions are not only the responsibility of the government, but also that of the people themselves.

The socioeconomic health and other development status of the world have changed rapidly and radically in recent years. Spectacular scientific advancement has led humans into outer space and also to apply such advanced knowledge and skill to health sciences, with which millions of lives have been saved. Yet, majority of people in over 150 countries around the world had a per-capita Gross National Income (GNI) of below US$10 725 in 2005, which are known generally, as the low- and middle-income (LMI) countries

as classified by the World Bank (World Bank 2006a). People in many LMI countries live in poverty with inadequate healthcare and low health status. The present chapter reviews the history and development of public health in LMI countries of which about one-third are classified as least-developed nations. It provides an insight that could contribute to the solution of present and future challenges and opportunities for health development which actually influence the health of the world. Learning from the experience of past developments in public health is an essential element in modern public health education. Some examples of public health development in LMI countries of Asia and the Pacific are highlighted.

The chapter firstly traces health systems development from the colonial period to the present century. It documents the post-independent efforts of LMI countries in their health development, within the context of socioeconomic and political development, including collaborative work at inter-country and international levels. In the next section, it briefly touches upon disease prevention and control, especially how LMI countries cope with the prevailing high morbidity and mortality conditions, and the major public health achievements and failures. The lessons in eradication and elimination efforts for preventing and controlling priority diseases provide a clear perception on the application of principles and practice of public health. It also highlights the links between the epidemiological, political, and financing aspects of disease control. The next section covers why and how there is a shift in major causes of deaths and diseases in LMI countries with an increasing burden of chronic non-communicable diseases. This has led to adoption of measures and interventions beyond the usual health-sector functions for reducing risks, such as legislative, environment, and educative actions. These include the reduction of tobacco and alcohol use, avoiding unhealthy diets and promoting physical activity, or adopting multisectoral measures for road safety and injury prevention.

At the turn of the twentieth century, many LMI countries moved towards another era of public health development, with new thinking from a narrow view of vertical disease control interventions to a wider perspective of multisectoral interventions. Besides the usual public health measures undertaken by governments, an increasing number of non-governmental organizations and the private sector agencies, both at the local and global levels, were involved in public health development. In addition to the international agencies dealing with health under the UN system, many intergovernmental and international bodies and philanthropic organizations, foundations, and alliances are supporting and complementing the global public health functions. In summary, public health essentially deals with the health of the population in its totality. The success of public health measures depends on adhering to the basic principles of equity, social justice, and partnerships.

Protecting people's health

Public health practices during the colonial period

From time immemorial, human beings have dealt with the spread of dreadful diseases like diarrhoeal diseases, smallpox, plague, or syphilis, through various aspects of personal hygiene and other public health practices, including civic duties on sanitation measures, which were enforced by royal decrees. Since those ancient periods, measures to promote and protect the health of the people remained as the dedicated actions of the statehood in many countries in Asia, Africa, the Americas, and Europe. Modern public health principles and practices were further developed during the so-called Victorian period of the eighteenth–nineteenth centuries. With increasing ability to identify the causal factors of the diseases and conditions, knowledge on the social, environmental, and political dimensions of the diseases and their prevention grew tremendously. In addition to the establishment of medical care facilities, a series of legislative measures similar to that of colonial countries were initiated in order to protect the health of their own people. Such legislative measures on public health matters—such as improved sanitation facilities and practices, installation of safe water supply systems, and the preventive and control responses to epidemics—might have varied according to the origin of the colonial powers, but were effective in reducing the outbreaks of communicable diseases. The definite imprints of these legislative measures—such as the Public Health Acts, Local Government and Municipality Acts, Vital Registration Act, Factory Act, Food Adulteration Act, Vaccination Act, Contagious Diseases Act, etc.—are still in existence in many LMI countries. Only a few years ago, some laws and acts were updated or replaced with newer legislation. Some health systems' practices like hospital care, maternity homes, sanatoria, and quarantine places are still functioning as they did for centuries. The European model of a national social health insurance scheme also spread to other countries, especially to those in East Asia.

Many missionaries with western education and an allopathic medical background had established education, medial care, and research institutions, the so-called western institutions. The introduction of western medicine by missionaries resulted in first exposure and increasing access by the local populace to the western way of allopathic medical practices. The infectious diseases were identified as tropical diseases, since they mainly existed in the tropical countries. The prevention, control, and management of tropical diseases became priority teaching subjects for medical professionals and public health workers who liked to work in the colonies (Uragoda 1987; Harrison 1994). Many researchers and public health professionals in Europe and America became well known after they did their practices and research studies on the epidemiology and control of infectious diseases in the tropical countries. During the late eighteenth century, education in public

health and tropical diseases flourished in Europe and North America with new institutions for undergraduate and postgraduate training. Many pioneer public health schools and tropical disease research institutions were established in the colonial home countries starting from the eighteenth century. These were institutions like Johns Hopkins School of Public Health in the United States, the London and Liverpool Schools of Tropical Medicine in Britain, and the School of Public Health in Spain. These institutions acted as home-based training institutions for research and development to spread the knowledge and information on the prevention and control of tropical diseases, and to train people who would like to serve in the tropical countries. Discoveries of causative organisms and ways of stopping transmission of malaria, sleeping sickness, and worm infestations, and also identification of nutritional disorders through clinical and public health research studies were initiated by these schools. These education and research practices were later spread to the people and institutions in the colonies and other countries. With technical and financial support of the Rockefeller Foundation and the technical support of the Johns Hopkins School of Public Health, the London School of Tropical Medicine was transformed into the London School of Hygiene and Tropical Medicine in 1920, expanding the scope of research and teaching in tropical medicine, public health administration, medical statistics, and epidemiology (Wilkinson & Power 1998). Spain established its National School of Public Health in 1924 and introduced a public health component into its comprehensive rural medical care network. The British authorities also established similar public health educational and research institutions in India starting from the early 1920s, such as the Institute of Tropical Medicine and the All-India Institute of Hygiene and Public Health in Kolkata (Calcutta) to undertake research in tropical diseases and to train local people on hygiene and public health. After that, a series of research and training institutions and laboratories were established for undertaking basic and applied research and training on specific diseases in India, which later became the exemplary institutions serving India and its neighbours for several decades (Jaggi 1979). Other colonial rulers also established similar medical and public health educational and research institutions in their respective colonies. Independent countries like Poland, China, Thailand, and Japan also followed similar developments. These educational institutions worked closely with their colonial counterparts to strengthen the skill, knowledge, and expertise on control of tropical diseases.

Actually, the development of public health and medical care services for the general public or natives in the colonies remained rudimentary. Local people were suffering from epidemic outbreaks not only from indigenous infectious sources but also from diseases imported through trade and migration routes. Moving millions of people to totally unfamiliar areas made them vulnerable to new diseases. Thousands of people died in new territories due to smallpox, malaria, yellow fever, typhus, typhoid, and cholera, or were disabled due to yaws, leprosy, and syphilis. Similarly, people who went for trade and commodities brought back infectious diseases to their homes in Europe and America. While the Americans initially launched the control of malaria and yellow fever campaigns in the eighteenth century, the British, French, and Dutch colonials initiated major international public health initiative for control of smallpox through vaccination, first among the people within the colonial administration and the workers employed, and later the general public. The colonials later launched community-based health interventions and research-cum-action projects for malaria control and worm infestation in some tropical countries, to have a better knowledge for the prevention and control that could be replicated in other parts of the world (Foster & Anderson 1978).

Foundation for international public health

Efforts in international public health were intensified in the mid-1800s, when the United States of America and the European nations started applying protective legislative measures to prevent the importation of diseases from trading ships and their cargo. An international sanitary conference, organized by a group of European nations in Paris in 1851, looking for solutions for protecting epidemic diseases coming from the tropics, drafted the international quarantine regulations, which was the precursor of today's International Health Regulations. Over the next 50 years, a series of international conferences held in Europe and America covered health and social issues including trafficking in liquor and opium. A major milestone at the eleventh international sanitary conference held in Paris in 1903 was the adoption of the first international sanitary convention for prevention and control of three tropical diseases, viz. plague, cholera, and yellow fever. Based on the recommendation of this convention, the French Government established in Paris in 1907 the first international health office—L'Office International d'Hygiene Publique (OIHP), whose main objective was to protect Europe from three tropical diseases (Howard-Jones 1974). Similar international health institutions were established in different parts of the world, mainly as regional bodies, responsible for reporting and controlling the outbreaks of diseases for cross-border transmission. One of the earliest institutions was the L'Conseil Sanitaire Maritime et Quarantenaire d'Egypte, situated in Alexandria since 1881. Following the decision of the 2nd international conference of American States, the International Sanitary Bureau for Americas was established in 1902, to facilitate the exchange of information on infectious diseases among the countries in the American continent. When the OIHP was established, this American sanitary bureau changed its name to the Pan American Sanitary Bureau (PASB), which later became the executive bureau of the Pan American Sanitary Organization (PASO). The PASO, under the agreement in 1949 as per WHO Constitution, acted as the Regional Organization of WHO for the Americas. The PASO was renamed as the Pan American Health Organization (PAHO) in 1957, with its headquarters in Washington, in the United States.

By 1911, just a few years before the outbreak of World War I, the task of OIHP in Paris was expanded, to become the first truly international health agency with the main responsibility of monitoring and reporting the outbreaks of the three tropical diseases occurring around the world, and providing information through a monthly bulletin to the general public, on health measures undertaken to combat these diseases (McNeill 1977). Around 1910–1920, major epidemics of infectious diseases due to plague, typhus, cholera, and the great influenza pandemic were rampant in many countries. After World War I, the countries formed an alliance for peace by establishing the League of Nations. Since the OIHP with its small staff and funding could not cope with major international public health crisis, the League of Nations in 1920 agreed to establish a new international health organization under its auspices. After intensive negotiations between the countries in the League and other independent nations, the League of Nations Health Organization (LNHO) was established

in 1923, while the OIHP continued its function (Howard-Jones 1977). The LNHO was assigned to handle international health matters including organization of conferences and symposia, provision of technical assistance to countries, and the clearing-house function. The Weekly Epidemiological Records published since then by the OIHP was continued to date by its successor, the World Health Organization. The LNHO also initiated a series of basic, clinical, and field research studies on medicine and public health. It organized a series of international conferences and meetings of various experts in a wide range of subjects, such as malaria, tuberculosis, leprosy, maternal and child health, health systems, and medical education. It also promoted international medical education, including postgraduate education in public health (WHO 1967).

As early as the 1930s, senior public health administrators from the colonies expressed their concerns at the health status of the population, especially those from rural areas, at the international health conferences organized by the LNHO. The Conference of Far-Eastern Countries on Rural Hygiene organized by the LNHO in 1937 at Bandung, the Netherlands East Indies (present-day Indonesia) was a cornerstone in public health and rural health development in Asia. At this Conference, while noting the rampant condition of communicable diseases and nutritional deficiency disorders in the rural areas, the senior health administrators had identified health as central to development and emphasized the need for integrating health and intersectoral actions. They also recognized that adoption of basic health service approaches by bringing maternal and child healthcare and basic medical care through hospitals and dispensaries nearer to the people could reduce the morbidity and mortality (LNHO 1937).

Many LMI countries became the battlefields and victims of the devastating war for about 6 years during World War II. They had experienced the destruction, destitution, and diseases as well as human misery and suffering with very heavy death tolls. The virtual non-existence of the basic health infrastructure or public utility distribution system had resulted in miserable conditions. The spirit of international peace, solidarity, security, and tranquillity was transcended immediately after the War. The original draft of the UN Charter did not include health. The UN General Assembly (UNGA) in June, 1946 approved to include health in its Charter, and also called for an international conference whose main purpose was to foster consensus in the establishment of a new international health organization in place of the OIHP and LNHO. On 22 July 1946, at the New York conference, a total of 61 nations, many of which were still under colonial rule, approved the Constitution of the World Health Organization (WHO). After ratification by the twenty-sixth Member State, the WHO Constitution came into force on 7 April 1948, the date being celebrated as World Health Day every year. The main functions assigned to WHO were: To direct and coordinate international health work and to cooperate with Member States and partners in international health development (WHO 1992). WHO is collaborating closely, with its Member States, for over 60 years, through its six regional organizations and its headquarters, as a leading international health organization.

Health systems in post-independence period

With the people's movements, democratic reforms, and international pressure, many LMI countries gained independence one after another within a few years from the end of World War II, and some only in the mid-1950s. These countries started reconstruction and rehabilitation activities in various sectors to achieve the rapid economic growth and social development, while catching up with the technological advances in the colonials. Only a few fortunate countries in Asia, the Pacific, and Africa entered the post-World War II period in a relatively calm and favourable condition that helped them in rapid growth and reconstruction. Some countries were challenged by their own internal ethnic conflicts, thereby delaying the development efforts. Even after a few decades of independence, healthcare facilities were very few, rudimentary, and mainly concentrated in urban areas. A number of paramedical training institutes, public health training and research institutions, and health development centres were established in the rural areas, with technical assistance from bilateral and UN agencies. The *Kalutara* rural health training unit in Sri Lanka, the *Aung San* health demonstration unit in Myanmar, and the *Singur* rural health centre in India were a few of them. Exactly two decades after the Bandung Rural Health Conference, another international rural health conference was held at New Delhi in India in 1957, at which the concept and functioning of basic health services in the rural areas in Asia were reviewed including the training and use of multipurpose health workers, enhancement in prevention and control of infectious diseases, promoting intersectoral action, and participation of the local community, including formation of village health committees. The conference highlighted the importance and the need for strengthening rural health centres which were the basic units where comprehensive healthcare was provided (WHO 1957).

Many LMI countries till the 1960s had weak health infrastructure in providing maternal and child health (MCH) care. While a few of them had the technical and managerial authoritative bodies for MCH matters at the central level, the MCH services were mainly provided by the briefly trained nurse-aids, midwives, or nurse-midwives at the hospitals and hospital-based clinics which existed mostly in the urban areas. After a few decades, it was realized that the vertical approach of opening MCH centres and deploying MCH workers alone did not serve the purpose of expanding MCH care. Various strategies were adopted to integrate and expand the MCH as part of the essential basic healthcare packages. In the 1960s, many LMI countries started adopting comprehensive population policies, which included family planning as part of MCH care, to address both demographic and maternal health problems. Even though simple and effective technology for the family planning services was available during the 1960s, only 9 per cent of women in LMI countries had access to contraceptive services.

According to the United Nations Millennium Development Goal (UN-MDG) Report in 2006, an estimated 824 million people in the developing countries were affected by chronic hunger as measured by the proportion of people lacking the food needed to meet their daily needs. The countries in sub-Saharan Africa and South Asia were the worst hit, with 20–30 per cent of the people living with insufficient food (UN 2006). Protein-energy malnutrition (PEM) is a major nutritional deficiency disease due to inadequate energy intake leading to wasting and stunting. The research studies in LMI countries especially in Asia in 1980s showed that PEM was in fact due to calorie deficiency (Gopalan 1992; WHO 1986). The highest levels were found in South Asia (46 per cent) and the lowest in Latin America (7 per cent) and the Caribbean (5 per cent). More than 20 million children were born with low birth weight in the developing world, and more than half of these children were in

South Asia. The risk of being malnourished as measured by weight was 1.2 times higher in Asia than in Africa, and 3 times higher in Africa than in Latin America. There has been little progress (from 20 per cent in 1990 to 17 per cent in 2000) of the prevalence of malnutrition among LMI countries. The percentage of children under 5 years with stunted growth or underweight in low income countries remained at 43 per cent; and the proportion of low birth weight babies was also around 20 per cent (World Bank 2005).

The hidden-hunger or micronutrient deficiency disease was more widespread than PEM. Around 1999, an estimated 5 billion people suffered from iron deficiency anaemia (IDA) alone, which had profound effects on overall health and development of the people. The IDA actually enhanced the morbidity and mortality of mothers and young children, and limiting the learning capacity, impairing the immune function, and reducing productive capacity. The vitamin A deficiency (VAD) is another micronutrient deficiency responsible for blindness among children. After extensive clinical trials in LMI countries, nutrition supplementation programme with vitamin A was introduced as part of activities for promotion of breastfeeding and dietary improvement, with the support of UN and bilateral agencies. Although there was an increase in coverage of vitamin A supplementation from 50 per cent in 1999 to 70 per cent in 2004, the VAD remains a public health problem of today (UNICEF 2006). The iodine deficiency disorders (IDD) is another important micronutrient deficiency disorder, which is widespread in Asia and Africa. While the universal iodization of salt and diversification of dietary intakes had successfully reduced the prevalence of IDD in the western and some Asian countries by 1980s, there were over 200 million people worldwide with goitre and 26 million people suffered from brain damage, associated with IDD, including 6 million children being identified as cretins. The IDD elimination policy and programme actions were proposed at the thirty-eighth World Health Assembly (WHA) in 1986 and later endorsed as an ambitious target in 1990 at the Global Summit for Children. By 1995, it was estimated that IDD was still a significant public health problem in 118 countries, affecting around 43 million people. Fortification of iodine in the widely consumed food and salt, and the advice on diversification of iodine-rich dietary intakes were promoted as main public health strategies in combating IDD. Bhutan, a land-locked Himalayan country, witnessed a remarkable reduction in the prevalence of IDD from 65 per cent in 1990 to 14 per cent in 2000, using a multisectoral approach including extensive availability and use of iodized salt to the whole population, monitoring by health staff on the iodine content of salt at various points of distribution and at the consumers' homes, and promoting social mobilization (WHO 1999a). A similar pattern of reduction in Myanmar, from 33 per cent of goitre rate among school children (6–11 years of age) in 1994 to less than 5.5 per cent (almost reaching the elimination target of 5 per cent) in 2004, was achieved through extensive publicity campaigns and rapidly expanded coverage of more than 90 per cent with universal iodization of salt (Ko Ko *et al.* 2005). By 2005, only 67 per cent of all types of salt consumed in LMI countries were fortified with iodine (World Bank 2005). The success with IDD elimination would depend upon the political commitment for sustained provision of iodine fortified salt for daily household use, promotion of diversified iodine-rich dietary intakes, and effective public education.

One of the key factors contributing to health development is having competent human resources for health or health workforce, i.e. the right numbers and mix of health professionals with the right knowledge, skills, and attitude at the right location and at the right time. As human resources for health consume as much as 60–70 per cent of the health budget, it is essential that they are fully developed and optimally utilized. Very often, health professionals have found it difficult to keep pace with new knowledge and skills. Hence, education and training of health personnel, whether pre-service, in-service, or continuing education, requires to equip them with the requisite knowledge, skills, and attitude, to effectively keep up with the rapid advancement in health and other technologies, as well as to keep responding to the changes in health needs. Almost all LMI countries have pre-service educational programmes for various health personnel to be deployed in their own national health systems. Each country is striving towards ensuring the quality and relevance of health personnel education. In the area of medical education, countries have established useful linkages for conducting collaborative training programmes among different institutions. The World Health Report 2006 provided a global situation analysis of the health work force in 2006 and identified effective strategies to strengthen allied health services and education (WHO 2006a).

Countries are still confronted with issues such as lack of clear national policies for health personnel development; inadequate norms and standards for health professionals resulting in an inappropriate mix of health personnel; lack of mechanisms for the exchange of information on health professionals' education and training; lack of common standards for health professionals' education and training; and absence of quality control mechanisms in health professionals' practices. Numerous strategies had been identified to strengthen the health workforce's services and education, which included among others: Development of comprehensive human resources for health; ensuring curriculum to meet changing service needs and technology and to provide evidence-based and cost-effective care; uniformity in education quality and products; establishing/strengthening national and regional centres of excellence that would address the changing health workers' needs.

Access to essential medicines continues to be the core element of healthcare. With technical advancement, more and more medicines and vaccines would be available and LMI countries need to strengthen their national medicines policies, including food and drugs quality control in order to improve access, promote rational use, and ensure quality, quantity, safety, and efficacy. Most LMI countries have developed national lists of essential medicines and vaccines, and enhanced the work of their Drug Regulatory Authorities to ensure safe, effective, and quality medicines. With the expansion of the private sector in healthcare, access to essential medicines has become an important issue. Most countries have long-standing price control mechanisms for essential medicines, but it is difficult to keep the medicines affordable and provide a sufficient return to the manufacturers. An information exchange mechanism between countries and evaluation of drug pricing systems has been established. The public health impact of the Trade Related Intellectual Property Rights (TRIPs) is being debated to find ways and means to solve the problems of countries, having been prevented from obtaining new medicines and vaccines essential for their public health needs in future. Intellectual property rights are important for innovation relevant to public health and are a factor in determining access to medicines. But neither innovation nor access depend on just intellectual property rights.

The work of the commission on intellectual property rights, innovation, and public health, established by WHO in 2005, focused on the interactions between intellectual property rights, innovation, and public health. Based upon the commission's report, further debate is continuing to identify possible policy interventions for innovations useful for public health development (WHO 2007a).

Environmental health promotion

The promotion of environmental health including personal hygiene and public sanitation has always been part of healthy public and personal practices since the early days of health development in Asia. The nineteenth century experience of the high-income and some LMI countries showed that improvement in personal hygiene, provision of adequate and safe water supply, and enhancement of environmental health had prevented and controlled many infectious diseases. The incidence of water- and food-borne diseases including cholera in these countries had reduced dramatically through improvement in the water supply and sanitation, even when effective medicines were not yet available. Environmental health promotion is a part of civic duties and a main function of public bodies such as municipalities and local administrative bodies. Despite these legislative measures supplemented by education campaigns and subsidy support, progress in environmental health promotion in the LMI countries was not satisfactory. By 2000, about 2.4 billion people around the world still lacked access to improved sanitation facilities. Figure 1.3.1 showed the proportion of population having access to improved sanitation facilities in the countries of Asia, an average of the least-developed countries and the world in 2004, comparing with those in 1990. More than 50 per cent of the vast population of China, India, and many other Asian countries and many of the least-developed countries have no access yet to improved sanitation facilities (UNDP 2006), which had actually aroused to call for at the UN Millennium Summit at 2000, to halve the proportion of people without sustainable access to safe drinking water and sanitation by 2015. It was a formidable challenge for LMI countries especially in Asia and Africa, with more than half of their population not having access to safe water supply and sanitation.

The provision of improved sanitation facilities is often regarded as the responsibility of individuals and family members rather than public bodies. It would not be possible for a rural community to build and run a community-based sewerage system (for a whole village of 1000 households), which would be an equivalent of a public water-supply system for urban population, due to the heavy investment and maintenance costs. Many national sanitation programmes thus promoted the use of an on-site sanitation facility at the household level. For many poor families, the benefit of having clean water from a single common water supply source with a little cost incurred by them seemed to have more visible impact than the long-term benefit of having improved latrine for each household with a similar small investment. A study in a few least-developed countries in Asia showed that it would take 20 days' wages to build a simple pit latrine. Asian Development Bank had estimated in 2005 that the annual value of time saved by having better access to clean, safe, and reliable water supply, and sanitation facilities would amount to US$54 billion for achieving the UN MDG target, and US$109 billion to improve water supply and sanitation for all in Asia alone (ADB 2005). Community involvement in local decision-making is also a key to success. People will demand more if they

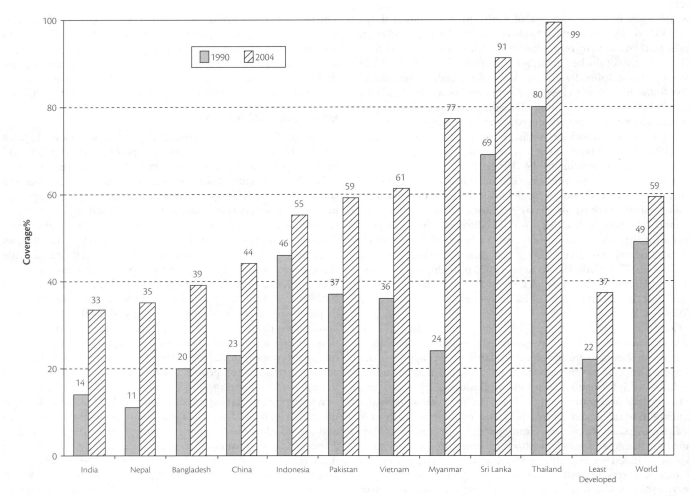

Fig. 1.3.1 Proportion of population with sustainable access to improved sanitation of the World, the least-developed countries and selected Asian nations, 1990 and 2004. *Source*: UNDP Human Development Report (2006).

know the benefits of having improved sanitary facilities. The use of public and private electronic and print media and the organization of national and sub-national sanitation campaigns are important strategies for promoting environmental sanitation, in addition to educating school children and mothers. With the existing economic growth, most middle-income countries could afford to invest a proportion of the national budget for initiating mass sanitation campaigns within the next decade to attain the UN MDG goal in this area. However, low-income countries may need additional financial support for achieving the target.

Reforming public health systems

Health-for-all movement

During 1950–60s, the LMI countries with the support of international agencies had made tremendous efforts to reduce the burden of communicable diseases with the establishment of nation-wide medical care and public health systems. Actually, the organized public health systems in the modern sense intended to benefit the whole population barely existed a century ago in these countries. Some countries adopted the so-called modern (allopathic-based) health systems as recently as the 1960–70s. Till date, the major works of the health systems in some LMI countries were run by the

charitable or non-governmental organizations (NGOs). Some forms of a social insurance system as part of the welfare schemes for employed workers were introduced in a few middle-income countries, copying the social welfare model from western countries. After 30 odd-years, countries started realizing that healthcare systems based on hospitals and health centres were a burden on the public due to the high costs of medicines, technological equipment, and staff, as well as other facilities. Rapid expansion of basic health centres without properly trained human resources could not provide essential healthcare to the vast majority of rural people. The integration of specialized disease control programmes into general health services also moved slowly, with many vertical disease control programmes continuing as autonomous bodies for more than 4–5 decades. There was little coordination in planning and management between various sections of the health ministry itself and between the health and health-related sectors. Much of the health planning was done at the central level without the close involvement of the people responsible for implementation (Djukanovic & Mach 1975; WHO 1978a).

By mid-1970s, there were glaring contrasts in health status between high-income and LMI countries as well as among LMI countries. The average life expectancy at birth in LMI countries was around 55 years, with many countries having infant and child mortality above 100 per 1000 live births. Most infant and young children's deaths were due to infectious diseases that were easily preventable and controlled. Despite these drawbacks, a few LMI countries showed significant improvement in health status with little investment in health. Examples of Cuba, Chile, Sri Lanka, Tanzania, Kerala state of India, and rural health in China were used as the best policies and practices for successful health achievements. The underlying factors of successes in many LMI countries were the national policies and programmes addressing equity, social justice, community involvement, appropriate technology, and multi-sectoral approaches. The need for closing the gaps between those who achieved good health and those who were not able to do so led to the adoption of a historic resolution at the World Health Assembly in 1977 which set the main social target of Member States and WHO, of the attainment by all the citizens of the world by the year 2000 of a level of health that would permit them to lead a socially and economically productive life. This universal social target was termed as—Health for All by the year 2000 or HFA2000. It was meant to be a political and social aspiration that people would use better approaches than they had before, individually and by the community as a whole, for preventing and controlling diseases and alleviating unavoidable illness and disability. It was conceived as a process leading to progressive improvement in the health of the people and not as a single finite target. Essential healthcare would be accessible to individuals and families in acceptable and affordable ways with their full involvement. These principles were further clarified at the International Conference on Primary Health Care (PHC) jointly organized by WHO and UNICEF at Alma-Ata in the then USSR in 1978 which adopted the path-breaking Declaration of Alma-Ata (WHO 1978b). This Declaration and the accompanying report of the Conference called for urgent action by all governments, health and development workers, and the world community to protect and promote the health of all the people of the world using primary healthcare as the key approach. LMI countries saw the outcome and recommendations of the Alma-Ata Conference as well as the principles of the Declaration as an opportunity for restructuring their health systems, using the PHC approach as a practical, scientifically sound, and socially acceptable public health measure. They had formulated new health policies and strategies, as well as plans of action to launch and sustain their healthcare systems within the common framework of global HFA strategies. The adoption of the universal goal helped many countries to recognize new ways of reaching a higher level of health status, and to place greater emphasis on adherence to health goals. Some countries concentrated on vertical types of healthcare interventions like immunization, family planning, and maternal care, while others tried to be as comprehensive as possible in their public health development. For example, UNICEF and many other development agencies initially introduced the vertical programmes like MCH and family planning, growth monitoring, oral rehydration, breast-feeding, and immunization. The accessibility of essential healthcare, in fact, improved in most countries, with over 80 per cent of population covered with basic healthcare by 1980s. However, the progress on some aspects of healthcare, like essential care for pregnant mothers and safe delivery, immunization to infants and children, or provision of adequate water supply and sanitation, remained very slow in some LMI countries, particularly the least-developed ones. Healthcare for pregnant mothers as measured by the coverage of attendance by trained health personnel during pregnancy and childbirth was less than 25 per cent in many countries. Despite widespread acceptance by national health authorities of the idea of integrated health systems since the early days of health system developments in the 1950s, there were practical operational constraints in transforming semi-autonomous vertical or selective health development programmes into the general health services. One of the main factors that slowed implementation of HFA strategies using primary healthcare as the key approach was lack of a full understanding of the fundamental policies and principles of PHC and HFA that were applicable to national health systems development. This led to achieving an insufficient level of universal access to essential healthcare. There was inadequate coordination and collaboration between specific health intervention campaigns and the development of basic health infrastructure (district health systems development). This further led to difficulties in involving communities in health action, and slowed the pace of integration of vertical disease control campaigns into the general health infrastructure. It was further compounded by weak planning and management of health development, especially at the operational levels, and the imbalance and irrelevance of human resources for health (Tarimo & Webster 1994).

The late 1990s saw an intense democratization process in many LMI countries, which, in turn, led to a certain amount of devolution/decentralization of power and responsibility to the people, thereby increasing their involvement in the planning and management of development programmes including health. The World Bank, IMF, and many other multilateral and bilateral donors used these changes in devolution as a condition for extending external assistance. Thus, many reforms for health systems initiated in LMI countries in the last few decades included devolution of authority to local bodies on health matters as an important strategy. The approach varied among countries depending on the extent of devolution and decentralization, division of responsibility and resources, and the management capacity at each level of the health systems. Most nationwide health development programmes promoted community awareness and the creation of active and effective mechanisms for community involvement. A few successful programmes in various parts of the world showed that the conventional approach of merely expanding basic health services had proved inadequate. It was proving impossible economically to bear the cost of expansion of basic healthcare services by the public sector to the entire population in the face of the existing resource constraints. Thus, many countries adopted to deploy a large number of community-level health volunteers, trained for short periods, who constituted as a third force of human resources for health. This proved to be a success for expanding essential healthcare coverage in many countries. With their involvement in health action, many essential public health interventions especially in disease prevention and control including epidemic control and immunization, health promotion, maternal and child healthcare including nutrition promotion, information gathering and surveillance, treatment of minor ailments, and environmental health promotion were undertaken. Such public health initiatives received international attention as well as recognition, and their movements had been promoted by instituting the Sasakawa Health Prize, the Health for All medals, and other forms of recognition.

A series of new health reforms, such as improving the content of essential packages for health and the way these were financed, were undertaken as the third generation of health reforms. Many models of health financing either at national scale or local level were developed in LMI countries, including reforms in expanding social health insurance. Another global trend in health development is the increasing role of the private sector both for profit and non-profit. The issue of an appropriate public and private mix in health systems had been extensively debated, that stemmed from the fact that the larger proportion of health expenditure came out of private sources mainly from out-of-pocket (OOP) payment, while the governments could not increase their expenditure on health. Fewer agencies of non-profit were involved in public health development and medical care to the unserved populations. It is not a simple solution of either private or not, but a balanced mix of both that can fit within the existing socioeconomic, political, and health situation of the country and also how far the national health plans would ensure that wider reforms would address the gaps in healthcare and create a pro-poor health system.

Health development in the twenty-first century could be achieved through a dynamic yet harmonious balance between health in terms of consumption and health as an investment. Bringing in theory and practices of economic and social sciences, health development programmes had been designed by introducing the cost-effective health intervention packages tailored to economic and social realities of each country. New generations of health reforms were undertaken within the framework of health for all policy for the twenty-first century, as adopted in the World Health Declaration in May 1998 (WHO 1998a). Many LMI countries, especially those receiving substantial external investments in health from multilateral financial institutions like the World Bank, had used essential healthcare packages as part of their national health sector-wide programmes.

Health policy and planning

After WHO had introduced the country health planning (CHP) process for health sector development in the 1980s as part of capacity strengthening for policy-making and health development planning, planning and budgeting in the health sector became the norm for national development in many LMI countries. The centrally directed planning framework using CHP process had moved many LMI countries to a higher level of health attainment. It was highly successful in the era when selective healthcare interventions like immunization, malaria or leprosy control, and MCH/Family Planning were promoted through federally or centrally controlled development projects. The development assistance by bilateral and multilateral financing institutions in the 1990s had enhanced the financing of vertical programmes and later that of integrated health sector programmes. Attempts were made from a wider socioeconomic perspective by fostering greater involvement of national and international stakeholders in sectoral policy development and planning, both for short- and long-term periods.

With the initiatives of the World Bank and other external donors, the national poverty reduction strategy papers had included health as an integral part of development efforts. The long- and medium-term national health sector development plans in line with the global goals, such as HFA goals, Child-Summit goals and UN-MDG were developed, using the Sector Wide Approach (SWAp). SWAp is a wider consultative process involving the civil society groups, public and private sectors, and external donors. A shared policy framework using SWAp and a common or pooled programme budget has allowed less duplication, better resource allocation, and more opportunity for working in partnership (Cassels 1997). The health development plans were much more results-oriented and outcomes focused, and the development activities and efforts are geared toward achieving health impacts. By pulling all health development plans together into one framework using SWAp, the national health planners and programme managers could better identify the strategies and activities needed to achieve national and global objectives with estimated resources. There was growing experience in using SWAp for health development in LMI countries, which suggested that SWAp represented an effective investment in health systems capacity and government ownership. The evidence also showed that the successes would depend upon how far specific and high priority objectives were embedded for targeting the poor in the health sector plans (WHO 2000a). The recent initiative in one team, one programme, and one budget, for the country's development as part of UN reforms also fits in this perspective.

Health financing

While the high-income countries continued to increase spending on health in response to growing expectations, LMI countries were struggling with major problems in managing and financing their health systems. In the poorer LMI countries, the health sector financing had stagnated or even contracted over the last 25 years, whilst the demands for health had grown exponentially. The investment in health in terms of the proportion of GNP spent on health ranged from 1 to 6 per cent in many LMI countries as compared to more than 10 per cent in the developed world. Due to relatively low public investment in health, people had to spend more from out-of-pocket for appropriate access to essential healthcare. In most of LMI countries especially least developed nations, the OOP payment constituted a major source of financing. For example, according to the World Health Report 2006, the OOP payment for Nepal accounted for 73 per cent of total health expenditure, while it was 75 per cent in Bangladesh and 66 per cent in China (WHO 2006a).

Many LMI countries in the mid-1980s had introduced user charges, with a view to cover some part of the public health expenditure. While some might support that the user fees would increase revenue that could be used to improve the quality of public health services and expand coverage, but the amount of revenue recovered was not high enough to recover the increasing amount of health expenditure. Moreover, the poor would not be able to afford the fee, and access the most essential necessary healthcare services. In some LMI countries, community financing is organized and managed by the community, with some form of Government subsidy or technical support. The main aim of universal coverage of health financing is to develop health systems that guarantee universal access to effective health services regardless of a person's income or social status (Kutzin 1998). While the coverage of social health insurance (SHI) was high in the Americas, it was very low in many LMI countries of Asia and Africa, and almost non-existent in some LMI countries. Those who had such social health insurance usually had the coverage for formally employed workers as part of social welfare schemes usually managed by the Ministry of Labour. The major challenge in all these countries was how to extend the coverage of social health protection from the formal sector to the non-formal sector of employment, to non-working spouses, or to the child dependants and other family members (Than Sein 2002). A health system predominately funded by public sources including general taxation and social health insurance provides more equitable access by all members to a wide range of health services. These types of prepayment-based financing arrangements reduce the undue financial burdens from medical care costs and contain costs of health services (WHO 2006b).

Health research and development

Health research and development have been progressive with advancements in science and technology, and health systems development. In the past, LMI countries relied on the results of research and development from the high-income countries. In practical terms, many scientific breakthroughs in health actually came from the experiences gained in LMI countries such as identification of causal organisms for communicable diseases and the way they are transmitted, immunization against smallpox and other infectious diseases, development and use of contraceptives, and multidrug therapy. Promotion of research capability in LMI countries was high on the development agenda for many years. With the support and strengthening of WHO Collaborating Centres and networks of national centres of excellence around the world, and with the establishment of regional and global advisory committees on health research by WHO during the 1960–70s, the scientific communities from LMI countries played significant roles in international research promotion and development. A series of research and development efforts were initiated in the area of prevention and control of tropical diseases including vaccines, promotion of human health and reproduction including contraception and other fertility control measures, strengthening of health systems, protection of environmental health, control of non-communicable diseases, and development of essential healthcare technologies.

In order to promote innovation and intensification of health reforms during the post Alma-Ata era, people realized that health systems research (HSR) was an important tool for innovation and programme development for strengthening health systems based on PHC and HFA principles, especially in setting priorities for health research (Nuyens 2007). Many countries established and strengthened their HSR units/sections within the ministries of health or as separate autonomous national institutes to conduct health systems and health policy research, and to provide appropriate scientific, evidence-based information to decision-makers. Considerable progress was made in capacity building and capability strengthening in promoting health systems research. The development works further pave the way for developing an effective national health research system. International exchanges of experiences of the countries on health research system development had been promoted through various forums and networks of institutions and expertise had been established in recent years such as Asia-Pacific Health Research System Network and African Health Research System Network. When compared with investment in basic science research, the budget allocation for HSR remained relatively small both at national or international levels. There has been an attempt to recommend that the developing countries need to invest at least 2 per cent of national health expenditures in health research and research capacity strengthening, and at least 5 per cent of the development aid for the health sector from external agencies has to be earmarked for the same purpose (WHO and World Bank 1990). The Ad Hoc Committee on Health Research established by WHO in 1996 concluded that the central problem in health research promotion and development was the '10/90' disequilibrium of investing in health research and development (WHO 1996). An estimated US$56 billion was invested globally for health research, yet only 5–10 per cent was spent on health research on issues that affected the large majority of the world's population. This concern became even more acute in the context of the public health challenges of the twenty-first century.

Improving performance

For over half a century, economic performance indicators, such as Gross Domestic Product (GDP), Gross National Product (GNP) or Gross National Income (GNI), and inflation rates, have been available to policy makers and political leaders accountable for economic management. Using the scientific development and evidence, WHO had attempted to introduce a framework for *health system performance assessment*, with relevant concepts, possible indicators, and an initial report on measuring performance for improving health systems for its 190 Member States in its World Health Report 2000 (WHO 2000b). The original purpose of the framework for measuring health system performance was to establish a foundation for a solid body of evidence on the relationship between the organization and outcomes of health systems, with a view to provide governments with information for health policy development and to enable users to understand better the functions of health systems, and to access information about the extent to which health system outcomes attained. The World Health Report 2000 had created an unprecedented level of interest and debate all over the world, though not necessarily with positive reactions. While some experts, researchers, and governments made formal protests and questioned the underlying theoretical basis, the statistical techniques selected, the reliability of the data, and the reliability of ranking the social outcomes using a composite index, others had expressed their support for further improving the methodology. WHO had attracted extensive media attention and contributed a much-needed debate, but such high visibility could run the risk of a counterproductive effect if technical mistakes remained uncorrected and resultant rankings unsupportable (WHO 2001; Jamaison & Sandhu 2001). A series of technical publications were brought out on various aspects of summary measures of health including development of a composite index for health development (WHO 2002a). A few countries have even attempted the application of such analytical tools either at national or sub-national levels with a view to identifying policy gaps in improving health system performance of respective countries (IIPS/WHO 2006; WHO 2007d). Although several countries expressed strong views on the methodology especially the ranking, the experts highlighted the need for a critical analysis with scientific rigour on the assessment of health system performance in individual countries. Further development and wider consultation would be required to develop acceptable, effective tools and methods for assessment of health system performance.

Disease eradication and elimination

Disease control campaigns

With the advancement and expansion in the application of science, technology, and knowledge immediately after World War II, a number of vaccines, pharmaceuticals, and diagnostic tools were developed and used for public health interventions. Vaccination campaigns against infectious diseases such as smallpox, tuberculosis, and poliomyelitis were started from early 1950s as nation-wide campaigns. Similarly, some tropical diseases were put under control through mass use of chemotherapy. High-income countries had assisted LMI ones to contain the spread of infectious diseases at their source.

Campaign for control of yaws was initiated in Africa, Asia, the Pacific, and Latin America almost immediately after World War II, since antibiotics became available. As early as 1948, WHO and UNICEF had initiated a campaign for global control of yaws by introducing mass treatment with long-acting penicillin. At that time, there were an estimated 20 million cases of yaws worldwide, half of them in Asia. Although yaws was almost eliminated in many LMI countries by the early 1970s, scattered foci of infection still persisted in some parts of Latin America, the Pacific and South and Southeast Asia. A resurgence of yaws cases occurred in India in the mid-1980s. Due to concerted efforts, the annual incidence of yaws in India steadily declined from a peak of 3500 in 1996 to 46 cases in 2003, and no more reported cases since 2004. The spectacular success of yaws control, using the early case identification and mass treatment strategy, provided a boost to the control of other diseases through campaign approach.

Malaria was a tropical disease aimed for control and later eradication since millions of people died during the 1940s. Assured of massive support from international and bilateral agencies, many governments launched large-scale malaria control campaigns in 1950s that expanded progressively in scope and coverage in later decades. Many LMI countries established national malaria research/vector control institutes to provide technical direction, research development and training related to malaria and vector control. Initiated by the World Health Assembly in May 1955, nearly all newly independent LMI countries around the world started launching national malaria eradication programmes, utilizing the strategies such as active case finding with treatment and controlling mosquitoes with DDT insecticide. The malaria eradication in its earlier years saw dramatic successes. The reduction in malaria caseload during 1950–60s was spectacular, as seen from the experience of the countries of WHO Southeast Asia. The malaria caseload in these countries declined from over 100 million cases in 1950 to as low as 230 000 in 1965. Through this global funding of Malaria Special Account in the 1960s, the insecticide—DDT and the anti-malarial medicines, being produced in the western countries, were supplied to the needy countries in Asia and Africa. This helped to solve to some extent, the deficit in national programmes in LMI countries especially in Asia. Substantial stocks for DDT insecticide and necessary spraying equipment, personnel, and transport for large-scale operations was beyond the means of LMI countries. The inadequate supply and irrational use of medicines for malaria also led to drug resistance. This situation was followed in many countries by reverting programmes for the eradication of malaria to those for control during the mid-1970s. Despite this drawback, there was the beneficial effect of the use of DDT spraying on the control of another infectious disease called kala-azar which was highly endemic in the same groups of countries, and the disease almost completely disappeared by the 1960s (WHO 1992). Many countries also tried to integrate the control programmes for all vector-borne diseases under one national programme. Conceptually as well as managerially, it might be possible to have all vector-borne diseases under one consolidated national programme, practically it had been difficult to implement successfully and effectively. Many vector-borne diseases are still prevailing in many LMI countries.

LMI countries recognized leprosy as a priority communicable disease for centuries. In the absence of effective control methods

earlier, people with leprosy and their families were isolated from others and this is still practised in some parts of the world. The discovery of dapsone (DDS) in 1943 and its immediate availability in the early 1950s for treatment of leprosy provided a major boost to leprosy control. The main strategies for leprosy control were mass screening, early detection and treatment with long-term dapsone therapy, case holding and release from control along with health education. Millions of leprosy cases were identified and registered and put under long-term treatment with dapsone. For numerous leprosy patients, dapsone therapy brought the long-denied hope and promise (Than Sein & Kyaw Lwin 2003).

During the eighteenth century, syphilis was usually regarded as the disease of the foreigners, and some Asians used to call it as *Farangi Roga*. Actually, limited information showed that syphilis had already been rampant among the populace in Asia earlier than those periods. Many LMI countries in the 1950s introduced national prevention and control programme for sexually-transmitted disease (STD) including syphilis, using strategies like early case detection, treatment with long-acting penicillin, and health education. Availability of treatment with penicillin actually conveyed a false sense of security, and the STD programmes totally ignored the increasing prevalence of prostitution, promiscuity, and homosexuality, which are the main social determinants. Since these main issues could not be addressed properly, newer STDs like HIV/AIDS, HBV infection, etc. are coming up and flourishing till date.

Cholera is one of the most feared infectious diseases in public health. The public health experience during the nineteenth century in Europe, the Middle-East, and Asia showed that adequate sanitation and safe water supply, as well as adequate personal and food hygiene practices could contain many local epidemics and the six global pandemics of cholera effectively in the past 10 decades. The use of new therapeutics and adequate rehydration therapy with early case detection demonstrated that many deaths from cholera could be averted. A series of cholera epidemics that occurred since 1991 due to the new O139 strain had affected more than 120 countries around the world. One of the serious concerns is that it would become the eighth cholera pandemic (Lee 2001). For LMI countries with more than 1 billion people without access to safe water supply and improved sanitation, it would be a major challenge to address the potential pandemic of cholera in the years to come.

Smallpox control—a public health success

Control of smallpox is to be recorded as the most successful public health intervention. Using the traditional technique of variolation—inoculation of pus taken from smallpox cases to healthy persons in Asia for many centuries—Edward Jenner in 1796 introduced a modified technique, not from human smallpox but from cowpox cases. The wider application of this method—vaccination—to the general population in Europe and the Americas had resulted in controlling smallpox within a shorter period (Henderson 1997). The spread of smallpox could not be controlled widely in other parts of the world, due to the variable purity and potency of the vaccine, poor vaccination techniques, and low coverage among the general population. In the early 1950s, nearly a million cases were reported in more than 100 countries/territories, with 58 per cent of cases being reported from British India alone. Lack of commitment and lack of broad humanitarian objectives by the colonial administration, limitation of technical and human resources, and lack of confidence in vaccination by the local populace were hindering the progress for control of smallpox through vaccination (Ko Ko *et al.* 2002). Thus, even more than a century after the discovery of small-pox vaccination, the disease continued to rage throughout the world. With the assurance of continued supply of freeze-dried smallpox vaccine, WHO, in 1958, advocated for worldwide small-pox control, through mass vaccination campaigns aiming at eradication. Initially, many LMI countries were sceptical on global campaign, since there was an inadequate supply of smallpox vaccine as well as inaccessibility of health facilities by a large segment of population. With intensive advocacy and support by international agencies, they later adopted smallpox control, organized through mass campaigns using basic health staff and institutions backed by legislation.

By the middle of the 1960s, several LMI countries achieved the smallpox eradication status (WHO 1964). However, smallpox still killed 2–3 million people annually worldwide as recently as 1967 and till the mid-1970s; and some countries in Asia and Africa had experienced sporadic outbreaks. Intensive case-detection and mass vaccination in affected areas successfully contained the disease, even in those countries where the incidence was high and relatively few people were vaccinated (Foege *et al.* 1971; Fenner *et al.* 1988). India launched a massive public health campaign called Operation Smallpox Zero in the early 1970s which led to the last case in May 1975 (Basu *et al.* 1979). Other neighbouring countries also followed suit leading to no more smallpox cases by 1975. The last naturally-acquired human smallpox case in the world was reported in Somalia in October 1977. After considering the final report of the global international commission on smallpox eradication, the 33rd World Health Assembly in May 1980 made a declaration that the world was free from natural transmission of smallpox. This was certainly the most spectacular public health achievement of the twentieth century. However, the final extinction of the smallpox virus itself has remained controversial from the scientific point of view. Especially after anthrax was used as a biological weapon in USA in 2001 and the occurrence of pandemic avian influenza in recent years, a consensus has not been reached on the timing for destruction of existing variola virus stocks. Currently, the decision for destruction of the variola virus has been deferred to 2010 (WHO 2006c).

The possibility of eradicating disease was mentioned by Thomas Jefferson in 1800 referring to the discovery of smallpox vaccine by Jenner. Eradication and elimination of infectious diseases such as the eradication of smallpox, yellow fever, and yaws or the elimination of soil-transmitted helminthes had been attempted for decades as public health goals. Achieving the eradication of smallpox by 1980 provided an impetus to develop acceptable public health strategies for eradication and elimination of many infectious and non-infectious diseases. A number of such diseases have been examined and identified as candidate diseases for possible global and local eradication or elimination. Accelerated development and rapid application of scientific and other technological knowledge in public health with increased access to healthcare in all corners of the world, has made a tremendous impact on disease prevention and control, especially prevention and control of immunizable diseases.

Expanded programme of immunization

By 1970, many safe, effective, and affordable vaccines, medicines and other chemicals, and diagnostic means were available to expand activities related to the prevention and control of both infectious and non-infectious diseases. While some diseases were aimed for elimination (to have zero cases, but the risk of disease remains), some were targeted for eradication (to have zero cases with zero risk) (Goodman & Foster 1998). With improved availability of vaccines for infectious diseases such as measles, poliomyelitis, diphtheria, tetanus, and others, many LMI countries initiated the Expanded Programme of Immunization (EPI) in the mid-1970s, in collaboration with WHO, UNICEF, and other partners, with the aim of controlling these diseases through the expansion of coverage of universal child immunization (immunizing at least 80 per cent of all 2-year-old children with essential vaccines). It took more than two decades for many LMI countries to improve the immunization coverage to the desired levels for elimination or eradication of vaccine-preventable diseases. Many LMI countries initially felt that the goal of universal child immunization might not be achievable, since they lacked human and financial resources to effectively deliver vaccines. Bilateral and multilateral donors, regional financial institutions, and UN system agencies provided large-scale assistance to LMI countries to improve immunization coverage through support of national EPI programmes. Within 10 years, nearly 80 per cent of all 2-year-old children globally were immunized against six major vaccine-preventable diseases. As an outcome, the lives of approximately 2 million children were saved from disability and deaths from six diseases. It is actually a concerted global effort with input of large financial and human resources to achieve and maintain a higher level of coverage. The EPI initiative was termed by many public health professionals as a silent revolution in public health in the twentieth century.

Figure 1.3.2 shows the immunization coverage of major childhood vaccines from 1980 to 2005, from the available data from the WHO Southeast Asia (SEA) Region. New vaccine for HepB was introduced as part of vaccines to be covered under routine EPI programme in late 1990s in several endemic countries, but the coverage does not yet reach to a higher level. GAVI initiative has provided necessary financial and material support to enhance this immunization programme. There was a parallel improvement in the production, transport, and storage of the EPI vaccines. Extensive training of health staff at various levels of the national health systems for programme management and epidemiology was undertaken. Similarly, the extended social mobilization efforts had boosted the increase in coverage of immunization (WHO 1993). Countries in the Americas, Europe, and some parts of Asia were able to achieve effective control of poliomyelitis by higher immunization coverage from 1980 onwards. This experience had led to a strong belief by many health policy makers and planners and public health professionals that the world might be ready to adopt plausible eradication and elimination strategies for prevention and control of diseases especially through effective immunization, both locally, nationally, regionally, and later globally. Community involvement in such extensive public health measures emerged as a significant strategy, together with improved mechanisms for bringing together the private and public sector agencies (WHO 1998b).

In 1988, the world community resolved to achieve global eradication of poliomyelitis by 2000 within the existing global EPI initiative, and also within the context of strengthening health systems and disease surveillance. This global call for poliomyelitis eradication provided LMI countries with challenges as well as opportunities, since they had to improve and sustain the expanded coverage

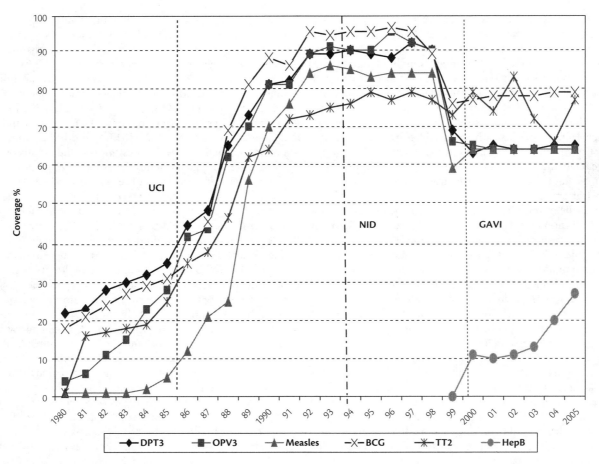

Fig. 1.3.2 Immunization coverage, WHO SEA Region, 1980–2005.
Source: WHO/SEARO, IVD Unit (UCI-Universal Child Immunization; NID-National Immunization Days).

of immunization, while they were improving their health infrastructure. At the start of the global poliomyelitis eradication campaign, the wild poliomyelitis virus was circulating in more than 125 countries in five continents, disabling more than 1000 children every day. While the average global coverage of poliomyelitis immunization had remained over 80 per cent since 1990, some LMI countries were not able to achieve that level and some were even less than 50 per cent. In order to improve this situation and also with the possibility of the interruption of transmission of wild virus by high coverage, an additional strategy was piloted in the Philippines and China, then followed as nation-wide campaigns in other polio-endemic countries. This new strategy was the adoption of a national immunization day (NID) by assigning a fixed date of a year as a special day for immunization. By the end of 1997, more than 450 million children under-5 years of age (almost half of the world's children) in at least 80 LMI countries were immunized with oral polio vaccine through NID campaigns, in addition to over 500 million children immunized through routine EPI programme. Surveillance of acute flaccid paralysis (AFP) in these countries was also intensified with additional human resources, proper case investigations, and prompt laboratory support.

Figure 1.3.3 shows the trends of polio immunization coverage by WHO regions in 1980, 1990, and 1996 to 2005, where the coverage of polio vaccine for infants is the lowest in the countries of Africa. With GAVI support, there was some improvement in coverage in

other regions, compared with Africa. By 2003, around 415 million children under-5 years in the 55 LMI countries were immunized with over 2.2 billion doses of oral polio-vaccine. Similarly, 14 previously polio-free countries in Africa and Asia were able to stop the epidemics of poliomyelitis that had occurred by importation of wild poliovirus from other countries in 2005. Egypt with indigenous polio transmission existed for more than 5000 years from the time of Pharaohs and was declared a polio-free status by January 2005. China, after two rounds of NID in 1993 and 1994, showed the reduction of poliomyelitis from 5000 cases in 1990 to almost zero in 1995. India has been implementing the NID campaigns for poliomyelitis elimination as part of its national EPI programme from 1993; however, the wild poliovirus is still circulating in certain parts of the country even in 2007.

By early 2007, only four countries—India, Afghanistan, Pakistan, and Nigeria—remain endemic with indigenous transmission of wild poliovirus. They accounted for 92 per cent of all new cases of poliomyelitis. The remaining 8 per cent of cases occurred in a few countries where local wild poliovirus transmission is controlled but being reintroduced. Surveillance on new polio cases and acute flaccid paralysis cases with timely and prompt response for control is crucial in these countries. A concerted effort to intensify the polio eradication by interrupting transmission of wild poliovirus is required by implementing the multiple rounds of supplementary immunization activities, and by limiting the risk of reintroducing

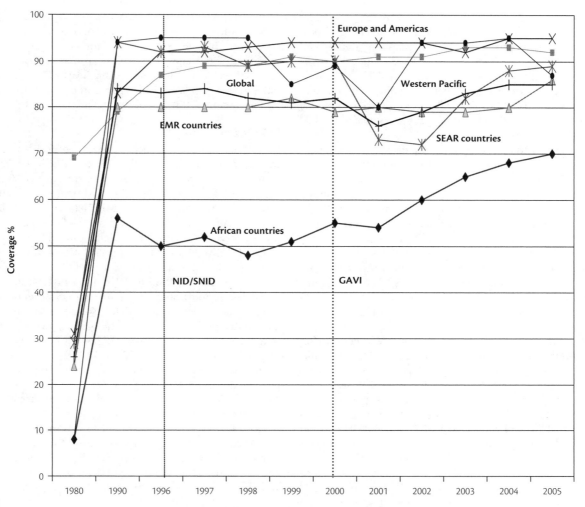

Fig. 1.3.3 Polio Immunization Coverage for < 1 year of age by WHO Regions, 1980, 1990, and 1996–2005.
Source: WHO/IVD Unit 2007.

wild poliovirus into poliomyelitis-free areas with stronger political will and support with national and international resources. An unprecedented level of financial support to the global polio eradication effort by the bilateral and multilateral donors, Rotary International and the Bill and Melinda Gates Foundation has ensured the intensification of polio elimination campaigns. By 2010, it is expected that all the countries around the world will be free from indigenous transmission of wild poliovirus (WHO 2006d). If and when, efforts to eradicate wild poliovirus from the world succeed by 2010, this would represent a major landmark in public health in this new Millennium.

Other immunizable diseases

While success on a global scale for polio elimination is imminent, there were disturbing declining trends in routine immunization during the last few years, especially among LMI countries. The donor-driven EPI programmes organized solely for the purpose of improved immunization coverage in the 1990s were short-lived and collapsed after the withdrawal of external inputs. Immunization coverage of women of child-bearing age with anti-tetanus vaccination had never reached the expected level of more than 80 per cent in most countries, and similar patterns were also seen for other vaccinations.

By 2003, more than 27 million children worldwide were still missed for immunization in their first year of life, and each year, around 1.4 million children under 5 years of age died from vaccine-preventable diseases. Intensified efforts for sustaining coverage through routine immunization services were necessary to achieve the desired reduction in mortality and morbidity.

Measles is an easily transmitted viral infection responsible for around 10 per cent of deaths from all causes among under-5 children globally. While more than 20 million children are affected by measles and nearly 800 000 children were dying annually, the routine measles coverage during the last decades globally was around 70–80 per cent. A majority (>95 per cent) of these deaths occurred in the low-income countries with GNP per capita less than US$1000. The main reason for high measles morbidity and mortality was the failure to deliver at least a single dose of measles vaccine to more than 90 per cent of infants. A concerted effort to boost the coverage of measles vaccination from around 70 per cent to a higher and sustained level of over 90 per cent of every birth cohort was required to interrupt transmission of measles especially among the children in these countries. Maintaining a high level of coverage over 90 per cent and the ultimate elimination of measles in the Americas in 2000 had prompted other developed and developing countries to follow suit. With additional resources from the GAVI Alliance, the Measles Initiative was launched by WHO in collaboration with other partners such as JICA, the Gates Foundation, and CIDA. The initiative had expanded financial and technical support to endemic countries to improve measles coverage. The world community in May 2005 agreed to implement the global immunization and vision strategy (GIVS) which called for countries to reduce global measles deaths in 2010 by 90 per cent as compared to 2000 estimates (WHO 2007b).

Neonatal tetanus (NNT) is a major cause of death among neonates, and providing tetanus toxoid (TT) immunization to all women of childbearing age is the simplest and most cost-effective way to reduce neonatal mortality. In 1989, the global community called for the elimination of neonatal tetanus by 2005. Actually, only 104 of 161 endemic LMI countries had achieved this target of less than one NNT case per 1000 live births in every district (www.who.int) by 2005. Around 90 per cent of the NNT cases were concentrated in the 27 remaining countries, which are mostly from Africa and Asia. The existing high incidence of NNT was not just because of inadequate coverage of TT vaccination, but was due to the poor access to good antenatal care and clean and safe delivery by trained personnel.

Hepatitis B virus (HBV) infection was known earlier as serum hepatitis, with the earliest outbreak recorded in 1883, when shipyard workers in Germany became sick with jaundice within weeks following inoculation with smallpox vaccine. The HBV was identified only in 1960, and known to be transmitted by percutaneous and mucosal exposure to infected blood or other body fluids (including sexual transmission) (Shepard *et al.* 2006). In 2004, an estimated 2 billion people worldwide would have the serological evidence of past or present HBV infection, and 360 million were at risk for chronic diseases. Approximately 60 per cent of the world's population live in geographical areas where HBV infection is highly endemic such as China, Indonesia, Nigeria, and much of Asia and Africa (WHO 2004a). More than 150 countries worldwide had adopted the immunization against Hepatitis B as part of national EPI programmes. With the recommendation of WHO for utilizing the plasma-derived Hepatitis B (HepB) vaccine, many endemic countries had introduced it since 1992. The plasma-derived vaccine was later replaced by the recombinant HepB vaccine. Countries that started HepB vaccination since mid-1980s showed that the sero-prevalence among children was reduced from 10 per cent to less than 1 per cent, and the annual incidence rate of hepatocellular carcinoma among children of 6–14 years had reduced by half after a decade. If properly managed, HepB infection would be eliminated within the next 20 years.

Since the early 1990s, some LMI countries started introducing new vaccines against mumps, meningitis, rubella, HepB and HepC infections, and haemophilus influenza. Acknowledging the decreasing trends of routine immunization coverage and also the non-availability of vaccines against major diseases that are still prevalent in LMI countries, the Global Alliance for Vaccines and Immunization (GAVI) was launched in 2000 as a public–private partnership, comprised of partners such as WHO, UNICEF, the Bill and Melinda Gates Foundation, the World Bank, the Rockefeller Foundation, the governments of the developing and developed countries, vaccine manufacturers, civil society groups, as well as the research and technical institutes. The GAVI provided 74 LMI countries with new vaccines and related equipment, technical and financial support to strengthen immunization services, through funding of nearly US$1.5 billion by the end of 2005. The second phase of the GAVI support from 2006 to 2010 with a total of US$5 billion has been mobilized with major proportion (around US$2 billion) already secured (www.gavialliance.org). An investment plan of US$500 million had been earmarked as part of the expansion of immunization programmes through health systems strengthening.

Leprosy elimination

Even though efforts had been made to control leprosy for more than four decades, it was still highly endemic in 1980 in over 120 countries with around 12 million leprosy cases. With the rapid expansion of early case detection and treatment of all registered cases, the multidrug therapy (MDT) (a combination of drugs consisting of rifampicin, dapsone, and clofazimine), a few million leprosy cases were cured, and another few millions had been prevented from the disability and social stigma, thus, reducing the total burden. The total leprosy case load was reduced significantly from 5.4 million in 1985 to 3.7 million in 1990 in the endemic countries of Southeast Asia alone. This experience had led the World Health Assembly in 1991 to resolve to attain the global elimination of leprosy as a public health problem, with a defined target of reduction of prevalence to a level below one case per 10 000 population by the year 2000 (WHO 1991).

Elimination of leprosy within a certain defined target date is possible due to the following unique opportunities and principles: An epidemiological situation where cases were accumulated over several decades; a technological opportunity of using highly effective MDT to cure the disease, and to control the infective cases, thus interrupting the transmission; strong political commitment in all endemic countries, ultimately forming a global alliance; readily and easily available resources provided by a number of national and international development partners; and need for setting a time-bound target since such a situation or opportunity may not last for long. WHO together with the Nippon Foundation of Japan, the International Federation of Anti-Leprosy Associations (ILEP), the Novartis Foundation for Sustainable Development, the UN and its specialized agencies, multilateral and bilateral donors and other philanthropic societies, and the endemic countries themselves, formed a Global Alliance on leprosy and the alliance had provided generous and sustained contributions, in terms of financial, material, and human resources to the global effort for leprosy elimination. As a result of joint national and international efforts within a decade or more, the coverage of MDT in endemic countries had improved tremendously, and the case load had decreased significantly. By 2001, 107 out of 122 endemic countries had achieved the global target of leprosy elimination, i.e. reducing the prevalence of leprosy to a level below one case per 10 000 population (WHO 2002b). While China achieved the global elimination target by 1981, Myanmar could achieve it in early 2003. India could reach that target only in 2005.

Globally, a total of 296 500 new cases were detected in 2005, which was almost half of the level in 2000. By early 2007, 117 endemic countries had achieved the global elimination target, with around 200 000 leprosy cases being still registered for treatment with MDT. There are five endemic countries (Brazil, Nepal, DR Congo, Mozambique, and Tanzania), which have yet to achieve the elimination target. Sustained efforts on early case detection, treatment with MDT, and strengthened routine and referral services still remain the cornerstone of leprosy control. The Global Alliance had intensified necessary financial and human resources and logistic support to make leprosy control services sustainable and to ensure quality care easily available to the population through an integrated approach (WHO 2005a). If the current trend in disease reduction is well sustained with the full support from global alliance, the global leprosy elimination goal could be achieved and the burden of the disease further reduced in all endemic countries in the near future. Leprosy elimination would be another case of a successful public health initiative in the twenty-first century.

Neglected tropical diseases

While efforts are made to prevent and control many tropical diseases around the world, some countries felt that there are some neglected tropical diseases (NTD), such as visceral leishmaniasis or kala-azar, onchocerciasis, dracunculiasis, soil-transmitted helminthic infections, lymphatic filariasis, trachoma, schistosomiasis, the Chagas' disease, African trypanosomiasis, and leprosy, because they are localized conditions or of low morbidity or mortality, or interventions may not yet be available or may be too expensive.

For example, visceral leishmaniasis first came to the attention of Western doctors in 1824 in India where it was initially thought to be a variant form of malaria. Local people gave the name 'kala-azar' to the disease, meaning a disease with high temperature and darkening of the skin on abdomen and extremities. Visceral leishmaniasis is a parasitic disease transmitted by infected sand flies. It is highly prevalent in various localities in Asia, Africa, and southern Europe. Due to the extensive use of residual insecticide DDT for the malaria campaigns during the 1960–70s, the prevalence of visceral leishmaniasis has reduced to a large extent. The new medicine *Miltefosine* as an oral medicine is currently available in India and in neighbouring countries. The Institute for OneWorld Health, an international public–private partnership charity organization, is piloting the visceral leishmaniasis control programme using paromomycin, which was originally identified as the drug of choice in the 1960s and abandoned because of non-profitability for production. Until newer drugs are available at affordable price and accessible means to the mass population in these endemic countries, the misery and suffering due to visceral leishmaniasis would continue.

Onchocerciasis also known as river blindness is another parasitic infection caused by the filarial worm (*Onchocerca volvulus*) and transmitted by female black flies (*Simulium*). Even after the launching of Global Onchocerciasis Control Programme launched in 1974 in partnership with WHO, FAO, UNDP, the World Bank, and a coalition of more than 20 donors and agencies, some 86 million people were at risk and about 18 million were infected, 99 per cent of whom were in Africa, by 1990. A million people were visually impaired and over 350 000 were blind as a consequence of infection. The onchocerciasis programme in the Americas was converted into an elimination campaign in 1991. Similar changes occurred in Africa in 1996. The renewed initiative for elimination of river blindness with additional support from Carter Center, the Bill and Melinda Gates Foundation, Merck & Co., Inc., Lions Clubs, and US-CDC was launched again in the early 2000s, to reduce severe pathological manifestations of the disease through wider use of case management with an effective microfilarial drug (*ivermectin*) (WHO 2006e).

Before 1980, more than 10 million cases of dracunculiasis also known as guinea worm disease, were reported in Africa and South Asia annually. A global campaign to eradicate dracunculiasis was initiated in 1980 by the Centres for Disease Control and Prevention (CDC), USA, taking into account the implementation of International Drinking Water Supply and Sanitation Decade (IWSSD), 1981–1990. Although no medicine was available for this disease, the world community in 1986 called for its elimination by disruption of transmission through improvement of water supply and sanitation as well as promoting personal hygiene. African ministers of health resolved in 1988 to eradicate dracunculiasis by the end of 1995. The endemic countries in Africa and Asia launched elimination campaigns using combined strategies such as clean and safe drinking water supply and sanitation as part of IWSSD activities, improved community awareness and involvement in personal hygiene, surveillance and case containment, and larval control, and also with some cash incentives to identify cases. With concerted effort, the number of cases had been reduced from 3.2 million in 1986 to less than a million in 1989, and subsequently, to around 10 000 cases by 2005 with almost 90 per cent of these remaining cases in Ghana and Sudan. Main reasons of failure to control in the latter two countries were inadequate human resources, poor sanitation and water supply, and the continuing civil war that hampered the implementation of eradication campaigns (WHO 2006f).

Trachoma was an infectious chronic eye disease affecting around 400 million people in 1980, of which more than six million people became blind. Trachoma affected more in poor people and children due to inadequate water supply and unhygienic personal practices. People living in the dry and un-arid zones of the endemic tropical countries were being affected most. Many endemic countries implemented the SAFE strategy (surgery, antibiotics, facial cleaning, and environmental health) under the integrated trachoma control programme, within the Vision 2020 strategy, and with the ultimate aim of elimination of the disease. WHO estimated that in 2002 there were 3.6 million cases of blinding trachoma worldwide, and the majority is in LMI countries. A Global Alliance called GET 2020 (Alliance for Global Elimination of Blinding Trachoma by 2020) was established in 1996 with the partnership of endemic countries, WHO, Helen Keller Worldwide, the Carter Center, the Conrad N. Hilton Foundation, *Christoffel Blinden Mission* (CBM), Pfizer's International Trachoma Initiative (ITI) among others. During the last 7 years, nearly 41 million antibiotic treatments have been administered, approximately 240 000 people have received sight-saving surgery, and a few million people in endemic countries have benefited from health education and improved access to water and sanitation. If the constraints on the availability of antibiotics and specialized surgical sets could be overcome through the efforts of international alliances, the elimination of trachoma could even be achieved by 2010, 10 years ahead of the target set under the GET 2020 campaign (Tun Aung Kyaw 2005).

Lymphatic filariasis (LF) is another parasitic disease aimed for elimination, which is a blood-borne infection by microscopic, thread-like parasitic worms—microfilariae. By 2005, an estimated 1.3 billion people in 83 endemic countries were at risk. Of these, around 80–100 million people are having the disease but no symptoms. Another 15–20 million people would suffer from elephantiasis (swelling of the legs, hands, and genital organs). An improvement in the environmental health could interrupt the transmission and reduce the parasitic levels. Since the 1960s, national LF control programmes were introduced in many countries by adopting mass blood surveys and treatment of cases with appropriate medicine, in combination with appropriate vector control. Despite these efforts for decades, the disease continues to be highly prevalent in many countries mainly in Asia, the Pacific, and Africa. The 50th World Health Assembly in 1998 called for the elimination of lymphatic filariasis as a public health problem (WHO 2000c). Later, endemic countries developed national LF elimination programmes, with an aim of reducing it to a cumulative incidence rate over 5 years of less-than one new case per 1000 susceptible individuals. All endemic countries joined WHO and the development partners, including multinational pharmaceutical corporations like SmithKline Beecham and Merck & Co., by launching a global programme for eliminating lymphatic filariasis (GPELF) with the main goals of interrupting the transmission of infection by providing appropriate mass drug administration (MDA), and alleviating and preventing both the suffering and disability caused by the disease by providing appropriate healthcare (Molyneux *et al.* 2000). By 2006, 42 of the 82 endemic countries were implementing the MDA programmes with over 250 million people being treated with multidrug therapy for mass population. Most of these countries had completed five rounds of mass treatment in the endemic districts and were assessing withdrawing the MDA (WHO 2006g). There is hope that it may be possible to eliminate LF in the near future in some LMI countries through sustained and concerted strategies.

The Global Network for Neglected Tropical Diseases Control (GNNTDC) was a public–private partnership launched in 2006 to raise the profile of neglected tropical diseases and to stimulate a paradigm shift in disease control efforts. This partnership will concentrate on the control of a single tropical disease, and will work in collaboration with WHO to design an integrated drug administration platform that would address the seven neglected tropical diseases such as trachoma, soil-transmitted helminthic infections, and other parasitic diseases. The aim of the global network was to contribute toward the achievement of the UN MDG by eliminating and controlling the neglected diseases through an integrated mass drug delivery approach. A synergistic approach will streamline operational activities, improve efficiencies, and ensure that the priority health needs of impoverished communities in LMI countries are met (www.gnntdc.org).

Since the idea for eradication was started with the efforts to eradicate yellow fever in the eighteenth century, the terms—eradication and elimination—were used extensively and loosely for prevention and control of communicable diseases and later even for non-communicable diseases. This led to a misunderstanding of the purposes and sometimes inappropriate adoption of public health strategies. As far back as 1988, when the global eradication and elimination campaigns against many infectious diseases were launched, the International Taskforce for Disease Eradication had clarified various terms: Control as reduction of disease morbidity or mortality to an acceptable level with continued control measures; elimination as reduction to zero of an incidence of a specified disease in a defined geographical area with concerted and continued control measures; and eradication as a permanent reduction to zero of the worldwide incidence of infection caused by a specified agent, such that control measures could stop (www.cartercenter.org). With the rapid advancement of science and technology, there is a possibility of eliminating or eradicating some of the existing candidate diseases. Newer candidates might also be added in the near future.

Enhancing healthy lives

Burden of chronic non-communicable diseases

In recent years, many public health experts are debating on the proxy indicators for measuring health status in addition to the usual morbidity and mortality statistics. No measure is still perfect for the purpose of summing up the health of a population. The introduction of a new measure in health science being much debated as advocated in the World Health Report 1999 was the disability-adjusted life expectancy-DALE or healthy life expectancy-HALE. In simple terms, it is most easily calculable and well understood, reflecting all states of health. It is the expected years of life at birth with the adjustment of time spent in poor health, and easily understood as the number of years in full health that a newborn can expect to live, based on current rates of ill-health and mortality. The Global HALE at birth for women in 1999 was 57.8 years, which was 2 years higher than that for men. While infectious diseases continue to be a major public health problem, there were ominous signs that chronic non-communicable diseases (NCD) became increasingly prevalent in LMI countries. Recent estimates of global burden of disease and risk factors showed that over 26 million people died (almost 53 per cent of all deaths) in 2001 in LMI countries, due to chronic non-communicable diseases, such as cardiovascular diseases, diabetes, cancer, mental disorders, injuries, and other disabled diseases and conditions (World Bank 2006a).

Cardiovascular diseases, diabetes, and cancers

Cardiovascular disease (CVD) is a group of disorders of the heart and blood vessels, consisting of hypertension (high blood pressure), coronary heart disease, cerebrovascular disease, rheumatic heart disease, congenital heart disease, cardiomyopathies, deep vein thrombosis, and other heart and blood vessel disorders. More than 60 per cent of the global burden of coronary heart disease occurred in LMI countries (WHO 2004b). With increasing adoption of the lifestyle of the high-income countries by the people in LMI countries, there is likely to be greater exposure to various risk factors such as increased use of tobacco and alcohol, high blood pressure, unhealthy diets with high saturated fat leading to elevated serum cholesterol level and physical inactivity (Reddy & Yusuf 1999). Many large-scale, well-designed clinical trials on reducing risk factors primarily conducted in the established market economies had shown that lowering common risk factors could reduce illness and death from CVD. The dual approach of screening and intervening in cases of relatively high risk of CVD and of fostering population-wide preventive activities is as appropriate in LMI countries as in the high-income countries (Lenfant 2001). Over the past 30 years, mortality from cardiovascular diseases has decreased considerably in the high-income countries due to concerted and sustained efforts of a combination of health promotion, legislative and policy action, prevention of risks, and better case management (NIH 2000). Necessary policy steps could easily be introduced in LMI countries to adopt population-based health promotion and prevention, in combination with management of high-risk cases with proven therapeutic agents. The promotion of healthy diets that limit the intake of saturated fats and sodium, effort to prevent people from use of tobacco and alcohol, and effort to encourage life-long physical activity could be done as a population-wide, large-scale, public health intervention programme for prevention and control of CVD.

Diabetes mellitus is another chronic non-communicable disease, either insulin dependent (Type 1) or non-insulin dependent (Type 2), affecting around 170 million people of over 20 years of age worldwide in 2000. Even though insulin was discovered in 1921 for the treatment of diabetes, many people suffering from insulin-dependent diabetes in LMI countries are not yet accessing it adequately. The people affected by diabetes may increase to 370 million by 2030 if a proper prevention and control strategy is not in place (Wild *et al.* 2004). LMI countries such as India, China, Indonesia, Brazil, and Bangladesh would have a majority of diabetic cases. Maintaining a balanced body weight by height, being physically active for at least 30 min of moderately intense exercise, and taking low sugar and high consumption of vegetables and fruits are the simple and effective strategies for preventing and controlling diabetes. With early screening, diagnosis, and effective management with diet, exercise, and essential medicines, diabetes and its complications can easily be controlled.

Cancer has been a well-known chronic non-communicable disease for many decades, and a leading cause of deaths worldwide with more than 70 per cent of all cancer deaths occurring in LMI countries. Cancer is absent or low on the health agendas of LMI countries. Cancer is actually a generic term used for a group of more than 100 diseases and conditions that affect mainly the liver, lungs, breast, colorectum, cervix, prostate, and stomach. Liver cancer affects approximately 5.5 million people, predominantly caused by the viral hepatitis. In countries of low endemic viral hepatitis, chronic alcoholism and high content of aflatoxins in food are major risk for liver cancer. Stomach cancer is another common cancer caused by *Helicobacter pylori* infection. High consumption of salt, and salted, smoked, pickled, and preserved food is also the common risk for stomach cancer. Introduction of refrigerators and adoption of better methods for food preservation have considerably brought down the incidence of stomach cancer in many countries. Cancer of the breast is another common disease among women which is intimately related to a high-calorie diet, lack of exercise, and reproductive factors. While early detection with proper screening and increasing improvement in therapy has reduced the mortality associated with breast cancer, it is unfortunately not accessible to large segments of the population in LMI countries. Early diagnosis and treatment could reduce mortality of breast cancer by 45 per cent in women above the age of 50 years. Cancer of the uterine cervix is another cancer prevalent among women of childbearing age, which is mainly due to sexually transmitted human papillomavirus (HPV) infection. Pap smear screening has significantly reduced mortality from cervical cancer, and it could bring down the incidence of cervical cancer to less than 5 per 100 000 population in some countries of Europe and North America. Broad implementation of this approach in LMI countries could be hindered by the financial constraints and poor health infrastructure. The introduction of HPV vaccine, especially in low-resource settings could be hindered by its high cost and other challenges in implementing vaccination programmes. All people with incurable cancers could also obtain appropriate palliative care. Most of the population in LMI countries has little access to radiotherapy or other modern oncological services. The rational use of medicines would improve affordability of cancer chemotherapy. Specialists and radiotherapy facilities are few and tend to be located in the metropolitan areas. In the absence of appropriate financial

mechanisms and protection, out-of-pocket payment for the diagnosis and treatment of cancer could devastate the affected families and individuals. The installation and maintenance of high-technology equipment stand in the way of equitable radiotherapy service. Cancer control plans should be developed in all LMI countries starting from now, in order to tackle effectively the silent epidemics.

Reducing tobacco and alcohol use

There was a major increase in tobacco-related illnesses and deaths worldwide during the last decades, with four million people killed every year, and if no proper control measures are instituted, the deaths may go up to 10 million. After the United States, four LMI countries, viz. China, Brazil, India, and Indonesia, are the highest producers of tobacco, and total production by these four countries is more than two-third of the tobacco produced globally in 2004 (Mackay *et al.* 2006). Among the various forms of tobacco used, cigarettes account for the largest share of manufactured tobacco products in the world. In addition, people used tobacco in various forms. Tobacco consumption among the youth is also increasing. With an intensive global campaign, WHO launched its global tobacco free initiative in 1998 to galvanize global political support for evidence-based tobacco policies, build and strengthen new and existing partnerships for action, accelerate national, regional, and global strategies for tobacco control, and mobilize resources. The initial focus was on developing the WHO Framework Convention on Tobacco Control (FCTC), the first health treaty initiated by WHO using its constitutional mandate. The WHO FCTC was approved by the World Health Assembly in May 2003, and became an international legal instrument by February 2005 after a mandated number of countries had ratified it. As of February 2007, a total of 168 countries are signatory to the Convention and 146 countries are parties to the Convention (www.who.int/tobacco). The WHO FCTC asserts the importance of national policies and strategies for reducing demand and addressing supply issues for tobacco use. The main provisions of the WHO FCTC includes the regulation of contents, packaging, and labelling of tobacco products, prohibition of sales to and by minors, illicit trade in tobacco products, and smoking in work and public places. It also called for a reduction in consumer demand by price and tax measures, a comprehensive ban on tobacco advertising, promotion and sponsorship, education, training, raising awareness and assistance with quitting, protection of the environment, and the health of tobacco workers. The Convention will help promote the economies that are not dependent on tobacco products, strengthening the women's roles in tobacco control, and supporting the countries by making people aware about the dangers of tobacco, and protecting most vulnerable communities. Several countries in the world now have comprehensive national tobacco control legislation, conforming to the provisions of the WHO FCTC. Under the leadership of the Conference of the Parties, the challenge is to build on the experience of the Convention and to develop strong national and international protocols on specific issues, as well as to support the countries, especially the least-developed nations, in implementing their obligations.

The World Health Report 2002 indicated that there were about 2 billion people worldwide who consume alcoholic beverages, and 76.3 million suffered from alcohol use disorders. A WHO sponsored study conducted in India that showed the financial losses to the state in the long-term were far greater than the immediate revenue (WHO 2006h). A wide range of policy options and interventions for reducing public health problems caused by harmful use of alcohol was advocated. One policy option proposed was to allocate part of the taxes generated from the sales of alcohol to support health promotion, including community education, sports, and recreational activities. Thailand has adopted, under its health promotion act, the use of sin tax on tobacco and alcohol, the proceeds being used for health promotion activities including reducing alcohol consumption and related problems. Other legislative measures adopted by many LMI countries included various measures on the limitation of physical availability of alcohol, by setting a minimum legal age limit, restricting the number, density and locations of sale outlets, or limiting hours and days of sale, and imposing some other restrictions on sale. In recent decades, community-level efforts to control harmful use of alcohol in some countries have been successful through enhanced partnerships and networks, involving public agencies and NGOs.

Other diseases and conditions

An estimated 400 million people worldwide suffer from mental and neurological disorders and other psychosocial problems including substance abuse. According to the World Health Report 2001, an estimated 12.3 per cent of all DALYs were attributable to mental and neurological disorders in 2000. Mental health disorders such as dementia, depression, and schizophrenia, generally affect the elderly. While many LMI countries have established national mental health policies, legislative measures, or mental health promotion programmes, some national policies, legislation, and programmes are based on outdated knowledge, concepts, and approaches (Rafei 2004). A major problem with the community-based approach was the lack of awareness among the community and lack of trained personnel, particularly community-level health workers who would be able to carry out basic essential mental healthcare services. Currently, many LMI countries are particularly affected by the problem of substance dependence. Most countries have developed policies to control substance abuse, with the focus on demand reduction and prevention of harm to substance abusers.

Injuries have emerged as a major public health problem worldwide, as estimated in World Health Report 2004, with almost 16 000 people dying from all types of injuries everyday worldwide. About 50 per cent of these deaths occurred in the countries of Asia and the Pacific. In LMI countries, 34 per cent of all deaths due to injuries are road traffic related. Road traffic injuries are the second leading cause of deaths among both children 5–14 years and young adults aged 15–29 years worldwide. The rapidly rising number of motor vehicles and motorcycles in the world and especially in LMI countries has seen an equally rapid increase in the number of injuries and deaths. Many countries have made progress in implementing national programmes to prevent and control injuries. Some have not yet put injury prevention on the public health agenda, since they considered injury as the problem to be tackled by sectors other than health such as the police, transport, education, and legal authorities. In a few LMI countries, injury prevention and control started with improving medical care services such as the establishment of accident and trauma centres, strengthening emergency ambulance services, and promoting the training on injury care and management. The first step of a public health approach to injury prevention and control is to have appropriate information in order to ascertain the magnitude and characteristics of injuries and their basic causes. An injury surveillance system provides relevant information on the kind of injuries suffered, on those affected, on places and time how people are injured, etc.

Healthy ageing

Many LMI countries have started giving attention to promoting the health of the elderly, focusing on partnerships and promotion of social welfare and healthcare at home and in the community, promotion of traditional family ties, making optimal use of existing healthcare delivery systems, and establishment of old-age homes. Some countries have formulated national policies on ageing and health. A few have started collection and analysis of related information for advocacy, policy and programme development, decision-making, dissemination to the general public, pensioners, healthcare professionals, and policy-makers to promote appropriate services, advice, and practice on healthy ageing. Efforts are also being made to develop an advocacy strategy in close collaboration with government agencies, NGOs, and the media, aiming at influencing public opinion and encouraging support for community-based programmes for healthy ageing. A few countries have also organized research studies related to epidemiology, patterns of the ageing population, and determinants of healthy ageing and improved the capacity of healthcare providers in the area of care of the elderly. The economic, social, and health status of the fast-growing elderly population poses a great challenge to all sectors. The major difficulties in developing appropriate healthcare for the elderly include the lack of reliable data for programme planning, a virtual absence of national policies and strategies for the care of the elderly, and an inadequate infrastructure to cope with their rapidly increasing health needs. The joint family system and family values are gradually being eroded in many countries. With regard to health status, around 6 per cent of the aged are immobile due to various disabling conditions. Approximately 50 per cent of the elderly suffer from chronic diseases. At the same time, health services for the elderly are inadequate. Knowledge among health workers on the specific needs of the elderly is also minimal.

Addressing risks

Since human behaviour occurs in a specific milieu, comprehensive policy interventions that improve the physical, social, and economic environments and modify the social norms of the population have proven to be far more effective in reducing the NCD burden and improving health, rather than a sole focus on behaviour change at the individual level. It is also uneconomical to promote unregulated growth of expensive specialized healthcare services focused on addressing individual patients, usually who come and seek services in an advanced stage of diseases. Healthy public policies are needed to change the physical and socioeconomic environment. Population-wide interventions aimed at reduction of tobacco and alcohol consumption, and promoting physical activity and healthy eating habits coupled with interventions targeting high-risk groups and individuals could greatly reduce the burden of NCD and improve public health outcomes with the potential to prevent at least 80 per cent of cardiovascular disease and diabetes, and 40 per cent of cancers (WHO 2005d). The costs of care and treatment of individual NCD cases are increasingly overstretching the public health systems, as well as the budgets of affected families. It could be considerably reduced by application of cost-effective interventions at the primary prevention level so that people may not even suffer from the diseases. Establishment of basic health facilities and community-based treatment, rehabilitative and palliative services no doubt contributed significantly in improving the quality of life of people with disabilities and those in the terminal stages of chronic diseases. A majority of effective public health interventions for prevention and control of NCD are primarily beyond the direct control of the health ministry.

Comprehensive NCD policies and programmes would require addressing the NCD prevention holistically. The measures include: Development and modification of healthy public policies and appropriate health legislation, regulations and financing mechanisms, modification of physical environment, and resource-sensitive organization and delivery of health services. National programmes need to select the interventions potentially feasible for implementation within existing resources and realistically increased resources in the short and medium term. The ministry of health should take a leadership role in coordinating and promoting partnerships that would involve stakeholders beyond government sectors such as the private sector, civil society groups, individual philanthropists, and international agencies. Governments also have a central role to play in establishing appropriate health financing mechanisms and models.

Health promotion as a core function of public health is effective in reducing the burden of both communicable and non-communicable diseases and in mitigating the social and economic impact of such diseases. It contributes to positive social and behavioural changes among individuals and communities resulting in the reduction of risks, premature deaths, and illness. The goal in promoting health is to mitigate the impact of risk factors associated with broad determinants of health leading to premature death and illness, and ultimately to improve the quality of lives of individuals and communities. To effectively address the identifiable determinants of health, health promotion requires strategic directions and policies to be formulated in addition to political commitment. The Bangkok Charter for Health Promotion in a Globalized World, 2006, confirmed the need to focus on health promotion actions to address the determinants of health. It encouraged stakeholders in all sectors and settings to advocate for health based on human rights and solidarity, to invest in sustainable policies, actions and infrastructure to address the determinants of health, to build capacity for policy development, leadership, health promotion practice, knowledge transfer and research, and health literacy, to regulate and legislate to ensure a high level of protection from harm and enable equal opportunity for health and well-being for all people; and to build alliances with public, private, non-governmental and international organizations, and civil society to create sustainable actions.

New paradigm of public health
Globalization of public health

The transformation of local societies to a global society resulted in the blurring of territories. An analysis on the impact of globalization and health is available in many health and development literature (Chen *et al.* 1999; Society for International Development 1999; Drager & Beaglehole 2001). It is accepted that globalization actually enhanced the opportunities for human advancement as well as economic and cultural growth of all peoples, through sharing of resources. Global markets, global finances, global technology, global knowledge, global solidarity, global governance, and global security—all of these entities have the ability to improve the health of people everywhere and achieve the target of health-for-all. The threats to and opportunities in public health were also analysed extensively within the context of globalization (Yach & Bettchnner 1998; Berlinguer 1999; Navarro 1999; UN 2003). Berlinguer used the term 'microbial unification of the world' as the phenomenon of the transmission of disease epidemics across countries and continents as part of globalization.

Today, the occurrence of a local epidemic of a disease has become a global issue. The rapidly increasing numbers of people travelling and migrating to neighbouring countries or across the world would pose the threat of spreading diseases. As disease agents could pass over any physical boundaries among nations and territories, transmission of disease could take place at any time anywhere in the world. A revised International Health Regulations had been adopted at the 58th World Health Assembly in 2005, in order to prevent, protect against, control, and provide a public health response to the international spread of disease, in ways that are commensurate with and restricted to public health risks, and avoid unnecessary interference with international traffic and trade (WHO 2005b).

The new measures adopted under IHR (2005) included among others: Immediate notification and verification of a public health emergency of international concern; internationally coordinated public health response; and provision of public health measures, including strengthening global surveillance. Certain infectious diseases could also be transmitted through food exports and tourism. If the preparations of food and food products are not carried out in accordance with good manufacturing practices, there are possible threats of spreading infectious diseases associated with the consignments. If proper manufacturing and export practices are followed, the export products could be consumed safely. Yet, there are many trade-related cases from Asia, the Americas, and Africa where exports from LMI countries are restricted or sanctioned by high-income nations, for the purpose of protecting from infectious diseases. Peru lost over US$770 million during the cholera outbreak in 1991, due to trade sanctions by several high-income countries by trade sanction on imports of Peruvian fishes and fishery products. Similarly, India lost around US$4000 million from export earnings due to the plague outbreak in 1994. Several African countries lost millions of dollars due to an embargo on certain fishery products during the cholera outbreaks in 1998 (Kinnon 1998; Miyagishima & Kaferstein 1998).

Emerging and re-emerging diseases

While many old scourges like tuberculosis, malaria, human plague, and leprosy remained or re-emerged as high burden diseases, a few new or previously unrecognized infections such as HIV-AIDS, ebola and other haemorrhagic diseases, SARS, and avian influenza are being reported both in the high-income and LMI countries. Main factors that aggravate this situation include: The change in human demography and job opportunities leading to mass migration; change of human behaviour, especially sexual relations; advancement in technology and industrial development such as air-conditioning, food processing, and preservation; environmental degradation; microbial adaptation and resistance; and the breakdown of public health infrastructure especially surveillance.

Acquired immunodeficiency disease syndrome (AIDS) was unknown before 1981 and its causal organism—the Human

Immunodeficiency virus (HIV) was discovered only in 1983. After a decade of a Global Programme on AIDS (GPA) launched by WHO, UNDP, the World Bank, and other partners, its work was consolidated into a UN AIDS Control Programme (UNAIDS). In the absence of an effective vaccine, the main strategies of prevention and control of HIV/AIDS were political advocacy, mass education on disease including sex education, behavioural intervention and social mobilization, and integrated social development. In industrialized countries, the number of deaths due to AIDS has dropped rapidly due to increasing accessibility of proper care and appropriate therapy. The impact on human development had gone beyond mortality as the epidemic had affected the sustainability of households and the socioeconomic resources of communities (UNDP 1998). An overwhelming majority of people with HIV infection or AIDS are living in LMI countries. The progress in improving life expectancy in the 1970–80s in many LMI countries, especially those in Africa, were reversed by the high burden of HIV/AIDS (WHO 1999b). An effective vaccine is still a long way off. With WHO advocacy in 2005 and support from the Global Fund, access to antiretroviral drugs (ARV) has improved tremendously in many endemic countries.

Tuberculosis (TB), an age-old scourge continues as a globally dangerous infection that led to adoption of a global Stop TB programme in 1991. The problem of TB is more complex than before since drug-resistant TB cases have increased and there is an increasing incidence of co-infection of TB and HIV. Effective case management and the vaccination of infants with BCG, and health education were the main control strategies. Improving socioeconomic conditions, access to good housing and reducing in-door and out-door pollution, and good personal hygienic practices played an important public health role in reducing TB morbidity and mortality. High-burden countries have been compelled to use the directly observed treatment, short-course (DOTS) strategy for effective management of infectious TB cases, thus reducing the infectious case load in a short period. A total of 183 countries and territories were implementing the DOTS strategy during 2004. More than 26 million TB patients were treated under the DOTS programmes over 11 years from 1995 to 2005 (WHO 2006i). The global prevalence of tuberculosis fell from 297 per 100 000 population in 1990 to 229 in 2004, partly as a consequence of DOTS expansion. This enhancement of coverage of TB treatment was accomplished with the support of the Stop TB partnership and the arrangement of the Global Drug Facility.

Even after initiating eradication campaigns during 1950–60s and implementing extensive control programmes in 1970–80s, malaria remains a major public health threat worldwide. Every year, over 3 billion people are at risk of contracting malaria and more than 500 million people suffer from acute disease resulting in more than 1 million deaths. Countries along the Mekong river in Asia and other high-malaria endemic countries in Africa joined together to fight the drug-resistant malaria. Many countries had introduced multidrug therapy as the first- and second-line therapy for malaria. Rapid deterioration in the malaria situation in many countries calls for greater efforts by governments of endemic countries and the full support of the international agencies. The global malaria control strategy was adopted at the Ministerial Conference on Malaria held at Amsterdam in 1992 and subsequently endorsed by the World Health Assembly and the UN General Assembly in 1993. In 1998, another global movement—Roll Back Malaria (RBM), was initiated as a global partnership between WHO, UNDP, UNICEF, and the World Bank, to combat malaria by using the strategies already adopted at the Ministerial Malaria Summit. The programme anticipated a 50 per cent reduction in the number of deaths from malaria within a decade through better access by all people in malaria-affected areas to a range of effective interventions (WHO 1999b). Development partners worked together with the malaria-affected countries to achieve this new goal. In recent years, through various funding mechanisms such as the Medicines for Malaria Venture, the Global Fund to Fight AIDS, Tuberculosis and Malaria, the malaria initiative of the President of USA, the World Bank Booster programme for malaria control and the Bill & Melinda Gates Foundation, many national programmes have enhanced their malaria prevention and control activities, especially in improving access to multidrug therapy including adoption of Artemisinin-based combination therapy (ACT), increasing coverage of selected indoor residual spraying and use of effective insecticide-treated bednets (ITN), and increasing availability of rapid diagnostic tests. Funds in millions of dollars were poured into malaria endemic countries to expand the coverage of treatment and use of ITN. Many countries had adopted revised malaria control strategies by scaling up coverage and proper use of ITN, expanding the coverage of diagnosis and treatment coverage with multidrug therapy, and promoting rapid diagnosis tests (RDT), revamping surveillance, and strengthening monitoring and evaluation, organizing advocacy, and launching malaria campaign weeks (WHO 2006j).

The Global Fund to Fight AIDS, Tuberculosis and Malaria (Global Fund) is a partnership between the governments, civil society, the private sector, and the affected communities to operate as a financial instrument to dramatically increase resources to fight three of the world's most devastating diseases. At the sixth round of proposal reviews in 2006, a total of US$846 million worth of proposals from 63 countries around the world had been approved, of which US$453 million was for HIV in 34 countries, US$202 million for malaria in 19 countries, and US$190 million for tuberculosis in 34 countries. Since 2001, the Global Fund has attracted US$4.7 billion for financing, through 2008. During its first two rounds of approving grants, it has committed US$1.5 billion in funding support for 154 programmes in 93 countries worldwide (www.globalfund.org). With this large-scale investment by the Global Fund, millions of people infected with HIV and suffering from AIDS, millions of tuberculosis cases especially multidrug-resistant cases, and millions of malaria cases had been identified and treated, and millions have been prevented from getting such diseases.

Human plague cases have dramatically declined in many LMI countries due to improvement in sanitary measures, use of antibiotics and insecticides, and proper handling of dead rats (rat falls). The total number of people who suffered from human plague during 1989–2003 was 38 310, with 2845 deaths, as reported in 25 countries. Sporadic cases of rat falls and annual reported human plague cases of about 1000–3000 occurred in many parts of Asia, Africa, and the Americas. After silent periods of about 30–50 years, human plague was reported in three geographical areas: India in 1994 and 2002, Indonesia in 1997, and Algeria in 2003 (WHO 2004c). The outbreak of plague in India in 1994 somehow created a wave of public panic, both within and outside the country. Inadequate sharing of information with the general population caused the country to lose billions of dollars in export earnings. Since pneumonic plague can kill a person in 3–4 days after infection, the potential for using the plague bacilli as a biological weapon is a threat. Current research is going on to address the preventive action against possible terrorist-caused plague disease outbreaks (www. niaiad.nih.gov/factsheets/plague.html).

About 90 per cent of an estimated 200 000 yellow fever (YF) cases occurred annually in Africa, where both the urban and jungle type of transmission existed (WHO 2003). The disease is still endemic in 34 African countries with several in Western and Eastern Africa reporting sporadic outbreaks every year since 1994. Some countries in South America are still at risk, predominated by the jungle type of YF. Even though the disease can be efficiently and effectively prevented and controlled through immunization, it is still persisted as a threat for international spread. Thousands of lives could easily be lost, unless a good surveillance system and higher immunization coverage in the countries at risk are sustained.

There is an annual worldwide incidence of 1.5 million cases of clinical viral hepatitis due to hepatitis A (HepA) virus, and if seroprevalence data were used, this annual incidence might be as high as tens of millions of people (WHO 2000d). The disease is most endemic in LMI countries where poor environmental conditions and inadequate hygienic practices facilitate the transmission especially among children with predominant asymptomatic infection. Essentially the entire population would have been infected before reaching adolescence. The disease is more serious in high-income and some LMI countries with a better standard of living and good hygiene, where the majority of population may not have any immunity to the HepA infection and could lead to sporadic community-wide outbreaks. Immunization against HepA has been an effective tool for protection of persons who travel to high-endemic countries and also in reducing incidence among the population in communities where annual incidence is rather high (Wasley 2006).

The advent of inexpensive and effective oral rehydration therapy (ORT) for diarrhoea and simplified case management for ARI and other childhood illnesses in the early 1970s resulted in conceivable progress in implementing effective clinical interventions as part of promoting the integrated management of childhood illness (IMCI). Poor sanitation and housing conditions including unclean and smoky kitchens, inadequate supply of safe water, and improper personal hygiene resulted in a high incidence of diarrhoeal diseases and ARI. The total number of ARI episodes in young children throughout the world has been estimated to be around 2000 million a year. The action to impart the knowledge and skill to basic health workers on IMCI has required a lot of professional and financial resources. Greater efforts are required to ensure that 80 per cent of the families in LMI countries have access to IMCI, in order to reduce the burden of diarrhoeal diseases and ARI. Not just developing more and more expensive medicines, research efforts need to be made on development of appropriate vaccines in the short-time span (e.g. expediting the development of rotavirus vaccination). Similarly political and financial investments have to be made in improving the water supply and sanitation, housing, reducing indoor and outdoor pollution, and also improving hygienic practices. These would ultimately lead to reducing the total burden of diarrhoeal diseases and ARI in the long run.

Dengue and dengue-haemorrhagic fever (D-DHF) have been major vector-borne diseases affecting the high mortality and morbidity among children in urban areas of Asia and the Pacific for many decades. Except in the improvement in management of the cases which had saved a lot of lives of children, the prevention and control of D-DHF concentrated only on active surveillance of the disease which is more of seasonal and cyclical in nature and effective reduction of mosquitoes in the immediate vicinity of where the epidemics occurred. The disease is further spreading in rural areas and also other continents such as Africa, Middle-East, and the Americas. Now, the disease is endemic in more than 100 countries with more than 2.5 billion people being at risk. Development of Dengue vaccine has been initiated since a few decades ago, but not yet been successful for wider use. Ebola is another haemorrhagic fever transmitted to humans by direct contact with the blood or body fluids of infected persons, mainly reported in a few countries of Africa since 1974. Except supportive intensive care being provided to the patient and precautionary infection control measures for health personnel who attended patients, there is no specific treatment or vaccine available for ebola (WHO 2004d). Another emerging viral haemorrhagic fever similar to ebola caused by Marburg virus infection mainly affected infants and young children in Africa reported as early as 1967 (www.itg.be/ebola). Japanese encephalitis (JE) is a vector-borne viral infection occurring in rural and peri-urban areas of Asia and the Pacific. There is no specific treatment, but JE vaccine is available now and a few countries have started including it as part of routine EPI programme.

Another seriously emerging disease is the avian influenza, caused by a highly pathogenic H5N1 virus which primarily causes diseases to domestic and migratory birds. It became a global alert in 2003 due to its potential rapid transmission around the globe. Only a little over 100 human cases with 70 per cent case-fatality rate were reported since December 2003 till January 2007 from nine countries. But, several countries around the world, mainly from Asia, Africa, Middle-East, and Europe, had confirmed existence of H5N1 virus in wild and domestic birds. Some countries have effectively controlled poultry outbreaks, but the virus may have been entrenched in domestic birds as shown by reported H5N1 outbreaks which re-emerged in these countries. Some countries in East Asia have introduced the poultry immunization on a large scale since 2004, and curtailed the poultry outbreaks significantly. Local preparedness and response to the epidemic control of both animal and human outbreaks of H5N1 infection are most crucial in determining the outcome, when the countries are challenged by the dreadful virus (WHO 2006k). There is a strong need to have global collaborative research to combat the avian influenza, since the H5N1 virus is a significant threat to animal and human health globally.

Health emergencies and health security

WHO's Constitution clearly states that the health of all peoples is fundamental to the attainment of peace and security. The terrorist attacks on the USA in September 2001, and countless terrorist acts against civilian populations in many parts of the world including use of biological weapons are in themselves threats to the health of the people. Communal violence and armed conflicts of long duration in many parts of the world have also caused psychosocial and other illnesses to the people and compounded by needlessly prolonged destruction of their health services. During the last 15 years, more than 10 000 events of natural and human-made disasters, including armed conflicts and complex emergencies occurred around the world, affecting around 4 billion people with nearly 2 million deaths, which cost more than US$1 trillion.

The most devastating disaster was the Asian Tsunami and earthquakes, which occurred on one single day on 26 December 2004, and affected several millions and took thousands of lives of the people around the countries of Southeast Asia (WHO 2005c). Since then, a series of natural disasters, like earthquakes, tsunami, and hurricanes, etc. had happened in various parts of the world with millions people dying or becoming homeless. Many actors at local, intercountry, and international levels are necessary to have quick responses to such catastrophic incidences, since health systems and other infrastructure in most cases also collapsed at the same time. A global system for surveillance and control of health and human security is required to protect the world public from any attack of infectious and other contagious threats, irrespective of national boundaries. Priorities include: Improving access to essential healthcare for vulnerable people; strengthening coordination among health partners; establishing and strengthening disease surveillance, early warning and response systems; supporting systems to reduce maternal, infant, and under-5 mortality and morbidity; and strengthening health and psychosocial support to victims. A global vision of health for all had instigated a climate of trust and improved the international relations. Governments of affected countries, majority of which are of LMI countries, in collaboration with multilateral financial institutions, international NGOs and foundations, donor agencies of high income countries, and WHO and other UN agencies had to respond to the death menace and saved countless lives and helped millions of victims.

Social medicine and public health

The initial ideas of social medicine or social dimension of public health had emerged around the early twentieth century (Ko Ko 1996). Professor Winslow defined public health as the science and art of preventing disease, prolonging life, and promoting physical health and efficiency through organized community efforts. This definition was debated for long as to whether it should fall in the area of preventive medicine or public health or beyond. The expansion of the concept of social medicine had emerged since the late 1940s as a new public health discipline. The leaders of both clinical medicine and public health questioned the polarization of curative and preventive medicine and specialization in each field, as if they were in water-tight compartments. Although new knowledge about causal factors, risks, and prevention and control of chronic noncommunicable diseases were available since 1950–60s, the application for development of healthy public policy and public health interventions were done in the 1980s. The social and behavioural aspects that influenced illness and well-being became recognized. and many social interventions were proposed as part of health promotion. Without in-depth consideration of the basic concept of social medicine, many medical universities and faculties converted their departments or schools of public health into those of preventive and social medicine. Instead of teaching social medicine or new public health, educational institutions considered public health equating with preventive and social medicine and teaching more of conventional public health. Most of the associated changes are more of a change in designation than in the evolving concept of public health.

Because of the political needs and demands of the community, the widening gaps between health needs and available resources, and the rising pressure of societal factors, many health planners come out strongly that the tasks before them required fitting clinical medicine into a social context. Socialized healthcare had become the most reasonable, workable, and acceptable approach. The relationships between health and poverty were highlighted in an effort to find appropriate solutions. People themselves became more aware of the social and economic determinants impacting health. Empirical evidences were studied from both parts of the world. The value of health as a fundamental human right and its attainment as an essential social goal were firmly recognized. Mahler, WHO Director-General Emeritus, said that without health, life had little quality, for even if health was not everything, without it, the rest was nothing (WHO 1992). As a result of debates on the linkages of health with social, environmental, economic, and political factors, there are more discussions now to give a political dimension to international public health.

Policy makers are increasingly becoming concerned about finding equitable, realistic, and sustainable approaches for improving health. Meanwhile, experience has shown that many governments in LMI countries regarded the health expenditure by the public sector as purely a commodity of consumption. The total spending on health as a percentage to GDP in these countries is still around or even below 5 per cent. International agencies have encouraged these LMI countries to set priorities and improve resource allocation. A new paradigm for public health emerged in the early 1990s that health was central to development and to the quality of life. After three decades since the Alma-Ata Conference, the analysis of global health situation revealed that sustained progress in health development using PHC as the main approach towards achieving universal goal of health for all was a complex and difficult task for many LMI countries. Despite these draw backs, a few countries in Asia, Latin America, and Africa could display to the world that they could achieve major improvements in health outcomes while keeping the total public health spending at the lowest or modest levels (Rannan-Eliya 2006). Governments in these countries have adopted consistent multi-sectoral policies and programmes reaching the poor and the vulnerable, with the most effective preventive, promotive, and curative health interventions, in addition to other social and economic development programmes. Extensive use of health volunteers in providing essential primary healthcare and also expanding health knowledge through mass media and school education were the success factors.

In spite of the rapid expansion and improvement in health systems development over three decades, not all citizens in LMI countries have access to minimum essential healthcare. Many children in some LMI countries have missed basic services like polio, measles, and tetanus immunization. A majority of TB, malaria, HIV/AIDS, or leprosy patients do not have access to multidrug therapy. The challenge during the next century is what kind of public health policies are needed to ensure universal access to healthcare by all citizens. WHO has advocated the new universalism in health meaning that universal coverage is aimed for all, but not of everything (WHO 1999a). Essential public health interventions could be efficient and effective with quality, and should not be dependent on who is providing. These essential interventions for each country may need to be defined based upon the health financing mechanisms, health systems infrastructure, social behaviour, and other aspects of socioeconomic development. Public health development in the last couple of centuries had explicitly shown the need for increasing interdependence between high-income and LMI countries, in order to promote the health of the citizens of the world. The health risks are shared by every citizen of the world and could also be seen as opportunities for improvement. Debates in recent years have been intensified on the issues of global public health development and global governance of health (Dodgson *et al.* 2002; Kickbusch & Payne 2004). During the last 50 years, many inter-country, intergovernmental, international, bilateral, and multilateral development agencies and organizations, as well as alliances have emerged out of necessity to deal increasingly with international developmental issues, both in policy and programme terms including health and other social development.

In November 2006, Chan, the newly-elected WHO Director-General, defined a new role for the World Health Organization that could be a step towards becoming a truly international as well as a global health organization (WHO 2006l). While the main mission of WHO continues to be attaining for all people the highest possible level of health, it further adopts a corporate strategic framework that will result in achieving greatest possible contribution to world health (WHO 2007c). LMI countries need to work in close collaboration with WHO and other partners by focusing the global efforts to build healthy populations and communities in addressing the excess burden of sickness and suffering resulting from both communicable and non-communicable diseases especially in poor and marginalized populations. Partnerships could be established to sustain and support health system development so that equitable health outcomes are achieved and peoples' demands are met.

Looking ahead

The final decades of the twentieth century witnessed a rapidly changing political situation and severe economic upheavals, especially towards the end of the Cold War in the 1990s. Strong demands were made for pluralistic democracy, good governance, social justice, and respect for human rights for a clearly defined role of the State and for economic globalization. Social expectations and awareness of social and economic development linked with health improvement were infused in many LMI countries. There was a dramatic change in international public health development, especially the global health governance and international health cooperation. The centrality of health to human development was charted in a wide range of national and international agreements and affirmed in action by a wide-ranging set of stakeholders. A multiplicity of new actors in national and international health had redefined the boundaries of health sector, each with its own unique expertise and vision. Groups of individuals united in a particular cause, such as patient groups or civil society groups, become major players for policies and programme development, by creating powerful lobbies and raising public awareness. Increased access to the Internet and other new communication tools has revolutionized the people's reach for information with a certain degree of freedom of choice. Growing involvement of more non-governmental organizations in direct delivery of healthcare had complemented the efforts of national health systems. They become influential players in policy development and decision-making in socioeconomic and health-related issues.

New mechanisms for health financing with public–private partnerships and the scale of resources brought in by new partners are changing the way health is externally funded in many countries. This new paradigm in public health development, especially in low-income countries who had to rely heavily on external aids, has led to a complex relationship among traditional and new players in international health and health-related development, planning and use for resources, and the need for delineation and harmonization of responsibilities. Partnerships could enhance the value of public health interventions that were previously dominated by the public sector. Partnerships offer opportunities for involving the private sector and civil society groups, in scaling up the response to global health issues. There were however some concerns that the partnerships might widen the gaps by increasing fragmentation of international cooperation in health, overwhelming the national capacity, distorting the national priorities, diverting the scarce human resources, and also marginalizing the UN system agencies.

Conclusion

Health is a cause rather than an effect of economic development. The history of public health development among the high-income and LMI countries showed that important breakthroughs in public health have led to great improvements in economic development, as witnessed by the rapid growth of Britain and Japan during the industrial revolution in the late eighteenth century, and some countries in Asia and Middle-East during 1960–70s. Health actually determines economic productivity, intellectual prosperity, physical and emotional well-being of the people. Disease burden slows economic growth that is presumed to solve the health problems. For example, more than half of Africa's growth shortfall relative to the high-growth countries of East Asia could be explained statistically by disease burden, demography, and geography, rather than by more traditional variables of macroeconomic policy and political governance (Bloom & Sachs 1998).

The population afflicted with a high infant mortality rate usually lacks the secure knowledge of its children's longevity, witnesses higher rates of fertility, and experiences the quality–quantity trade-off in child rearing. The efforts of national and international communities should be aimed at promoting healthy living, reducing the double burden of disease, and making essential healthcare accessible to all. Ever since the HFA movement initiated over three decades ago, health, equity, and social justice remain the main themes of social and health policy. These values and principles of solidarity, social justice, and ethics for primary healthcare and health for all continue to be relevant and will continue in the future. It is essential for all public health professionals and the international community to sustain these values.

References

Asian Development Bank (ADB) (2005). *Asia Water Watch 2025: Are countries in Asia on track to meet target 10 of the Millennium Development Goals?* ADB, Manila.

Basu, Z. *et al.* (1979). *Eradication of smallpox from India*, Regional Publication Series No. 5, WHO, New Delhi.

Beaglehole, R. and Bonita, R. (1997). *Public health at the crossroads.* Cambridge University Press, Cambridge.

Berlinguer, G. (1999). Globalization and global health. *International Journal of Health Services*, **29**, 579–95.

Bloom, D.E. and Sachs, J. (1998). *Geography, demography, and economic growth in Africa.* Revised October 1998, pp. 36–8. (www.clas.ufl.edu/ users/bbsmith/Sachs_Geography.pdf)

Cassels, A. (1997). *A guide to health sector-wide approach: Concepts, issues and working arrangement.* WHO, Geneva (WHO/ARA97.12).

Chen, L.C. *et al.* (1999). Health as a global public good. In (eds. I. Kaul *et al.*) *Global public goods*. Oxford University Press, New York.

Dodgson, R. *et al.* (2002). *Global health governance: A conceptual review*. WHO, Geneva and London School of Hygiene and Tropical Medicine.

Detels, R. and Breslow, L. (2000). Current scope and concerns in public health. In (eds. Detels *et al.*) *Oxford textbook of public health*, 4th edition, Vol. 1. p. 3, Oxford University Press, New York.

Drager, N. and Beaglehole, R. (2001). Globalization: Changing the public health landscape. *Bulletin of World Health Organization*, **79** (9), 803.

Djukanovic, V. and Mach, E.P. (eds.) (1975). *Alternative approaches to meeting basic health needs in developing countries*. A joint UNICEF/WHO study. WHO, Geneva.

Fenner, F. *et al.* (1988). *Smallpox and its eradication*, pp. 473–516. WHO, Geneva.

Foege, W.H. *et al.* (1971). Selective epidemiologic control in smallpox eradication. *American Journal of Epidemiology*, **94**, 311–5.

Foster, G.M. and Anderson, B.G. (1978). *Medical anthropology*, pp. 224–5. John Wiley & Sons, New York.

Goodman, R.A. and Foster, K.L. (eds.) (1998). Global disease elimination and eradication as public health strategies, Proceedings of a conference held in Atlanta, Georgia, USA, February 1998, pp. 23–25, *Bulletin of the World Health Organization*, 1998, **76** (Suppl 2), 5–162.

Gopalan, C. (1992). *Nutrition in developmental transition in South-East Asia*. Regional Health Paper No. 21, pp. 9–11, WHO, New Delhi.

Harrison, M. (1994). *Public health in British India: Anglo-Indian preventive medicine 1859–1914*, Cambridge University Press, Cambridge.

Henderson, D.A. (1997). Edward Jenner's vaccine. *Public Health Reports*, **112**, 116–21.

Henderson, D.A. (1998). Smallpox eradication—a cold war victory, *World Health Forum*, **19**, 113–9.

Howard-Jones, N. (1974). The scientific background of the international sanitary conferences 1851–1938. *WHO Chronicle*, **28**, 159–71 and 455–70.

Howard-Jones, N. (1977). International public health: The organizational problems between the two World Wars (2). *WHO Chronicle*, **31**, 449–60.

International Institute for Population Sciences (IIPS) and World Health Organization (WHO) (2006). *Health system performance assessment: World health survey, 2003: India*, WHO-India, New Delhi.

Jaggi, O.P. (1979). *History of science, technology and medicine in India*, Volume XIII, Western Medicine in India: Medical Education and Research, Atma Ram & Sons, Delhi.

Jamaison, D.T. and Sandhu, M.E. (2001). WHO Ranking of health system performance. *Science*, August, **293**, 1595–6.

Kickbusch, I. and Payne, L. (2004). *Constructing global public health in the 21st century*. Lecture delivered at the meeting on global health governance and accountability, 2–3 June 2004, Harvard University, USA.

Kinnon, C.M. (1998). World trade: bringing health into the picture, *World Health Forum*, **19**, 397–406.

Ko Ko (1986). *Public health: Myth, mysticism and reality*. WHO, New Delhi.

Ko Ko (1996). *Closing the gaps in health care—A holistic approach to medical education*. In SEA Regional Conference on Medical Education, February 7–9, pp. 152–67, Bangkok.

Ko Ko *et al.* (2002). *Conquest of scourges in Myanmar*, pp. 51–2. Myanmar Academy of Medical Science, Yangon.

Ko Ko *et al.* (2005). *Conquest of scourges in Myanmar: An update*, p. 238, 309. Myanmar Academy of Medical Science, Yangon.

Kutzin, J. (1998). Enhancing the insurance function of health systems: A proposed conceptual framework. In (eds. S. Nitayarumphong and A. Mills) *Achieving universal coverage of health care*. Office of Health Care Reform, Ministry of Public Health, Nonthaburi, Thailand.

Lee, K. (2001). The global dimensions of cholera. *Global change and human health*, Vol. 2, No. 1, pp. 6–17.

Lenfant, C. (2001). Can we prevent cardiovascular diseases in low and middle income countries? *Bulletin of the World Health Organization*, **79** (10), 980–2.

League of Nations Health Organization-LNHO (1937). *Report of the intergovernmental Conference of Far-Eastern countries on rural hygiene*, held at Bandoeng (Java), August 3–13, Geneva.

Mackay, J. *et al.* (2006). *The tobacco atlas*, 2nd edition. American Cancer Society.

McNeill, W.H. (1977). *Plagues and peoples*. Basil Blackwell, Oxford.

Miyagishima, K. and Kaferstein, F.K. (1998). Food safety in international trade. *World Health Forum*, **19**, 407–11.

Molyneux, D.H. *et al.* (2000). Elimination of lymphatic filariasis as public health problem- lymphatic filariasis: Setting the scene for elimination. *Transactions of the Royal Society of Tropical Medicine and Hygiene*, **94**, 589–91.

National Institutes of Health (NIH) (2000). *Morbidity & mortality: 2000 chart book on cardiovascular, lung and blood diseases*. National Heart, Lung, and Blood Institute, Bethesda, MD, USA.

Navarro, V. (1999). Health and equity in the world in the era of globalization, *International Journal of Health Services*, **29**, 215–26.

Nuyens, Y. (2007). Setting priorities for health research: Lessons from low- and middle-income countries. *Bulletin of the World Health Organization*, April, **85** (4), 319–21.

Rafei, U.M. (2004). *Health development in the South-East Asia Region: An overview*, (SEARO Regional Publications No. 44) pp. 34–6, WHO, New Delhi.

Rannan-Eilya, R. (2006). Sri Lanka's health miracle, *South Asia Journal*, October–November, No. 14: pp. 63–73.

Reddy, K.S. and Yusuf, S. (1998). Emerging epidemic of cardiovascular disease in developing countries. *Circulation*, **97**, 596–601.

Society for International Development (1999). Responses to globalization: Rethinking health and equity. *Development*, **42** (4), 1–158.

Shepard, C. *et al.* (2006). Hepatitis B virus infection: Epidemiology and vaccination, *Epidemiology Reviews*, **28**, 112–25.

Tarimo, E. and Webster, E.G. (1994). *Primary health care concepts and challenges in a changing world: Alma-Ata revisited*. Current Concerns: SHS Paper No. 7 (WHO/SHS/CC/94.2), WHO, Geneva.

Than Sein (2002). *A policy brief on health care financing reforms in WHO South-East Asia Region*, (unpublished internal document). WHO, New Delhi.

Than Sein and Kyaw Lwin (2003). A million smiles: Elimination of leprosy in South-East Asia. *Regional Health Forum*, Vol. 7, No. 1. pp. 11–25. WHO, New Delhi.

Tun Aung Kyaw (2005). Control of trachoma in Myanmar. In (eds. Ko Ko *et al.*) *Conquest of scourges in Myanmar: An update*, p. 187. Myanmar Academy of Medical Sciences, Yangon.

UN (United Nations) (2003). *Human security now: Commission on human security*, pp. 95–112. New York.

UN (United Nations) (2006). *The UN report on millennium development goals 2006*, pp. 4–5, New York (http://mdgs.un.org/).

UNDP (United Nations Development Programme) (1998). *Human development report 1998*. UNDP, New York.

UNDP (United Nations Development Programme) (2006). *Human development report (HDR) 2006; Beyond scarcity: Power, poverty and the global water crisis*. UNDP, pp. 119–20.

UNICEF (United Nations Children's Fund) (2006). *States of the world's children 2006*. Oxford University Press, New York.

Uragoda, C.G. (1987). *A history of medicine in Sri Lanka–from the earliest times to 1948*. Sri Lanka Medical Association, Colombo.

Wasley, A. *et al.* (2006). Hepatitis A in the era of vaccination. *Epidemiological Review 2006*, **28**, 101–11.

Wilkinson, L. and Power, H. (1998). The London and Liverpool Schools of tropical medicine 1898–1998. *British Medical Bulletin*, **54**, 281–92.

Wild, S. *et al.* (2004). Global prevalence of diabetes: Estimates for the year 2000 and projections for 2030, *Diabetes Care*, **27** (5), May, 1047–53.

WHO (World Health Organization) (1957). *Report on rural health conference*, held during 14–26 October 1957. Document SEA/RH/9, WHO, New Delhi.

WHO (World Health Organization) (1964). *WHO expert committee on smallpox: First report*. WHO Technical Report Series No. 283, pp. 7, 9–11, 15, 24, 31.

WHO (World Health Organization) (1967). *Twenty years in South-East Asia: 1948–1967*. WHO, New Delhi.

WHO (World Health Organization) (1978a). *A decade of health development in South-East Asia 1968-1977*. WHO, New Delhi.

WHO (World Health Organization) (1978b). *WHO Alma-Ata 1978: Primary health care*. HFA Series No.1, WHO, Geneva.

WHO (World Health Organization) (1986). *Regional advisory committee on medical research for South-East Asia: Proceeding of the special session commemorating the tenth anniversary*. Held on 12 April 1985, Regional Publications Series No.15, WHO, New Delhi.

WHO (World Health Organization) (1991). *Resolution WHA44.9 on leprosy elimination*. WHO, Geneva.

WHO (World Health Organization) (1992). *WHO Collaboration in Health Development in South-East Asia: 1948–1988, Fortieth Anniversary publication (updated)*. WHO, New Delhi.

WHO (World Health Organization) (1993). *Implementation of global strategy for health for all by the year 2000: Eight report on the world situation*. Volume 1, WHO, Geneva.

WHO (World Health Organization) (1996). *Investing in health research and development: Report of the Ad hoc committee on health research relating to future intervention options*. WHO, Geneva (TDR/Gen/96.1).

WHO (World Health Organization) (1998a). *Health for all in the 21st century* (Document A51/5) and *World Health Declaration annexed to Resolution WHA51.7*, WHO Geneva.

WHO (World Health Organization) (1998b). *The World health report 1998: Life in the 21st century: A vision for all*. WHO, Geneva.

WHO (World Health Organization) (1998c). *Evaluation of the implementation of the global strategy for health for all by the year 2000, 1979–1996*. WHO, Geneva (Document WHO/HST/98.2).

WHO (World Health Organization) (1999a). *Health situation in the South-East Asia Region 1994–1997*, p. 155. WHO, New Delhi.

WHO (World Health Organization) (1999b). *The World health report 1999: Making a difference*. WHO, Geneva.

WHO (World Health Organization) (1999c). *Nutrition for health and development: Progress and prospects on the eve of the 21st century*. (WHO/NHD/99.9), WHO, Geneva,

WHO (World Health Organization) (2000a). *Sector-wide approaches for health development, a review of experience*, by Mike Foster *et al.* (WHO/GPE/00.1), WHO, Geneva.

WHO (World Health Organization) (2000b). *The World Health Report 2000, Health systems: Improving performance*. WHO, Geneva.

WHO (World Health Organization) (2000c). *Eliminate filariasis: Attack poverty. Proceedings of the First Meeting of The Global Alliance to eliminate lymphatic filariasis*, Spain, 4–5 May 2000 (CDS/CEE/200.5). WHO, Geneva (http://www.filariasis.org/) and International Filaria Journal (http://www.filariajournal.com/).

WHO (World Health Organization) (2000d). Hepatitis A Vaccines, *Weekly Epidemiology Record*, February, **75** (5): pp. 38–44, WHO: Geneva.

WHO (World Health Organization) (2001). *Assessment of health systems performance*, (EB107/9 and Resolution EB107.R8), WHO, Geneva.

WHO (World Health Organization) (2002a). *Summary measures of population health: Concepts, ethics, measurements and applications*, by Murray *et al.* (eds.). WHO, Geneva.

WHO (World Health Organization) (2002b) Leprosy control. *Weekly Epidemiology Record*, 77, pp. 1–8, WHO, Geneva.

WHO (World Health Organization) (2003). Yellow fever vaccine, *Weekly Epidemiology Record*, October, **78** (40): pp. 349–360, WHO: Geneva.

WHO (World Health Organization) (2004a). Hepatitis B vaccines. *Weekly Epidemiology Record*, July, **79** (28), pp. 255–63. WHO, Geneva.

WHO (World Health Organization) (2004b). *The atlas of heart disease and stroke*. pp. 18–19, WHO Geneva.

WHO (World Health Organization) (2004c). Human plague. *Weekly Epidemiology Record*, August, **79** (33), pp. 301–8, WHO, Geneva.

WHO (World Health Organization) (2004d). Ebola haemorrhagic fever. *Fact Sheet No. 103*, May. WHO, Geneva (http://www.who.int/).

WHO (World Health Organization) (2005a). *Global strategy for further reducing the leprosy burden and sustaining leprosy control activities (2006–2010)*, (WHO/CDS/CPE/CEE/2005.53). WHO, Geneva.

WHO (World Health Organization) (2005b). *Resolution WHA58.3 revision of international health regulations*. WHO, Geneva.

WHO (World Health Organization) (2005c). *Moving beyond the tsunami: The WHO story*. WHO, New Delhi.

WHO (World Health Organization) (2005d). *Global report: Preventing chronic diseases: A vital investment*. WHO, Geneva.

WHO (World Health Organization) (2006a). *World health report 2006: Health workforce*. WHO, Geneva.

WHO (World Health Organization) (2006b). *Strategy on health care financing for countries of the Western Pacific and South-East Asia Regions (2006–2010)*. WHO, New Delhi.

WHO (World Health Organization) (2006c). *Smallpox eradication: Destruction of variola virus stocks*. (EB120/11 and Resolution EB120.R8), WHO, Geneva.

WHO (World Health Organization) (2006d). *Poliomyelitis eradication*. (EB120/4 Rev.1), WHO, Geneva.

WHO (World Health Organization) (2006e). Onchocerciasis Control. *Weekly Epidemiology Record*, July, No. **30**, pp. 293–6, WHO, Geneva.

WHO (World Health Organization) (2006f). Dracunculiasis. *Weekly Epidemiology Record*, May, **18**, pp. 173–188. WHO, Geneva.

WHO (World Health Organization) (2006g). Global programme to eliminate lymphatic filariasis, *Weekly Epidemiology Record*, June, **81** (22): pp. 221–232, WHO: Geneva.

WHO (World Health Organization) (2006h). *Public health problems caused by harmful use of alcohol in South-East Asia: Gaining less or losing more?* WHO, New Delhi (Alcohol Series No. 4).

WHO (World Health Organization) (2006i). *Global tuberculosis control: Surveillance, planning and financing: WHO report 2006*, p. 27, WHO, Geneva.

WHO (World Health Organization) (2006j), *The revised Malaria Control Strategy: South-East Asia Region 2006–2010*, (SEA-MAL 243) pp. 8–11, WHO, New Delhi.

WHO (World Health Organization) (2006k). *Report by the Secretariat on avian and pandemic influenza: developments, response and follow-up, and application of IHR (2005)*. (EB120/15), WHO, Geneva.

WHO (World Health Organization) (2006l). *Speech to the special session of World Health Assembly by the Director-General Elect Dr Margaret Chan on 9 November 2006*. WHO, Geneva, accessed at (http://www.who.int/dg/speeches/) on 12 February 2007.

WHO (World Health Organization) (2007a). *Public health, innovation and intellectual property: Towards a global strategy and plan of action*, (EB120/Inf.Doc./1), and *Public health, innovation and intellectual property: towards a global strategy and plan of action: Follow-up to the first session of the Intergovernmental Working Group*, (EB120/Inf.Doc/5), WHO, Geneva.

WHO (World Health Organization) (2007b). *Fact Sheet No. 286 on Measles*, January 2007. (http://www.who.int/).

WHO (World Health Organization) (2007c) *Medium Term Strategic Plan for 2008-2013 and Programme Budget for 2008–2009*. WHO, Geneva.

WHO (World Health Organization) (2007d). *Sub-national Health System Performance Assessment, Country Report on Indonesia*, WHO, Jakarta, Indonesia, April 2007. (http://www.who.or.id/eng/products/ow6/sub2/indexsub.asp?id=5).

WHO and UNICEF (2000). *Report on the global water supply and sanitation assessment*, WHO, Geneva and UNICEF, New York.

WHO and World Bank (1990). *Commission on health research for development: Essential link to equity in development*. Oxford University Press, New York.

World Bank (2005). *World development indicator 2005*. p. 114, Table 2.17.

World Bank (2006a). *The World development report 2007: Development and the Next Generation*, Washington, p. 285.

World Bank (2006b). *Global burden of disease and risk factors: Disease Control Priorities Project*, Lopez *et al.* (eds.), Oxford University Press, New York.

Yach, D. and Bettcher, D. (1998). The globalization of public health: Threats and opportunities. *American Journal of Public Health*, **88**, 735–43.

1.4

The development of the discipline of public health in countries in economic transition: India, Brazil, China

Puja Thakker and K. Srinath Reddy

Abstract

The three low- and middle-income countries (LMICs) profiled in this chapter are countries which together constitute nearly 45 per cent of the global population. These countries represent societies wherein the economies are on the upswing and are accompanied by demographic and epidemiological transitions profoundly influencing the agenda of public health as well as the level of resources available to address it. The dominant ideologies of both the state and society of the time, as can be seen in the social, political, and economic histories of these countries, have significantly influenced the development of public health.

As these countries focus on establishing strong systems for the delivery of health care, the role of the state has undergone substantial changes over time. The increasing dominance of market economics even in the health-care sector has substantially shaped the role of the private sector, and thus, the health-seeking behaviour of the population. Although a progressing economy has significantly increased national income per capita, the transition has varying impacts on the health system, especially raising concern over the quality of care delivered and the widening inequities in access to care.

Public health in LMICs has not succeeded in drawing upon interdisciplinary research and multisectoral action to the extent needed. Presently, the capacity for developing and implementing intersectoral policies is missing, and the active engagement of public health academia and health workers with the health system and policymakers is suboptimal. Although promising signs of a change are visible in some of these countries, the extent to which the discipline will advance further over the next two decades will be a critical determinant of health and development in the high-velocity transitional period that lies ahead.

Introduction

An overwhelming majority of the world's population presently resides in low- and middle-income countries (LMICs). The three LMICs profiled in this chapter are countries that together have a population size of 2.6 billion and constitute nearly 40 per cent of the global population. Hence, the development of public health in these countries, both as an academic discipline and as a delivery system, is of great importance to the state of global health. Key health indicators of these countries are summarized in Table 1.4.1.

The evolution of public health as a discipline in populous LMICs, such China, India, and Brazil, has been influenced by multiple interactive factors. These include the following:

1. Changing global and national perceptions, over time, of the ambit of public health as an academic discipline and its contribution as an application pathway for improving the health of the population.

2. Growing recognition of the multiple determinants of health, demanding interdisciplinary amalgamation of academic learning and directing public health practice into multisectoral action channels.

Table 1.4.1 Key health indicators for India, China, and Brazil (2007)

	Under-5 mortality (per 1000 live births)	MMR (per 100 000 live births)	Underweight children under 5 years of age (%)	Vaccination coverage* (%)
India	74	301	44	55–78
China	27	48	6	91–94
Brazil	33	260	3.7	92–99

* Estimates for BCG, DPT1, DPT3, polio, tetanus, MCV vaccines.
Source: CIA World Factbook: https://www.cia.gov/library/publications/the-world-factbook/ (accessed on 3 November, 2007); WHO/UNICEF: Immunization Profile, India. Website: http://www.who.int/vaccines/globalsummary/immunization/countryprofileresult.cfm?C='IND' (accessed on 31 October, 2007); Immunization Profile, China. Website: http://www.who.int/vaccines/globalsummary/immunization/countryprofileresult.cfm?C='CHI' (accessed on 31 October, 2007); Immunization Profile, Brazil. Website: http://www.who.int/vaccines/globalsummary/immunization/countryprofileresult.cfm?C='BRA' (accessed on 31 October, 2007).

3. The relative balance between preventive- and clinical-care components of public health services, as reflected in policymaker priorities and fiscal allocations.

4. The composition and characteristics of the health system, including the public–private–voluntary mix, the roles and responsibilities of different categories of health-service personnel, the size of the public health workforce, and the nature and strength of linkages between health services and educational/training institutions, which are charged with the task of creating the capacity of public health professionals and functionaries.

5. Economic transitions influencing the growth patterns and distributional dynamics of income and opportunity within the global and national settings.

6. Demographic and social transitions propelled by relatively late industrialization, recent but rapid urbanization, and fast-paced globalization.

7. Epidemiological and health transitions which are reordering the principal public health challenges, in terms of disease burdens, and rearranging priorities for public health action

8. The levels of access to the enlarging pool of global knowledge and expanding array of technological innovations which advance the precept and practice of public health.

9. National capacity for knowledge creation and knowledge management as well as the ability to identify and overcome barriers in knowledge translation.

10. National and international partnerships that are available to strengthen the intellectual as well as institutional resources needed for advancing public health.

11. Collaborative agreements with international agencies, such as the World Health Organization (WHO) and the World Bank as well as bilateral and multilateral development partners, which influence the overall agenda of public health programmes as well as determine the level of technical and financial resources available for specific programmes.

This chapter profiles some of these determinants, as generally applicable to these selected LMICs, and briefly describes the evolution of public health in each of them.

Defining public health

The debate on what defines the discipline of public health and what delineates the ambit of public health policies and programmes has witnessed several paradigm shifts over the past century. From an initially restricted mandate of ensuring public sanitation, safe water supply, and food safety, public health expanded to include services aimed at individual protection (such as immunization and contraception) and health promotion (mainly through health education). In recent years, recognition of the need to influence the upstream social determinants (which impact on group and individual behaviours, and thereby alter the biology of individuals to produce disease or promote health) has led to public health also adopting social legislation and regulation in areas such as tobacco control and nutrition.

The disciplinary mandate of public health has, therefore, expanded from providing essential hygienic services and disease-preventive personal protection to broader social-engineering efforts, which combine public education and policy interventions that have a

population-wide effect, for health promotion. This global trend has also influenced the evolution of the discipline in LMICs, although the speed and scale of change have varied across countries.

Determinants of health

The course of public health has also been influenced by a growing understanding of the multiple determinants of health, their independent and interactive contributions to the health of societies and their constituent individuals, as well as the need for planned interventions to influence these determinants. The initial preoccupation with factors operating at the individual level (an interplay of beliefs, behaviours, and biology) gave way to greater recognition of determinants that operate at family and community levels (perceptions, priorities, and pathways). In recent years, awareness of the social and economic determinants that operate at national levels has increased, along with the recognition that these upstream factors are increasingly becoming dominant in the wake of globalization and economic liberalization rapidly rewriting social and trade policies. The factors that operate at the national and global levels, such as development, distribution, and demand–supply levers of trade, now impact profoundly on the health of the community, the family, and the individual. The evolution of public health as a discipline needs to integrate an understanding of all of these determinants (Fig. 1.4.1) as well as the underpinnings in society in order to influence each of them through appropriate interventions.

In LMICs, non-personal policy interventions, which have a population-wide impact (e.g. tobacco taxes and food prices), are likely to have a greater impact than education, in a short time frame, in promoting individual behaviour change. Public health leaders in LMICs have not yet realized the full potential of such policy interventions, and consequently, transdisciplinary research, multisectoral action, and multi-stakeholder advocacy have so far remained slow and subdued in their response to the rapid changes to the social determinants of health. Even as scientific advances in molecular genetics tend to swing the pendulum of causation discourse to individual susceptibility, the profound impact of social and environmental determinants remains inadequately addressed. This imbalance needs to be corrected if public health has to evolve to its full potential.

Determining the balance between preventive and clinical medicine

Even as definitional debates on the scope of public health have continued, the key factor influencing the evolution of public health in

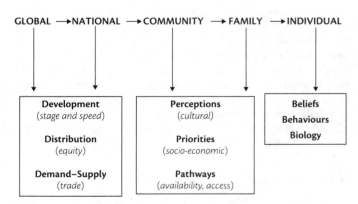

Fig. 1.4.1 Cascade of health determinants.

LMICs has been the level of resource allocation for preventive and promotive public health programmes, in comparison with that provided for public-sector clinical services. In resource-constrained economies, the emphasis was initially on providing essential clinical services, especially in primary health care. Public health programmes were resourced at lower levels and mainly involved immunization, disease control for major infectious diseases, and in the case of India, population control. Public health was more often viewed as the vehicle for extending the outreach of personalized clinical interventions across the population rather than as a pathway for promoting the health of the population. Even in terms of individual health protection, public health systems were used to deliver sporadic interventions at select points in an individual's life, in staccato style, rather than adopt a lifespan approach to the protection, preservation, and promotion of health at all stages of life. It is only in recent years, with a spurt in the growth of national economies, that public health is being better supported through increased financial allocation and is beginning to adopt a broader agenda of action. As public spending on health increases, public health is beginning to get greater attention within the health sector, even though clinical care is likely to continue as the major area of health expenditure.

Designing of health systems

Because the design and operation of efficient health systems which provide a mix of health-promotive, disease-preventive, diagnostic, and clinical services to all sections of the population is considered to be within the mandate of public health, the individual and collective contributions of public, private, and voluntary sectors become relevant to the evolution of this field. In many LMICs, the public sector was the principal provider of health services, at all levels, in the early stages of health-system development. Later, the role of the private sector grew, covering not only a large segment of tertiary care but also extending into secondary care. Private health care now also caters to much of urban primary health care in countries such as India. The not-for-profit voluntary sector has become actively engaged in health care at various levels in India, but the extent of its coverage remains limited.

The size of the workforce in the health sector overall, and in public health services in particular, has determined the level of efficiency of the health system. The misdistribution of health personnel, with urban preponderance and rural paucity, as well as chronic shortages of qualified health personnel, aggravated by migration to richer nations, have affected the performance of the health systems in India and Brazil. The lack of medical personnel also spurred on the creation of other categories of health-service personnel, such as 'barefoot doctors', community health workers, and volunteers (with varied nomenclature), and sustained the presence of traditional health-system practitioners as care givers to large segments of the population. The evolution of health systems in LMICs has yet to fully assimilate and accommodate these varied contributors into an integrated framework.

Disconnect between public health education and health-system operations

Ideally, institutions engaged in public health education and research should have been closely connected to the health systems. This would have been mutually beneficial, with the needs of the health systems and learnings from the reality of 'field' experiences influencing the curriculum and pedagogical methods of public health educational programmes and the academic institutions. This, in turn, could have invigorated the health systems through policy- and programme-relevant research as well as contributed to training programmes. However, public health training institutions, whether located in medical colleges or in university settings, remained largely distanced from the general health system. They also played a limited role in influencing the organization and performance of the health systems. This disconnect is especially visible in countries such as India, where the lack of such engagement has adversely affected the evolution of public health.

Development and rights perspectives

Against this background, the economic transitions of the past two decades have rapidly changed the way in which health is perceived by countries and the manner in which health services are provided. In resource-constrained economies, social-sector spending was initially considered a lower priority than 'growth' and infrastructure spending, and it was assumed that health would passively benefit from economic development. It became clear during the 1990s that investments in health are essential for accelerated economic growth. This 'human capital' approach, wherein the productivity of the workforce was linked to their health status, was complemented by a 'rights' approach, whereby the right to health became ably articulated as an essential right by increasingly assertive civil-society groups. The setting up of the National Commission on Macroeconomics and Health and the growth of the People's Health Movement (with public hearings on the 'right to health' organized by it in concert with the National Human Rights Commission), in the past decade in India, are illustrative of this convergent advocacy for health both as a developmental imperative and an inalienable human right.

Dangerous fallout of structural reforms

At the same time, the integration of LMIC economies into the global market posed several challenges. While promising increased growth opportunities, it also made them more vulnerable to the vagaries of the global market. The influence of international agencies promoting economic liberalization led to 'structural reforms' in the health system, wherein the role of the public sector became diminished, and several public health services such as water and sanitation were labelled as not being cost-effective (World Bank 1993). As a result, public health services suffered a setback in several LMICs. For example, the rapid shift from state-provided health care to limited availability of insured health care or private purchased health care has had an adverse impact on rural health services in China, in the post-liberalization phase, and correctives are now being applied. In India too, out-of-pocket (OOP) health expenditure has reached a level of 77 per cent, despite the state's commitment to the public sector as the primary provider of free health services.

Disparities

The economic growth of China, India, and Brazil has brought about an increase in per-capita incomes. Although this increase is expected to have a favourable impact on health states, the skewed distributional patterns of the wealth created during this growth phase have aggravated socioeconomic inequalities within these societies, resulting in major disparities in health outcomes. To illustrate, Table 1.4.2 showcases the urban–rural inequality that exists

Table 1.4.2 Socioeconomic inequalities exacerbate risk factors

	Access to improved drinking water sources (%)		Access to improved sanitation (%)	
	Urban	**Rural**	**Urban**	**Rural**
India	89	48	59	22
China	93	67	69	28
Brazil	96	57	83	37

Source: World Health Organization. World health statistics 2007. Geneva: World Health Organization; 2007 and National Council of Applied Economic Research (2000). *Rural Households Survey.*

in access to improved sanitation and clean drinking water within these three countries.

Health expenditure

The evolution of public health in LMICs has to be understood against the backdrop of these profound changes accruing in their economies and the resultant impact on health financing, health services, and health indicators. Figures 1.4.2.1–1.4.2.3 show the recent changes in the government's share (as a percentage) of the total health spending against the increase in gross national product (GNP) per capita.

Governmental contributions to total health expenditures are indicative of the political will and commitment towards health. A higher commitment from the government, in general, reduces out-of-pocket expenditures, and protects the poor from the financial risk associated with a health accident. Although several studies have shown that government spending on health benefits the middle and affluent class the most, it nevertheless serves as an essential safety net for the poorest segment of the population. Brazil (Fig. 1.4.2.3) has shown consistently upward trends in government spending on health as the GNP per capita has increased over the last decade. Government health expenditure in China (Fig. 1.4.2.2) has continually declined in recent years, despite its rapid economic growth. In India (Fig. 1.4.2.1), government health spending has been more erratic, and is currently at 17.3 per cent of the total health spending (Government of India 2005). With recent schemes such as the National Rural Health Mission, launched in 2005, and the National Urban Health Mission, launched in April 2008 , the government aims to increase this spending to 25 per cent of the total health spending by 2010.

A positive relationship between national income and health trends has long been observed across the globe. The lower national incomes of LMICs leave their populations disadvantaged in terms of their health states. Developing countries account for 84 per cent of the global population but 90 per cent of the global disease burden. Due to severe budget constraints, they also tend to spend much less on health. Developing countries account for 20 per cent of global gross domestic product (GDP) but only 12 per cent of all health spending. Even after adjusting for differences in the cost of living, high-income countries spend 30 times more on health per capita than low-income countries (Gottret & Schieber 2006). Further, a large percentage of health expenditure in LMICs tends to be OOP, as a consequence of missing safety-net policies within the health system and low overall public spending on health, leaving the poorest segment unprotected from catastrophic health spending.

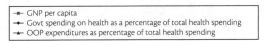

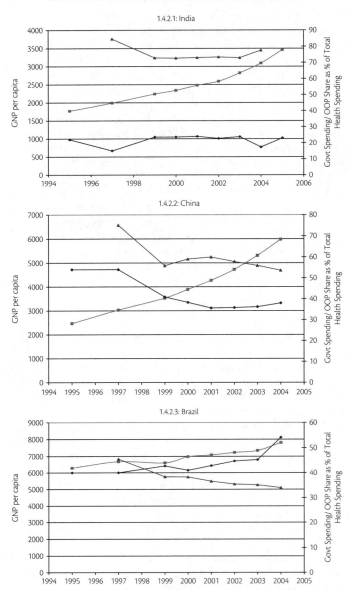

Fig. 1.4.2 Government spending on health as a percentage of the total health spending compared with changes in gross national product (GNP) per capita: (1.4.2.1) India, (1.4.2.2) China, and (1.4.2.3) Brazil.

Garg and Karan (2006) estimated that 32.5 million people fall below the national poverty line due to OOP payments in India each year.

The percentage of OOP expenditure is indicative of how equitably health services are being financed within a state. The general trend shows that greater government spending on health decreases OOP spending. OOP spending trends in India and China have remained virtually unchanged since 1999, still high at 77 per cent and 53 per cent in 2004, respectively (World Health Organization 2007). OOP expenditures in Brazil have declined marginally since 1999, to 34 per cent in 2004 (World Health Organization 2007). Rising OOP spending in recent years also reflects a shift in emphasis towards

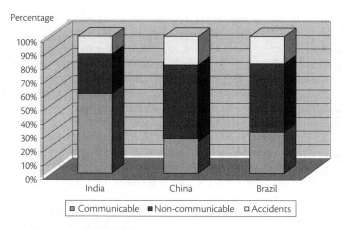

Fig. 1.4.3 Years of life lost (YLL), by cause.

curative care, with the declining role of the state in the provision of health-protecting and health-promoting activities.

The relationship between economic reform and public health has been salient from the time of the Great Depression in the 1930s. In the preceding decades, most spending by the state was limited to sectors which were direct drivers of economy, such as industry, agriculture, and infrastructure. It was only after World War II that the role of the state became significant for the delivery of several social functions such as health, education, etc. To execute such an undertaking, taxation was increasingly used and the concept of social welfare became more clearly defined among governments.

Historically, economic or political crises have often been the drivers behind economic reform. As a consequence of budget cuts during economic crises, government expenditures on health, education, and other 'soft sectors' are usually compromised first. Countries with low incomes have thus been unable to prioritize health as a critical investment. Confronted with changing disease burdens and socio-demographics as part of the development process, health systems are faced with new challenges that they are not adequately equipped to handle.

As countries progress across the development spectrum from low-income to middle-income, or from middle-income to high-income, they are escorted by large demographic and epidemiological changes that are reflected in the health of the population absorbing the economic growth. Economic growth of a country brings about several changes in the health states of its population. Juxtaposed with globalization, this recent economic growth has lead to rapid urbanization in countries in transition. Urbanization has brought about profound changes in living habits. Exposure to risk factors of non-communicable diseases such as obesogenic foods, alcohol, and tobacco in addition to reduced physical activity and augmented stresses associated with modern-day living have become increasingly prevalent. Urbanization itself has also brought about a greater number of deaths due to injuries (including homicide, suicide, and traffic accidents).

As population segments within LMICs witness morbidity and mortality shifts towards non-communicable diseases, as predicted with the advancement of the epidemiological transition, they continue to carry a high burden of infectious and other poverty-related diseases as well. As a consequence, countries in economic transition battle a dual burden: The rising share of non-communicable diseases such as cardiovascular illnesses, cancer, diabetes, and depression, and the traditional problems of infectious disease and malnutrition. Figure 1.4.3 shows the growing trend of non-communicable diseases in the three countries. While communicable diseases such as malaria, tuberculosis, cholera, and AIDS still persist in these countries, non-communicable diseases account for 56 per cent and 50 per cent, respectively, of the years of life lost (YLL) in China and Brazil today (World Health Organization 2007). Escalating at rates parallel to economic growth, non-communicable diseases have grown to become major contributors to premature death and disability. In India, 29 per cent of the YLL are to non-communicable causes.

The evolution of public health in LMICs has also to be understood in the context of the epidemiological transition that accompanies economic and demographic transitions.

In 1971, Omran (2005) broadly explained epidemiological transition as occurring mainly in three stages:

◆ Era of *pestilence* and *famine*, characterized by high mortality rates, short life expectancy, and no population growth.

◆ Era of *receding pandemics*, characterized by declining mortality due to large epidemics and stable population growth.

◆ Era of *degenerative* and *man-made diseases*, characterized by a sharp decline in mortality, a higher life expectancy and demographic growth as determined by fertility, and a shift to chronic (non-communicable) diseases as the major cause of mortality.

In 1985, Olshansky and Ault (1985) proposed a fourth era:

◆ The era of *delayed degenerative disease*, in which degenerative and man-made diseases are still the major killers, but whose distinguishing characteristic is the delayed *age* at which most of the deaths due to them occur.

Based on the experience of Russia and other post-Soviet republics in Eastern Europe, Yusuf *et al.* in 2001 proposed a fifth era:

◆ The era of *health regression* and *social upheaval*, in which war or other causes of social upheaval lead to increases in alcoholism and violence, increased ischaemic and hypertensive diseases in the young, as well as increased infectious disease caused by the breakdown of social and health structures. This regressive stage is marked by decreased life expectancy due to the resurgence of diseases from the first two eras, while diseases from the third and fourth stages continue to persist.

The onset of globalization in the twenty-first century has presented LMICs with new health challenges brought on by economic development. Increased rates of urbanization and industrialization marked by rapid deforestation, exponential vehicular growth, and loss of biodiversity have led to a sharp increase in ambient levels of air pollution. Further, the effects of climate change have compromised agricultural yields, thus contributing further to the risk of poor nutrition. The Food and Agricultural Organization (2007) has estimated that, in sub-Saharan Africa, climate change could reduce yields of major crops by 40 per cent over the next 25 years.

The increasing use of agricultural products in the quest for newer sources of energy has also raised concerns about food security and its consequences on nutrition levels. The expanding demand for biofuels such as biodiesel and ethanol, produced from crops such as maize and sugarcane, has also hiked the price of these crops, making them unavailable to the poor. For example, only 10 per cent of the global sugar harvest going into the production of ethanol has caused the price of sugar to double (Integrated Regional Information Network 2007). Brazil, the world's largest sugar producer and exporter, is now converting half of its sugar harvest into ethanol fuel. Such commercial farming is also leading to increased deforestation. Thus, both direct and indirect outcomes of changes in the environment have direct implications for the health of the population.

Characterized by the early onset of respiratory-related conditions in the short term and rising mortality due to several cancers and natural disasters in the long run, worsened by direct risks to nutritional status, a sixth era has presented itself as a new phase of the epidemiological transition:

◆ The era of *environmental degradation*, which is marked by acute deaths from natural calamities and infectious diseases from their aftermath, as well as chronic conditions such as cancers, emphysema, and asthma due to changes in the surrounding environment. Indirect effects of climate change on health also present issues such as the lack of food security and increased risks of malnutrition. The effects of degradation of the ambient and global natural environment may cause regression into any of the previous five eras, bringing about declines in life expectancy for all age groups.

Epidemiological transitions do not necessarily occur in a linear or unidirectional manner. Countries in economic transition continuously face the risk of regression due to resurgence of a condition that persisted in a previous phase of the epidemiological transition. The sequence of these phases may vary greatly, depending upon the developmental cycle of a country. The rate at which it transitions from one phase to another also depends upon the rate at which it develops economically, and is unique from other countries. In fact, due to persistent regional inequalities, the rate of transition, and the prevalent phase of transition, may even vary within different parts of the same country, as is seen in the case of urban and rural China.

The mid-phase of the epidemiological transition marks an overall shift in the leading causes of mortality from communicable to non-communicable diseases. This shift, juxtaposed with substantial gains in life expectancy, now pose a serious challenge to the health systems in economies in transition, which are still to be reconfigured to respond to these new threats.

Knowledge generation and management

In an increasingly globalizing world, not only are the agents of disease transmitted across nations (be they microbes or tobacco) but also knowledge and technologies integral to the advancement of public health become disseminated rapidly. The ability of LMICs to access these is also a factor that influences the speed at which public health can gain strength from science and technology for overcoming major challenges. Proprietary science and patent-restricted access to technologies become barriers to countries that are resource-constrained. Growth in national capacity for knowledge generation, through strengthening of academic institutions and networks engaged in research, and development of indigenous capacity for technological innovation are essential for LMICs to ensure that these barriers do not limit the growth of public health. Countries such as India, China, and Brazil are increasingly investing in building such capacity.

Partnerships

Partnerships with other countries and with international organizations such as the WHO are also useful in providing access to technical,

and in some cases, financial resources to strengthen national capacities in public health. This engagement also influences the public health agenda, when donors or development partners set the agenda, or when the WHO calls for national participation in global programmes such as polio eradication or surveillance for avian influenza. Assistance for national capacity-building is often more forthcoming when the health programmes are part of a global agenda, but this should not unduly distract national authorities from conducting a well-informed priority-setting exercise in the national context. National capacity-building, in an era of increasing global cooperation, is the way forward for public health in countries such as China, India, and Brazil.

India

Public health in India has undergone several changes during its periods of political, social, and economic transition. From the time of British colonization, there has existed an organized framework for the delivery of public health services. The British first established their presence in India in the 1600s. In those times, much emphasis was placed on sanitation, waste management, and outbreak control, similar to the sanitary movements in England that had just occurred. However, these services and measures were in place largely to protect British civilians and their army cantonments, with an emphasis on the early detection of contagious diseases, such as cholera and plague, to prevent their spread to the ruling class (Das Gupta 2005).

The public health system established by the British had several strengths. They put into place the Indian Medical Service (IMS) in the 1760s, which despite its predominantly military orientation, laid the foundation for future health developments in years to come. The British also established medical colleges in Calcutta, Bombay, and Madras in 1835.

The continued interest of the British in the development of preventive health services was rooted in the high mortality of their soldiers during the uprising in 1857, which claimed hundreds of thousands of combatant and civilian lives. It is noted that as many as 69 out of every 1000 soldiers sent from Britain died during their first year of arrival (Harrison 1994), and became a huge cause for concern back in Britain. A commission was set up to investigate the high number of deaths of British soldiers and to evaluate hygiene standards within in its cantonments, the result of which was the setting up of separate establishments for British soldiers and civilians. It was ultimately recognized that the health of British civilians and soldiers could not be seen in isolation from that of the Indian people as they regularly interacted with Indian civilians, despite their deliberately distant habitations from them.

The plague outbreak in the early twentieth century reiterated the need for further investments and attention to public health. The British rulers undertook the establishment of several high-quality academic institutes for training and research, such as the Malaria Institute of India, the Haffkine Institute at Bombay, the Vaccine Research Laboratories at Kasauli, and the King Institute of Preventive Medicine at Madras (Banerji 1997). The School of Tropical Medicine and the All India Institute of Hygiene and Public Health in Calcutta were established shortly thereafter in the 1920s. These institutes of medical training and research were, however, symbols of elitist western civilization in India, and still did not serve the vast needs of the indigenous people.

During the decades preceding independence in 1947, health conditions of the masses were especially poor. Malnutrition and undernutrition rates were high, and communicable diseases were on a constant rise. According to the National Planning Committee (NPC) of 1948, malaria—the most predominant of all infectious diseases at the time—accounted for 100 million cases each year, of which a million proved to be fatal (Banerji 1997). Other infectious diseases such as tuberculosis, cholera, smallpox, dysentery, and diphtheria took a heavy toll of life, and cases of leprosy, filariasis, worm infestations, and venereal disease were also prevalent. Widespread disease and impoverishment were exacerbated by weak access to health care because western systems of medicine were mostly available only to the affluent class.

Further, as methods of western medicine gained popularity, the demand for indigenous medical practices also gradually diminished within the affluent class. Because the indigenous systems had historically thrived on their contributions, this decrease in demand undermined the financial sustainability of these systems. The underprivileged masses, who earlier relied almost exclusively on them, suffered the consequences of their withering. High taxation and exploitation by the colonial regime added substantially to the burden of indigenous families. These miserable conditions led to widespread discontentment and ultimately provided the impetus for a movement demanding health services for the people, and added fuel to the already existing fervour for independence from the British.

On the forefront of the public health movement were eminent medical professionals who were also prominent activists in the struggle for freedom. They were generous in envisioning a health system for India which was vast in scope. One of the main aspirations of the movement was to put in place a system that would serve the people of India, which was something the British rulers had notoriously neglected. The Indian National Congress (an organized opposition against the British empire, which later became the nation's dominant political party for several decades), played a significant role in this movement. Subhash Chandra Bose, President of the Congress in 1938, set up an NPC to be headed by Jawaharlal Nehru (soon to become the first prime minister of independent India). In order to evaluate the existing health conditions and systems, the NPC set up a national health subcommittee (also known as the Sokhey committee).

Concurrently, the British established a health survey and development committee chaired by Sir Joseph Bhore. Although colonial in origin, this committee—later known as the Bhore committee—was greatly influenced by the objectives of the national movement through the assessment and actions recommended by the Sokhey committee. The Bhore committee was eclectic in its constitution, drawing upon experts from various health-science institutions of India, officials such as the Minister of Health, the Director General of the Indian Medical Service, and the Director of the Medical Council of India; other experts from the United States, Britain, and the Soviet Union; and most importantly, representatives of the Indian civil society. The report of the Bhore committee is one of the founding doctrines of health policy in India even today.

Guided by principles that were remarkably similar in essence to the Alma Ata Declaration of 1972, the Bhore committee's recommendations strived for equity in access and health for all. First, the Bhore committee emphasized the need for improved access to primary health services through the setting up of primary health centres (PHCs) throughout rural areas. The establishment of five PHCs and one secondary health unit (SHU) per district in 1952, soon after independence, was perhaps the most direct outcome of this recommendation. It was also planned that these would be increased to 25 PHCs and two SHUs over a 10-year period (Banerji 1997). The Committee also emphasized that preventive and curative services must be well-integrated at all levels of administration. At the lowest level, it recommended the involvement of the community for the implementation of national health programmes. The setting up of a village health committee consisting of residents of the village, who would practice health promotion, was envisaged. Third, the Committee recognized the importance of addressing the social causes of disease, and therefore, recommended the social reorientation of physicians and medical graduates. Recognizing the lack of adequate educational institutes for public health, the Committee also recommended the setting up of centrally sponsored institutes for high-quality research and training programmes in the health sciences, at the graduate and postgraduate level. The All India Institute of Medical Sciences (AIIMS), set up in 1956, was a result of this recommendation. Even though some of the recommendations of the Committee were considered to be ambitious, they set the benchmark for policymakers in the decades to come.

One clear failure of the Bhore committee was that, despite its futuristic response to the public health challenges of the time, it overlooked the potential role of non-clinical researchers and professionals, and as a result excluded them completely from the formal practice of public health. Much emphasis was placed on the social reorientation of physicians by significant modification of the curriculum in medical colleges, as well as through an additional short three-month training course in public health, or preventive and social medicine (PSM) as it was then known. Doctors training doctors left little scope for the inclusion of non-medical personnel such as social scientists, economists, managers, and activists in training and research areas, and public health education remained this way for several decades. It was only in the 1990s that institutes such as the Sree Chitra Tirunal Institute for Medical Sciences and Technology in South India began to offer public health training programmes for the non-clinical community, but these have been few and far between, with only a small number of public health professionals being trained in multidisciplinary settings.

Even within the medical fraternity, PSM was limited in its scope and slow in its development. With a sudden surge in the number of medical colleges in the country post independence, quality control and standardization of education became a challenge. Authoritarian ways of curriculum development, and hierarchical administrations within these institutions did not exhibit any flexibility for change (Narayan 1984). The minimal requirements set by the Medical Council of India did little to promote excellence. Within medical colleges, PSM departments were often neglected and starved of resources. Often considered poor alternatives to clinical medicine, they suffered from low prestige and failed to attract the best talent into the PSM stream.

Fifteen years later, the Mudaliar committee (1961) was appointed to assess the performance of the health sector since the submission of the Bhore committee report. This Committee found the conditions in PHCs to be unsatisfactory and recommended the strengthening of already existing PHCs before the establishment of new ones. The Committee also pressed for the development of an Indian cadre of public health professionals along the lines of the

Indian Medical Service that existed during the British rule. In order to build capacity for the same, it recommended the establishment of a school of public health, in each state, that would grant degrees in public health and train both medical and non-medical personnel. Several other committees in later years also recommended the augmentation of trained public health workforce in the country.

Several of these recommendations, however, did not get the political attention they deserved. In fact, national plans in the initial years post independence have shown regressive policy trends, which have had serious repercussions on the development of the public health system and health policy, which would have potentially benefited from the operationalization of the Bhore and Mudaliar recommendations (Narayan 1984). It was not until the late 1990s that flaws of the public health education system, and the weak influence that it has had on practice, were beginning to be recognized. Poor health outcomes of public health programmes have attested to this neglect. Public health education in India has been too disease-oriented rather than determinants-oriented, and too programme-oriented rather than systems-oriented, lacking a multidisciplinary approach to public health analysis. This is perhaps a consequence of the exclusion of non-medical personnel during the early years of the development of public health training and services in India, as well as policy trends that prevented the convergence of clinical and non-clinical professionals on public health issues.

The paradigm of public health has essentially evolved according to the dominant ideology of both the state and society of the time. The period immediately following independence, namely from 1947 to 1970, was the era of centralized planning characterized by state-led growth of the economy. The state was socialist in its conceptualization, as was reflected in the setting up of its egalitarian health system. Public health developments were centred around the prioritization of primary health services, especially for the rural population, through the setting up of the PHCs. The state became the dominant provider of health at that time.

The first two decades post independence from 1947 to 1967 have been referred to as the golden decade of public health in India (Banerji 1997). Several disease-specific vertical programmes were created; PHCs were established; the state-sponsored Family Planning (later Family Welfare) programme was initiated; steps were taken to promote indigenous systems of medicine; water supply and sanitation was given emphasis in rural areas under the community development programme; and the Integrated Child Development Services (ICDS) was initiated to address malnutrition and undernutrition of children in the preschool years. Human resources for health also developed considerably: A large number of multipurpose workers (MPWs) were trained and recruited, through a scheme launched in 1971, and community health volunteers, later the village health workers, were also trained and recruited within the health system.

It was only a decade later that recommendations similar to the Bhore and Mudaliar committees were made once again in the Alma Ata Declaration of 1978. The declaration urged all governments and health workers to take urgent action to work towards achieving health for all by the year 2000. As one of the signatories, India seized the opportunity to deliberate upon its recent trends in health policy, and revisit the recommendations of the Bhore and Mudaliar committees. The western models of education, training, research, and practice of public health, which had been so predominant,

were found 'inappropriate and irrelevant' to the needs of the population (Government of India 2002) . The Indian government also realized that the disease-oriented approach to health-care delivery was benefiting the upper class and urban populations the most. Several programmes, existing and new, attempted to augment the goals of the declaration thereafter.

During the first four decades after independence, the country adopted a 'mixed economy' model, consistent with the dominant political ideology of 'democratic socialism'. This allowed the private sector to flourish, along with state control of key infrastructure, industries, and major public services. In health too, private health-care providers were widely represented, from individual general practitioners to secondary-care hospitals. The indigenous systems of medicine continued to have a presence, especially in the rural areas.

The health sector was jolted by the economic reforms that began in 1991. These reforms led to extensive liberalization of the economy. After half a century of inward orientation, India's contribution to world trade and industry grew substantially. It witnessed a large increase in foreign direct investment and began its journey on the path to becoming one of the largest economies of the world. Unfortunately, the health sector benefited little from these economic developments. Government spending on health as a percentage of the GDP plummeted from 1.3 per cent in 1990 to 0.9 per cent by 2000. As central spending on health steadily declined, more of the financial responsibility was transferred to the states.

In recent years of the post-reform period, the role of the central government in the health sector has diminished greatly, under the influence of neoliberal economics, structural reform, and the spectacular liberalization of India's markets. The central government divested itself of a lot of social responsibility during its transition from a socialist to a capitalist economy. Such patterns of development have had a significant impact on the health sector. Since then, the private sector has grown phenomenally in the health-care delivery arena over the past two decades, mostly at the tertiary- and secondary-care levels. The public sector has begun to adopt practices such as 'user fees', making access more difficult for the poor, and has also begun to divest the management of public-sector health facilities to the private sector under ill-defined 'public–private partnerships'.

Public health systems, unlike most personal medical services, produce 'public goods', and are of high priority and assure good health outcomes for a nation. Although the government was expected to play a critical role in the effective planning and equitable delivery of central health agencies in a large federated union of states such as India, it has performed inadequately ever since India became independent. The nation has faced heavy economic costs for this neglect. For instance, the WHO estimated that the 1994 plague epidemic in Surat resulted in losses totalling US$1.7 billion due to the lack of an adequate public health system. The lack of timely public health action to prevent chronic (non-communicable) diseases has led to high costs of productivity losses and health-care expenditures caused by these neglected diseases. The WHO also estimated that India suffered a loss of US$9 billion in 2005 due to cardiovascular diseases, cancers, and diabetes. These losses are expected to cumulatively lead to US$237 billion by 2015 (World Health Organization 2005).

Due to demographic and epidemiologic transitions, the public health challenges of the country have expanded in recent decades, but have remained largely unmet by the weak response attempted by the national health system, the political leadership, and the academia at large. Unevenly distributed infrastructure, human resource constraints, and low budgetary allocations have significantly contributed to this failure. It is no surprise that efforts of the past have had little impact on health outcomes, despite having a well-developed administrative system, good technical skills in many fields, and an extensive network of medical institutions for research, training, and diagnostics. Although policy priorities have overlooked fundamental public health functions, the system also has deep management flaws that hinder effective use of resources (Das Gupta & Rani 2004).

The public health system as it exists today is an extensive network of district-level hospitals, block-level community health centres, cluster-level PHCs, and subcentres at the village level. Central to the rural public health system is the PHC. Each PHC covers approximately five to six villages, with a subcentre in each village to serve as the first point of access. Patients are referred to a higher tier when more elaborate treatment is required. Similar to a PHC, urban areas have urban health centres (UHCs) or urban family welfare centres and a general hospital (GH) serving a larger population.

The rural population is increasingly reliant on private health care or has no option but to resort to amateur 'doctors' and faith healers, even to treat deadly diseases such as tuberculosis (TB) and malaria. Often, because of the cost of travel and the fear of losing income while they are away, the rural sick tend to use the moderately better health-care services that are located in urban areas only when they are gravely ill. Conditions that could be easily treated, and at little expense, often prove fatal because they have reached an advanced stage by the time they can seek adequate treatment. Kala azar (black fever), for instance, is known by public health workers as an 'epidemic rooted in poverty'. Even though it is curable, it claimed the lives of 60 000 rural poor due to their lack of access to adequate health care (Parwini & Woreck 2004).

A dearth of critical health manpower has only exacerbated the problem of inequities in access to quality care. Despite the presence of over 250 medical colleges in the modern system of medicine and over 400 in traditional Indian system throughout the country, there is a serious shortage of trained health-care providers, particularly in rural areas, and a considerable drain of human resources due to migration of doctors and nurses to other countries.

To address the largely unmet needs of the rural population, the central government launched the National Rural Health Mission (NRHM) in April 2005 and proposed to increase its total health spending on health from 0.9 per cent of the GDP to 2–3 per cent of the GDP by 2012. Since its implementation, current health spending has increased to 1.13 per cent of the GDP (The Economist 2007). The focus of the NRHM is to improve rural health conditions, with a special focus on states with weak public health infrastructure and poor health indicators. The NRHM is improving access to the public health delivery system by the most marginalized segments of the population, including women and children, thereby reducing urban–rural disparities.

The NRHM was launched simultaneously with the Reproductive and Child Health (RCH) programme phase II. The NRHM is a larger and integrative health programme that encompasses all programmes in the area of family welfare, reproductive and child health, and others that are partially or entirely centrally funded, including vertical health programmes for specific diseases such as malaria, filariasis, blindness, etc.

Originally, the RCH-I was launched as a five-year project within the framework of fifty-year-old nationwide National Family Planning programme. Post-Alma-Ata, the Government of India, in its national health policy (NHP), envisaged Health for All by 2000. A mid-decade evaluation of the NHP revealed the need to restrategize in order to achieve certain reproductive health indicators. It was thought that the goals envisaged in the new RCH approach may coincide with the ninth five-year plan of the country. The RCH-I programme introduced a new approach of managing population growth by eliciting more community participation, especially the empowerment of women to take care of their own reproductive health. The RCH-II is now being implemented over the period of 2005–2010, and is a large component of the NRHM. Central to the NRHM is the positioning of at least one accredited social health activist (ASHA) in each village. The main task of this community health worker is to liaise between people of her village and the health facility. She serves as the primary contact of the public health system with the population. Not just a provider of basic curative medicines and first aid, an important part of her role is to facilitate preventive care via certain interventions as well as health education. The presence of the ASHA has caused a decline in fatalities due to unsafe motherhood in several states.

The central government also launched an urban analogue to this scheme, called the National Urban Health Mission (NUHM), in April 2008 (The Economist 2007). Urban social health activists (USHAs), urban counterparts of the ASHAs, will be trained and recruited to promote urban health, especially for homeless and street children, focusing on decreasing the levels of malnutrition and prevention of infectious disease through improved vaccination coverage.

Although financial allocations to the health sector are increasing and new national health programmes are being implemented to increase the outreach of health services, public health has not adequately engaged with policies that are traditionally considered outside the health sector but do exercise a profound impact on the health of the population, often more than policies in the health sector do. Policies related to agriculture, food processing, water resources, urban design, environment, trade, and education are among such policies, which need to become sensitive to and supportive of public health. Taxation and regulation too are measures that, when used judiciously, can influence the determinants of health. Tobacco control is a public health imperative requiring such multisectoral action. India's response to the growing epidemic of non-communicable diseases has now begun to evolve, commencing with a comprehensive legislation on tobacco control (2003) and now has extended to a new national programme for cardiovascular diseases, diabetes, and stroke (2008). This commitment must now extend to policies and actions outside the health sector. Public health must evolve to involve all of the government in policymaking for health and all of society in advancing health action.

In order to infuse greater public health expertise into the health system and broaden the scope of cross-cutting sectors such as public health to extend beyond the health sector, recent initiatives, such as the Public Health Foundation of India (PHFI), have come into existence. The mandate of this not-for-profit organization, created through a public–private partnership, includes the setting up of several institutes of education and training for public health programmes at the graduate and postgraduate level, the establishment of pathways for public health action that are truly multisectoral, and the advancement of a transdisciplinary research agenda which would inform policy and empower programmes. The attainment of such goals would necessitate that public health education be truly interdisciplinary in including subject areas such as epidemiology, biostatistics, behavioural sciences, health economics, health-services management, environmental health, health inequities and human rights, gender and health, health communication, and ethics of health care and research. Initiatives such as the PHFI are attempting to establish synergistic links between these diverse disciplines and the health system to improve the design and delivery of health care.

The Indian government needs to play a proactive role in developing a health policy that ensures equitable access of health resources to all strata of society. Although health is enlisted as a state subject under the Indian constitution, the central government needs to ensure good management of state health systems and oversight in addition to providing financial support, with checks and balances in place. Health financing is an area that needs to ensure equity and affordability while assuring the sustainability of health services. These policy challenges need to be addressed quickly to develop a robust framework for the further evolution and advancement of public health in India.

China

Public health practices in China date back several centuries into a rich history of traditional medicine. The formal practice of public health as a modern academic discipline can be traced back to the 1920s and 1930s, with the establishment of the Peking Union Medical College following the pneumonic plague outbreak in Manchuria in 1911. The college had a formal department of public health, which did some groundbreaking work in the establishment of a primary health-care network, and conducted studies to address the problems of insufficient drug supply in rural China. Guided by the principles of health for all, the university made recommendations for the provision of primary health care (Lee 2004). However, public health academics and health-systems development soon forked from each other, and it is only in recent years that convergence has been sought once again.

Public health in China has also been deeply influenced by its long social and political history over several centuries. These developments have been unique in that no other country (besides Russia) has undergone a political and economic transition so dramatic. The shift from autocratic to decentralized politics, from a closed economy to open markets, and from a predominantly agrarian to an increasingly industry-driven economy (Grant Thornton International Business Report 2008) have had a drastic impact on the health sector. The following paragraphs describe a brief history of China's social and political changes over the second half of the twentieth century and the influence of these changes on the development of the public health system in the decades that followed.

In 1949, Mao Zedong proclaimed the establishment of the People's Republic of China in a victory over imperialism and the Kuomintang (KMT), the opponent party of social democrats. Mao's regime marked a major era in Chinese history. He was one of the founding members of the Chinese Communist Party (CCP), formed in 1921. A revolutionary by conviction, Mao was a radical thinker. Even though his successors deviated from Mao's radical thoughts, 'Maoism', or Marxism as it was interpreted by Mao, is the guiding philosophy of the government even today. The political and socioeconomic changes brought about by the Mao regime had several implications for the health sector.

Before the founding of the People's Republic of China in 1949, very few health facilities existed apart from traditional Chinese medicine clinics and dispensaries, and preventive medicine was virtually non-existent. In the first National Health Congress of 1950, four basic guidelines for the health system were specified, stating that (i) medicine should serve the workers, peasants, and soldiers; (ii) preventive medicine should be emphasized over curative services; (iii) traditional medicine practices should be integrated with western medicine; and (iv) health-related work should be combined with mass movements (Beaglehole & Bonita 2004). Mass campaigns were launched several times a year, and were very effective in the control of infectious diseases. Another outcome of the Congress was the mandate of the Ministry of Health requiring all local governments to establish health centres in rural areas and assign health workers to them. Policies and guidelines such as this promoted the establishment and development of an institutional framework for public health across the nation, particularly benefiting rural China.

To understand the development of the Chinese public health system, it is pertinent to understand the social administration of the time. China was primarily agrarian, with 85 per cent of its population living in rural areas and employed in agriculture (Liu & Wang 1991). The CCP's attempt to speed up the socialization of China through a planned economy led to the practice of collectivization of agriculture in China. Mao implemented the organization of people into 'communes', and made them official state policy in 1958. Communes were essentially cooperatives comprising smaller agricultural units, and were integral to the social fabric of the nation. Communes were an effort to create a truly egalitarian society where everything was shared, and equality was sought in all aspects of life. The cooperatives controlled the prices and production of agricultural goods. Under the communal way of life, produce was merged and redistributed according to household size, and most public services were collectively financed. Health expenses in communes were met by the Cooperative Medical Scheme (CMS), a prepaid mechanism that would provide reimbursements for most medical expenses to its contributors. The CMS inherently increased equity within the system, by making health care affordable and accessible to all.

The period from 1949 to 1976 was an era of centrally planned and managed health services. A three-tier health-care network was established in 1957, which was constituted by village, town, and county in rural China, as part of its social welfare system. Village health clinics providing basic preventive and curative care at the local level served as the first point of access to health care, township health institutions served as the intermediary unit providing primary and secondary health services between the village clinics and the larger county hospitals, and county hospitals, in addition to providing tertiary care, also served as technical guidance centres for personnel and technical training to the lower-tier institutions. These institutions were well-coordinated at each level. They were mutually reliant and supported one another for the provision of comprehensive preventive and curative care through a bottom-up referral system.

There was also an elaborate system for the provision of preventive care through the setting up of epidemic prevention stations (EPSs) at each level of administration, which were closely knit with clinical services. In addition to the preventive services offered within the three-tier health system, there also existed maternal and child health centres, and specialized disease prevention and treatment centres for specific diseases such as TB, malaria, schistosomiasis, leprosy, and other endemic diseases. At the county and provincial level, there were as many as 3600 EPSs for epidemic control and disease prevention, which were responsible for several preventive services such as the early detection and control of infectious disease, inspections for environmental and food hygiene in industrial worksites and schools. All of these were united by the Academy of Preventive Medicine, the national-level institution responsible for research in preventive medicine, which provided technical support to all the other public health institutions at lower levels (Liu & Mills 2002).

Before the establishment of the People's Republic of China, most health expenditures were met by OOP spending of households. With the establishment of the three-tier network and the CMS, households were no longer burdened with health-care costs. However, inequalities still persisted because of an urban bias in the postings of physicians. The severe shortage of skilled medical personnel affected the quality of care delivered to rural areas the most. The unmet demand for providers resulted in the formation of a cadre of minimally trained health personnel, or 'barefoot doctors' in rural China. Barefoot doctors were typically agricultural workers themselves, and provided clinical care to their agricultural units and cooperatives (which later became villages) on a part-time basis. Plenty of resources were allocated by the central government towards the development of the CMS and for the training of barefoot doctors. Although they were only able to provide very basic health services to the peasant class, they existed in large numbers and were widely available (more than one per 1000 members of the population). By 1976, 96 per cent of the agricultural production teams were covered by the service of barefoot doctors (Guangpeng *et al.* 2007).

Although this was a period of relatively lower individual income, China witnessed stellar gains in the health of its people during this egalitarian period. The average life expectancy of the Chinese rose from 35 to 68 years, infant mortality decreased from 250 to 40 deaths per 1000 live births, and the prevalence of malaria was slashed from 5.5 per cent to 0.3 per cent of the population (Hsiao 1995). However, these remarkable gains in health outcomes could not be sustained because of the political and economic changes that took place with the advent of the Cultural Revolution in 1966.

The Revolution was a period of immense social upheaval with the dismissal of several civil rights—a tremendous setback to economic development. China fell even further behind industrialized powers of the world. It was only under the leadership of Deng Xiaoping, post 1978, that the party and the government relaxed control over people, and granted them certain civil rights in a new constitution that was adopted in 1975. In this new phase of reform and development, China went through a remarkable transition from an inward-looking closed economy to an open market-oriented economy, exhibiting immense growth. Global trade increased, diplomatic relations improved, and participation in international organizations was assumed. China became one of the fastest growing economies of the world.

With the end of the Cultural Revolution in the mid-1970s and the economic changes that followed, collective farming was abolished and individual household responsibility was introduced. This drastic change in agricultural policy led to the reorganization of the social structure, and therefore of the health system that was built around it. The breakdown of collective farming led to the collapse of the collectively financed CMS. Health centres sustained by contributions from the communes were now turned into self-financing township, county, and village health centres (Schuchend & Suzhen 2007). The effects of the economic reforms of the 1980s on the rural Chinese population and their health status were paradoxical. On one hand, as the rural economy developed, individual household incomes increased. Rural areas also witnessed the creation of a variety of institutes such as the county maternal and child health centres, county specialized disease prevention and treatment institutes , county centres for disease control, and county health supervision institutes (Gu & Tang 1995). Despite the increase in the number of institutions, the health of the population suffered and health gains from the previous decades started to erode. Inequities in affordability, accessibility, and availability of health services set in and rapidly escalated. There were three chief reasons for this:

1. Reduced government subsidies: The government cut subsidies to health institutions to an amount that accounted for just about 25 per cent of their revenue, covering only basic wages for their staff (Dummer & Cook 2007). In order to remain financially sustainable, health facilities were made to generate additional revenue from charging user fees and dispensing of drugs.

2. Fiscal decentralization: There was tremendous decentralization of the fiscal system to the provinces. Health spending was further decentralized from provincial to county and township governments. As a consequence of diminished government control, the vertical lines of communication within the health system became significantly weakened (Liu 2004).

3. Privatization: Liberalization of the public sector allowed private dispensaries to fill the unmet health needs of the population on the basis of their ability to pay. The increased availability of health services was offset by decreased affordability.

The consequences of these changes on health outcomes were profound:

1. User fees: Introduction of user fees into the health system, in addition to the collapse of the CMS, changed the health-seeking behaviour of those it was meant to serve. The unaffordable fees led to a reduction in the utilization of health services by the poorer segment of the population, creating greater disparities in health outcomes. OOP expenditures as a percentage of the total health spending increased dramatically, and remain high even today. In recent decades, OOP spending has risen from 38 per cent in 1991 to nearly 60 per cent in 2000. Although this number was 53 per cent in 2003, the decline has only been marginal (The Economist 2007).

2. Fragmentation of health system: When health centres were left to generate their own revenue, there was a loss of coordination within the three-tiered system. Health facilities started competing for patients rather than working together through referrals to provide comprehensive care.

3. Inequitable redistribution of health facilities: Centres that were located in poor neighbourhoods and were unable to generate sufficient revenue from user fees and drug prescriptions had to close down and merge with a neighbouring facility (Gao *et al.* 2002).

This redistribution exacerbated hardships in accessing health facilities for the poor.

4. Poor quality care: Health facilities in higher-income areas that generated sufficient revenues were able to pay higher wages to staff, thus attracting professionals of higher calibre. Health facilities in poor areas, if they managed to stay afloat, were unable to attract highly skilled physicians and health workers, as was reflected in the quality of care delivered.

5. Overprescription of drugs and services: There has been growing evidence that patients were prescribed unnecessary drugs and procedures such as X-rays (*The Economist* 2007) in an effort to generate higher revenue (Hsiao 1995; Akin *et al.* 2005; Collins *et al.* 2000), which has negatively impacted the health of the population. In some areas, drug resistance has risen as a dangerous consequence of the consumption of unnecessary drugs.

6. Marginalization of preventive services: EPSs were also adversely affected during the decades following the economic reforms and the consequent changes in government subsidies. The changed financing mechanisms led them to focus more on activities that were revenue-generating, rather than on preventive services, which were essentially free. Whereas in 1985, government subsidies accounted for nearly 80 per cent of their total income, this number was reduced to only 40 per cent in 1997 (Liu *et al.* 1999).

Government spending on health in China has since progressively declined (Fig. 1.4.2.2). More than 50 per cent of the total health spending came from government funds in 1991, but declined to 38 per cent by 2004, and OOP expenses rose from 38 per cent to 60 per cent during the same period (World Health Organization 2007).

There are multiple challenges that the health system must address, and adapt to the altered health needs due to changing disease patterns and demography. China's success in curtailing its fertility rate over the recent years, juxtaposed with major gains in life expectancy, presents it with the real problem of a large aging population. The unique and demanding health needs of this age group further burden a health system that is already pressed for resources.

The Chinese public health system has evolved into a vast establishment, with institutions at each level of the government involved with preventive care, curative care, and surveillance, and overseen by the Academy of Preventive Medicine at the centre. In recent years, the focus of the Academy has been primarily on activities that are hygiene-related and on other preventive services delivered through the EPSs, based on a biomedical model. China has since invested vast resources for the establishment of disease surveillance systems, especially after the recent SARS and avian flu epidemics. The establishment of the China Centre for Disease Control and Prevention (China CDC) in 2004 has been a milestone in the history of Chinese public health. Based on the Academy model, the China CDC's mandate extends to include a more broad-based approach to public health. Some of its main functions are disease surveillance and prevention, emergency response, health promotion and health education, training and applied research, and international cooperation (China Center for Disease Control 2008). It consists of an elaborate four-tiered network for disease control. It is also considered to be multisectoral in nature, through its partnerships with several ministries at the central level, universities, and

research institutions. Collaborations with professional and non-governmental organizations make the China CDC a cross-cutting body with a key role in influencing policymaking.

Health-systems research has also been given increasing importance among policymakers, with the setting up of the Health Policy Advisory Board within the Ministry of Health in mid 1980s, and the founding of the China Health Economics Network shortly thereafter (Zhang & Zou 1998). After the SARS outbreak in 2003, research institutes and universities have been increasingly engaged in health policy and systems research, and their expertise for health-systems development has been sought at different levels of the government (Lei 2005). The establishment of the Health Policy and Regulation department within the Ministry of Health in 2004 is a result of such collaborations. While there is an increasing demand for public health researchers within the system, human resources are lacking and vacancies are plentiful. Although pathways for their close integration into the health sector are being paved, China has yet to see adequate investments in capacity-building for public health professionals.

Other challenges to the health sector

Uneven economic growth

China's growth rate of >9 per cent of the GDP for the last two decades has led to significant overall economic development of urban and rural populations. However, urban segment areas, especially in the 'Gold Coast' and the eastern provinces, have benefited much more. Rural areas such as the Yunnan, Guizhou, and Hunan provinces are still developing at a much slower pace than urban China, and will continue to lag behind for quite some time. The widening gap between urban and rural socioeconomic positions has only exacerbated disparities in health outcomes.

Technological barriers

China's open markets have brought in high-quality medical equipment, advanced biotechnological interventions, modern medical amenities, and the latest drugs. However, their availability depends largely on a persons ability to pay, and is concentrated in urban areas. With the diminishing role of the government in health-care delivery and increasing role of market forces, inequalities in access to health care and health status have continued to rise in recent years. Further, secondary translational barriers have prevented the health system from making technological advancements in health widely available to the masses. In the past, as resources for health have increased, government investment in public health has been skewed towards vaccination programmes and clinical care, with preventive and promotive care subsequently marginalized. Developing countries have realized in recent years that interventions need to be more evidence-based, context–specific, and resource-sensitive, and that following western models of public health need not lead to successful outcomes.

Human resources

After reforms in medical education, barefoot doctors were required to earn a certification and practice as a 'village doctor'. This deterred several barefoot doctors from practising, resulting in the loss of several trained health workers. Further, an urban bias in the preferences of medical graduates for employment has left the void created by the loss of several barefoot doctors unfilled. The lack of adequate public health personnel is also a lacuna that needs to be addressed.

Stark disparities in health outcomes

Disparities in maternal and infant mortality rates between urban and rural areas have been widening. Official data from the Ministry of Health and the WHO report that the infant mortality rate in urban areas is 10.1 per 1000 live births and in rural areas is 24.5 per 1000 live births. Maternal mortality indicates a similar disparity, with rates of 26.1 per 100 000 live births in urban areas and 63 per 100 000 live births in rural areas. Non-communicable diseases are simultaneously on the rise, affecting both rural and urban areas. Rural areas also face an increased risk of infectious diseases. According to Ministry of Health estimates, 80 per cent of the TB patients in China live in rural areas, particularly in the less-developed western regions, where the epidemiological transition is still in the early stages (Dummer & Cook 2007). Although levels of risk factors for chronic disease are higher in urban areas, the very low chances of detection and treatment of those with risk factors in rural areas leaves them highly vulnerable to adverse events such as stroke and heart disease.

Environmental degradation

Rapid industrialization and urbanization has increased the ambient air pollution in urban areas, which is an inherent risk factor for several respiratory illnesses. The lack of urban planning and unregulated vehicular growth further contribute to this. After the United States, China is the second largest contributor to environmental pollution in the world. Deforestation and decline in the number of open spaces in cities is damaging the biodiversity of these areas considerably, often beyond reversal. The short-term gains in health from the effects of globalization have long been replaced by the ill-effects of mass consumerism, such as depletion of natural reserves and deterioration of the natural environment. The World Bank estimates that by 2020, China will be paying US$390 billion (13 per cent of its projected GDP) to treat diseases indirectly caused by coal burning (Dummer & Cook 2007). Policymakers will have to proactively take measures to ensure the regulated and planned growth of new cities and intervene with environmental standards to protect, conserve, and restore China's natural resources, with active involvement of the public health community.

The Chinese experience shows that economic growth does not necessarily translate into better health outcomes. Progressive health-sector policies have often been left outside the purview of economic developments in transitional economies under the influence of neoliberal structural reforms. The Chinese experience also shows that the provision of health services cannot be left to the mercy of market economics. Meng *et al.* (2004) estimated that nearly 50 per cent of the village clinics in rural areas were privately owned. Excessive privatization without adequate government regulation and planning has compromised the quality of care. The role of the state in the assurance of, if not the provision of, health services has not been clearly defined. The resurgence of infectious diseases such as TB and schistosomiasis attests to the weak role of the state in the provision of preventive care.

Brazil

The development of public health, or *collective health*, as it is known in Brazil, has been markedly different from India and China, and any other country in Latin America. The development of the health system and the civil movement for political stability have played a mutually influential role in each other's development.

Development of the health system

State-provided health care in Brazil dates back to 1923, as a component of the social security system that was a promulgation of the Eloy Chavez law. Under this social welfare system, urban workers employed in the private sector received coverage for health care through compulsory contributions to pension and retirement funds (CAPS), later organized into institutes by professional category (IAPs), through payroll deductions and employer contributions. By default, workers in excluded professional categories, the unorganized sector, the unemployed, and the rural population were almost entirely devoid of health coverage from this system. These centrally regulated social security funds in turn provided reimbursements for health services provided by the private sector. For several decades, this system was financed by employers and employees, with very little involvement of the government in setting of health priorities. Government funds were used mainly to contract-out services to the private sector, or as subsidies for the construction of private hospitals and clinics. Further, most facilities that existed were concentrated in the more developed south and south-east, and further exacerbated issues off access to health-care facilities among poorer segments and those living in less developed areas.

The government during that period was known for its policies propagating rigid centralization and prioritization of economic development over social services (Cortes 2006). Until the 1960s, the social welfare system was centred on the provision of medical care to workers in the private sector, and the Ministry of Health, formed in 1953, was involved mainly with issues of community health and vaccine distribution through various campaigns and disease-specific vertical programmes. Although its mandate also included the provision of basic medical care to low-income populations where adequate services did not exist, it owned very few hospitals, which mainly specialized in contagious diseases and psychiatry (Medici 2007). Issues related to universal access to care were not prioritized on the agenda of policymakers. It has been estimated that barely 30 per cent of the country received coverage from an IAP by the end of the 1950s (Oliveira 2008).

However, significant changes occurred in this structure with the unification of these institutes to form the National Social Welfare Institute (INPS) in 1966, and brought about a growing trend towards expanding health-care coverage for categories not previously covered. The authoritarian government that came into power in 1964 recognized the lacunae existing within the fragmented health system and attempted to expand health-care delivery by contracting services to a larger network of private establishments in order to meet the greater demand for health care. A large portion of public funding was, thus, provided for the expansion of the private sector. Although several minor institutional and structural changes took place over the next couple of decades, the welfare system remained practically unchanged until the mid-1980s when a new constitution was adopted. This new constitution redefined social security to be inclusive of the rights to welfare, health, and social assistance, providing coverage to the entire population, independently of their professional job or any affiliation. A new unified national health-care system was established in 1988.

The public health reform movement

The development of public health in Brazil has been strongly influenced by the Latin American Social Medicine (LASM) movement which began in 1966. Inspired by similar historical social movements and political processes in France, Germany and England, led by Rudolf Virchow and others in mid-nineteenth century, the movement was deep-rooted in the economic and political changes that Brazil was witnessing. By the 1970s, what began as the struggle for democratization of health services had taken the shape of a much larger nationwide struggle against military rule. Drawing participation from across groups, professions, and communities such as health-services researchers, political party representatives, and health workers' organizations (Elias & Cohn 2003), the public health reform movement expressed itself through several symposia, conferences, and academic gatherings.

Although democracy was not established in Brazil till 1985, the Movement was able to exert an important influence over the post-dictatorial reforms (Collins *et al.* 2000). Many of the leaders of the Movement came from academic backgrounds. Its forerunners were protesting university students, especially those in health-related fields, who became involved in the political movement for democracy. As a result, they chose practices that promoted political change even after they had graduated. Given the heavy involvement of students and professionals in the political movement, their orientation towards social justice and politics in turn influenced curricula within educational institutes, which initially led to the introduction of social medicine in medical schools. Pioneered by the University of Rio de Janeiro in Brazil, separate graduate-level master's programmes in preventive and social medicine were offered across several countries in Latin America over the next decade (Waitzkin *et al.* 2001).

With the adoption of the new constitution in 1988 in democratic Brazil, health care was specified as a constitutional right and a responsibility of the state. During the same period, several Latin American countries were implementing neoliberal reforms, propagated by the World Bank, that encouraged privatization and the limiting of the state's involvement in the provision of health services to regulation only (Homedes & Ugalde 2005). Contrariwise, Brazilian health reforms aimed to increase the role of the state not only in health-service delivery but also in research and training, and largely curbed the dominance of the private sector. The role of the state was finally confirmed. Inspired by Italian health reforms of the 1960s and 1970s, Brazilian health reforms propagated decentralization, or *municipalization* as a means of de-concentrating power at the centre and strengthening the public sector. This was done through the establishment of the Unified Health System or the Sistema Único de Saúde (SUS) in 1988, which consisted of a three-tier network of primary health centres and hospitals owned by the central, state, and municipal governments (known as *municipios*). The SUS was to be nationally coordinated by the state and jointly implemented with local and state authorities. Health-care delivery by the private sector existed as a supplementary health network known as the SSAM, and was complementary to and coordinated with government services. The federal government would, through the Ministry of Health, play a larger regulatory role in the creation and implementation of the national health policy, and in national programmes for communicable diseases and nutrition. Public health activities such as disease surveillance, health promotion, and immunizations would also be delivered through the SUS (Buss & Carvalho 2007). Some of the key features of the democratization of the health sector were community participation, the decentralization of health services, and fiscal devolution at each level of the government (Medici 2007).

Before the establishment of the SUS, health-care delivery relied exclusively on centrally regulated social security funds, and the care delivered was largely dependent on the private sector. Now, it is almost entirely funded by local state and regional governments, and the role of the government in the provision of services has increased, but inequities still persist. Today, the SUS stretches nationwide and strives to provide a complete medical package, covering more than 70 per cent of Brazil's population (Schmidt & Duncan 2004). The complementary private system, or SSAM, provides care to the remaining population consisting of lower-risk individuals in the higher- and middle-income groups. As a result, expensive procedures not covered by the private SSAM network, and costs for high-risk individuals, are left entirely for the SUS to meet.

Through the 1990s, health services continued to be increasingly decentralized—both in terms of fiscal devolution and decision-making authority. Decentralization was facilitated through the transfer of power and funds to local municipalities to use on health services at their discretion. Fiscal devolution to the regional- and local-level authorities gave greater flexibility to the local governments to respond more appropriately to the needs of the population, as they were better informed about ground realities. This was managed by the members of two commissions—the Tripartite commission at the national level, consisting of representatives from all three levels of government, and the Bipartite commission at the state level, consisting only of state and municipal representatives. However, it also introduced competition between local and state governments for central government funding and further exacerbated inequities in access to quality health care.

Community participation, an important aspect of Brazil's health-reform policies, was mandated by law for state and local governments to be eligible for central funding. Civil society was involved by the creation of health councils at each level of the government. These were essentially advisory bodies that assisted with policy decisions regarding the implementation of the SUS. The councils were constituted such that they involved participation from several actors within the community, including members of civil society, the users as well as providers of health services. Although the actual distribution of power among the stakeholders within the councils has been skewed towards government representatives, the very existence of these councils made decision making a diverse and inclusive process (Tajer 2003). The establishment of a participatory forum helped the democratization of Brazilian institutions, empowering social sectors that were traditionally excluded from direct representation in the political system. Presently, under the PRO-SAUDE programme, Brazil's institutions providing training to the health workforce receive financial support for projects aimed at realigning the health system to the needs of the community.

Decentralization and devolution have been central to the debate on health-sector reform for decades, and Brazil duly illustrates its pros and cons. Although decentralization is meant to bring about greater equity and efficiency within the system, the varying levels of development and performance of local governments may also lead to greater disparities in health outcomes and fragmentation of the system. The attainment of equity and assured quality are challenges that Brazil's SUS faces today.

New developments

The Ministry of Health initiated the Family Health Programme (PSF) in 1992 in an effort to enhance the provision of basic health services including preventive services to underserved populations. The core of the PSF is the placement of a team of providers and specialists in a certain geographic area that serves roughly 1000 families. This programme currently serves 47 per cent of Brazil's population (Medici 2007). The PSF focuses on several health-promoting activities such as child development, vaccinations, prenatal examinations, promotion of personal hygiene, breastfeeding campaigns, and water and sanitation requirements within communities. It is currently one of the most effective programmes being carried out in the country (Buss & Carvalho 2007). In 2006, the National Commission on Social Determinants of Health (CNDSS) was also launched within the Ministry of Health. This commission consists of state and municipal health council representatives as well as ministers from cross-cutting sectors.

Several intersectoral programmes extending beyond the Ministry of Health have also been launched in recent years: The Family Grant Programme (PBF), managed by the Ministry of Social Development, offers financial support to families below the poverty line; the Family Agriculture Programme, managed by the Ministry of Agriculture, promotes family agriculture instead of industrial agriculture, thus improving nutritional levels and ensuring sustainable agriculture; the National Programme of Food and Nutrition (PNAN), tied closely to the PSF, sets nutritional guidelines for the Brazilian population and takes on several health-education campaigns to disseminate information on health-promoting dietary practices; the Healthy Cities/Communities initiative (CCS) is a network of municipal governments and universities and schools of public health, existing entirely at local levels, without the involvement of the central government; the Health Promoting Schools programme (EPS) is another intersectoral initiative between the Ministry of Health and the Ministry of Education to promote healthy practices within schools among teachers, students, and their families.

Brazil has been one of the most advanced countries for scientific theory and research generation in Latin America, with plenty of state support since the 1990s. An increasing number of graduate programmes in preventive and social medicine, extending beyond the medical community, have helped to shape the public health movement as a tool for political and social justice. The Brazilian health sector has significantly advanced due to thriving health-services research and the coming together of several professional and political organizations. The national health service now depends on academic support for various functions such as programme planning, implementation, monitoring, and evaluation (Schmidt & Duncan 2004). The CNDSS recommendations, in 2006, to the Ministry of Health resulted in the allocation of significant funding towards research on social determinants and inequity in health . A consortium of several public health education and research-based organizations such as FIOCRUZ, the Brazilian Association of Postgraduation in Collective Health (ABRASCO), and Canadian Public Health Association (CPHA) are currently carrying out the intersectoral Actions for Health project, which aims at capacity-building and knowledge exchange between different institutions across the country. Prizes for academic excellence and funding for health-systems research related to issues within the SUS are being increasingly awarded to researchers to build synergies between research outputs and the requirements of the health system. In 2007, 90 medical, nursing, and dental colleges received grants for making curricular changes that would promote

engagement between different faculties of health-care professionals, primary care, and action learning (Global Health Workforce Alliance 2008). The case of Brazil exemplifies how academia and policymakers mutually benefited from one another and together contributed to the development of the national health system and strengthened the practice of public health.

Conclusion

The three countries profiled in this chapter (China, India, and Brazil) represent societies wherein the economies are on the upswing and are accompanied by demographic and epidemiological transitions, profoundly influencing the agenda of public health as well as the level of resources available to address it. Despite growth in their economies and increasing urbanization, they also have large segments of rural or otherwise disadvantaged populations, posing challenges not only to health equity but also presenting diversity in dominant disease burdens.

All of these countries have focused on developing health systems which will extend health care to all sections of the population. In doing so, clinical care was prioritized over preventive and promotive measures by all of them. It is only in recent years that countries such as China and India are paying greater attention to building broader public health capacity and looking at multisectoral interventions for promoting population health. In Brazil, the political discourse that shaped popular movements and governmental policies, over the past two decades, has accorded a high priority to public health. As the value of better health as an accelerator of economic development and its relevance to human rights gain greater recognition in each of these societies, public health is likely to grow in its influence and impact.

Even as the focus has been on establishing strong systems for delivery of health care, the role of the state has undergone substantial changes, over time, in these countries. China has dramatically shifted from universal state-supported and communitized models of health care to a mixed model of state-/employer-supported care and private purchased care. India, which always had a mixed model, has substantially reduced the role of the state in the supply of health services and has allowed an unregulated private sector to emerge as a major provider, increasing market distortions in the availability, quality, and pricing of health care. The rising out-of-pocket expenditures on health care in these countries are a cause for concern, because the poor may be deprived of affordable health care. Brazil, on the other hand, has emphasized the primary responsibility of the state in extending health care to all sections of the people and has clearly defined a small but supplementary role for the private sector.

Although decentralization has been accepted by each of these countries as essential for efficient operationalization of public health programmes, it has not been implemented with an equal measure of success everywhere. China's shift to decentralization has reduced state support for services. India's commitment to decentralization is becoming more manifest in new national programmes such as the National Rural Health Mission, but the serious gaps in the availability of health workforce, lack of public health expertise, and limited coordination among multiple vertical programmes raises concerns about the limited ability of local stakeholders in taking full advantage of a decentralized system. Brazil, on the other hand, has built a robust model of well-coordinated but adequately decentralized health-care system. As these countries develop further, they have to carefully balance local autonomy and central support so that the public health system is operationally unchained but not left rudderless. Even as democratic devolution and efficiency are promoted though decentralized systems, central coordination would be needed for ensuring commitment to goals, quality of services, and to provide for early recognition of and rapid response to emerging or exacerbated inequities.

In an era of rapid globalization, the pressures to free the markets will see these LMICs move towards greater privatization in all sectors, including health. However, the need for a strong role for the state in planning for universally available and affordable health care, and its predominant position in advancing policies and programmes for public health should not be overlooked. The state must act as the guarantor of services for the vulnerable sections of the people and a promoter of policies that protect the health of the entire population. Access to adequate and affordable health services must be fully assured by the state, even if not fully provided by it.

Even as the role of public health is enhanced in the priorities and programmes of these economically advancing countries, capacity-building for public health needs greater attention. Adequately trained and motivated human resources as well as strong institutional structures and networks for advancing public-health-related education and research are needed. As schools of medicine, nursing, and dentistry must upscale the public health components of their curriculum, schools of public health which provide interdisciplinary learning to medical as well as non-medical public health professionals must be developed. The limited biomedical model of health sciences must be replaced, through such education and research, with a trans-disciplinary model of applied public health sciences that integrates knowledge and perspectives from life sciences, social sciences, economics, quantitative sciences (such as epidemiology and biostatistics), and management sciences.

At the same time, public health education and research must become more closely connected to the development, evaluation, and strengthening of health systems. Public health will evolve into a stronger discipline with a greater ability to make a substantial societal contribution if it moves along these new directions of growth in the LMICs. Although promising signs of such a change are visible in some of these countries, the extent to which the discipline will advance further over the next two decades will be a critical determinant of health and development in the high-velocity transitional period that lies ahead.

Key points

◆ The disciplinary mandate of public health, globally and nationally, has expanded from providing essential hygienic services and disease-preventive personal protection to broader social-engineering efforts, which combine public education and policy interventions that have a population-wide effect, for health promotion.

◆ Health systems have been influenced by many of the economic and social changes that have occurred in LMICs, and have developed within that context.

◆ Economic transitions have been accompanied by profound demographic and epidemiological changes. The rapidly increasing burden of non-communicable (chronic) diseases juxtaposed with gains in life expectancy and lowered fertility rates are challenging present health systems in new ways.

◆ Skewed distributional patterns of the wealth created during this growth phase in the LMICs have aggravated socioeconomic inequalities, resulting in major disparities in health outcomes.

◆ A clearly defined role of the state in setting health priorities and assuring health services is key to improving health outcomes, especially among the poorer segments.

◆ Adequate engagement of public health researchers, policymakers, and practitioners is vital for the development of the discipline to its full potential.

References

Akin J.S., Dow W.H., Lance P.M. *et al.* Changes in access to health care in China, 1989–1997. *Health Policy and Planning* 2005;**20**(2):80–9.

Banerji D. *Landmarks in the development of health services in the countries of South Asia.* Delhi, India: Consul Press; 1997.

Beaglehole R., Bonita R. *Public health at a crossroads—achievements and prospects.* 2nd ed. London: Cambridge University Press; 2004. pp. 227–32.

Berman P., Ahuja R. (2008). Government Health Spending in India. *Economic and Political Weekly,* June–July. Vol. 43 (26, 27) pp. 209–216.

Buss P., Carvalho A. Health promotion in Brazil. *Promotion and Education* 2007;**14**(4):209.

China Center for Disease Control. People's Republic of China; 2008. Available from: http://www.chinacdc.net.cn

Collins C., Araujo J., Barbosa J. *et al.* Decentralising the health sector: issues in Brazil. *Health Policy* 2000;**52**:113–7.

Cortes S.M.V. Building up user participation: councils and conferences in the Brazilian health system. *Sociologias* 2006;**1**:1–23.

Das Gupta M., Rani M. India's public health system: how well does it function at the national level? Policy Research Working Paper 3447. Washington (DC): World Bank; 2004. p. 1–24.

Das Gupta M. Public health in India: an overview. Policy Research Working Paper 3787. Washington (DC): World Bank; 2005. p. 1–12.

Dummer B., Cook G. Exploring China's rural health crisis: processes and policy implications. *Health Policy* 2007;**83**(1):1–16.

Economic and Social Data Service. World Bank Data – China. Website: http://ddp.ext.worldbank.org (Accessed November 15th, 2007).

Elias P., Cohn A. Health reform in Brazil: lessons to consider. *American Journal of Public Health* 2003;**93**(1):44–8.

Food and Agricultural Organization. Paying farmers for environmental services. In: The state of food and agriculture. Rome, Italy: Food and Agricultural Organization; 2007.

Gao J., Qian J., Tang S. *et al.* Health equity in transition from planed to market economy in China. *Health Policy and Planning* 2002;**17** Suppl 1:20–9.

Global Health Workforce Alliance. *Scaling up, saving lives.* Geneva: World Health Organization; 2008.

Gottret P., Schieber G. Health transitions, disease burdens, and expenditure patterns. In: *Health financing revisited: a practitioner's guide.* Washington (DC): World Bank; 2006.

Government of India. National health accounts. Mumbai, India: Reserve Bank of India; 2005.

Government of India. *National health policy.* India: Ministry of Health; 2002.

Government of People's Republic of China. The Chinese statistical yearbook. People's Republic of China: Ministry of Health.

Grant Thornton International Business Report. Emerging markets: Brazil, Russia, India, China (BRIC). 2008.

Gu X., Tang S. Reform of the Chinese health care financing system. *Health policy* 1995;**32**:181–91.

Guangpeng Z., Xiaoyan L., Junhua Z. *et al.* The history and development of three-tier health care network in rural China. People's Republic of China: Health Human Resources Development Center (HHRDC), Ministry of Health; 2007.

Harrison M. *Public health in British India*. Cambridge: Cambridge University Press; 1994.

Homedes N., Ugalde A. Why neo-liberal health reforms have failed in Latin America. *Health Policy* 2005;**71**:83–96.

Hsiao W. The Chinese health care system: lessons for other nations. *Social Sciences and Medicine* 1995;**41**(8):1047–55.

Integrated Regional Information Network (IRIN). Combustion or consumption? Balancing food and biofuel production. UN Office for the Coordination of Humanitarian Affairs; 2007 Apr 25.

Lee L. The current state of public health in China. *Annual Review of Public Health* 2004;**25**:327–39.

Lei H. *Health systems research in China: macro situations*. Peoples Republic of China: Department of Health Policy and Regulation, Ministry of Health; 2005.

Liu X., Mills A. Financing reforms of public health services in China: lessons for other nations. *Social Science and Medicine* 2002; **54**:1691–8.

Liu X., Wang J. An introduction to China's health care system. *Journal of Public Health Policy* 1991 Spring:105–17.

Liu Y., Hsiao W.C., Eggleston K. *et al.* Equity in health and health care: the Chinese experience. *Social Science and Medicine* 1999; **49**:1349–56.

Liu Y. China's public health care system: facing the challenges. *Bulletin of the World Health Organisation* 2004;**82**:532–8.

Medici A. Structure of the health system. Brazil: Ministry of Foreign Affairs. Available from: http://www.mre.gov.br/cdbrasil/itamaraty/web/ingles/polsoc/saude/estsist/index.htm [accessed 2007 Dec].

Meng Q., Shi G., Yang H. *et al. Health policy and systems research in China*. Geneva: World Health Organization; 2004.

Narayan R. 150 years of medical education rhetoric and relevance. *Medico Friend Circle Bulletin* 1984;**97–98**:1–9.

O'Donnell O., Doorslaer E., Rannan-Eliya R. *et al.* Explaining the incidence of catastrophic expenditures on health care: comparative evidence from Asia. EQUITAP Project; 2005. Working paper 5.

Oliveira F. Social welfare. Brazil: Ministry of Foreign Affairs. Available from: http://www.mre.gov.br/CDBRASIL/ITAMARATY/WEB/ingles/polsoc/previd/apresent/index.htm [accessed 2008 Feb].

Olshansky S., Ault A. The fourth stage of the epidemiological transition: the age of delayed degenerative disease. In: *Should medical care be rationed by age?* Lanham (MD): Rowman and Littlefield; 1985.

Omran A. The epidemiologic transition: a theory of the epidemiology of population change. *The Milbank Quarterly* 2005; **83**(4):731–57.

Parwini Z., Woreck D. Black fever in India: an epidemic rooted in poverty 30th December, 2004. *The World Socialist Web* 2004.

Schmidt M., Duncan B. Academic medicine as a resource for global health: the case of Brazil—improving population health demands stronger academic input. *British Medical Journal* 2004;**329**(2):753–4.

Schuchend W., Suzhen F. The history, current status, and future prospects of barefoot doctors in China. People's Republic of China: Health Human Resources Development Centre, Ministry of Health; 2007.

Tajer D. Latin American social medicine: roots, development during the 1990s and current challenges. *American Journal of Public Health* 2003;**93**:2023–7.

The Economist (2007). Missing the barefoot doctors. October 2007. Website: http://www.economist.com/world/asia/displaystory.cfm?story_id=9944734 (accessed November 2, 2007).

Waitzkin H., Iriart C., Estrada A. *et al.* Public health then and now. *American Journal of Public Health* 2001;**91**:1952–1601.

World Bank. Investing in health: world development indicators. In: *World development report*. Washington (DC): World Bank; 1993.

World Health Organization. *WHO report 2006: working together for health*. Statistical Annexe; 2006.

World Health Organization. *World health report 1995: bridging the gaps*. Statistical Annexe; 1995.

World Health Organization. *World health report 1996: fighting disease, fostering development*. Statistical Annexe; 1996.

World Health Organization. *World health report 1997: conquering suffering, enriching humanity*. Statistical Annex; 1997.

World Health Organization. *World health report 1998: a life in the 21st century—a vision for all*. Statistical Annexe; 1998.

World Health Organization. *World health report 1999: making a difference*. Statistical Annexe; 1999.

World Health Organization. *World health report 2000: health systems—improving performance*. Statistical Annexe; 2000.

World Health Organization. *World health report 2001: mental health—new understanding, new hope*. Statistical Annexe; 2001.

World Health Organization. *World health report 2002: reducing risks, promoting healthy life*. Statistical Annexe; 2002.

World Health Organization. *World health report 2003: shaping the future*. Statistical Annexe; 2003.

World Health Organization. *World health report 2004: changing history*. Statistical Annexe; 2004.

World Health Organization. *World health report 2005: make every mother and child count*. Statistical Annexe; 2005.

World Health Organization. *World health report 2006: health workforce*. Statistical Annexe; 2006a

World Health Organization. *World health statistics 2007*. Geneva: World Health Organization; 2007.

Xinhua News Agency. TB tops list of China's killer diseases. 2006 May 10.

Yusuf S., Reddy K.S., Ounpuu S. *et al.* Global burden of cardiovascular diseases: Part I: general considerations, the epidemiologic transition, risk factors, and impact of urbanization. *Circulation* 2001;**104**:2746–53.

Zhang T., Zou H. Fiscal decentralization, public spending, and economic growth in China. *Journal of Public Economics* 1998;**67**:221–40.

SECTION 2

Determinants of health and disease

2.1

Globalization

Kelley Lee

Abstract

Globalization, defined as the closer integration or interconnectedness of human societies across national borders through spatial, temporal, and cognitive changes, is creating wide ranging impacts on public health. This interconnectedness is characterized by cross-border flows of people, other life forms, goods and services, capital, and knowledge to an unprecedented degree in terms of intensity and extensity (geographical reach). The emergence of a global economy, for example, has led to the restructuring of many health-related industries such as pharmaceuticals, food, and tobacco. Other global changes taking place, such as the increased movement of populations, environmental change, and financial transactions, have had indirect yet profound impacts on health determinants and outcomes.

To date, the public health community has played a limited role in influencing the nature of the changes taking place, which have been largely driven by powerful economic and political interests. Contemporary globalization, as a result, has been characterized by an inequitable distribution of costs and benefits within and across countries. For the public health community, there is a need to better understand the linkages between globalization and health, and the possible interventions available to protect and promote public health. A review of key activities in public health practice suggests the need for a 'global public health' approach which seeks to minimize the costs, and maximize the benefits, to public health arising from globalization. Recent developments in infectious disease outbreak control, environmental health, health promotion, and monitoring of health status provide examples of the challenges faced. These include opposition by powerful vested interests to stronger regulation, the need for effective collective action across all societies to tackle crossborder public health issues, and the current weaknesses of global health governance. Nonetheless, there are opportunities for the public health community to influence globalization by demonstrating the shared benefits to be gained. Greater attention to the public health impacts of globalization, through redistributive policies, greater attention to health equity, and appropriate social and environmental protections will, in turn, contribute to more sustainable forms of globalization.

Introduction

'Globalization' is a term associated with complex and varied changes to the world around us, and has received substantial research and policy attention in a wide range of fields. While scholars, policy makers, and practitioners continue to debate the benefits and drawbacks of these changes, there is agreement that better understanding of the nature of these changes, and their specific impacts on human societies, is much needed.

There is now a substantial body of scholarship on globalization and public health which seeks to explain how contemporary flows of people, other life forms, goods and services, capital, and knowledge are influencing the determinants of health and health outcomes (Lee 2003b; Lee & Collin 2005; Kawachi & Wamala 2006). The unprecedented scale of these flows, in some cases rendering the national borders of individual countries irrelevant, has posed three major challenges for the public health community: How can the evidence base on globalization and health be strengthened; what effective policy responses are needed to optimize the benefits, and minimize the costs to public health, arising from globalization; and how can these policy options be practically and effectively implemented?

This chapter is concerned with how globalization is influencing public health. It begins by defining globalization, and how it is a distinct and contemporary phenomenon. This includes the increasingly used concept of 'global public health'. The key drivers of globalization are described, alongside an understanding of the types of changes occurring as a result. The chapter then focuses on the implications raised by globalization for key functions of public health policy and practice. Many of the issues raised in this chapter are addressed in more detail elsewhere in this textbook, a reflection of the importance of global forces now at play in so many aspects of public health. The chapter concludes by considering the governance issues raised. While the public health community has found itself at the frontline of many of the impacts resulting from globalization, and needing to adapt to many of the changes taking place, it remains somewhat in the background when it comes to shaping and managing globalization. The public health community must increase its capacity to influence such decisions if globalization is to prove a positive force for human health.

What is globalization?

The popular and widespread use of the term 'globalization' has led to considerable variation, and at times lack of clarity, of what it actually means. In many cases, the term has been used to replace 'international', denoting subjects that concern two or more countries. Alternatively, the term is defined more narrowly to refer to increased international trade, the spread of Hollywood films or other relics of western culture, or the greater movement of people across borders. Alongside definitional vagueness lie marked differences in how globalization is normatively assessed. Some writers see globalization as a unifying and progressive force, bringing unprecedented economic growth and prosperity (Dollar & Kraay 2000; Feachem 2001). Others believe that globalization is a new form of colonialism which serves to reinforce inequalities of wealth and power, and consequently health and other social conditions, within and across countries (Cornea 2001; Labonte *et al.* 2005). These differences in perspective are reflected in the highly contested nature of scholarship in this field.

While it is beyond the scope of this chapter to review these debates in detail, including the substantial evidence now accumulating of the costs and benefits of globalization, it is an important starting point to approach the term critically. In the broadest sense, globalization has become widely understood as the closer integration or interconnectedness of human societies across national borders. Different societies have long interacted across vast distances (e.g. migration of the human species out of Africa in one million BC, the Silk Road trade route, and the Age of Discovery from the fifteenth century). Globalization can thus be recognized as an historical process. At the same time, we can see that there are contemporary forms of globalization in which there has been intensified flows of people, other life forms, goods and services, capital, and knowledge across borders to an unprecedented degree since the mid to late twentieth century. In recent decades, not only has there been a vast increase in the quantity of social interaction across populations, but the reach of those linkages to virtually all parts of the world is also new. Held *et al.* (1999) write that it is this greater intensity and extensity of linkages across human societies that define globalization today.

Three types of changes to human societies are occurring as a result of globalization (Lee 2003a). The *spatial dimension* refers to changes to how people organize and interact with physical or territorial space. The now clichéd image of globalization as a shrinking world or 'global village' refers to the extension of economic, political, and social linkages to a worldwide scale. E-mail, long-haul package holidays, cyberspace, and the global operations of transnational corporations are all examples of the restructuring of social space. For the most part, our experience of the world is that it is 'shrinking' because of a greater capacity to access distant locations. In other cases, novel ways of organizing social interactions are emerging, largely through new information and communication technologies. The creation of virtual communities, such as YouTube™ and Facebook®, for example, allow individuals to communicate, and form social connections and networks, irrespective of geographical location.

The *temporal dimension* concerns changes to how we think about and experience time. The contemporary world is largely characterized by an acceleration of the timeframe which things can be, and are expected to be, done. For instance, financial transactions involving currency trading, buying and selling of equities (stocks and shares), and the securing of credit can take place in a matter of seconds through global information and communication systems, even when involving parties located in different parts of the world. Similarly, advances in transportation technology have enabled larger numbers of people to travel greater distances in shorter amounts of time (e.g. bullet train, supersonic jets). Modern life has been one of time pressures to 'multi task', speed dial and 'drive through'.

Third, the *cognitive dimension* concerns changes to how we think about ourselves and the world around us. The dissemination and adoption of knowledge, ideas, values, and beliefs have become worldwide in scale through the global reach of the mass media (including the advertising industry), research and educational institutions, consultancy firms, religious groups, and political parties. The ascendance of English, as the leading language for diplomacy, science, air transportation systems, and entertainment is also a result of cognitive globalization. Some argue that this is leading to the marginalization of local cultures and languages, and corresponding domination by Western values and beliefs defined by individualism and consumerism (Barber 2003). Huntington (2002) warns of a potential 'clash of civilizations' as competing ideologies and value systems come together to cause religious or political conflict. However, others believe cognitive globalization is progressively spreading shared ideas and principles which support human rights, gender equity, environmental and labour standards, and democracy. In public health, Benatar *et al.* (2003) write of the development of global health ethics such as the human rights based approach. Overall, the three types of changes taking place as a result of globalization—spatial, temporal, and cognitive—are closely intertwined, and together are leading to a mixture of positive and negative impacts.

Another point of substantial debate surrounding globalization is an understanding of what is driving these change processes. Globalization is clearly enabled by technological advances which make flows across borders possible. As the capacity of these technologies expands, and the cost of using such technologies decline, they have become more accessible to larger numbers of people. For example, the industrial policies pursued by many governments since the 1970s has emphasized the achievement of increased economic competitiveness through promoting access to cheaper transport and fuel. This has led to a decline per ton of sea and air freight which, in turn, has encouraged the rapid growth of international trade (US Department of Transport 2000; Teitel 2005). Overlooking the environmental impacts, the advent of low cost air travel amid fierce competition has made holidays abroad accessible for the first time to millions of people (Swan 2007). Communication costs have declined even more rapidly. When desktop computers (microcomputers) became commercially available in the late 1970s, a desktop computer cost around US$5000, putting them out of reach of most private users. By 2007, the cost had declined to a few hundred dollars for many times the processing power of the original machines (Lee & Collin 2005). Not surprisingly, information and communication technologies have been frequently cited as the major force behind globalization (Hundley *et al.* 2003).

For some writers, however, technology is an enabler, but not the driver, of globalization. The real factors driving technological developments and their application are, it is argued, economic in nature. The global spread of capitalism has been driven, on the one hand, by untold thousands of producers seeking access to the cheapest inputs (i.e. raw materials, labour, research and development, transport and communications), most efficient (and greatest) economies of scale, and largest potential markets. Millions of consumers around the world, on the other hand, fuel this process by demanding the highest quality and quantity of goods and services at the lowest possible price. The millions of economic transactions that result, what eighteenth century economist Adam Smith called the 'invisible hand' of the market, is seen as the real force behind globalization (Dicken 1999).

A further perspective rejects globalization as an essentially technological or economically driven process which implies a degree of rationality and progress. Instead, some scholars point to current and dominant forms of globalization as driven by certain ideologically-based values and beliefs broadly referred to as neoliberalism. It has been the global spread of this ideology that has, for instance, defined the industrial policies facilitating the development of such technologies (e.g. the promotion of an information economy through deregulation and privatization of telecommunications sector), and their dissemination for particular purposes (e.g. deregulation of financial markets). It is argued that neoliberalism has also defined economic policies which encourage international trade (e.g. trade negotiations), market driven competition, and foreign investment (e.g. tax incentives, and a minimal role for the state at the expense of social welfare and environmental protections (Falk 1999).

Not surprisingly, differences in perspective about the drivers of globalization reflect variation in views about whether, on balance, such changes are beneficial or costly to human societies. So-called globalists (supporters of contemporary globalization) predict a world of closer integration, shared identities, greater efficiency and productivity, more rapid economic growth, and increased prosperity. While there may be bumps to negotiate along the way, such as temporary inequalities in wealth within and among countries, it is believed that the globalization path is progressive in the longer term, and will bring largely benefits for the greatest number of people. In sharp contrast, the opponents of contemporary globalization, who see its associated changes as largely driven by a neoliberal defined agenda, do not agree that the resultant changes taking place are mainly positive. A broad range of individuals and organizations, often referred to as the anti-globalization movement, see fundamental flaws inherent within the assumptions underpinning current globalization processes. Of particular note are stark imbalances in power and influence within the emerging global order, dividing the world into winners (those with access to technology, capital, knowledge and gainful employment) and losers (i.e. poor, unskilled), with the latter far greater in number. Although globalization may generate increased aggregate wealth, critics challenge the assumption that this wealth will eventually 'trickle down' to those at the bottom of the global pecking order. Rather, anti-globalists cite substantial evidence which is strongly suggestive that, without strong commitment to redistributive policies, along with appropriate social and environmental protections, neo-liberal globalization will lead to a widening gap between haves and have-nots including health inequities (Kim *et al.* 2000; Mittelman 2002). Moreover, if allowed to continue unabated, many critics argue that current forms of globalization are socially and environmental unsustainable in the longer term.

This chapter is broadly located within the latter perspective. From a public health perspective, globalization is leading to diverse and complex changes to health determinants, resulting in both positive and negative health outcomes. For the protection and promotion of public health, and to ensure the longer-term sustainability of globalization, these changes must be actively managed to ensure that the positive outweigh the negative impacts, and that any costs to health are equitably and fairly shared across societies. In order to develop effective responses to the public health implications raised by globalization, it is useful to consider in greater detail what changes are taking place.

Features of contemporary globalization

Current forms of globalization can be seen as dominated by the integration and convergence of systems of economic production, distribution and consumption on a worldwide scale. While economist have varied opinions on the precise timing of when these processes began to emerge, most agree that the creation of the Bretton Woods Institutions—the World Bank, International Monetary Fund (IMF) and General Agreement on Tariffs and Trade (GATT) after the Second World War laid its institutional and normative foundations. Each has played an important role in facilitating the emergence of a global economy defined by the liberalization of capital flows, and opening of national markets to trade and investment.

The first major pillar of the global economy, liberalization of capital flows, was introduced in the US from the mid 1970s which, in turn, precipitated a complete restructuring of financial markets across the world. Historically, banks, insurance companies, investment companies, and brokerage firms have been subject to heavy governmental regulation. Deregulation of financial markets, such as the removal of restrictions on the types of securities that financial institutions could trade, levels of interest that could be paid on specific types of securities and bank accounts, and types of institution entitled to act as financial intermediaries, was introduced to increase competitiveness within the market and encourage greater capital flows within and across countries. Information and communication technologies enabled high-speed electronic-based transactions which eventually linked financial markets across countries. The result has been the creation of a globally integrated financial market capable of 24-hour trading in foreign exchange and related money markets, the international capital markets, the commodity market, and the markets for forward contracts, options, swaps, and other derivatives (Valdez 2006). The scale of capital flows has correspondingly boomed. The world's financial assets totaled US$136 trillion in 2005, and will exceed US$228 trillion by 2010. Global crossborder capital flows reached a record US$6 trillion in 2006, more than double their level in 2002. Foreign exchange trading increased from US$17.5 trillion/year to US$1.5 trillion/day between 1979 and 2002 (OECD 2005; McKinsey & Company 2007).

A second key pillar of the global economy is the trade of goods and services. While trade has been the lifeblood of commerce for thousands of years, it is the restructuring and integration of production processes across the world, accompanied by the growth in scale and scope of trade, which characterizes the global economy of recent decades. Historically, trade among countries has been dominated by raw materials and natural resources (e.g. oil, timber), commodities (e.g. grains, metals) or manufactured products (e.g. textiles and clothing, food products). In 1948, the GATT was established as an agreement under which signatories could negotiate reductions in tariffs on traded goods. Originally, the GATT was to become an international organization like the World Bank or IMF. However, without consensus among member states, this could not be achieved. Instead, the GATT remained an agreement under which eight trade rounds were carried out between 1948 and 1994 through which thousands of concessions on tariff reductions were reached. During this period, membership grew from 23 countries in 1947 to 125 countries in 1994, thus establishing a worldwide trading system.

The boom in traded goods and services since 1945 led to renewed support for a permanent organization. In 1995, following the conclusion of the Uruguay Round of trade negotiations, the GATT was replaced by the World Trade Organization (WTO). Membership has since increase to 150 member states, with many more countries seeking accession. Moreover, the scope of the world trading system has broadened to embrace trade in services, agriculture, intellectual property rights, government procurement and other areas (Wilkinson 2006). The overall effect has seen a growth in the scale and range of international trade. Since 1948, world trade has consistently grown faster (6 per cent annually in real terms) than world output (3.9 per cent). In 2006, this trend continued with world merchandise exports increasing by 15 per cent to US$11.76 trillion, and commercial services exports growing by around 11 per cent (US$2.71 trillion) compared with global gross domestic production (GDP) growth of 3.7 per cent (WTO 2007).

The global restructuring of production and exchange processes has been an integral part of the boom in international trade over the past half century. In many sectors, transnational corporations (TNCs) have emerged which have geographically relocated components of their business to different parts of the world (Dicken 1999). Thus, resource extraction may take place in one country, manufacturing in another, and research and marketing in still others. The targeted consumers have also changed, with TNCs increasingly seeing the world as a single marketplace. According to the *Forbes Global 2000*, a ranking of the world's top corporations by sales, profit, assets and market value, the increase in so-called 'global brands' has been a key feature of a restructured world economy. In 2005, *BusinessWeek* ranked the top five global brands (measured as the 'most valuable') as Coca-Cola, Microsoft, IBM, General Electric and Intel (Anon 2005).

While global restructuring has not occurred in all industrial sectors, it can be observed in many sectors with direct or indirect impacts on public health. One important example is the pharmaceutical industry which, as a result of mergers and acquisitions, is today dominated by a small number of large companies. Pharmaceutical companies ranked among the largest 100 global corporations in 2006 led by Pfizer (35), Johnson and Johnson (57), Sanofi Aventis (58), GlaxoSmithKline (82), Novartis (83), Unilever (87), and Roche (97) (Forbes 2006). Table 2.1.1 describes the largest companies in 2004 by sales, growth and market share, all of which are headquartered in major industrialized countries. Table 2.1.2 lists the leading pharmaceutical trading countries, led by Switzerland with a trade surplus of £5561 million in 2004. The overall trend in the sector has been towards larger and fewer companies, controlling a growing share of the market. In 1992, the 10 largest companies accounted for one-third of world revenue (Tarabusi & Vickery 1998). By 2002, this share had increased to one-half (Busfield 2005). The trend towards larger pharmaceutical companies has been driven by global competition. The cost of

Table 2.1.1 Top world pharmaceutical corporations (2007)

	Country	Sales (£) million	Growth* (%)	Market share** (%)
Pfizer	USA	22 292	−2	6.7
GlaxoSmithKline	UK	18 847	1	5.6
Novartis	SWI	17 154	9	5.1
Sanofi Aventis	FRA	16 788	8	5.0
Astrazeneca	UK	15 010	9	4.5
Johnson & Johnson	USA	14 478	5	4.3
Roche	SWI	13 814	18	4.1
Merck & Co	USA	13 631	8	4.1
Abbott	USA	9570	8	2.9
Lilly	USA	8335	13	2.5
Leading 10		**149 920**	**6**	**44.9**
Amgen	USA	8188	1	2.5
Wyeth	USA	7949	8	2.4
Bayer	GER	7020	13	2.1
Bristol-Myers Squibb	USA	6519	6	2.0
Boehringer Ingelheim	GER	6277	11	1.9
Schering-Plough	USA	6181	10	1.9
Takeda	JAP	5479	9	1.6
Teva	ISR	5300	12	1.6
Novo Nordisk	DEN	3336	18	1.0
Daiichi Sankyo	JAP	2925	7	0.9
Leading 20		**209 093**	**7**	**62.6**

* Calculated in US$
** IMS audited markets
Source: Reprinted with permission by the Association of the British Pharmaceutical Industry (ABPI). Available at http://www.abpi.org.uk/statistics/section.asp?sect=1.

research and development (R&D), large-scale manufacturing, and worldwide marketing and distribution, means that successful companies need to be of a certain size with considerable resources. For example, the industry estimates that developing and launching a new drug product onto the world market costs around US$403 million in 2000 (DiMasi *et al.* 2002). The desire to gain access to overseas markets and 'pipeline' products has further encouraged mergers and acquisitions with local companies.

As industry ownership has become more concentrated, and so-called 'Big Pharma' has pursued the most profitable products to recover associated costs, concerns have been raised within the public health community about the neglect of certain diseases and populations deemed to offer insufficient financial returns. For conditions where there are a relatively small number of sufferers, or the potential market is a population unlikely to afford available treatment, companies have not invested resources (Trouiller *et al.* 2002). Another major concern is the assertion of intellectual property rights (IPRs) by pharmaceutical companies over new drugs. Patent protection entitles companies to exclusive marketing rights and to charge higher prices in order to recover R&D investment.

Table 2.1.2   World trade in pharmaceuticals, 2007

	Exports (£)	Imports (£)	Balance (£)
Switzerland	20 206	9336	10 870
Ireland	9664	1520	8144
Germany	24 395	18 810	5586
UK	14 567	10 291	4276
France	13 675	10 135	3540
Sweden	4726	1731	2995
Netherlands	7439	7276	163
Italy	7607	8466	−859
Spain	4142	5227	−1085
Japan	1736	4625	−2889
USA	17 491	35 801	−18 310

Source: Reprinted with permission by the Association of the British Pharmaceutical Industry (ABPI). Available at: http://www.abpi.org.uk/statistics/section.asp?sect=1.

Higher prices, however, has meant reduced access to new drugs by the poor. The need to improve access to essential medicines, such as second line anti-retroviral drugs, to treat major public health problems led to the Doha Declaration on IPRs and Public Health in 2003. Tensions between trade and public health policy, however, persist as practical implementation of the declaration's provisions in low-income countries remains a major challenge (Kerry & Lee 2007).

The food industry has undergone similar pressures to 'go large', with the ascendance of TNCs increasingly controlling food production from 'plow to plate'. The history of food production and consumption is closely linked to the migration of human populations, raising and exchange of food crops, and domestication of animals. The distinct feature of contemporary globalization is the industrialization of food production and consumption into a complex of global businesses (excluding subsistence farming). Among the Fortune Global 500 are food retailers Wal-Mart (2), Carrefour (25), Metro (55), and Tesco (59), and manufacturers Nestlé (53), Unilever (106), and PepsiCo (175), all of which command sizeable proportions of the world market. As global food brands have gained ground, local and small-scale producers have become increasingly marginalized in the name of economies of scale and efficiencies.

The globalization of the food industry raises a wide range of public health issues. The rapid rise in rates of obesity, as discussed further below, has led to concerns about the global trend towards diets high in fat, salt and sugar intake (Cassels 2006). In a follow-up to WHO's Global Strategy on Diet, Physical Activity and Health (WHO 2004), Lang *et al.* (2006) assessed compliance by 25 of the world's largest food manufacturers and retailers to recommendations concerning such factors as ingredients, advertising, portion size, and labelling. The report found only a small proportion of companies acting to reduce salt, sugar, and fats from their products, four (Cadbury Schweppes, Danone, Nestlé, and Unilever) had any policies on advertising, two (Kraft and McDonalds) were acting to reduce portion sizes, and 11 were improving labelling. While the public health community has pushed for stronger

regulation of this hugely powerful industry, governments to date have largely resisted in favour of voluntary codes.

The tobacco industry offers a further example of the public health implications arising from the global restructuring of the world economy. As smoking prevalence has steadily declined in high-income countries, the tobacco industry has turned its efforts to so-called 'emerging markets' in Asia, Africa, Eastern Europe, and Latin America. Consequently, the industry has consolidated through numerous mergers and acquisitions into four transnational tobacco companies (TTCs) which control around 75 per cent of the world cigarette market: Philip Morris, British American Tobacco, Japan Tobacco International, and Imperial Tobacco. This excludes the Chinese National Tobacco Corporation, a state monopoly which supplies 98 per cent of the 300 million smokers in China, the world's largest tobacco market. Importantly, globalization has facilitated the tobacco industry's expansion into emerging markets through trade liberalization, overseas manufacturing, marketing and advertising, and economies of scale (Bettcher & Yach 2000; Callard *et al.* 2001). Consequently, based on current trends, it is predicted that deaths from tobacco use will rise from 5 million in 2006 to 8.4 million by 2020, with 70 per cent occurring in the developing world (WHO 2002b).

Finally, the global economy has a dark underbelly of illicit activity with important implications for public health. Of particular note is the growing problem of smuggled and counterfeit goods. The trade in illegal psychoactive drugs is a serious worldwide problem, with 200 million people (or 5 per cent of the global population age 15–64) having used illicit drugs at least once in the last 12 months. In recent decades, the trade has become global in the number of countries in which (producers and consumers are located), and the transnational network of criminal organizations involved. In 2003, the retail (street) value of the trade was estimated at US$322 billion (United Nations Office on Drugs and Crime 2006). The global nature of cigarette smuggling, representing around 20–25 per cent of total consumption, also poses a major problem by supplying the market with cheaper priced products and thus undermining national tobacco control policies. Counterfeit goods now comprise 5–7 per cent of world trade. Many counterfeits, notably medicines, food products and cigarettes, are of dubious quality and content, and can pose direct risks to public health. WHO estimates that counterfeit drugs account for 10 per cent of all pharmaceuticals, with the number rising to as high as 60 per cent in developing countries. For example, a survey in Nigeria found 80 per cent of drugs distributed in major pharmacies in Lagos to be counterfeit (WHO 2006a). Counterfeit baby milk powder in rural China caused the deaths of 50 children and acute malnutrition in hundreds of others (Watts 2004).

As well as the restructuring of economies, globalization has contributed to unprecedented levels of population mobility in terms of frequency and distance travelled. Population movements are not new—humankind has been on the move since *Homo erectus* migrated out of Africa in one million BC. Mass migrations, both voluntary and forced, have been prompted by the search for food, water, and arable land, and to escape hardship, conflict, and natural disasters. The migration of Europeans to the Americas from 1492 marked a period of large-scale movement of populations over the next 500 years. For example, 15 million slaves were transported from Africa to the Americas during the eighteenth and nineteenth centuries. More than 30 million people moved as indentured workers after the abolition of slavery in 1850. Around 59 million people migrated from Europe to the Americas, Australia, New Zealand, and South Africa between 1849 and 1939 in search of economic opportunities (ILO 2000). Global migration is thus part of an ongoing historical process.

What have characterized population movements since the mid twentieth century are the unprecedented volume, speed, and geographical reach of travel. All regions of the world have seen increasing numbers of people on the move. International migration now accounts for approximately 130 million people (2 per cent of the world's population) per year. Two million people cross international borders daily, and 500 million people cross borders on commercial airlines annually. Between 1995 and 2010, an increase of 80 per cent in long haul travel is predicted (Anon 2007). Total international tourist arrivals reached 842 million in 2006, growing by 20 per cent since 2002. International refugees receiving UN assistance increased from 1.4 million in 1961 to 9.2 million in 2004. It is estimated that 900 000 people were trafficked internationally in 2003. For all of these reasons above, by 2006 up to 200 million people (1 in 33 people) were living outside their country of birth, compared with 75 million in 1965 (UNFPA 2003). Furthermore, internal migration (movement within a single country) has occurred at an even greater magnitude. In the mid-1980s, one billion people, or about one-sixth of the world's population, moved within their own countries (Castles & Miller 2003).

The International Labour Organisation (ILO 2007) reports that, although more people globally are working than ever before, the number of unemployed remained at an all time high (195.2 million) in 2006. For the relatively educated, highly skilled, and mobile, globalization has created new employment opportunities. For the poorly educated and low skilled, globalization has brought employment insecurity. For healthcare, the most direct impact has been the accelerated migration of health workers. While the migration of health workers from poor countries, notably sub Saharan Africa, to the industrialized world has received much needed attention, migration patterns are recognized to be more widespread. The decision to migrate is an individual one, based on personal circumstances and employment prospects, but broader forces shaped by globalization, affecting work and living conditions are also at play (Bach 2003). The *World Health Report 2006* (WHO 2006c) estimates that there are 59.2 million full-time paid health workers worldwide, and an estimated shortage of almost 4.3 million doctors, midwives, nurses, and support workers. The shortage is most critical in 57 countries, especially in sub-Saharan Africa and parts of Southeast Asia. The African region has 24 per cent of the global health burden but only 3 per cent of health workers commanding less than 1 per cent of the world health expenditure. The so-called 'brain drain', caused by the flow of health workers from low- to high-income countries, has gravely worsened this problem. On average one in four doctors and 1 in 20 nurses trained in Africa is working in OECD countries.

The implications of globalization for public health

The Institute of Medicine (1997) defines 'global health' as 'health problems, issues, and concerns that transcend national boundaries, may be influenced by circumstances or experiences in other countries, and are best addressed by cooperative actions and solutions'.

Public health is concerned with improving the health of whole populations, rather than the health of individuals (Walley *et al.* 2001: 19). The US Health and Human Services Public Health Service (1995) identifies 10 core activities of public health:

1. Preventing epidemics

2. Protecting the environment, workplace, food, and water

3. Promoting healthy behaviour

4. Monitoring the health status of the population

5. Mobilizing community action

6. Responding to disasters

7. Assuring the quality, accessibility, and accountability of medical care

8. Reaching out to link high-risk and hard-to-reach people to needed services

9. Researching to develop new insights and innovative solutions

10. Leading the development of sound health policy and planning

Global public health, in this sense, concerns how globalization is impacting on each of these core activity areas. Globalization is not only leading to public health issues transcending national boundaries, but to the need for collective efforts across countries to help shape more socially just and sustainable forms of globalization. The remainder of this chapter examines some of these key functions of public health, how globalization may impact on their practice, and how the public health community might effectively respond to these impacts.

Globalization and the control of infectious disease outbreaks

The prevention, control, and response to, infectious disease outbreaks are a core activity in public health. Historically, disease-causing microbes have travelled across vast distances for as long as mobile human populations have come into contact with each other and other animal species. For example, the shift from hunting-gathering to agrarian societies and the domestication of animals, between 8000 and 3500 BC, led to the emergence and spread of new zoonotic diseases (Swabe 1999). The so-called 'Columbian exchange', following the arrival of Christopher Columbus in the Americas, is noted by historians for the widespread exchange of plants, animals, foods, human populations (including slaves), and ideas that followed. Diseases, such as bubonic plague, cholera, influenza, measles, malaria, smallpox and tuberculosis, were also exchanged, resulting in the decimation of up to 90 per cent of the indigenous American population (Crosby 1972). Another notable example is the influenza pandemic of 1918–1919 at the end of the First World War, which killed around 25 million people. The pandemic similarly demonstrated the capacity of infectious disease to spread across the world amid large-scale human migration and weakened social structures.

Contemporary globalization, characterized by unprecedented volume, speed, and geographical reach of population mobility, is leading to growing evidence that infectious disease outbreaks have a greater capacity to emerge and spread more rapidly and further afield. This is because globalization, in its current forms, potentially influences a broad range of biological, environmental, and social factors that influence human infections.

First, globalization may alter what populations are at risk of certain infections. The Global Burden of Disease Study estimates that infectious diseases were responsible for 22 per cent of all deaths and 27 per cent of disability-adjusted life years worldwide in 2000 (Lopez *et al.* 2006). Many infections continue to disproportionately affect the poor within and across countries, and globalization can worsen their vulnerability by, for example, contributing to rapid urbanization without sufficient attention to basic needs such as water, sanitation, gainful employment, and healthcare. This lesson was gradually recognized in nineteenth-century Europe during the Industrial Revolution, which prompted social reforms that eventually led to a decline in infectious diseases, and vast improvements in health status, during the first half of the twentieth century. Today, it is no coincidence that infectious diseases still account for a large proportion of death and disability among those who have been excluded from, and in many cases bear a disproportionate share of the costs associated with, globalization processes.

At the same time, globalization can 'democratize' certain infectious diseases, making all populations vulnerable to them. While tuberculosis and cholera are diseases historically associated with poverty, because of the role of poor quality housing and sanitation in their spread, other infections do not discriminate by socioeconomic class. Some infections, such as measles, diphtheria, and tetanus, can be caught by any population, but vaccination reduces their reach. Where prevention is not possible, such as pandemic influenza, the consequences for whole populations, regardless of socioeconomic status, can be devastating. The rapid and extensive reaction to the outbreak of severe acute respiratory syndrome (SARS) in 2002–2003 was due to the perceived vulnerability of all populations, rich or poor (Woollacott 2003). Moreover, the rapid spread of SARS from China to around 25 countries within weeks, illustrated how quickly infectious diseases can spread within a globalized world. There are similar concerns about the potential for avian influenza to cause a human influenza pandemic of unprecedented proportions amid globalization.

Second, globalization may influence the *prevalence* (number of people with a disease within a given population) and *incidence* (number of new cases of a disease in a specified period of time per total population) of infectious diseases. De Vogli and Birbeck (2005) argue that vulnerability to HIV/AIDS, tuberculosis, and malaria is closely linked to poverty, gender inequality, development policy, and health sector reforms that involve user fees and reduced access to care. Dorling *et al.* (2006) similarly argue that 'global inequality in wealth will have compounded the effects of AIDS on Africa', notably caused by globalization-related policies such as structural adjustment programmes.

Third, globalization may influence the emergence of novel infections or re-emergence of diseases previously in decline. Environmental degradation, such as the felling of rainforests or dumping of toxic wastes, can increase contact with new sources of infection or lead to mutation of existing infectious agents (e.g. cholera Bengal). Perhaps the most worrying potential 'public health emergency of international concern' is an influenza pandemic involving a highly pathogenic strain such as H5N1. Intense animal rearing practices, alongside human populations, is believed to be contributing to an increased risk of antigenic shift of the influenza virus. The prospect of an influenza pandemic spreading across continents today has led to unprecedented efforts to prepare and coordinate across countries and regions (Lee & Fidler 2007).

The SARS outbreak provided a worrying example, not only of the speed and reach of outbreaks, but the weak capacity by public health systems around the world to cope with a large-scale outbreak of this kind.

A cautionary note should be appended here. To prove that globalization is responsible for the increasing prevalence of a specific infection would require standardized monitoring of the exposure (the process of globalization being studied), the outcome (incidence of a particular infectious disease), and other determinants of disease (e.g. immunity, treatment, socioeconomic factors) over many years. The necessary studies would be extremely difficult to construct, and highly vulnerable to confounding due to new and unforeseen factors developing out of the enormous transformations occurring in most aspects of contemporary political, economic and cultural life. In addition, surveillance systems describing the incidence and prevalence of infectious diseases over time are very rare, particularly for populations in low-income countries, who are often the most likely to experience the adverse health effects of global transformations. Even if a causal association were detected, there would likely be considerable dispute over whether the relevant process, for instance global warming, was in fact caused by globalization. Thus, the assessment of health risks associated with globalization must accommodate much unavoidable uncertainty (Saker *et al.* 2006). This does not mean that no conclusions should be drawn on the influence of global processes on past, present and future disease patterns. Indeed, poor or absent supportive evidence of the benefits of globalization has not dissuaded proponents of unregulated economic globalization from arguing forcefully for its introduction. The need to respond in situations where we do not have full and incontrovertible evidence for our actions is well expressed by the precautionary principle: 'Where there are threats of serious or irreversible damage, lack of full scientific certainty shall not be used for postponing cost-effective measures' (UN Conference on the Environment and Development 1992).

The perceived heightening of infectious disease risks from a globalizing world has prompted actions to develop more effective public health responses. Alongside risks, globalization brings opportunities to improve the capacity of public health institutions to respond more effectively to infectious disease outbreaks. Foremost is the advent of new information and communication technologies which, in principle, enable faster, cheaper, and more efficient gathering and sharing of knowledge. ProMED-mail (see Box 2.1.1) and regional disease surveillance networks have sprung up to facilitate the collection and reporting of epidemiological data. The lessons learned from SARS led to renewed efforts to revise the International Health Regulations (IHR), which came into effect in 2007, to harness a broader range of information sources. Another change is the expansion of the scope of the IHR beyond named diseases, notably plague, yellow fever, and cholera, to the broader term 'public health emergencies of international concern'. This may include human or natural disasters. Beyond surveillance, technological advances are also permitting faster development, such as drugs, vaccines, because of the capacity for more rapid development and testing, and potential dissemination of new knowledge within the medical research community (WHO 2005).

Protecting environmental health in a global context

The discipline of environmental health concerns 'the theory and practice of assessing, correcting, controlling, and preventing those

---

Box 2.1.1 Programme for Monitoring Emerging Diseases (ProMED-mail)

The Programme for Monitoring Emerging Diseases (ProMED)—mail was established in 1994, with the support of the Federation of American Scientists and SatelLife, as an Internet-based reporting system dedicated to rapid global dissemination of information on outbreaks of infectious diseases and acute exposures to toxins that affect human health, including those in animals and in plants grown for food or animal feed. Electronic communications enable ProMED-mail to provide up-to-date and reliable news about threats to human, animal, and food plant health around the world, seven days a week.

By providing early warning of outbreaks of emerging and re-emerging diseases, public health precautions at all levels can be taken in a timely manner to prevent epidemic transmission and to save lives.

ProMED-mail is open to all sources and free of political constraints. Sources of information include media reports, official reports, online summaries, local observers, and others. Reports are often contributed by ProMED-mail subscribers. A team of expert human, plant, and animal disease moderators screen, review, and investigate reports before posting to the network. Reports are distributed by email to direct subscribers and posted immediately on the ProMED-mail Web site. ProMED-mail currently reaches over 30 000 subscribers in at least 150 countries.

A central purpose of ProMED-mail is to promote communication amongst the international infectious disease community, including scientists, physicians, epidemiologists, public health professionals, and others interested in infectious diseases on a global scale. ProMED-mail encourages subscribers to participate in discussions on infectious disease concerns, to respond to requests for information, and to collaborate together in outbreak investigations and prevention efforts. ProMED-mail also welcomes the participation of interested persons outside of the health and biomedical professions.

Source: International Society for Infectious Diseases. About ProMED-mail. http://www.promedmail.org/pls/promed/f?p=2400:1950:17 654933971171386906 (accessed 12 March 2007)

---

factors in the environment that can potentially affect adversely the health of present and future generations' (Pencheon *et al.* 2001: 206–207). Environmental threats to public health range from local, small-scale factors (e.g. household exposures) to widespread exposures affecting whole populations. Protecting against a perceived environmental health threat involves identifying the hazard, determining the relationship between the hazard and the effect (dose-response assessment), exposure assessment, and risk characterization.

The possible impacts of globalization on environmental health are wide-ranging, going beyond global-scale threats to potentially affecting populations at the regional, community, occupational and household levels. Impacts from globalization can be direct, such as through the transport and dumping of hazard waste across borders, relocation of hazardous occupations (such as ship breaking in low-income countries), or damage caused by acid rain or a nuclear accident. Economic globalization, in which companies compete on a worldwide scale to increase returns, are raising concerns that there are incentives to undermine environmental health. Governments, seeking to attract foreign direct investment to fuel economic growth and employment, may engage in a so-called 'race to the bottom' by offering reduced taxation rates, low wages, or weak environmental, health and safety protections (Brecher & Costello 1994). As stated by the environmental organization, the Sierra Club (2000), 'By promoting economic growth without adequate environmental safeguards, trade increases the overall scale and pace of resource consumption; promotes adoption of high-consumption, high-polluting lifestyles; and prompts countries to seek international advantage by weakening, not raising, environmental protections'. China's rapid integration into the global economy, for example, has come at the cost of severe environmental degradation:

Scores of rivers have dried up in northern China over the past 20 years. More than 75 per cent of river waters are not suitable for drinking or fishing. China's cities are an environmental

disaster, since urban infrastructure has not kept up with the influx of people. Many cities face serious sanitation problems, with sewage and wastewater going straight into rivers. Large cities, including Beijing, are smothered in smog. Old and weak people are often warned to stay indoors. Between 2001 and 2020 almost 600 000 people in China are expected to suffer premature death every year due to urban air pollution. (Lovgren 2005)

The World Bank (2000) argues that '[e]very society has to decide for itself on the relative value it places on economic output and the environment'. Others argue, however, that there can be substantial inequity in who bears the environmental costs. In addition, many of the environmental impacts can affect more than one country and can even be global in scope. More commitment is thus needed to better balance the 'tradeoffs' between economic growth and environmental protection, including a fuller understanding of environmental health risks.

In managing this trade-off, the indirect effects of globalization on environmental health must also be recognized. A change in investment or lending policy by a global financial institution, such as the IMF, can have health consequences for local communities. For example, policy conditions set by the World Bank, or requirements to repay substantial sums of foreign debt, can restrict the public expenditure of borrowing countries on environmental protection or investment in basic infrastructure, such as water and sanitation. A cholera outbreak in South Africa in 2000–2001, which led to around 120 000 cases and 265 deaths, has been blamed on the introduction of user fees following the privatization of water utilities as part of the country's structural adjustment programme. As water supplies were cut to poor people unable to pay for the new charges, many resorted to using polluted river water (Anon 2006). Today, more than 2.6 billion people—over 40 per cent of the world's population—do not have access to basic sanitation, and more than one billion people still use unsafe sources of drinking water

(WHO/UNICEF 2006). Predictions of the growing scarcity of fresh water supplies globally, and the continued trend towards the privatization of water utilities with ownership dominated by large TNCs, is likely to worsen this situation.

The capacity of the public health community to correct, control, and prevent environmental health risks can be affected by globalization. For example, globalization poses additional challenges for identifying a hazard. In a more interconnected world, causal relations can become more extended and complex. The tasks associated with identifying a hazard must take account of factors that extend far beyond national borders, a greater range of stakeholders, and jurisdictions that lie beyond the reach of public health authorities. A good example is the increase in reported outbreaks of foodborne illnesses involving more than one country which has been linked, in part, to the globalization of the food industry (Kaferstein et al. 1997; Hall 2002). Tracing the source and cause of such an outbreak can be hindered by inadequate recordkeeping in some countries, lack of timely sharing of information, inconsistency in labelling, or lack of access to production facilities abroad. The work of environmental health workers can be made even more difficult by hazards arising from illicit activities such as dumping, counterfeiting or smuggling across borders (Kimball 2006).

The undertaking of risk assessment, defined as 'the process of estimating the potential impact of a chemical, physical, microbiological, or psycho-social hazard on a specified human population or ecological system under a specific set of conditions and for a certain timeframe' (Pencheon et al. 2001: 208), is also made more challenging by globalization. The population of interest may be widely dispersed, because of their mobility or transience, and identifying and measuring a suspected hazard requires large-scale analysis. Weiland et al. (2004) study 650 000 subjects as part of the International Study of Asthma and Allergies in Childhood. A collaboration with 155 participating centres worldwide, it is the first study 'to take a global view [of] . . . the relationship between asthma and eczema and climate' (Graham 2004).

Global health promotion

The rapid growth of the health burden from non-communicable diseases (NCDs) worldwide in recent decades, such as ischemic heart disease, cancer, and diabetes (Beaglehole & Yach 2003; Matthews & Pramming 2003) has led to growing attention to the need for global approaches to health promotion (Lee 2007). NCDs are the leading causes of death and disability worldwide. Disease rates from these conditions are accelerating globally, advancing across every region and pervading all socioeconomic classes. The *World Health Report 2002: Reducing risks, promoting healthy life*, indicates that the mortality, morbidity, and disability attributed to the major chronic diseases currently account for almost 60 per cent of all deaths and 43 per cent of the global burden of disease. By 2020, their contribution is expected to rise to 73 per cent of all deaths and 60 per cent of the global burden of disease. Moreover, 79 per cent of the deaths attributed to these diseases occur in the developing countries. Four of the most prominent chronic diseases—cardiovascular diseases (CVD), cancer, chronic obstructive pulmonary disease, and type 2 diabetes—are linked by common and preventable biological risk factors, notably high blood pressure, high blood cholesterol and overweight, and by related major behavioural risk factors: Unhealthy diet, physical inactivity, and tobacco use. Action to prevent these major chronic diseases should focus on controlling these and other key risk factors in a well-integrated manner.

Health promotion is the process of enabling people to increase control over, and to improve, their health (WHO 1986). Interventions address three areas of activity in order to prevent disease and promote the health of a community: Communication, service delivery, and structural (enabling factor) components (Walley et al. 2001: 147). A global approach to health promotion takes into account the ways in which globalization may be influencing the broad determinants of health, and health behaviours, as well as offering opportunities for providing appropriate interventions. The adoption of the Bangkok Charter for Health Promotion in a Globalized World in 2005 was in recognition of the major challenges, actions, and commitments needed to address the determinants of health in a globalized world by reaching out to people, groups, and organizations that are critical to the achievement of health. How this might be achieved can be understood in relation to two key issues—obesity and tobacco control.

The rapid increase in the incidence of overnutrition and obesity, among both adults and children, has attracted substantial public health concern in recent years (Taubes 1998). According to WHO and the International Obesity Taskforce (IOTF), around 300 million people worldwide are obese (BMI > 30), with levels continuing to rise rapidly in the early twenty-first century. At least 155 million school-age children are overweight or obese, with 30–45 million classified as obese. This accounts for 2–3 per cent of the world's children aged 5–17 years. In the EU, childhood obesity is described as 'out of control':

> The number of children affected by overweight and obesity is now rising at more than 400 000 a year and already affects almost one in four across the entire EU, including accession countries in 2002. The new prevalence of 24 per cent in 2002 is five points higher than had been expected based on original trends in the 80s and is already higher than the predicted peak for 2010. (IOTF 2004)

Also, the obesity epidemic is not limited to high-income countries. Changes in diet, levels of physical activity, and nutrition (known as the 'nutrition transition') have led to sharp increases in rates of obesity in such wide ranging countries as India, Thailand, Brazil, and China. As Drewnoski and Popkin (1997: 32) write:

> Whereas high-fat diets and Western eating habits were once restricted to the rich industrialized nations . . . the nutrition transition now occurs in nations with much lower levels of gross national product (GNP) than previously. . . . First, fat consumption is less dependent on GNP than ever before. Second, rapid urbanization has a major influence in accelerating the nutrition transition.

Similarly, Prentice (2006) links the trend to globalization of food production and lifestyles:

> The pandemic is transmitted through the vectors of subsidized agriculture and multinational companies providing cheap, highly refined fats, oils, and carbohydrates, labour-saving mechanized devices, affordable motorized transport, and the seductions of sedentary pastimes such as television. This trend has been linked

to the globalisation of sedentary lifestyles alongside changes in food production and consumption.

Many interventions to address the obesity epidemic have focused on the modification of individual behaviours, such as healthy eating initiatives and the promotion of physical activity. Global health promotion, however, must also seek to tackle the structural factors that constrain or enable lifestyle choices. This includes what and how food is produced and marketed by an increasingly globalized food industry. For example, the Institute of Medicine (2005) report, *Food Marketing to Children and Youth: Threat or Opportunity?* recognizes that dietary patterns begin in childhood and are shaped by an interplay of many factors—genetics and biology, culture and values, economics, physical and social environments, and commercial media environments. Importantly, the report provides the most comprehensive review to date of the scientific evidence on the influence of food marketing on diets and diet-related health of children and youth. It argues that environments supportive of good health require leadership and action from the food, beverage, and restaurant industries; food retailers and trade associations; the entertainment industry and the media; parents and caregivers; schools; and the government.

Global-level regulation of food-related industries, however, remains problematic. The process of adopting the WHO Global Strategy on Diet, Physical Activity and Health was fraught with efforts by the food industry to avoid the setting of explicit recommendations on healthy levels of salt, sugar, and fats intake, amid calls for binding regulation of marketing, labelling and other industry activities by public health advocates (Lang *et al.* 2006). In the US, the politically powerful food industry has instead succeeded in promoting self-regulation. As Kelly (2005) writes:

> *The global hegemony of the United States in the production and marketing of food, while a marvel of economic success, has contributed to the epidemic of obesity that is particularly afflicting children. So far the U.S. government has declined to regulate the aggressive ways in which food producers market high-energy, low-nutrition foods to young people. That public-health responsibility has been left to an industry-created scheme of self-regulation that is deeply flawed; there is a compelling need for government involvement.*

Lessons for global health promotion can also be drawn from efforts to strengthen tobacco control worldwide. As described above, the globalization of the tobacco industry has led to a rise in tobacco consumption, facilitated by the industry's consolidation, greater economies of scale, and aggressive marketing strategies to gain entry to emerging markets (Bettcher & Yach 2000). WHO initiated negotiations for a Framework Convention on Tobacco Control (FCTC) in the mid 1990s in recognition of the need to globalize tobacco control policies (Reid 2005). Referring to the impact of globalization on the tobacco pandemic, then WHO Director-General Gro Harlem Brundtland stated:

> *[O]ver the past fifteen years, we have seen that modern technology, has limited the effectiveness of national action. Tobacco advertising is beamed into every country via satellite and cable. Developing countries are the subject of massive marketing campaigns by international tobacco companies. In the slipstream of increasing global trade, new markets are opened to international tobacco companies which see these emerging markets as their main opportunity to compensate for stagnant or dwindling markets in many industrialized countries.* (Brundtland 2000)

As the first multilaterally negotiated public health treaty, the FCTC negotiation process encompassed regional consultations, public hearings, contributions by civil society organizations, and old-fashioned diplomacy among WHO's 192 member states. The process also faced extensive efforts by the powerful tobacco industry to undermine negotiations through seeking representation on some national delegations, lobbying of tobacco producing countries and farmers, orchestrated criticism of WHO for neglecting other public health priorities, and even challenges to long established science on tobacco and health (Lynn & Lerner 2002; Waxman 2002; Hammond & Assunta 2003).

Despite persistent industry opposition, public health advocates prevailed in successfully adopting a comprehensive treaty which sets out measures to address both the supply of and demand for tobacco. As of October 2008, 168 countries have signed, and 160 countries have fully ratified the treaty. Importantly, the FCTC represents a collective effort across WHO member states to address a clear global public health challenge. The involvement of a broad spectrum of stakeholders, notably civil society organizations, was critical to raising public awareness and support at the regional, national and local levels. The mobilization of public health advocates, led by the Framework Convention Alliance, was greatly facilitated by the use of the Internet (focused on the *Globalink* network) which allowed groups to keep abreast of negotiations, organize advocacy activities, and share experiences to an unprecedented degree (Collin *et al.* 2004). While weaker on some aspects of globalization, such as international trade, than initially hoped, the treaty will accommodate other transborder issues such as smuggling and marketing (e.g. sports sponsorship, satellite broadcasting) through the negotiation of additional protocols.

Initiating high-profile policies, such as the Global Strategy on Diet, Physical Activity and Health and the FCTC, can raise the profile of health promotion and be effective vehicles for addressing the global aspects of the challenges faced. The experiences of established campaigns, such as the WHO/UNICEF International Code on the Marketing of Breastmilk Substitutes and Health Cities Initiative, and more recently initiatives such as the Public–Private Partnership for Handwashing, shows that adoption of agreements is a starting point. Implementation requires longer term mobilization of political will, resources and technical capacity to translate commitments into effective action. In the context of globalization, trade flows, information and communication technologies, and marketing strategies are beginning to be harnessed for health promotion purposes. For example, the tobacco control community has developed countermarketing campaigns to challenge the use of advertising imagery associating cigarette smoking with glamour and excitement in emerging markets (Box 2.1.2). Worldwide consumer boycotts of TNCs, such as Nestlé and McDonalds, have been organized to pressure companies to change their marketing practices or unhealthy product ranges (Yach & Beaglehole 2003).

In summary, the global spread of unhealthy lifestyles and behaviours pose new challenges for health promotion. In many cases,

Box 2.1.2

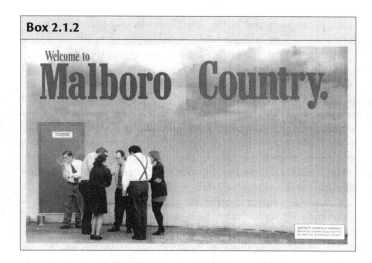

powerful vested interests within key sectors of the global economy have facilitated this process through foreign investment, production, trade and marketing practices. There is accumulating evidence that these practices are resulting in a sharp increase in NCDs. The public health community faces major challenges in influencing these practices, as well as opportunities to harness aspects of globalization to promote healthier lifestyles and behaviours. Collective efforts across countries to appropriately regulate harmful aspects of the global economy is clearly needed.

Monitoring the health status of the population

Assessing the health of a given population is the starting point for a wide range of public health activities such as policy reviews, programme development, goal setting and resource allocation. There are well recognized steps for assessing population health status:

◆ Define the purpose of the assessment

◆ Define the population concerned and any comparator population

◆ Define the aspects of health to be considered

◆ Identify and review existing data sources

◆ Select the most appropriate existing data (Gentle 2001)

In assessing the linkages between globalization and population health status, two challenges are presented. First, there is variable capacity across countries to collect and manage basic health data. Data remains of poor quality or limited in availability in many low- and middle-income countries. According to WHO (2006b):

A country health information system comprises the multiple sub-systems and data sources that together contribute to generating health information, including vital registration, censuses and surveys, disease surveillance and response, service statistics and health management information, financial data, and resource tracking. The absence of consensus on the relative strengths, usefulness, feasibility, and cost-efficiency of different data collection approaches has resulted in a plethora of separate and often overlapping systems. Too often, inappropriate use is made of particular data collection methods, for example, the use of household surveys to produce information on adult mortality.

The WHO Health Metrics Network (HMN) is a global partnership working to strengthen and align health information systems around the world. The partnership is comprised of countries, multilateral and bilateral development agencies, foundations, global health initiatives, and technical experts that aim to increase the availability and use of timely, reliable health information by catalysing the funding and development of core health information systems in developing countries. As described by WHO:

HMN partners agree to align around a common framework that sets the standards for health information systems. The HMN framework will serve to define the systems needed at country and global levels, along with the standards, capacities and processes for generating, analysing, disseminating, and using health information. It links the normative framework for measurement in health with participatory assessment, planning, and implementation modalities that are objective, transparent, and include all stakeholders. Thus, it focuses the inputs of donors and technical agencies around a country-owned plan for health information development, thereby reducing the overlap and duplication. At both the country and global level, the HMN framework will enable access to and use of health information, thereby serving the needs of individual countries while also generating global public goods.

In seeking to improve health information systems, a second challenge is the limitations of existing data sources in capturing health needs that cut across the national level (i.e. transnational). For each country, health data is collected and managed by a department of health and associated institutions. The WHO Statistical Information System (WHOSIS), in turn, collects and coordinates data on core health indicators, mortality and health status, disease statistics, health system statistics, risk factors and health service coverage, and inequities in health from its 192 member states. This is compiled in the *World Health Statistics*. By definition, globalization is eroding, and even transcending, national borders so that health and disease patterns may be emerging that do not conform to such delineations. As a result, national level data may need to be aggregated and disaggregated in novel ways to reveal these new patterns.

A good example is the above discussed increase in obesity rates. Improving data on trends in different countries reveal a complex picture. In high-income countries, obesity is rising rapidly across all social classes but is particularly associated with social deprivation. In the UK, for example:

Obesity is linked to social class, being more common among those in the routine or semi-routine occupational groups than the managerial and professional groups. The link is stronger among women. In 2001, 30 per cent of women in routine occupations were classified as obese compared with 16 per cent in higher managerial and professional occupations. (UK Office of National Statistics Office)

In France, Romon *et al.* (2005) found that genetic predisposition influences the prevalence of obesity and changes in body mass index (BMI) among children from the higher social class. For children within the lowest social class, which has seen an increase in BMI across the whole population, environmental factors appear to have

Table 2.1.3 Per cent of population that is overweight, selected countries, 2002 and 2010 (Projected)

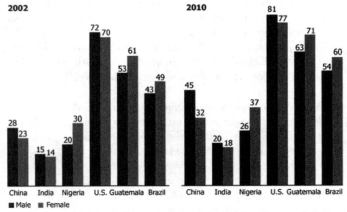

Note: 'Overweight' is defined as having a body mass index (weight in kilograms divided by height in metres squared) of between 25 and 30. 'Obese' is defined as having a body mass index of 30 or more.

Source: Reprinted with permission from the Population Reference Bureau.

played a more important role. In contrast, in low- and middle-income countries, the total number of obese or overweight people is projected to grow by 50 per cent by 2015 alongside the persistence of undernutrition (Table 2.1.3). Social class is one factor. In such diverse countries as Kenya, China, India, and Brazil, obesity among an increasingly affluent middle class has been observed (McLellan 2002). A high BMI may even be considered socially desirable as a sign of affluence. At the same time, some populations within the lower social classes are also experiencing rising rates of overweight and obesity. For example, Monteiro *et al.* (2004) find that a country's level of wealth is an important factor, with obesity starting to fuel health inequities in the developing world when the GNP reaches a value of about US$2500 per capita. Trends in over/undernutrition, in other words, are complex and changing over time, and require sufficiently detailed and comparable data across population groups defined along additional variables (e.g. gender, socioeconomic status, occupation).

The need to improve available data on the health of populations affected by globalization is illustrated by a wide range of other examples. The outsourcing of manufacturing to the developing world by TNCs, for example, has led to the employment of hundreds of thousands of workers. What public health needs to these workers have and are they addressed by local occupational health policies? Similarly, the greater movement of people across national borders may require increased attention to the health needs of different types of migrants. Alternatively, what public health issues arise for populations from global environmental change? All of these examples suggest the need to redefine new population groups within a global context, and to develop data sources that measure population health patterns which do not conform to national borders.

The governance of global public health

Governance broadly concerns the agreed actions and means adopted by a society to promote collective action and solutions in pursuit of common goals. Governance takes place whenever people seek to organize themselves to achieve a shared end through agreed

rules, procedures, and institutions. This can take place at different levels of decision-making and action. In public health, if a local community decides to initiate a campaign to slow traffic speed and improve road safety, this requires some form of governance to organize the effort. If a global campaign is initiated to strengthen tuberculosis control, an agreed form of governance is needed to take decisions, for example, on agreed treatment, resource mobilization, and implementation of agreed actions across countries. To what extent is there need for more effective governance to protect and promote global public health? What rules, procedures, and institutions do we need to improve the protection and promotion of public health within an increasingly globalized context.

The existing institutional architecture for global health development and cooperation traces its historical roots to the International Sanitary Conferences of the nineteenth century. This series of meetings, largely dominated by European countries, focused on protecting trading interests from certain epidemic diseases such as cholera and plague. The institutions eventually created, such as the *Office International d'Hygiène Publique*, were primarily concerned with collecting and disseminating epidemiological data on these diseases (Fidler 2001). The creation of the WHO as a specialized agency of the United Nations in 1948 was intended to universalize the membership, and broaden the scope of, international health cooperation. Its objective, 'the attainment by all peoples of the highest possible level of health', was reflected in the vast array of programmes initiated under WHO's auspices.

Recent decades have seen challenges to WHO's designated role as 'the directing and co-ordinating authority on international health work' [WHO Constitution, Article 2(a)]. In part, this has arisen from differences in perspective on whether WHO should be biomedically (disease) focused, or whether the organization should address the broad determinants of 'health for all'. These debates have been accompanied by rapid changes in WHO's operating environment, with the ascendance of new institutional players and ideological perspectives. From the 1980s, the World Bank became a major influence as the biggest source of financing for health development (Buse 1994), while other UN bodies such as the UN Children's Fund and UN Development Programme (UNDP) expanded their health portfolios. The 1990s saw the creation of numerous global public-private partnerships for health which attracted additional resources, but rendered the policy environment far more complex and crowded (Buse & Walt 2000). In recent years, charitable foundations led by the Gates Foundation, have also become major players in the funding of health projects in the developing world (Birn 2005). This influx of institutions and resources has, on the one hand, reflected the higher priority to health development given by governments, corporations and civil society organizations. On the other hand, there is substantial evidence of overlapping mandates, duplication of effort, and, above all, a lack of collective strategic thinking about how to effectively tackle the public health challenges posed by globalization.

The governance of global public health can thus be presently seen as undergoing a period of transition. In principle, the formal institutions governing public health remain focused on governments. Public health authority lies within the ministries of health of each WHO member state, and collaboration across countries and regions takes place on a wide range of functions through governmental bodies. However, as described in this chapter, intensified flows of people, other life forms, goods and services, capital, and knowledge are influencing the determinants of health and health outcomes in diverse ways. Effective regulation of these flows can require collective action across governments and, in some cases, the participation of institutions beyond government. Many scholars of global governance point to the need for new institutional arrangements, a kind of political globalization, to enable more effective action. As Homedes and Ugalde (2003) write, 'If international health problems are to be solved, political, cultural, and social interdependence need to be built with the same impetus by which policymakers promote international trade'. Examples described in this chapter—such as tobacco control, food and nutrition, and infectious disease outbreaks—demonstrate the need for innovation.

What can the public health community do to foster such innovation? Globalization is now an established subject of discussion and debate at public health meetings around the world, and there has been no shortage of commitments to address its impacts. The Final Communiqué of the 13th Commonwealth Health Ministers Meeting (2001) included attention to the 'Impact of Globalisation on Health' as follows:

In discussing globalisation, Ministers identified poverty as the main obstacle to development. Poverty prevents countries from exploiting the potential benefits of globalisation, which has the effect of widening the gap between rich and poor countries. Ministers urged the Commonwealth to develop structured responses to globalisation that would promote positive impact on health. These responses should acknowledge the inextricable links between health and the wider socio-economic development agenda. They should take account of moral and ethical considerations relating to equity in resource distribution.

Ministers expressed strong views about the imposition of conditions linked to development assistance, such as the removal of public subsidies. This militates against the development efforts of poorer countries, and is unfair if not applied in the same way to the more developed countries. Ministers urged the Commonwealth to work for fairness in financing and ensure that the rules apply to developing and developed countries alike.

In 2001, the World Federation of Public Health Associations issued a Call to Action which commits itself to work with WHO 'to clarify areas of emerging public health risk associated with globalization, ranging from infectious and occupational diseases to diseases which are a product of the growing world-scale of anti-health forces' (World Federation of Public Health Associations 2001). The Mumbai Declaration of the People's Health Movement, agreed in 2004, calls for an end to 'corporate-led globalization' (People's Health Movement 2004). The Sixth Global Conference on Health Promotion in 2005 issued the Bangkok Charter which identifies actions, commitments and pledges required to address the determinants of health in a globalized world through health promotion.

Given widespread recognition of the need to address the impacts of globalization within the public health community, the essential next step is to seek influence within those policy communities which drive contemporary globalization. Public health representation within ongoing trade negotiations, for example, is critical. WHO and other public health institutions have so far remained marginal observers in the WTO and other key decision-making forums.

The controversy surrounding intellectual property rights and access to medicines, the substantial concern by consumers about the social and environmental harms of globalization, and the potential costs to the global economy of a major infectious disease pandemic demonstrate the scope for greater collaboration across sectors. Lee *et al.* (2007) describe the potential role of health impact assessment for informing non-health-policy proposals. The global public goods for health approach addresses the growing globalization of health from an economic perspective. The concept identifies where a good or service (such as knowledge of an infectious disease outbreak), which would be of benefit globally, will not be produced or disseminated if left to the market because no one can be excluded from accessing the good, and thus no charge can be levied for its use and no costs recouped. At the national level, the production of these goods is usually ensured by government intervention, but at the global level there remains no 'global government' to undertake this role. Certain functions of public health may be classed as global public goods (e.g. immunization programmes, disease surveillance), which require collective action to overcome market failures (Smith *et al.* 2003). The concept might thus be an appealing rationale to non health policy makers shaping global change.

Conclusion

This chapter has described key ways in which globalization is relevant to the theory and practice of public health. There are both threats and opportunities arising from the complex and diverse changes created by globalization, although current forms of globalization is clearly characterized by an inequitable distribution of winners and losers. For the public health community, there is a need to understand and contribute to more effective management of the rapid changes taking place. Greater attention to these public health impacts will, in turn, contribute to more socially and environmentally sustainable forms of globalization.

References

Anon (2005). Global Brand Scorecard, The 100 Top Brands. *BusinessWeek*, 1 August.

Anon (2006). Report: Water problems remain in rural areas. *Guardian* and *Mail*, 12 July.

Anon (2007). World tourism marks another record year with 842 million arrivals, UN agency reports. *UN News Service*, 30 January. http://www.un.org/apps/news/story.asp?NewsID=21383&Cr=tourism&Cr1=# (accessed 26 March 2007).

Bach, S. (2003). International migration of health workers: labour and social issues. Working Paper, Sectoral Activities Programme, ILO, Geneva. http://www.ilo.org/public/english/dialogue/sector/papers/health/wp209.pdf (accessed 26 March 2007).

Barber, B. (2003). Jihad vs McWorld. In *The Globalization Reader* (eds. H. Lechner and J. Boli), pp. 21–26. Blackwell Publishing, London.

Beaglehole, R., and Yach, D. (2003). Globalisation and the prevention and control of non-communicable disease: the neglected chronic diseases of adults. *Lancet*, **362**, 903–6.

Benatar, S., Daar, A.S., and Singer, P.A. (2003). Global health ethics: the rationale for mutual caring. *International Affairs*, **79**(1), 107–38.

Bettcher, D.W., and Yach, D. (2000). Globalisation of tobacco industry influence and new global responses. *Tobacco Control*, **9**(2), 206–16.

Birn, A.E. (2005). Gates's grandest challenge: transcending technology as public health ideology. *Lancet*, **366**(9484), 514–9.

Brecher and Costello (1994), *Global Village or Global Pillage, Economic Reconstruction from the Bottom Up*, South End Press, Cambridge, MA.

Brundtland, G.H. (2000). Opening Statement. First Meeting of Intergovernmental Negotiating Body, Framework Convention on Tobacco Control, Geneva, 16 October. http://www.who.int/director-general/speeches/2000/english/20001016_tobacco_control.html (accessed 27 March 2007).

Buse, K. (1994). Spotlight on international organizations: The World Bank. *Health Policy and Planning*, **9**, 95–9.

Buse, K., and Walt, G. (2000). Global public-private partnerships: Part I – a new development in health? *Bulletin of the World Health Organisation*, **78**(4), 549–61.

Busfield, J. (2005). The globalization of the pharmaceutical industry. In *Global change and health* (eds. K. Lee and J. Collin), pp. 94–110. Open University Press, Maidenhead.

Callard, C., Chitanondh, H., and Weissman, R. (2001). Why trade and investment liberalisation may threaten effective tobacco control efforts. *Tobacco Control*, **10**, 68–70.

Castles, S., and Miller, M. (2003). *The Age of Migration, International Population Movements in the Modern World, 3rd edition*. Macmillan, London.

Collin, J., Lee, K., and Bissell, K. (2004). Negotiating the Framework Convention on Tobacco Control: The politics of global health governance. In *The Global Governance Reader* (eds. R. Wilkinson and C. Murphy), pp. 254–73, Routledge, London.

Commonwealth Health Ministers Meeting (2001). *13th Commonwealth Health Ministers Meeting Final Communiqué*, 25–29 November, Christchurch, New Zealand. http://www.thecommonwealth.org/document/34293/35232/35242/13th_commonwealth_health_ministers_meeting_final_c.htm (accessed 20 June 2007).

Cornea, G.A. (2001). Globalization and Health: results and options. *Bulletin of the World Health Organization*, **79**(9), 834–41.

Crosby, A. (1972). *The Columbian Exchange: Biological & Cultural Consequences of 1492*. Greenwood Press, Connecticut.

De Vogli, R., and Birbeck, G.L. (2005). Potential Impact of Adjustment Policies on Vulnerability of Women and Children to HIV/AIDS in Sub-Saharan Africa. *Journal of Health Population and Nutrition*, **23**, 105–20.

Dicken, P. (1999). *Global Shift, Transforming the World Economy*. Paul Chapman Publishing, London.

diMasi, J.A., Hansen, R.W., and Grabowski, H.G. (2002). The price of innovation: new estimates of drug development costs. *Journal of Health Economics*, **22**, 151–85.

Dollar, D., and Kraay, A. (2000). Growth is good for the poor. *Research Paper*, World Bank, Washington DC.

Dorling, D., Shaw, M., and Davey Smith, G. (2006). Global inequality of life expectancy due to AIDS. *BMJ*, **332**, 662–4.

Drewnoski, A., and Popkin, B. (1997). The Nutrition Transition: New Trends in the Global Diet. *Nutrition Reviews*, **55**(2), 31–43.

Falk, R. (1999). *Predatory globalization, a critique*. Polity Press, London.

Feachem, R. (2001). Globalisation is good for your health, mostly. *BMJ*, **323**, 504–6.

Fidler, D. (2001). The globalization of public health: the first 100 years of international health diplomacy. *Bulletin of the World Health Organization*, **79**(9), 842–9.

Forbes (2000). *The world's biggest public companies*. http://www.forbes.com/lists/2006/18/Rank_1.html (accessed 20 June 2007).

Gentle, P. (2001). Assessing health status. In *Oxford handbook of public health practice* (eds. D. Pencheon, C. Guest, D. Melzer and J.A. Muir Gray). Oxford University Press, Oxford.

Graham, S. (2004). Global Study Links Climate to Rates of Childhood Asthma. *Scientific American*, 21 June. http://scientificamerican.com/article.cfm?chanID=sa003&articleID=000624A7-66A2-10D3-A6A283414B7F0000 (accessed 27 March 2007).

Hall, G., D'Souza, R.M., and Kirk, M. (2002). Foodborne disease in the new millennium: out of the frying pan into the fire? *MJA*, **177**(11/12), 614–8.

Hammond, R., and Assunta, M. (2003). The Framework Convention on Tobacco Control: promising start, uncertain future. *Tobacco Control*, **12**(3), 241–2.

Held, D., McGrew, A., Goldblatt, D., and Perraton, J. (1999). *Global transformations*. Stanford University Press, Stanford.

Homedes, N., and Ugalde, A. (2003). Globalization and Health at the United States-Mexico Border. *American Journal of Public Health*, **93**(12), 2016–22.

Hundley, R.O., Anderson, R.H., Bikson, T.K., and Neu, C.R. (2003). *The Global Course of the Information Revolution, Recurring Themes and Regional Variations*. RAND National Defense Research Institute, Washington DC.

Huntington, S. (2002), *The Clash of Civilizations and the Remaking of World Order, 2nd edition*. Free Press, New York.

ILO (2007). *Global Employment Trends Brief 2007*. International Labour Organisation, Geneva. http://www.ilo.org/public/english/employment/strat/download/getb07en.pdf (accessed 20 June 2007).

ILO (2000), *Workers without Frontiers - The Impact of Globalization on International Migration*. International Labour Organization, Geneva.

IMF (2005). The IMF and the Fight against Money Laundering and the Financing Of Terrorism. *Fact Sheet*, September, Washington DC. http://www.imf.org/external/x10/changecss/changestyle.aspx (accessed 13 March 2007).

Institute of Medicine (1997). *America's Vital Interest in Global Health*. National Academy Press, Washington DC.

Institute of Medicine (2005). *Food Marketing to Children and Youth: Threat or Opportunity?* National Academy Press, Washington DC.

IOTF (2004). EU childhood obesity 'out of control'. *Press Release*, International Obesity Taskforce, Geneva. http://www.iotf.org/popout.asp?linkto=http://www.iotf.org/media/IOTFmay28.pdf (accessed 28 March 2007).

Kaferstein, F.K., Motarjemi, Y., and Bettcher, D.W. (1997). Foodborne disease control: A transnational challenge. *Emerging Infectious Diseases*, **3**(4), 503–10.

Kawachi, I., and Wamala, S. (eds.) (2006). *Globalization and Health*. Oxford University Press, Oxford.

Kelly, D. (2005). To quell obesity, who should regulate food marketing to children? *Globalization and Health*, 1(9). http://www.globalizationandhealth.com/content/1/1/9

Kerry, V.B., and Lee, K. (2007). TRIPS, the Doha declaration and paragraph 6 decision: what are the remaining steps for protecting access to medicines? *Globalization and Health*, **3**(3), 1–12.

Kim, J.Y., Irwin, A., Millen, J., and Gershman, J. (2000). *Dying for Growth: Global inequality and the health of the poor*. Common Courage Press, Monroe ME.

Korten. D. (1995) *When Corporations Ruled the World*. Kumerian Press and Berrett-Koehler, Bloomfield, Connecticut.

Kimball, A.M. (2006), *Risky Trade Infectious Disease in the Era of Global Trade*. Ashgate, London.

Labonte, R., Schrecker, T., and Sen Gupta, A. (2005). *Health for some: death, disease and disparity in a globalizing world*. Centre for Social Justice, Toronto.

Lang, T., Rayner, G., and Kaelin, E. (2006). *The Food Industry, Diet, Physical Activity and Health: a Review of Reported Commitments and Practice of 25 of the World's Largest Food Companies*. Centre for Food Policy, City University, London. http://www.city.ac.uk/news/press/The%20Food%20Industry%20Diet%20Physical%20Activity%20and%20Health.pdf (accessed 13 June 2007).

Lee, K. (2003a). *Globalization and health, an introduction*. Palgrave Macmillan, London.

Lee K. ed. (2003b). *Health impacts of globalization, towards global governance*. Palgrave Macmillan, London.

Lee, K. (2007). Global health promotion: How can we strengthen governance and build effective strategies? *Health Promotion International*, **21**(1), 42–50.

Lee, K., and Collin, J. (eds.) (2005). *Global change and health*. Open University Press, Maidenhead.

Lee, K., and Fidler, D. (2007). Avian and pandemic influenza: Progress and problems for global governance. *Global Public Health*, **2**(3), 215–34.

Lee, K., Ingram, A., Lock, K., and McInnes, C. (2007). Bridging health and foreign policy: The role of health impact assessment? *Bulletin of the World Health Organization*, **85**(3), 207–11.

Lopez, A., Mathers, C.D., Ezzati, M., Jamison, D.T., and Murray, C.J.L. (2006). *Global burden of disease and risk factors*. World Bank Publications, Washington DC.

Lovgren, G. (2005). China's Boom is Bust for Global Environment, Study Warns. *National Geographic*, 16 May. http://news.nationalgeographic.com/news/2005/05/0516_050516_chinaeco.html (accessed 23 March 2007).

Lynn, P., and Lerner, D. (2002). NGOs release new hard-hitting evidence of global tobacco industry tactics to subvert public policy. *Press Release*, 20 March, Corporate Accountability International, Boston. http://www.stopcorporateabuse.org/cms/page1294.cfm (accessed 15 June 2007).

Matthews, D., and Pramming, S. (2003). Diabetes and the global burden of non-communicable disease. *Lancet*, **362**(9397), 1763–4.

McKinsey Global Institute (2007). *Mapping the global capital markets, third annual report*. McKinsey & Company, San Francisco.

McLellan, F. (2002). Obesity rising to alarming levels around the world. *Lancet*, **359**(315), 1412.

Mittelman, J.H. (2002). Making globalization work for the have nots. *International Journal on World Peace*, **19**(2), 3–25.

Monteiro, C.A., Conde, W.L., Lu, B., and Popkin, B.M. (2004). Obesity and inequities in health in the developing world. *International Journal of Obesity*, **28**(9), 1181–6.

OECD (2005). *Measuring Globalisation, OECD Economic globalisation indicators*. Organisation for Economic Cooperation and Development, Paris.

Pencheon, D., Guest, C., Melzer, D., Muir Gray, J.A. (2001). *Oxford handbook of public health practice*. Oxford University Press, Oxford.

People's Health Movement (2004). *The Mumbai Declaration from the 3rd International Forum for the Defence of People's Health*. 14–15 January, Mumbai, India. http://www.phmovement.org/files/md-english.pdf (accessed 15 June 2007).

Prentice, A. (2006). The emerging epidemic of obesity in developing countries. *International Journal of Epidemiology*, **35**(1), 93–9.

Reid, R. (2005). *Globalizing Tobacco Control, Anti-smoking campaigns in California, France, and Japan*. Indiana University Press, Bloomington.

Romon, M., Duhamel, A., Collinet, N., and Weill, J. (2005). Influence of social class on time trends in BMI distribution in 5-year-old French children from 1989 to 1999. *International Journal of Obesity*, **29**, 54–59.

Saker, L., Lee, K., and Cannito, B. (2006). Globalization and infectious disease. In *Globalization and Health* (eds. I. Kawachi, I., and S. Wamala), pp. 19–38, Oxford University Press, Oxford.

Sierra Club (2000). *Comments to the Trade Policy Staff Committee, United States Trade Representative*, 20 May, Washington DC. http://www.sierraclub.org/trade/summit/testimony2.asp (accessed 20 June 2007).

Smith, R., Beaglehole, R., Woodward, D., and Drager, N. (eds.) (2005). *Global public goods for health, Health economic and public health perspectives*. Oxford University Press, Oxford.

Swabe, J. (1999). *Animals, disease, and human society: human-animal relations and the rise of veterinary medicine*. Routledge, London.

Swan, W. (2007). Misunderstandings about airline growth. *Journal of Air Transport Management*, **13**(1), 3–8.

Tarabusi, C., and Vickery, G. (1998). Globalization in the pharmaceutical industry. *International Journal of Health Services*, **28**(1), 67–105.

Taubes, G. (1998). As obesity rates rise, experts struggle to explain why. *Science*, **280**(5368), 1367–8.

Teitel, S. (2005). Globalization and its disconnects. *Journal of Socio-Economics*, **34**(4), 444–70.

Trouiller, P., Olliaro, P., Torreele, E., Orbinski, J., Laing, R., and Ford, N. (2002). Drug development for neglected diseases: a deficient market and a public-health policy failure. *Lancet*, **359**(9324): 2188–94.

UK Office for National Statistics (2001). *Obesity among adults: by sex and NS-SeC, 2001: Social Trends 34*. London. http://www.statistics.gov.uk/STATBASE/Product.asp?vlnk=11130&More=Y (accessed 15 June 2007).

UN Conference on the Environment and Development (1992). Rio Declaration on Environment and Development. Rio de Janiero, Brazil. http://www.un.org/documents/ga/conf151/aconf15126-1annex1.htm (accessed 20 June 2007).

UN Office on Drugs and Crime (2006). *2006 World Drug Report*. New York. http://www.unodc.org/pdf/WDR_2006/wdr2006_volume2.pdf (accessed 13 June 2007).

US Health and Human Services Public Health Service (1995). *For a healthy nation: returns on investment in public health*. US Government Printing Office, Washington DC.

Valdez, S. (2006). *An introduction to global financial markets*. Palgrave Macmillan, London.

Walley, J., Wright, J., and Hubley, J. (2001). *Public Health, an action guide to improving health in developing countries*. Oxford University Press, Oxford.

Watts, J. (2004). Chinese baby milk blamed for 50 deaths. The Guardian, 21 April. http://www.guardian.co.uk/china/story/0,7369,1196996,00.html (accessed 13 June 2007).

Waxman, H. (2002). The Future of the Global Tobacco Treaty Negotiations. *New England Journal of Medicine*, **346**(12), 21 March, 936–9.

Weiland, S.K., Hüsing, A., Strachan, Rzehak, P., Pearce, N., and the ISAAC Phase One Study Group (2004). Climate and the prevalence of symptoms of asthma, allergic rhinitis and atopic eczema in children. *Occupational and Environmental Medicine*, **61**(7), 609–15.

Wilkinson, R. (2006). *The WTO, Crisis and the governance of global trade*. Routledge, London.

World Bank (2000). Is Globalization Causing A 'Race To The Bottom' In Environmental Standards? *Briefing Papers*, April, PREM Economic Policy Group and Development Economics Group, Washington DC. http://www1.worldbank.org/economicpolicy/globalization/documents/AssessingGlobalizationP4.pdf (accessed 27 March 2007).

World Federation of Public Health Associations (2001). Public Health and Globalization. Proposed by the Resolutions Committee, WFPHA 35th Annual Meeting, 14 May, Washington DC. http://www.wfpha.org/pdf/01.23%20Public%20Health%20and%20Globalization.pdf (accessed 15 June 2007).

WHO (1986). *The Ottawa Charter for Health Promotion*. First International Conference on Health Promotion, Ottawa, 21 November 1986.

WHO (2002a). *Global Crises – Global Solutions, Managing public health emergencies of international concern through the revised International Health Regulations*. International Health Regulations Revision Project, Geneva.

WHO (2002b). WHO Atlas maps global tobacco epidemic. *Press Release*, 15 October, Tobacco Free Initiative, Geneva. http://www.who.int/mediacentre/news/releases/pr82/en/ (accessed 13 June 2007).

WHO (2004). *Global strategy on diet, physical activity and health*. WHA57.17, 57th World Health Assembly, Geneva.

WHO (2005). The World Health Assembly adopts resolution WHA59.2 on application of the International Health Regulations (2005). to strengthen pandemic preparedness and response. Epidemic and Pandemic Alert and Response, Geneva. http://www.who.int/csr/ihr/wharesolution2006/en/index.html (accessed 20 June 2007).

WHO (2006a). Counterfeit medicines. *Fact Sheet No. 275*, 14 November, Geneva. http://www.who.int/mediacentre/factsheets/fs275/en/print.html (accessed 13 June 2007).

WHO (2006b). *Health Metric Network (HMN) Workshop – better health information systems.* Health Metrics Network, Geneva. http://www.who.int/healthmetrics/news/20061027/en/index.html (accessed 20 June 2007).

WHO (2006c). *World Health Report 2006 – Working together for health.* Geneva.

WHO/International Obesity Taskforce (2000), *Obesity – Preventing and Managing the Global Epidemic.* WHO, Geneva.

WHO/UNICEF (2006). *Meeting the MDG drinking-water and sanitation target: the urban and rural challenge of the decade.* Water, Sanitation and Health, Geneva. http://www.who.int/water_sanitation_health/monitoring/jmpfinal.pdf (accessed 27 March 2007).

WHO/WTO (2002). The WTO Agreements relevant to health. In *WTO Agreements and Public Health* (Geneva: WHO/WTO).

Woollacott, M. (2003). The new killer threatening rich and poor alike. The Guardian, 25 April. http://www.guardian.co.uk/comment/story/0,,943179,00.html (accessed 20 June 2007).

WTO (2007). Risks lie ahead following stronger trade in 2006, WTO reports. *Press Release*, 472, Geneva. http://www.wto.org/english/news_e/pres07_e/pr472_e.htm (accessed 13 June 2007).

Yach, D., and Beaglehole, R. (2003). Globalization of Risks for Chronic Diseases Demands Global Solutions. *Perspectives on Global Development and Technology*, **3**(1–2), 1–21.

Overview and framework

Orielle Solar, Alec Irwin, and Jeanette Vega

Introduction

This chapter presents a conceptual framework within which to understand the multiple determinants that shape patterns of disease and well-being in populations. This provides a basis for evaluating where and how public health can intervene most effectively to improve health, particularly for vulnerable groups. This chapter starts from the premise that the central challenges for public health today include not just improving average health indicators, but reducing the unfair differences in health that currently exist among social groups, between and within countries. In other words, public health practice must be concerned with strengthening health equity. Getting to grips with this challenge requires finding answers to three fundamental problems:

1. Where do health differences among social groups originate, if we trace them back to their deepest roots?

2. What pathways lead from root causes to the stark differences in health status observed at the population level?

3. In light of the answers to the first two questions, where and how should we intervene to reduce health inequities?

This chapter seeks to provide a framework that can establish responses to the first two of these questions, in particular. Later chapters will investigate specific health determinant topics in greater detail. Our discussion here paints in the 'big picture' within which the more detailed analyses reveal their full meaning.

We begin by defining key concepts. We then review influential paradigms for understanding health determinants. Subsequent sections present a conceptual framework for analysis and action on the determinants of health, paying special attention to the determinants of health inequities. A final section sketches implications of this model for public health policy and practice. This chapter reflects work undertaken from 2004 to 2007 within the former Department of Equity, Poverty and Social Determinants of Health[1], World Health Organization, in connection with the WHO-sponsored Commission on the Social Determinants of Health (Solar & Irwin 2007).

Key concepts

Clarity on the meaning of a number of basic concepts is required for the arguments developed in this chapter, and for understanding

how this discussion relates to later chapters in this volume and to ongoing debates in public health.

Health equity

Recent decades have seen broad gains in life expectancy and other average health indicators in most regions of the world. At the same time, however, gaps in health status between population groups are increasing, within and between countries. During the past two decades, some regions, in particular sub-Saharan Africa and parts of the former Soviet Union, have experienced stagnation or even reversals of earlier progress in population health indicators. In turn, the impact of these reversals has been unevenly distributed across social groups within the countries and regions concerned. In light of these trends, *health equity* has emerged as a defining challenge for public health practice in the early twenty-first century.

The WHO Department of Equity, Poverty and Social Determinants of Health defines health equity as 'the absence of unfair and avoidable or remediable differences in health among population groups defined socially, economically, demographically, or geographically' (WHO 2004). In essence, health inequities are health differences which are: Socially produced; systematic in their distribution across the population; and unfair (Dahlgren & Whitehead 2006). Identifying a health difference as inequitable is not an objective description, but necessarily implies an appeal to ethical norms (Braveman & Gruskin 2003).

Awareness of health inequities is hardly a new phenomenon. Historians have found evidence of lucid observation of the inequitable impacts of occupation and social status on health in Egyptian papyri written thousands of years before the Common Era (Sigerist 1943; Berlinguer 2006). In recent times, public health and political leaders' concern with inequities has tended to rise and fall somewhat cyclically. The Alma-Ata Declaration on Primary Health Care (1978) and the Ottawa Charter on Health Promotion (1986) were moments in which the special health needs of poor and vulnerable populations, and hence health equity as a policy goal, emerged strongly in international debates. The Alma-Ata Declaration laid out a vision of equitable health improvement based on 'development in the spirit of social justice' (WHO and UNICEF, 1978). Primary healthcare as defined at Alma-Ata included the creation of healthy living and working conditions through intersectoral programmes. It was expected that such programmes would favour rapid health gains among poor and vulnerable populations.

---

[1] Now the Department of Ethics, Equity, Trade and Human Rights.

During the later 1980s and 1990s, in contrast, equity as a guiding principle for health and social policy receded, arguably as the result of neoliberal economic models emphasizing market-based solutions in health and a reduced redistributive role for the state, within a geopolitical context marked by the collapse of communism and the ascendancy of corporate-driven globalization (see Chapter 2.1).

Epidemiological research has clarified the nature and scope of health inequities through investigations revealing the existence of persistent *social gradients in health* for a wide variety of health indicators. The Whitehall Study of health outcomes among British civil servants was pioneering in this regard (Marmot *et al.* 1978). The Whitehall Study went beyond confirming the long-standing perception that the rich live longer, healthier lives than the very deprived. It showed that, even among relatively well-off members of society, a social gradient in health exists, with the most privileged category showing better outcomes than the group immediately below, which in turn enjoys better health than the category just beneath it, and so forth. Similar patterns have since been documented in numerous contexts around the world. The gradient effect is observed for practically all diseases and health status measures and across all segments of the socioeconomic spectrum. Action on health equity must grapple explicitly with the challenges posed by the social gradient (Graham & Kelly 2004).

During the late 1990s and early 2000s, evidence accumulated that existing global and national health policies had failed to reduce inequities, and indeed that substantial progress in average health indicators had been accompanied by widening health gaps between privileged and disadvantaged groups. Momentum for new, equity-focused approaches grew, at first primarily in wealthy countries. In recent years, public health's responsibility to confront health inequities at global, national, and local levels has been increasingly recognized (Evans *et al.* 2001).

Determinants of health

The determinants of health include all those factors that exert an influence on the health of individuals and populations. Classically, several major categories of health determinants have been identified, including: Genetic determinants; the impact of the natural environment; behavioural factors; and social, economic, cultural, and political arrangements. The many important factors that fall under the latter category are grouped together under the concept of 'social determinants of health'.

The concept of social determinants of health has been defined broadly to include the full set of social conditions in which people live and work, summarized in Tarlov's phrase as 'the social characteristics within which living takes place' (Tarlov 1996). Within the field encompassed by this concept, not all factors have equal importance. Causal hierarchies can be ascertained. The factors that directly determine individual health outcomes are not the same as the forces that shape the distribution of disease and well-being across populations. The conceptual framework elaborated in this chapter is fundamentally concerned with clarifying these distinctions and making explicit the relationships between underlying determinants of health inequities among social groups and the more immediate determinants of individual health.

Paradigms for understanding health determinants

In the contemporary context, several quite different paradigms coexist and inform public health policy and practice. These paradigms can be complementary. However, they may also lead to contradictory options. Here, we discuss three influential paradigms, which respectively emphasize biomedical interventions; individual lifestyle and behavioural factors; and a more comprehensive social approach to health.

The biomedical paradigm emerged in the late 1800s based on bacteriological discoveries and has been strengthened by advances in pharmacology and medical technology throughout the past century. This paradigm is essentially focused on deploying technological responses to disease at the level of the individual human body and its constituent organs. Primary emphasis tends to be on treating and when possible curing existing pathologies, rather than on preventive or promotive strategies. The current concern with genetic factors in disease processes is an outgrowth of the biomedical model, with distinctive long-term prospects for both curative and preventive techniques (see Chapter 2.4). The biomedical approach continues to constitute the dominant paradigm in health action today. The continued primacy of the biomedical model cannot be separated from economic motives and the high profits generated by the pharmaceutical industry and other components of the 'medical-industrial complex' (cf. Chapter 2.1).

An approach to health based on so-called 'lifestyle' and other behavioural determinants gained increased attention beginning in the 1970s. The 1974 Lalonde Report to the Canadian government acted as an important trigger. Lalonde argued that health for the majority of the population could not be attained through a concentration of public resources on personal medical services. The report described four major influences on the health field: Human biology, environment, lifestyle, and healthcare organization. In some respects, this analysis offered a welcome challenge to the biomedical model. Unfortunately, however, Lalonde's emphasis on health risks linked to individual lifestyle choices downplayed the differential impact of socioeconomic structures and political processes on people's opportunities for health. Instead, Lalonde's analysis lent itself to an interpretation of health as largely a matter of personal decision-making and hence private responsibility. In the international arena, this argument unintentionally played into the hands of neoliberal constituencies pressing for curtailment of state responsibility in the health sector, accompanied by aggressive privatization. While this was not Lalonde's intention, the report set precedents for a narrow, decontextualized understanding of 'lifestyle' and personal risk factors detached from social and political analysis (Colgrove 2002; Szreter 2002). This tendency has been dominant in many subsequent health promotion programmes.

In contrast to the narrow focus on individual behaviours and lifestyle choices, traditions in critical public health have developed more comprehensive paradigms that analyse the effects of a complex array of social and political factors on health outcomes. An understanding of the impact of structural social forces on health informed the work of some of the nineteenth century pioneers of modern public health. Rudolf Virchow (1985 [1848]), for example, wrote: 'Do we not always find the diseases of the populace traceable to defects in society?' This concept does not refer only to the direct impact on population health of the organization of the labour market and of social policy, including welfare state policies.

Rather, this structural perspective recognizes that a given model of social organization determines and shapes to a significant extent the options individuals have and their possibilities for changing their behaviour. During the twentieth century, traditions of social medicine developed in several global regions, from the Nordic countries to Latin America. These traditions have analysed the impact of socioeconomic structures on health and linked health progress for disadvantaged groups to community self-empowerment and movements for political and social change (Tajer 2003).

Different theories on the social patterning of disease

Epidemiological research has shown with increasing clarity that patterns of disease within populations are socially produced. This is already an important basic step towards answering the question of the origins of health differences among population groups. However, this insight leaves many questions still unanswered. Over recent years, various theoretical models have emerged to explain the processes through which social conditions and people's experience of life in society translate into differential health outcomes.

Among epidemiologists who acknowledge the primary shaping impact of social arrangements on health and illness, two major schools of thought have emerged. These can be labelled as: (1) Psychosocial approaches; (2) approaches that emphasize the social production of disease through the lens of what can be termed the political economy of health. These theoretical directions are not mutually exclusive. Both approaches seek to elucidate principles capable of explaining social inequalities in health, and both represent what Krieger has called theories of disease distribution, which presume but cannot be reduced to mechanism-oriented theories of disease causation. These approaches differ in their respective emphasis on particular social and biological factors that influence population health, how they integrate social and biological explanations, and thus in their recommendations for action (Krieger 2001, 2005).

The first school places primary emphasis on *psychosocial factors*, and is associated with the view that people's 'perception and experience of personal status in unequal societies lead to stress and poor health' (Raphael 2006; Raphael & Bryant 2006). This school traces its origins to a classic study by Cassel (1976), in which he argued that stress from the 'social environment' alters host susceptibility, affecting neuroendocrine function in ways that increase the organism's vulnerability to disease. More recent researchers, prominently including Richard Wilkinson, have sought to link altered neuroendocrine patterns and compromised health capability to people's perception and experience of their place in social hierarchies. According to these theorists, the experience of living in social settings of inequality forces people constantly to compare their status, possessions, and other life circumstances with those of others, engendering shame and anger in the disadvantaged, along with chronic stress that undermines health. At the level of society as a whole, meanwhile, steep hierarchies in income and social status weaken social cohesion, with this disintegration of social bonds also seen as negative for health. This research has inspired a substantial literature on the relationship between (perceptions of) social inequality, psychobiological mechanisms, and health status

(e.g. Lynch *et al.* 2001; Marmot & Wilkinson 2001; Lobmayer & Wilkinson 2002; Marmot 2004; Wilkinson & Pickett 2006).

The contrasting *social production of disease/political economy of health* framework is sometimes also described as a materialist or neomaterialist position. Researchers adopting this approach do not deny negative psychosocial consequences of income inequality. However, they argue that interpretation of links between income inequality and health must begin with the structural causes of inequalities and emphasize inequality's material aspects, instead of focusing primarily on perceptions of inequality. Under this interpretation, the effect of income inequality on health reflects both lack of resources held by individuals, and systematic under-investments across a wide range of community infrastructure (Kaplan *et al.* 1996; Lynch *et al.* 1998). Economic processes and political decisions condition the private resources available to individuals and shape the nature of public infrastructure—education, health services, transportation, environmental controls, availability of food, quality of housing, occupational health regulations—that forms the 'neomaterial' matrix of contemporary life. Thus, income inequality per se is but one manifestation of a cluster of material conditions that affect population health (Davey Smith 2003).

Recently, some innovative theoretical approaches have opened new perspectives. Krieger's 'ecosocial' approach and other emerging multilevel frameworks have sought to integrate social and biological reasoning and a dynamic, historical, and ecological perspective to develop new insights into determinants of population distribution of disease (Krieger 2001, 2002, 2005). Krieger's notion of 'embodiment' is a suggestive concept 'referring to how we literally incorporate biologically influences from the material and social world in which we live, from conception to death; a corollary is that no aspect of our biology can be understood absent knowledge of history and individual and societal ways of living'. Armed with such constructs, Krieger (2001) argues, 'we can begin to elucidate population patterns of health, diseases, and well-being as biological expressions of social relations'.

These alternative theoretical directions in social epidemiology have given rise to strident polemics, but they can largely be reconciled. All contribute to an understanding of social differences in health. In order to draw full benefit from their respective insights, the contributions of these models must be situated within a comprehensive framework enabling us to visualize the complete causal chain of determinants that engender health inequities.

A framework for analysis and action on the determinants of health

Our goal is to present a framework that can provide clear answers to the first two questions that guide our discussion in this chapter: i.e. What causes health inequities, and what pathways lead from root causes to measured differences in health status among population groups. In addition, the framework described below defines levels of policy intervention on health determinants and helps suggest the potential scope and limits of policy action in each area. This aspect will be taken up more extensively in later sections. A comprehensive health determinants framework should achieve the following:

(a) Identify the determinants of health and the determinants of inequities in health

(b) Show how major determinants relate to each other

(c) Clarify the mechanisms by which social determinants generate health inequities

(d) Provide criteria for evaluating which determinants are the most important to address

The framework presented below draws substantially on the contributions of many previous researchers, prominently including Finn Diderichsen. Diderichsen's and Hallqvist's 1998 model of the social production of disease was subsequently adapted by Diderichsen, Evans, and Whitehead (2001). The concept of social position is at the centre of Diderichsen's interpretation of 'the mechanisms of health inequality' (Diderichsen 1998). In its initial formulation, Diderichsen's model emphasized the pathway from society through social position and specific exposures to health status. The framework was subsequently elaborated to give greater emphasis to 'mechanisms that play a role in stratifying health outcomes', including 'those central engines of society that generate and distribute power, wealth and risks' (Diderichsen *et al.* 2001) Diderichsen's model showed that these 'engines' give rise to social stratification that in turn engenders differential exposure to health-damaging conditions and differential vulnerability, depending on where people are placed within the social hierarchy. The concept of differential vulnerability includes both health conditions per se and people's ability to access material resources to respond to health problems. Social stratification likewise determines differential consequences of ill health for more and less advantaged groups. An injury or episode of illness is likely to have very different consequences for the life of a person living precariously at the bottom of the socioeconomic scale than for someone belonging to a more privileged category, with easier access to material resources and support options. The unequal results of ill health include economic and social consequences, as well as differential health outcomes as such.

Power as a factor in the social production of disease

Before examining in detail the proposed framework for the analysis of health determinants and health equity, it is important to discuss explicitly an underlying factor sometimes ignored in such discussions: Power. As a critical factor shaping social hierarchies and thus conditioning health differences among groups, power demands careful analysis from researchers concerned with health equity and the determinants of health. Understanding the causal processes that underlie health inequities, and assessing realistically what may be done to alter them, requires understanding how power operates in multiple dimensions of economic, social, and political relationships. On the other hand, while power is 'arguably the single most important organizing concept in social and political theory' (Ball 1992), this central concept remains contested and subject to diverse and often contradictory interpretations.

Recent social theory, particularly feminist theory, has shown the importance of distinguishing among several fundamental types of power: (1) 'Power over' (the ability to influence or coerce); (2) 'power to' (understood as the capacity to organize and change existing hierarchies in society); (3) 'power with' (power from collective action); and (4) 'power within' (power from individual consciousness) (Luttrell & Quiroz 2007). The coercive aspect of political, economic, and social power obviously has considerable relevance for analysing the forces undermining health opportunities for oppressed social groups. On the other hand, the dimension of power as collective action also carries promise for alternative models of public health action based on the empowerment of vulnerable communities.

An understanding of power as collective action connects suggestively with a model of social ethics based on human rights. As one commentary has argued: 'Throughout its history, the struggle for human rights . . . has consisted of one basic reality: A demand by oppressed and marginalized social groups and classes for the exercise of their social power' (Instituto de Estudios Politicos para America Latina y Africa 2005). Understood in this way, a human rights agenda means supporting the collective action of historically dominated communities to analyse, resist, and overcome oppression, asserting their shared power and altering social hierarchies in the direction of greater equity.

Theories of power remind us that any serious effort to reduce health inequities will involve changing the distribution of power within society to the benefit of disadvantaged groups. Changes in power relationships can take place at various levels, from the 'micro' level of interpersonal dynamics within individual households or workplaces to the 'macro' sphere of structural relations among social constituencies, mediated through economic, social, and political institutions. Power analysis makes clear, however, that micro-level modifications will be insufficient to reduce health inequities unless micro-level action is supported and reinforced through structural changes. By definition, then, action on the social determinants of health inequities is a political process that engages both the agency of disadvantaged communities and the responsibility of the state.

The emphasis on state action and the significance for marginalized groups of expressing their power politically takes on added importance, given the recent spread of largely de-politicized models of 'empowerment' in mainstream international development discourse and practice. Critics have observed how the idea of empowerment, originally generated in the context of grassroots movements pressing for redistribution of social, economic, and political power to marginalized groups, has been increasingly appropriated by mainstream development actors, such as the World Bank. In some contexts where these organizations have exerted influence, 'community empowerment' has arguably been reinterpreted as a substitute for substantial political and economic change, rather than a means to achieve it (Luttrell & Quiroz 2007). In practice, 'empowerment' of civil society and community groups often functions as a code word sanctioning government withdrawal from responsibility for service provision in health and social protection. Communities are 'empowered' to tackle their own health and underlying socioeconomic problems—meaning that they are given sole responsibility for doing so, but often without the financial and institutional resources needed to exercise this responsibility. For this reason, it is vital that those planning and implementing public health agendas be specific about what they mean by terms like 'empowerment', and about how public health policies will contribute to vulnerable people's capacity to control the factors that influence their health.

Introduction to the framework

The framework illustrated in Fig. 2.2.1 defines the major domains that must be differentiated and analysed in order to arrive at satisfactory answers to our guiding questions. This section offers an initial overview of the major components of the framework. Subsequent sections will analyse each specific component in detail.

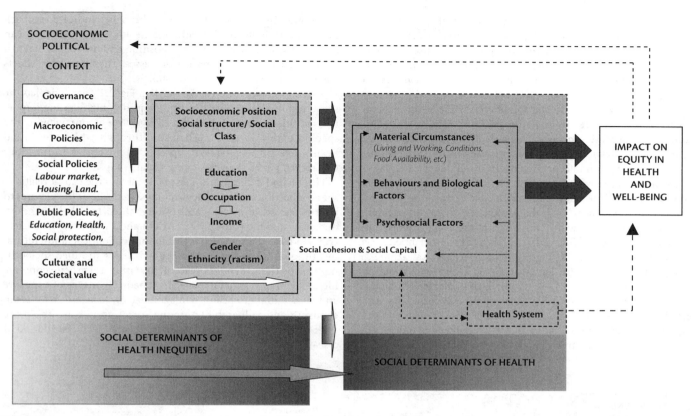

Fig. 2.2.1 Framework for understanding social determinants of health and health inequities.
Source: WHO Department of Equity, Poverty and Social Determinants of Health (Solar and Irwin 2007).

The framework defines two major domains. The first is that of *structural determinants*, which include people's socioeconomic position as well as relevant characteristics of the socioeconomic and political context. The second is that of *intermediary determinants*. This concept embraces what are often referred to as proximal determinants of health, and which at the individual level are termed risk factors, such as diet and exercise habits, smoking, or conditions of exposure to environmental pollutants in neighbourhoods, workplaces, and homes. A key aim of the framework is to clarify the relationship between structural and intermediary determinants.

In the far left column, the diagram shows the main *contextual factors that affect inequities in health*, e.g. governance, macroeconomic policies, social policies, public policies in other relevant areas, culture and societal values, and epidemiological conditions. 'Socioeconomic and political context' is a deliberately broad term that refers to the spectrum of factors in society that cannot be directly measured at the individual level. Context therefore encompasses a broad set of structural, cultural, and functional aspects of a social system whose impact on individuals tends to elude quantification but which exert a powerful formative influence on patterns of social stratification and thus on people's health opportunities. Within the context in this sense will be found those social and political mechanisms that generate, configure, and maintain social hierarchies.

Moving to the right, the next column of the diagram highlights the essential expression of social hierarchy, i.e. *socioeconomic position*, which reflects social structure and class relationships. People's socioeconomic position locates them with respect to the differential distribution of power, prestige, and resources in society. Since variables like 'power', 'prestige', and 'access to resources' may be difficult to measure, studies and evaluations of equity frequently use income, education, and occupation as proxies for these domains. When we refer to prestige and the related category of social discrimination, we find them strongly related to gender, ethnicity, sexuality, and education. Thus these latter factors are also included in the second column of the model, as factors linked to socioeconomic position.

Moving to the right once more, we reach the next stage in the social 'production chain' of health inequities (Diderichsen *et al.* 2001). Socioeconomic position influences people's health by acting through more specific, intermediary determinants. Those intermediary factors include: *Material circumstances*, such as neighbourhood, working and housing conditions; *psychosocial circumstances*, and also *behavioural, and biological factors*. Strenuous debates have characterized public health scientists' efforts to describe the interrelationships among these intermediary factors, with some groups giving relatively greater importance to psychosocial dynamics, others insisting on the primacy of the material dimension. The model presented here highlights material circumstances as the more fundamental area for action, while recognizing that material, psychosocial, and behavioural/biological factors influence each other through complex interactive patterns. Science has yet to understand the full set of mechanisms in play in these interactions. The fundamental point, however, is that all three categories of intermediary factors are shaped at a deeper level by the structural processes that assign individuals to different position in the socioeconomic hierarchy.

Accordingly, the model incorporates the fact that members of lower socioeconomic groups live in less favourable material circumstances than higher socioeconomic groups, and also the widely observed pattern whereby people closer to the bottom of the social scale more frequently engage in health-damaging behaviours and less frequently in heath-promoting behaviours than do the more privileged. The unequal distribution of intermediary factors (associated with differences in exposure and vulnerability to health-compromising conditions, as well as with differential consequences of ill-health) constitutes the primary mechanism through which socioeconomic position generates health inequities.

The framework gives attention to the concepts of *social cohesion* and '*social capital*', which occupy an unusual (and contested) place in public health debates. Over the past decade, these concepts have been among the most widely discussed in the social sciences and social epidemiology. Influential researchers have proclaimed social capital a key factor in shaping population health (Kawachi *et al.* 1997; Putnam 2000, 2001; Ferguson 2006). However, critiques of the utility of the concept of social capital have emerged (Muntaner *et al.* 1999; Muntaner 2004). These issues will be discussed in greater detail below. The model also includes the *health system* as an intermediary social determinant of health. This chapter will touch upon some implications of this perspective for health policymaking.

The dotted blue lines at the top of the figure indicate feedback processes through which health and health equity outcomes can affect individuals' socioeconomic position and broader contextual features, such as labour market processes. These feedback effects will be discussed in greater detail shortly.

A second version of the framework in Fig. 2.2.2 again depicts the social production chain of health inequities, highlighting important additional aspects. Figure 2.2.2 sharpens our view of the specific pathways and mechanisms through which the broad health-determining factors represented in Fig. 2.2.1 produce differential health impacts among social groups.

This second diagram more explicitly shows the causal relationship connecting structural determinants (left side of the picture) to intermediary determinants and, through them, to individual health outcomes and the patterning of health and sickness across society (right side of the model). Socioeconomic, political, and cultural institutions and processes give rise to a set of stratified socioeconomic positions. People's placement within this socioeconomic hierarchy in turn generates specific, unequal patterns of exposure and vulnerability to health-damaging factors. These differences in exposure and vulnerability among social groups are the more directly observable triggers of the socially patterned distribution of disease.

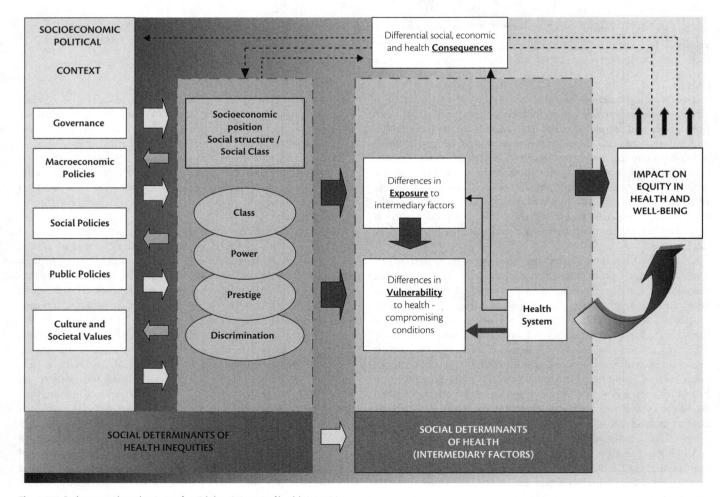

Fig. 2.2.2 Pathways and mechanisms of social determinants of health inequities.
Source: Solar and Irwin (2007).

Under the heading of 'socioeconomic position', Fig. 2.2.2 gives added emphasis to the concept of social class. As an inherently relational variable, class is able to shed particular light on the mechanisms associated with the social production of health inequities. By definition, class position is connected with the economic base and people's ability to access and control resources. Class is also linked with people's degree of power in society. The structures and mechanisms through which power is exercised, and the capacity of individuals and groups to wield power and exert control over decisions that affect their well-being, are in turn influenced by the political context (including functioning democratic institutions or their absence, corruption, access to media and information, etc.).

The inclusion of 'prestige' and 'discrimination' as facets of the social production of health/disease underscores that, in each society, the distribution of resources and power among groups is entwined with a hierarchical status system that assigns some groups higher social rank and greater respect than others. Though closely related to the unequal distribution of wealth and power, social status rankings are not identical with these other forms of hierarchy. Evidence suggests that forms of social prestige and/or systematic discrimination directed towards selected groups may exert health effects independent of wealth and material living conditions, as when studies show persistent differentials in life expectancy and other key health indicators between ethnic majority and minority groups, even when factors such as income and education are controlled for (Gee 2002).

The dotted lines at the top of Fig. 2.2.2, leading back from the right towards the left side of the diagram, illustrate significant 'feedback' effects that reveal an additional dimension of the dynamic interrelation between social conditions and health. Socioeconomic inequalities in health can in fact be partly explained by the impacts of health and sickness on socioeconomic position, e.g. when someone experiences a drop in income because of a work-induced disability or the medical costs associated with major illness. Persons who are in poor health less frequently move up and more frequently move down the social ladder than healthy persons. It may be noted, in addition, that some specific diseases can impact people's socioeconomic position not only by undermining their physical capacities, but also through associated stigma and discrimination, e.g. in the case of HIV/AIDS.

These observations help clarify why it is useful to view the health system itself as a social determinant of health. The model suggests the capacity of the heath sector to influence the social production of health/disease in at least three ways, by acting upon: Differences in exposures; differences in vulnerability; and differences in the consequences of illness for people's health and their social and economic standing. This is in addition to the health sector's key role in promoting and coordinating policy action across government sectors to address other social determinants of health.

Because of their magnitude, certain diseases, such as HIV/AIDS and malaria, can also impact key components of the socioeconomic and political context directly, e.g. the labour market and governance institutions. This effect is illustrated by the blue arrow in the diagram. The whole set of 'feedback' mechanisms just described is brought together under the heading of 'differential social, economic, and health consequences'. The framework includes the impact of existing social position on these mechanisms, indicating that path with a red arrow.

The following sections will discuss in greater detail each of the major components of the framework.

First element of the framework: Socioeconomic and political context

The model of health determinants developed in this chapter differs from some others in the importance attributed to the *socioeconomic and political context*. Political institutions and processes have been largely ignored in a substantial portion of the recent literature on health determinants. Population health researchers now routinely acknowledge that the health of individuals and populations is strongly influenced by social determinants. However, as Navarro and others have argued, it is much less common for public health scholars to recognize that the quality of determinants is in turn shaped by the policies that guide how societies (re)distribute material resources among their members (cf. Esping-Andersen 2002). In the growing area of determinants research, a subject rarely studied is the impact on social inequalities and health of political movements and parties and the policies they adopt when in government (Navarro & Shi 2001). Chung and Muntaner (2006) find similarly that few studies have explored the relationship between political variables and population health at the national level, and none has included a comprehensive number of political variables to understand their effect on population health, while simultaneously adjusting for economic determinants. As an illustration of the powerful impact of political variables on health outcomes, these researchers concluded in a recent study of 18 wealthy countries in Europe, North America, and the Asia-Pacific region that 20 per cent of the differences in infant mortality rate among countries could be explained by the type of welfare state they have adopted. Similarly, different welfare state models among the countries accounted for about 10 per cent of differences in the rate of low-birth-weight babies.

In general, the construction/mapping of context should include at least six points: (1) *Governance* in the broadest sense and its processes, including definition of needs, patterns of discrimination, civil society participation, and accountability/transparence in public administration; (2) *macroeconomic policy*, including fiscal, monetary, balance of payments and trade policies, and underlying labour market structures; (3) *social policies* affecting factors such as labour, social welfare, land and housing distribution; (4) *public policy* in other relevant areas such as education, medical care, water, and sanitation; (5) *epidemiological conditions*, particularly in the case of major epidemics such as HIV/AIDS, which exert a powerful influence on social structures and must be factored into global and national policy-setting; (6) *culture and societal values*.

While the category of culture and societal values includes a wide range of factors, one especially relevant aspect is the value placed on health and the degree to which health is seen as a collective social concern. This differs greatly across regional and national contexts. Elsewhere, following pioneering work undertaken by Kleczkowski *et al.* (1984), we have argued that the social value attributed to health in a country constitutes an important and often neglected aspect of the context in which health policies must be designed and implemented (Solar *et al.* 2004). In constructing a typology of health systems, Roemer and Kleczkowski have proposed three domains of analysis to indicate how health is valued in a given society:

◆ The extent to which health is a priority in the governmental/societal agenda, as reflected in the level of national resources allocated to health.

◆ The extent to which the society assumes collective responsibility for financing and organizing the provision of health services.

In maximum collectivism (also referred to as a state-based model), the system is almost entirely concerned with providing collective benefits, leaving little or no choice to the individual. In maximum individualism, ill health and its care are viewed as private concerns.

◆ The extent of societal distributional responsibility. This is a measure of the degree to which society assumes responsibility for the distribution of its health resources. Distributional responsibility is at its maximum when the society guarantees equal access to services for all.

Among many aspects of culture that operate as contextual determinants of health, the social value attributed to health may carry especially important consequences, not only by moulding individual and group behaviour, but also because this underlying valuation influences society's willingness to invest in public policies to address the determinants of health and health equity.

Second element of the framework: Socioeconomic position

The concept of 'socioeconomic position' locates people within complex, interpenetrating systems of social hierarchy. The two major variables used to operationalize socioeconomic position in studies of social inequities in health are *social stratification* and *social class*. The term stratification is used in sociology to refer to social hierarchies in which individuals or groups can be arranged along a ranked order of some attribute. Income or years of education provide familiar examples. Measures of social stratification are important predictors of patterns of mortality and morbidity. 'Social class', meanwhile, is defined by relations of ownership or control over productive resources (i.e. physical, financial, organizational) (Muntaner *et al.* 2003). Social class has important consequences for the lives of individuals. Class, in contrast to stratification, indicates the employment relations and conditions of each occupation. The task of class analysis is precisely to understand not only how macro structures (e.g. class relations at the national level) constrain micro processes (e.g. interpersonal behaviour) but also how micro processes can affect macro structures (for example, through collective action) (Muntaner *et al.* 1999).

Adler *et al.* (1994) observe that social class is among the strongest known predictors of illness and health and yet is, paradoxically, a variable about which very little systematic research has been conducted. Muntaner and colleagues have likewise noted that, while there is substantial scholarship on the psychology of racism and gender, little research has been done on the effects of class ideology (i.e. classism). This asymmetry could reflect that in most wealthy democratic capitalist countries, income inequalities are perceived as acceptable while gender and race inequalities are not (Muntaner *et al.* 1999). The concept of class adds significant value and should be included as a distinct component in discussions of socioeconomic position.

Historically, two central figures in the study of socioeconomic position were Karl Marx and Max Weber. For Marx, socioeconomic position was entirely determined by social class, whereby an individuals are defined by their relation to the 'means of production' (for example, factories, land). Social class and class relations are characterized by the conflict between exploited workers and the exploiting capitalists who control the means of production. This underscores that class is not an inherent property of individual human beings, but a relational characteristic generated by a social structure.

Weber developed a different view of class and social location. Weber saw differential societal position as incorporating three dimensions: Class, status and party (or power). Class has an economic base. It implies ownership and control of resources and is indicated by measures of income. Status is considered to be prestige or honour in the community. Weber considers status to imply 'access to life chances' based on social and cultural factors such as family background, lifestyle and social networks. Finally, power is related to a political context (Liberatos *et al.* 1988). In this chapter, we use the term 'socioeconomic position', acknowledging the three separate but linked dimensions of social class reflected in the Weberian conceptualization.

More recently, Krieger, Williams, and Moss (1997) have treated socioeconomic position as an aggregate concept that includes both resource-based and prestige-based measures. Resource-based measures refer to material and social resources and assets, including income, wealth, and educational credentials; terms used to describe inadequate resources include 'poverty' and 'deprivation'. Prestige-based measures refer to individuals' rank or status in a social hierarchy. Given distinctions between resource-based and prestige-based aspects of socioeconomic position and the diverse pathways by which they affect health, epidemiological studies should state clearly how measures of socioeconomic position are conceptualized. Educational level creates differences between people in terms of access to information and the level of proficiency in benefiting from new knowledge, whereas income creates differences in access to scarce material goods. Occupational status includes both these aspects and adds to them benefits accruing from the exercise of specific jobs, such as prestige, privileges, power, and social and technical skills.

Socioeconomic position can be usefully measured at three complementary levels: Individual, household, and neighbourhood. Each level may independently contribute to distributions of exposure and outcomes. Also, socioeconomic position can be measured meaningfully at different points of the lifespan: e.g. infancy, childhood, adolescent, adult (current, past 5 years, etc.). Relevant time periods depend on presumed exposures, causal pathways, and associated aetiologic periods. Today it is also vital to recognize gender, ethnicity, and sexuality as social stratifiers linked to systematic forms of discrimination (Krieger *et al.* 1993).

A close relationship exists between the social–political context and what we term the structural determinants of health inequities. The framework posits that *structural determinants* are those that generate or reinforce social stratification in the society and that define individual socioeconomic position. These mechanisms configure the health opportunities of social groups based on their placement within hierarchies of power, prestige, and access to resources (economic status). We prefer to speak of *structural determinants*, rather than 'distal' factors, in order to capture and underscore the causal hierarchy of social determinants involved in producing health inequities. Structural social stratification mechanisms, joined to and influenced by institutions and processes embedded in the socioeconomic and political context (e.g. redistributive welfare state policies), can together be conceptualized as *the social determinants of health inequities*. In all cases, structural determinants present themselves in a specific political and historical context. At the same time, the context forms part of the origin and foundation of a given distribution of power, prestige, and access to material resources in a society and thus of the pattern of social stratification and social class relations existing in that society. The positive significance of this relationship is that it is possible to address the effects of the structural determinants of health inequities through purposive action on contextual features, for example through public policy measures addressing the education system, the labour market, land ownership, social protection and redistribution, and other mechanisms impacting stratification at a structural level.

Third element of the framework: Intermediary determinants

Structural determinants operate through a series of *intermediary social factors* or *social determinants of health*. The structural determinants or social determinants of health inequities are causally antecedent to these intermediary determinants, which are linked, on the other side, to a set of individual-level influences, including health-related behaviours and physiological factors. The intermediary factors flow from the configuration of underlying social stratification and, in turn, determine differences in exposure and vulnerability to health-compromising conditions. A recent revision of Diderichsen's model sheds additional light on the processes (Diderichsen 2004). Both *differential exposure* and *differential vulnerability* may contribute to the relation between social position and health outcomes, as can be tested empirically (Whitehead *et al.* 2000). Ill-health has serious social and economic consequences due to inability to work and the cost of healthcare. These consequences depend not only on the extent of disability but also on the individual's social position and on the society's environment and social policies. At the most proximal point in the models, genetic and biological processes are emphasized, mediating the health effects of social determinants (Graham 2004). The social and economical consequences of illness may feed back into the aetiological pathways and contribute to the further development of disease in the individual.

The main categories of intermediary determinants of health are: Material circumstances; psychosocial circumstances; behavioural and/or biological factors; the health system itself as a social determinant, and social cohesion. These elements are reviewed in turn.

Material circumstances

These include determinants linked to the physical environment, such as housing (relating both to the dwelling itself and its location), consumption potential, i.e. the financial means to buy healthy food, warm clothing, etc., and the physical working and neighbourhood environments. Depending on their quality, these circumstances both provide resources for health and contain health risks. In the model, material circumstances are highlighted as fundamental, exercising a strong causal influence on the other categories of intermediary determinants. Patterns of interaction among intermediary determinants are complex, however. Much remains to be understood about the interrelationships among material, psychosocial, and behavioural/biological factors in different contexts.

Social-environmental or psychosocial circumstances

These include psychosocial stressors (for example, negative life events, job strain), stressful living circumstances (e.g. high debt) and (lack of) social support, coping styles, etc. Different social groups are exposed to different degrees to experiences and life situations that are perceived as threatening, frightening, and difficult to deal with. This partly explains the long-term pattern of social inequalities in health. Stress may be a direct causal factor in triggering forms of illness. Additionally, a background condition of ongoing, long-term stress may be part of the causal complex behind other illnesses. A person's socioeconomic position may itself be a source of long-term stress, and will also affect the opportunities to deal with stressful and difficult situations.

Behavioural and biological factors

These include smoking, diet, alcohol consumption, and physical exercise. Such factors can be either health protecting and enhancing (like exercise) or health damaging (cigarette smoking and obesity). Biological factors, including genetic factors, are situated at this same level of analysis.

Social inequalities in health have also been associated with social differences in behaviours, or what are often referred to as 'lifestyle' factors. Such differences are found in nutrition, physical activity, tobacco, and alcohol consumption. This indicates that differences in behaviour could partially explain social inequalities in health, but researchers do not agree on their importance: Some regard differences in personal behaviour as a sufficient explanation without further elaboration; others regard them as contributory factors that in turn result from more fundamental causes. For example, Margolis *et al.* (1992) found that the prevalence of both acute and persistent respiratory symptoms in infants showed dose–response relationships with socioeconomic position. When risk factors such as crowding and exposure to smoking in the household were adjusted for, relative risk associated with socioeconomic position was reduced but still remained significant (cf. Marmot *et al.* 1984).

Cigarette smoking is strongly linked to socioeconomic position, including education, income, and employment status, and it is significantly associated with morbidity and mortality, particularly from cardiovascular disease and cancer (e.g. Marmot *et al.* 1991). A linear gradient between education and smoking prevalence was also shown in a community sample of middle-aged women: Additionally, among current smokers the number of cigarettes smoked was related to socioeconomic position. Significant employment grade differences in smoking were found in the Whitehall II study, which examined a new cohort of 10 314 subjects from the British Civil Service beginning in 1985 (Marmot *et al.* 1991). Moving from the lowest to the highest employment grades, the prevalence of current smoking among men was 33.6, 21.9, 18.4, 13.0, 10.2, and 8.3 per cent, respectively. For women, the comparable figures were 27.5, 22.7, 20.3, 15.2, 11.6, and 18.3 per cent, respectively. Social class differences in smoking are likely to continue because rates of smoking initiation are inversely related to socioeconomic position, while rates of cessation are positively related to people's socioeconomic rank (e.g. Escobedo *et al.* 1990; Kaprio & Koskenvuo 1988).

Behavioural factors are relatively accessible and measurable for research. Partially as a result, a large literature on behavioural or so-called 'lifestyle' influences on health has developed. The existence of a body of research in this area does not mean, however, that behavioural factors are the most important causes of social inequalities in health. Other, more fundamental factors may be at the root of variations in both personal behaviours and health—a crucial consideration when it comes to planning appropriate interventions (see Macintyre 2007). Some surveys indicate that differences in lifestyle can only explain a small proportion of social inequalities in health (Marmot *et al.* 1978). For instance, material factors may act as a source of psychosocial stress, and psychosocial stress may influence health-related behaviours. Each of them can influence health through specific biological factors. For example a diet rich in saturated fat will lead to atherosclerosis, which will increase the risk of a myocardial infarction. Stress will activate hormonal systems that may increase blood pressure and reduce the immune response. Adoption of health-threatening behaviours is a response to material deprivation and stress. Environments determine whether individuals take up tobacco, use alcohol, have poor diets, and engage in physical activity. Tobacco and excessive alcohol use, and carbohydrate-dense diets, are means of coping with difficult circumstances (Mackenbach & Bakker 2002).

The health system as a social determinant of health

Many models have paid insufficient attention to the health system as a social determinant. The health system can directly address socially conditioned differences in people's exposure and vulnerability to health damage not only by improving equitable access to care, but also in the promotion of intersectoral action to improve health status. Examples would include food supplementation through the health system and transport policies and intervention for tackling geographic barriers to healthcare access. A further aspect of great importance is the role the health system plays in mediating the differential consequences of illness in people's lives. The health system is capable of ensuring that health problems do not lead to a further deterioration of people's social status, and of facilitating sick people's social reintegration. Examples include programmes for the chronically ill to support their reinsertion in the workforce, as well as appropriate models of health financing that can prevent people from being forced into (deeper) poverty by the costs of medical care.

A crosscutting determinant: Social cohesion/social capital

Bernales (2006) has recently provided a review of debates on this topic. In the most influential recent discussions, three broad approaches to the characterization and analysis of social capital can be distinguished: Communitarian approaches, network approaches, and resource distribution approaches. The *communitarian approach* defines social capital as a psychosocial mechanism, corresponding to a neo-Durkheimian perspective on the relation between individual health and society (Popay 2000). The *network approach* considers social capital in terms of resources that flow and emerge through social networks. It begins with a systemic relational perspective; in other words, an ecological vision is taken that sees beyond individual resources and additive characteristics. This involves an analysis of the influence of social structure, power hierarchies and access to resources on population health (Moore *et al.* 2006). This approach implies that decisions that groups or individuals make, in relation to their lifestyle and behavioural habits, cannot be considered outside the social context where such choices take place. Finally, the *resource distribution approach,* adopting a materialistic perspective, suggests that there is a danger in promoting social capital as a substitute for structural change when facing health inequity. Some representatives of this group openly criticize psychosocial approaches that have suggested social capital and cohesion as the most important mediators of the association between income and health inequality (Lynch *et al.* 2000). The resource distribution approach insists that psychosocial aspects affecting population health are a consequence of material life conditions (Lynch 2000).

Recent work by Szreter and Woolcock (2004) has enriched the debates around social capital and its health impacts. These authors distinguish between bonding, bridging, and linking social capital. *Bonding social capital* refers to the trust and cooperative relationships between members of a network that are similar in terms of their social identity. *Bridging social capital*, on the other hand, refers to respectful relationships and mutuality between individuals and groups that are aware that they do not possess the same characteristics in socio-demographic terms. Finally, *linking social capital* corresponds with the norms of respect and trust relationships between individuals, groups, networks, and institutions that interact from different positions along explicit gradients of institutionalized power. Collaborative relationships between civil society or community-based organizations and state institutions provide one example.

Impact of determinants on equity in health and well-being

According to the analysis we have developed, the structural factors associated with the key components of socioeconomic position are at the root of health inequities measured at the population level. This relationship is confirmed by a substantial body of evidence.

Socioeconomic health differences are reflected in general measures of health, like life expectancy, all-cause mortality, and self-rated health (Kubzansky *et al.* 2001; Mackenbach *et al.* 2002). Differences correlated with people's socioeconomic position are found for rates of mortality and morbidity from almost every disease and condition (Antonovsky 1967; Illsley & Baker 1991). Socioeconomic position is also linked to prevalence and course of disease and self-rated health. Socioeconomic health inequalities are evident in specific causes of disease, disability, and premature death, including lung cancer, coronary heart disease, accidents, and suicide. Low birth weight provides an additional important example. This is a sensitive measure of child health and a major risk factor for impaired development through childhood, including intellectual development (Graham 2005). There are marked differences in national rates of low birth weight, with higher rates in the US and UK and lower rates in Nordic countries like Sweden, Norway, and the Netherlands. These rates vary in line with the proportion of the child population living in poverty (in households with incomes below 50 per cent of average income): At their lowest in low-poverty countries like Sweden and Norway, and at their highest in high-poverty countries like the UK and US (Emerson 2004).

Impact along the gradient

There is evidence that the association of socioeconomic position and health occurs at every level of the social hierarchy, not simply below the threshold of poverty. Not only do those in poverty have poorer health than those in more favoured circumstances, but those at the highest level enjoy better health than do those just below (e.g. Marmot *et al.* 1984, 1991). The effects of severe poverty on health may seem obvious through the impact of poor nutrition, crowded and insanitary living conditions, and inadequate medical care. Identifying factors that can account for the link to health all across the socioeconomic hierarchy may shed light on new mechanisms that have heretofore been ignored because of a focus on the more readily apparent correlates of poverty. The most notable of the studies demonstrating the SEP-health gradient is the Whitehall study of mortality (Marmot *et al.* 1984). Similar findings emerge from census data in the United Kingdom (Susser *et al.* 1985).

Despite the demonstrated important impact of socioeconomic position on health, disconcertingly little is known about how socioeconomic position operates to influence biological functions that determine health status. Part of the problem may be the way in which socioeconomic position is conceptualized and analysed. Socioeconomic position has been almost universally relegated to the status of a control variable and has not been systematically studied as an important aetiologic factor in its own right. It is usually treated as a main effect, operating independently of other variables to predict health.

Life course perspective

A life course approach explicitly recognizes the importance of time and timing in understanding causal links between exposures and outcomes within an individual life course, across generations, and in population-level diseases trends (e.g. Lynch & Smith 2005). Adopting a life course perspective directs attention to how social determinants of health operate at every level of development—early childhood, childhood, adolescence, and adulthood—both to immediately influence health and to provide the basis for health or illness later in life. The life course perspective attempts to understand how such temporal processes across the life course of one cohort are related to previous and subsequent cohorts and are manifested in disease trends observed over time at the population level. Time lags between exposure, disease initiation, and clinical recognition (latency period) suggest that exposures early in life are involved in initiating diseases processes prior to clinical manifestations. However, the recognition of early-life influences on chronic diseases does not imply deterministic processes that negate the utility of later-life intervention.

Two main mechanisms are identified. The 'critical periods' model is when an exposure acting during a specific period has lasting or lifelong effects on the structure or function of organs, tissues, and body systems which are not modified in any dramatic way by later experiences. This is also known as biological programming, and is also sometimes referred to as a latency model. This conception is the basis of hypotheses on the foetal origins of adult diseases. This approach does recognize the importance of later life effect modifiers, for example in the linkage of coronary heart disease, high blood pressure, and insulin resistance with low birth weight (e.g. Frankel et al. 1996).

The 'accumulation of risk' model suggests that factors that raise disease risk or promote good health may accumulate gradually over the life course, although there may be developmental periods when their effects have greater impact on later health than factors operating at other times. This idea is complementary to the notion that as the intensity, number, and/or duration of exposures increase, there is increasing cumulative damage to biological systems. Understanding the health effects of childhood social class by identifying specific aspects of the early physical or psychosocial environment (such as exposure to air pollution or family conflict) or possible mechanisms (such as nutrition, infection, or stress) that are associated with adult disease will provide further aetiological insights. Circumstances in early life are seen as the initial stage in the pathway to adult health but with an indirect effect, influencing adult health through social trajectories, such as restricting educational opportunities, thus influencing socioeconomic circumstances and health in later life. Risk factors tend to cluster in socially patterned ways, for example, those living in adverse childhood social circumstances are more likely to be of low birth weight, and be exposed to poor diet, childhood infections, and passive smoking. These exposures may raise the risk of adult respiratory disease, perhaps through chains of risk or pathways over time where one adverse (or protective) experience will tend to lead to another adverse (protective) experience in a cumulative way.

Ben-Shlomo and Kuh (2002) argue that the life course approach is not limited to individuals within a single generation but should intertwine biological and social transmission of risk across generations. It must contextualize any exposure both within a hierarchical structure as well as in relation to geographical and secular differences, which may be unique to that cohort of individuals. Recently the potential for a life course approach to aid understanding of variations in the health and disease of populations over time, across countries, and between social groups has been given more attention. Davey Smith (2003) suggests that explanations for social inequalities in cause-specific adult mortality lie in socially patterned exposures at different stages of the life course.

Children born into poorer circumstances are at greater risk of the forms of developmental delay associated with intellectual disability, including speech impairments, cognitive difficulties, and behavioural problems (Maughan et al. 1999; Power & Hertzman 2004). Some other conditions, like stroke and stomach cancer, appear to depend considerably on childhood circumstances, while for others, including deaths from lung cancer and accidents/ violence, adult circumstances play the more important role. In another group are health outcomes where it is cumulative exposure that appears to be important. A number of studies suggest that this is the case for coronary heart disease and respiratory disease, for example (Davey Smith 2003).

Selection processes and health-related mobility

People with weaker health resources, allegedly, have a tendency to end up or remain low on the ladder of socioeconomic position. According to some analysts, the status of research on selection processes and health-related mobility within the socioeconomic structure can be summarized in three points: (1) variations in health in youth have some significance for educational paths and for the kind of job a person has at the beginning of his or her working career; (2) for those who are already established in working life, variations in health have little significance for the overall progress of a person's career; (3) people who develop serious health problems in adult life are often excluded from working life, and often long before the ordinary retirement age (see e.g. Manor et al. 2003). One might assume such effects to be inevitable. But they are in part due to discriminatory practices, in part also to failures to adapt educational institutions and working life to special needs. To the extent that this is the case, social selection is neither necessary, nor inevitable, nor fair. This phenomenon particularly affects persons with disabilities, persons from immigrant backgrounds and, to a certain extent, women (Graham 2004).

Impact on the socioeconomic and political context

From a population standpoint, we observe that the magnitude of certain diseases can translate into direct effects on features of the socioeconomic and political context, through high prevalence rates and levels of mortality and morbidity. The HIV/AIDS pandemic in sub-Saharan Africa can be seen in this light, with its associated plunge in life expectancy and stresses on agricultural productivity, economic growth, and sectoral capacities in areas such as health and education. The magnitude of the impact of epidemics and emergencies will depend on the historical, political, and social contexts in which they occur, as well as on the demographic composition of the societies affected. These are aspects that must be considered when analysing welfare state structures, in particular models of health system organization that may be considered to respond to such challenges.

Distinguishing determinants of health from determinants of inequities in health

Hilary Graham (2004) has rightly observed that the central concept of 'social determinants' remains ambiguous in much of the relevant public health literature. The term is used to refer simultaneously to the determinants of health and to the determinants of inequalities in health. Graham notes that: 'Using a single term to refer to both the social factors influencing health and the social processes shaping their social distribution would not be problematic if the main determinants of health—like living standards, environmental influences, and health behaviours—were equally distributed between socioeconomic groups'. But the evidence points to marked socioeconomic differences in access to material resources, health-promoting resources, and in exposure to risk factors. Furthermore, policies associated with positive trends in health determinants (e.g. a rise in living standards and a decline in smoking) have also been associated with persistent socioeconomic disparities in the distribution of these determinants (marked socioeconomic differences in living standards and smoking rates) (e.g. Howden-Chapman *et al.* 2000). We have attempted to resolve this linguistic ambiguity by introducing additional differentiations within the field of concepts conventionally included under the heading 'social determinants'.

We adopt the term *structural determinants* to refer specifically to the components of people's socioeconomic position. Structural determinants, combined with the main features of the socioeconomic and political context described above, together constitute what we call the *social determinants of health inequities*. This concept corresponds to Graham's notion of the 'social processes shaping the distribution' of downstream social determinants. Our term *intermediary determinants of health* refers to these more downstream factors. As noted, the vocabulary of 'structural' and 'intermediary' seeks to emphasize the causal linkage between the two categories and the priority of structural factors (Graham 2004).

Graham argues that what is obscured in many previous treatments of these topics 'is that tackling the determinants of health inequalities is about tackling the *unequal distribution of health determinants*'. Focusing on the unequal distribution of determinants is important for thinking about policy. This is because policies that have achieved overall improvements in key determinants such as living standards and smoking have not reduced inequalities in these major influences on health. When health equity is the goal, the priority of a determinants-oriented strategy is to reduce inequalities in the major influences on people's health. Tackling inequalities in social position is likely to be at the heart of such a strategy. For, according to Graham, social position is the pivotal point in the causal chain linking broad determinants to the risk factors that directly damage people's health. Graham emphasizes that policy objectives will be defined quite differently, depending on whether our aim is to address determinants of health or determinants of health inequities:

◆ *Objectives for health determinants* are likely to focus on reducing overall exposure to health-damaging factors along the causal pathway. The UK, for example, has focused on raising educational standards and living standards (important constituents of

socioeconomic position) and reducing rates of smoking (a major intermediary risk factor).

◆ *Objectives for health inequity determinants* are likely to focus on levelling up the distribution of major health determinants. How these objectives are framed will depend on the health inequities goals that are being pursued. One example would be progressive tax structures to redistribute income (Graham 2004).

Implications for public health policies

Three key policy orientations can be derived from the framework presented in this chapter:

◆ Arguably the single most significant lesson of the framework is that interventions and policies to reduce health inequities must not limit themselves to intermediary determinants, but must include policies crafted to tackle structural determinants. Interventions addressing intermediary determinants can improve average health indicators while leaving health inequities unchanged. For this reason, policy action on structural determinants is necessary. To achieve solid results, determinants policies must be designed with attention to contextual specificities, which should be rigorously characterized using methodologies developed by social and political science.

◆ Cross-sectoral or intersectoral policymaking and implementation are crucial for progress on health equity. This is because structural determinants can only be tackled through strategies that reach beyond the health sector. The health sector's work with other sectors can involve different levels: From simple coordination of objectives and strategies among different sectors, through more substantive cooperation, up to genuine integration of policies. Policy integration is required to tackle the structural determinants of health.

◆ Participation of civil society and affected communities in the design and implementation of policies to address health determinants is essential to success. Social participation is an ethical obligation for governments. In addition, the empowerment of civil society and communities and their ownership of the determinants agenda could build a sustained global movement for health equity.

Figure 2.2.3 summarizes the policy implications of the determinants framework in a visual representation. It highlights the need to promote context-specific strategies to address structural as well as intermediary determinants. Such strategies will necessarily include cross-sector and intersectoral policies, through which structural determinants can be most effectively addressed, and will aim to ensure that policies are crafted so as to engage and ultimately empower civil society and affected communities. These broad directions for policy action can utilize various entry points or levels of engagement, represented in the image by the cross-cutting horizontal bars.

Moving from the lower to the higher bars (from more 'downstream' to more structural approaches), these entry points include: Seeking to palliate the differential consequences of illness; seeking to reduce differential vulnerabilities and exposures for disadvantaged social groups; and, ultimately, altering the patterns of social stratification. At the same time, policies and interventions can be targeted at the 'micro' level of individual interactions; at the 'meso'

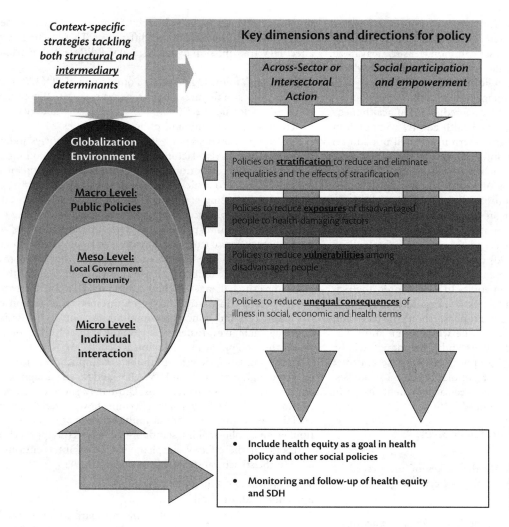

Context-specific strategies tackling both structural and intermediary determinants

Key dimensions and directions for policy

Across-Sector or Intersectoral Action

Social participation and empowerment

Globalization Environment

Macro Level: Public Policies

Meso Level: Local Government Community

Micro Level: Individual interaction

Policies on **stratification** to reduce and eliminate inequalities and the effects of stratification

Policies to reduce **exposures** of disadvantaged people to health-damaging factors

Policies to reduce **vulnerabilities** among disadvantaged people

Policies to reduce **unequal consequences** of illness in social, economic and health terms

- Include health equity as a goal in health policy and other social policies
- Monitoring and follow-up of health equity and SDH

Fig. 2.2.3 Framework for policy action on social determinants of health and health equity.
Source: Solar and Irwin (2007).

level of community conditions or local government; or at the broadest 'macro' level of universal public policies and the global environment.

Individual vs. population approaches in epidemiology and public health policy

Modern epidemiology has been heavily oriented to the study of risk factors for chronic non-communicable and communicable emergent diseases (McMichael 1999). The primary concern has been to understand disease occurrence in individual terms, looking at aspects such as consumer behaviour, individual exposures, metabolic factors and genetic effects. Epidemiology has become adept at determining which individuals are at increased risk of disease, looking at factors that are measurable at the individual level, but it has not been as successful at understanding the distribution of diseases within and between populations. Factors that are important causes of diseases in an individual within a population may be very different from the factors that primarily determine disease rates in the whole population (Rose 2001).

Implicit in the focus on proximate risk factors is the assumption that the individual is the site of aetiologic actions and, therefore, the natural unit of epidemiological observation. Larger scale variables that affect whole groups or populations, such as poverty and

cultural disruptions, are only viewed as important because and to the extent that they translate into individual-level risk factors. Poverty affects diet; cultural disruptions (such as economic transitions, rural-to-urban migration) spur increases in alcoholism, etc. However, this population vs. individual distinction needs careful examination, in light of the framework explored in this chapter. Are we distinguishing between structural and intermediary determinants and their proximate manifestations? Or is there a category of risk factor that, in some collective way, influences the health of the population at large via processes that do not have direct, proximate manifestations? Further, complex entities such a poverty, for example, can have very different meanings and can measure qualitatively different constructs at the individual and population levels (Schwartz 1994).

These distinctions are not only important for building appropriately comprehensive theoretical frameworks. They also have far-reaching implications for all aspects of public health policy. Individual and population-based approaches yield very different strategies for practice in both prevention and curative care. The individual approach seeks to identify high-risk, susceptible individuals and to offer them forms of personalized protection or treatment. In contrast, the population strategy seeks to control the determinants of incidence in the population as a whole. The 'high-risk individual' strategy is the traditional biomedical approach to prevention and cure. The population strategy attempts to remove the underlying causes that make the relevant diseases common. This strategy has a large potential for improving health in the population as a whole, but it raises new challenges for public health action.

Moreover, improvements in average health levels for the population are not necessarily associated with a reduction in health inequities. If the objective is to improve health equity, a population approach focused on intermediary determinants will not suffice. The strategy must also include intervention on the factors that determine health inequities, which we have termed structural determinants. Traditional forms of health promotion, whether adopting individual or population-based approaches, may actually widen health gaps between well-off and disadvantaged sectors of society, if policies do not incorporate measures to address structural factors. This is especially clear in the case of individualized interventions. As Macintyre (2000) notes: 'The capacity to benefit from individualized risk management and health education may be least among more disadvantaged people'. In other words, the rich are more likely to attend to and benefit from traditional forms of health promotion than are the poor. Emphasis should be placed on policies that can reduce risks across the whole population. For example, focusing on transport policies and urban design will be more useful that the traditional emphasis on exercise and diet alone. However, even in the case of population-based strategies, the groups in greatest need will not necessarily benefit first, and inequities will not necessarily be reduced.

Public health research and policy choices: Concrete examples

Specific examples will help clarify the stakes of the preceding discussion for public health research and policymaking.

The example of HIV/AIDS

Early studies of the human immunodeficiency virus/acquired immunodeficiency syndrome (HIV/AIDS) focused on individual characteristics and behaviours in determining HIV risk, a classic case of 'biomedical individualism' (Fee & Krieger 1993). Biomedical individualism is the basis of risk factor epidemiology; by contrast, social epidemiology emphasizes social conditions as fundamental causes of disease. Social epidemiologists examine how persons become exposed to risk or protective factors and under what social conditions individual risk factors are related to disease. Social factors are thus the focus of analysis and are not simply adjusted for as potentially confounding factors or used as proxies for unavailable individual-level data.

Social factors are critical to understanding non-uniform infectious disease patterns that emerge as a result of the dependent nature of disease transmission, incorporating the idea that an outcome in one person is dependent upon outcomes and exposures in others. Applying the vocabulary developed in this chapter, structural social determinants must be examined along with the intermediary determinants connected to individual factors—including biological, demographic, and behavioural risk factors—that may influence the risk of HIV acquisition and disease progression. Structural determinants are central to understanding the diffusion and differential distribution of HIV/AIDS in population subgroups. Structural determinants include people's socioeconomic position, as well as the legal and policy environment. Laws and policies can mitigate

the differential exposure, vulnerability, and consequences people face as a result of socioeconomic differences. These factors, in turn, affect HIV transmission dynamics and the differential distribution of HIV/AIDS.

Table 2.2.1, following work by Poundstone et al. (2004), summarizes the main features of approaches to HIV/AIDS based on: (1) a risk-factor perspective and (2) social epidemiology oriented to action on the determinants of health inequities.

This comparison does not imply an 'either/or'. Policies and interventions based on risk-factor analysis and responsive to individual needs are vital in confronting a major epidemic. However, the table emphasizes that, to achieve maximum results in combating HIV/AIDS while reducing equity gaps between more and less advantaged social groups, specific policies focused on underlying structural factors are indispensable. Policies informed by this social analysis are different from measures guided by a concern with individual risk factors; the objectives of the former cannot be met by simply doing more of the latter. This has consequences for the way public health challenges such as scaling up HIV/AIDS treatment are addressed—in particular, the requirement that responses be designed to expand vulnerable communities' control over decisions affecting their lives, fostering a genuine redistribution of social power through public health action.

These points of view have important implications for future epidemiological research on HIV/AIDS and for the design of more effective HIV/AIDS interventions. Ultimately, social epidemiology research in HIV/AIDS will help determine how we can design more effective sets of interventions at multiple levels of social organization. From a policymaking standpoint, cross-sector approaches are required for the effective implementation of interventions that address the structural social aspects of HIV/AIDS.

The examples of skilled birth attendance and child malnutrition

Two additional examples analyse the comparative impacts of the conceptual framework's main components—including socioeconomic position and intermediary determinants—on specific forms of health inequity. The analysis highlights the powerful impact of socioeconomic position in determining inequities across a broad spectrum of health challenges. At the same time, these examples show that the effects of specific categories of intermediary determinants, such as health system factors, vary considerably when we consider different areas of health action. This has important implications for public health policymaking, as well as for the monitoring systems needed to provide evidence for policymaking and programme management.

The pervasive impact of socioeconomic position

Figure 2.2.4 shows the results of analyses carried out by the WHO Department of Equity, Poverty and Social Determinants of Health[2] in 2007, based on data from the Demographic and Health Surveys (DHS) in a group of countries in Africa. This work generated an equity analysis grounded in the determinants framework presented in this chapter. The researchers identified items on the DHS survey that could provide information on each of the main framework components: Structural determinants (including socioeconomic–political context and socioeconomic position) and intermediary

---

2   Now the Department of Ethics, Equity, Trade and Human Rights.

Table 2.2.1 HIV/AIDS epidemiology and intervention strategies using different paradigms (adapted from Poundstone *et al.* 2004)

Research paradigm	Key research questions	Understanding of determinants of health	Intervention model and strategy

Risk factor epidemiology	What individual characteristics are associated with development of AIDS and disease progression?	1. Risk of HIV/AIDS is manifest at the individual level.
		2. To change unhealthy or risky behaviours, individual responsibility and choice are sufficient.
			1. Interventions focus on the individual
			   a) Behaviour change to prevent HIV transmission
			   b) Access to clinical AIDS care
			Strategy based on tackling intermediary determinants

Social epidemiology incorporating social determinants of health inequities	How do economic and political determinants help establish and perpetuate inequalities in HIV/AIDS distribution within and between populations? How do social factors influence psychology or behaviour to place persons at higher risk of HIV infection?	1. Limited access to resources places persons at risk of HIV infection and AIDS disease progression. 2. Psychosocial factors are conditioned and modified by the larger social context in which they occur. 3. Social determinants affect HIV/AIDS risk by shaping patterns of population susceptibility and vulnerability.	1. Interventions focus on policies and programmes to address structural social factors, enabling large reductions in HIV/AIDS at the population level and gains in equity 2. Interventions focus on creating space for vulnerable groups to gain greater control over their own lives: redistribution of social power *Strategy based on tackling structural determinants*

determinants (including behavioural factors and health system factors). An analysis was performed using a decomposable health concentration index. The purpose was to quantify the contributions of the different social determinants of health to the total wealth-related inequity in the area of skilled birth attendance. In all

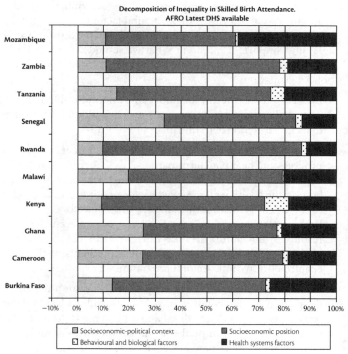

Fig. 2.2.4 Contributions of social determinants to inequities in skilled birth attendance in several African countries. Analysis performed by the former WHO Department of Equity, Poverty and Social Determinants of Health (Hosseinpoor *et al.* 2007).

countries analysed, socioeconomic position plays a fundamental role, accounting for between 50.3 and 77.6 per cent of the observed inequities in skilled birth attendance. Intermediary factors, such as living and working conditions and behaviours, play a minor role, not more than 7 per cent in the countries studied. The health system itself was found to cause between 11.5 and 33.3 per cent of inequities. Across all countries and all public health indicators for which comparable analyses has been performed, socioeconomic position regularly emerges as the most powerful determinant of inequities in health among social groups. The arguments developed in this chapter suggest that this is because socioeconomic position reflects people's level of power in society.

Different health challenges show different profiles

Figure 2.2.5 compares the relative causal impact of determinants on equity in two different key health indicators in Mozambique: Skilled birth attendance and child malnutrition. The results confirm that socioeconomic position plays the major role in shaping inequities in both these areas, accounting for 51 per cent of the observed inequities in malnutrition and 48 per cent in skilled birth attendance. Intermediary factors, such as living and working conditions and behaviours, play a minor role in connection with skilled birth attendance, although they constitute a somewhat more important determinant of inequities in malnutrition.

Significant differences between malnutrition and skilled birth attendance emerge when the impact of health systems factors on inequities is considered. Public health policy to address these issues will look very different, as monitoring and evaluation processes are configured to provide information on a wide spectrum of social determinants of health—in this case, especially the respective impacts of health systems factors on inequities. In the case of child malnutrition, the health system accounts for only 9 per cent of observed inequities. In skilled birth attendance, the proportion of inequities directly linked to health system factors rises to almost 38 per cent.

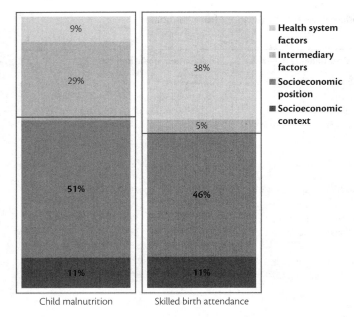

Fig. 2.2.5 Contribution of social determinants to health inequities in malnutrition and skilled birth attendance in Mozambique. Data source: DHS 2003. Analysis: WHO Department of Equity, Poverty and Social Determinants of Health (Hosseinpoor *et al.* 2007).

This suggests very different opportunities for the health sector to reduce inequities through direct action in these two areas.

At the same time, even in the case of skilled birth attendance, in the best case scenario, actions that can be undertaken directly by the health system still leave more than 60 per cent of health inequities untouched, given that the largest determinants of inequity lie beyond the reach of the health sector. This finding constitutes an argument that can be used to engage other sectors in work towards health equity. The bulk of inequities remain rooted in areas that must be addressed through coordination, cooperation, and integration of health policies and programmes with those of other sectors.

The picture emerging from these examples implies major differences in the nature of policy priorities to address equity challenges connected with different health problems, and in the degree of autonomy health officials enjoy to directly implement measures that can be expected to have a significant positive impact on health equity in these various areas. An approach sensitive to these differences is only possible when researchers and programme managers incorporate a social determinants perspective into their analyses, and when managers and policymakers recognize the causal hierarchy of determinants, as regards their origins, interrelationships, and respective impact. This highlights the need to develop health monitoring systems that provide information on social determinants of health, as a complement to more conventional population health indicators.

Conclusion

This chapter opened with three questions:

1. If we trace health differences among social groups back to their deepest roots, where do they originate?

2. What pathways lead from root causes to the stark differences in health status observed at the population level?

3. In light of the answers to the first two questions, where and how should we intervene to reduce health inequities?

The framework presented in these pages has been developed to provide responses to these problems. To the first question, on the origins of health inequities, we have answered as follows. The root causes of health inequities are to be found in the social, economic, and political mechanisms that give rise to a set of hierarchically ordered socioeconomic positions within society, whereby groups are stratified according to income, education, occupation, gender, race/ethnicity, and other factors. The fundamental mechanisms that produce and maintain (but that can also reduce or mitigate effect) this stratification include: Governance; the education system; labour market structures; and redistributive welfare state policies (or their absence). We have referred to the component factors of socioeconomic position as *structural determinants*. Structural determinants, together with the features of the socioeconomic and political context that shape their impact, constitute the *social determinants of health inequities*. The structural mechanisms that configure social hierarchies according to key stratifiers are the root cause of health inequities.

Our answer to the second question, about pathways from root causes to observed inequities in health, was elaborated by tracing how the underlying social determinants of health inequities operate through a set of what we call *intermediary determinants of health* to shape health outcomes. The main categories of intermediary determinants of health are: Material circumstances; psychosocial circumstances; behavioural and/or biological factors; and the health system itself as a social determinant. The vocabulary of 'structural determinants' and 'intermediary determinants' underscores the causal priority of the structural factors.

This chapter provides only a partial answer to the third and arguably most important question: What we should do reduce health inequities. However, the framework suggests three fundamental policy orientations:

♦ Efforts to reduce health inequities must not limit themselves to intermediary determinants, but must include policies crafted to tackle structural determinants.

♦ Intersectoral policymaking and implementation are crucial for progress on health determinants. This is because structural determinants can only be tackled through strategies that reach beyond the health sector. A key task for public health research is to: (1) identify successful examples of intersectoral action on health determinants in jurisdictions with different levels of resources and administrative capacity; and (2) characterize in detail the political and management mechanisms that have enabled effective intersectoral programmes.

♦ Participation of civil society and affected communities in the design and implementation of policies to address health determinants is vital, both on ethical and on pragmatic grounds. Real social participation in public health action works as an instrument to redistribute power in society, because it forces political authorities to listen to the voices and demands of excluded communities. In this sense, authentic participation can change the structural determinants of health inequities and give sustainability to these changes.

Subsequent chapters in this section will explore the role of specific determinants in greater detail. Chapters 3.2, 3.3, and 4.2, in particular, will delve further into the challenges of public health policy.

References

Adler, N.E., Boyce, T., Chesney, M.A. *et al.* (1994). Socioeconomic status and health: The challenge of the gradient. *American Psychologist*, **49**, 15–24.

Antonovsky, A. (1967). Social class life expectancy and overall mortality. *Milbank Memorial Fund Quarterly*, **45**, 31–73.

Ball, T. (1992). New faces of power. In (ed. T. Wartenberg) *Rethinking power*, pp. 11–24. SUNY Press, Albany.

Ben-Shlomo, Y. and Kuh, D. (2002). A life course approach to chronic disease epidemiology: Conceptual models, empirical challenges and interdisciplinary perspectives. *International Journal of Epidemiology*, **31**, 285–93.

Berlinguer, G. (2006). The social determinants of disease. Unpublished manuscript.

Bernales, P. (2006). Social capital review. Unpublished background study for the WHO conceptual framework on social determinants of health. WHO Department of Equity, Poverty and Social Determinants of Health, Geneva.

Braveman, P. and Gruskin, S. (2003). Defining equity in health. *Journal of Epidemiology and Community Health*, **57**, 254–58.

Cassel, J. (1976). The contribution of the social environment to host resistance. *American Journal of Epidemiology*, **104**, 107–23.

Chung, H. and Muntaner, C. (2006). Political and welfare state determinants of infant and child health indicators: An analysis of wealthy countries. *Social Science and Medicine*, **63**, 829–42.

Colgrove, J. (2002). The McKeown thesis: A historical controversy and its enduring influence. *American Journal of Public Health*, **92**, 725–9.

Dahlgren, G. and Whitehead, M. (2006). *Levelling up (part 1): A discussion paper on European strategies for tackling social inequities in health*. WHO EURO, Copenhagen.

Davey Smith, G. (2003). *Health inequalities: Lifecourse approaches*. Policy Press, Bristol.

Diderichsen, F. (1998). Towards a theory of health equity. Unpublished draft manuscript.

Diderichsen, F. (2004). *Resource allocation for health equity: Issues and methods*. The World Bank, Department of Health, Nutrition and Population (HNP), Washington.

Diderichsen, F., Evans, T., and Whitehead, M. (2001). The social basis of disparities in health. In *Challenging inequities in health* (eds. T. Evans, M. Whitehead, F. Diderichsen, A. Bhuiya and M. Wirth). Oxford University Press, New York.

Emerson, E. (2004). Poverty and children with intellectual disabilities in the world's richer countries. *Journal of Intellectual and Developmental Disability*, **29**, 319–37.

Escobedo, L.G., Anda, R.F., Smith, P.F. *et al.* (1990). Sociodemographic characteristics of cigarette smoking initiation in the United States: Implications for smoking prevention policy. *Journal of the American Medical Association*, **264**, 1550–5.

Esping-Andersen, G. (2002). *Why we need a new Welfare State*. Oxford University Press, New York.

Evans, T., Whitehead, M., Diderichsen, F. *et al.* (eds.)(2001). *Challenging inequities in health*. Oxford University Press, New York.

Fee, E. and Krieger, N. (1993). Understanding AIDS: Historical interpretations and the limits of biomedical individualism. *American Journal of Public Health*, **83**, 1477–86.

Ferguson, K. (2006). Social capital and children's wellbeing: A critical synthesis of the international social capital literature. *International Journal of Social Welfare*, **15**, 2–18.

Frankel, S., Elwood, P., Sweetnam, P. *et al.* (1996). Birthweight, body-mass index in middle age, and incident coronary heart disease. *Lancet*, **348**, 1478–80.

Gee, G.C. (2002). A multilevel analysis of the relationship between institutional and individual racial discrimination and health status. *American Journal of Public Health*, **92**, 615–23.

Graham, H. (2004). Social determinants and their unequal distribution. *Milbank Quarterly*, **82**, 101–24.

Graham, H. (2005). Intellectual disabilities and socioeconomic inequalities in health: An overview of research. *Journal of Applied Research in Inequalities*, **18**, 101–11.

Graham, H. and Kelly, M.P. (2004). *Health inequalities: Concepts, frameworks and policy*. NHS Health Development Agency Briefing Paper. NHS Health Development Agency, London.

Hosseinpoor, A., Prasad, A., and Vega, J. (2007). *WHO report on inequities in maternal and child health in Mozambique*. Mission report, Department of Equity, Poverty and Social Determinants of Health, WHO, Geneva.

Howden-Chapman, P., Blakely, T., Blaiklock, A.J. *et al.* (2000). Closing the health gap. *New Zealand Medical Journal*, **113**, 301–2.

Illsley, R. and Baker, D. (1991). Contextual variations in the meaning of health inequality. *Social Science and Medicine*, **32**, 359–65.

Instituto de Estudios Politicos para America Latina y Africa (2005). Curso sistematico de derechos humanos. Online training course. Available at: <http://www.iepala.es/curso_ddhh/ddhh27.htm>. Accessed 8 December 2007.

Kaplan, G.A., Pamuk, E.R., Lynch, J.W. *et al.* (1996). Inequality in income and mortality in the United States: analysis of mortality and potential pathways. *British Medical Journal*, **312**, 999–1003.

Kaprio, J. and Koskenvuo, M. (1988). A prospective study of psychological and socioeconomic characteristics, health behavior and morbidity in cigarette smokers prior to quitting compared to persistent smokers and non-smokers. *Journal of Clinical Epidemiology*, **41**, 139–50.

Kawachi, I., Kennedy, B.P., Lochner, K. *et al.* (1997). Social capital, income inequality, and mortality. *American Journal of Public Health*, **87**, 1491–8.

Kleczkowki, B.M., Roemer, M., and Van Der Werff, A. (1984). *National health systems and their reorientation toward health for all: Guidance for policymaking*. WHO, Geneva.

Koopman, J.S. and Longini, I.M. (1994). The ecological effects of individual exposures and nonlinear disease dynamics in populations. *American Journal of Public Health*, **84**, 836–42.

Krieger, N. (2001). Theories for social epidemiology in the 21st century: An ecosocial perspective. *International Journal of Epidemiology*, **30**, 668–77.

Krieger, N. (2002). A glossary for social epidemiology. *Epidemiological Bulletin*, **23**, 7–11.

Krieger, N. (2005). Embodiment: A conceptual glossary for epidemiology. *Journal of Epidemiology and Community Health*, **59**, 350–5.

Krieger, N., Williams, D.R., and Moss, N.E. (1997). Measuring social class. *Annual Review of Public Health*, **18**, 341–78.

Krieger, N., Rowley, D.L., Herman, A.A. *et al.* (1993). Racism, sexism and social class, implications for studies of health, diseases and well being. *Annual Journal of Preventive Medicine*, **9**, 82–122.

Kubzansky, L.D., Sparrow, D., Vokonas, P. *et al.* (2001). Is the glass half empty or half full? A prospective study of optimism and coronary heart disease in the normative aging study. *Psychosomatic Medicine*, **63**, 910–16.

Lalonde, M. (1974). *A new perspective on the health of Canadians*. Ministry of Health and Welfare, Ottawa.

Liberatos, P., Link, B.G., and Kelsey, J.L. (1988). The measurement of social class in epidemiology. *Epidemiology Review*, **10**, 87–121.

Lobmayer, P. and Wilkinson, R.G. (2002). Inequality, residential segregation by income, and mortality in US cities. *Journal of Epidemiology and Community Health*, **56**, 183–7.

Luttrell, C. and Quiroz, S. (2007). *Understanding and operationalising empowerment*. Joint electronic publication by: poverty-wellbeing.net/ Swiss Agency for Development and Cooperation/Inter-Development/ Overseas Development Institute.

Lynch, J. (2000). Income inequality and health: expanding the debate. *Social Science and Medicine*, **51**, 1001–5.

Lynch, J., Due, P., Muntaner, C. *et al.* (2000). Social capital: Is it a good investment strategy for public health? *Journal of Epidemiology and Community Health*, **54**, 404–8.

Lynch, J.W., Kaplan, G.A., Pamuk, E.R. *et al.* (1998). Income inequality and mortality in metropolitan areas of the United States. *American Journal of Public Health*, **88**, 1074–80.

Lynch, J. and Smith, G.D. (2005). A life course approach to chronic disease epidemiology. *Annual Review of Public Health*, **26**, 1–35.

Lynch, J., Smith, G.D., Hillemeier, M. *et al.* (2001). Income inequality, the psychosocial environment, and health: Comparisons of wealthy nations. *Lancet*, **358**, 194–200.

Macintyre, S. (2000). Modernizing the NHS: Prevention and the reduction of health inequities. *British Medical Journal*, **320**, 1399–1400.

Macintyre, S. (2007). *Inequalities in health in Scotland: What are they and what can we do about them?* MRC Social and Public Health Sciences Unit Occasional Paper No. 17. Medical Research Council Social and Public Health Sciences Unit, Glasgow.

Mackenbach, J.P. and Bakker, M.J. (eds.) (2002). *Reducing inequalities in health: A European perspective*. Routledge, London and New York.

Mackenbach, J.P., Bakker, M.J., Kunst, A.E. *et al.*(2002). Socioeconomic inequalities in health in Europe: An overview. In *Reducing inequalities in health: A European perspective* (eds. J.P. Mackenbach and M.J. Bakker). Routledge, London and New York.

Manor, O., Matthews, S., and Power, C. (2003). Health selection: The role of inter- and intra-generational mobility on social inequalities in health. *Social Science and Medicine*, **57**, 2217–27.

Margolis, P.A., Greenberg, R.A., Keyes, L.L. *et al.* (1992). Lower respiratory illness in infants and low socioeconomic status. *American Journal of Public Health*, **82**, 1119–26.

Marmot, M. (2002). The influence of income on health: views of an epidemiologist. *Health Affairs* (Millwood), **21**, 31–46.

Marmot, M. (2004). *The status syndrome: How social standing affects our health and longevity*. Henry Holt, New York.

Marmot, M.G., Rose, G., Shipley, M. *et al.* (1978). Employment grade and coronary heart disease in British civil servants. *Journal of Epidemiology and Community Health*, **32**, 244–9.

Marmot, M.G., Shipley, M.J., and Rose, G. (1984). Inequalities in death—specific explanations of a general pattern? *Lancet*, May 5, 1(8384), 1003–6.

Marmot, M.G., Smith, G.D., Stansfeld, S. *et al.* (1991). Health inequalities among British civil servants: the Whitehall II study. *Lancet*, **337**, 1387–93.

Marmot, M. and Wilkinson, R.G. (2001). Psychosocial and material pathways in the relation between income and health: A response to Lynch *et al. British Medical Journal*, **322**, 1233–6.

Maughan, B., Collishaw, S., and Pickles, A. (1999). Mild mental retardation: Psychosocial functioning in adulthood. *Psychological Medicine*, **29**, 351–66.

McMichael, A.J. (1999). Prisoners of the proximate: Loosening the constraints on epidemiology in an age of change. *American Journal of Epidemiology*, **149**, 887–97.

Moore, S., Haines, V., Hawe, P. *et al.* (2006). Lost in translation: a genealogy of the "social capital" concept in public health. *Journal of Epidemiology and Community Health*, **60**, 729–34.

Muntaner, C. (2004). Commentary: Social capital, social class, and the slow progress of psychosocial epidemiology. *International Journal of Epidemiology*, **33**, 674–80.

Muntaner, C., Borell, C., Benach, J. *et al.* (2003). The associations of social class and social stratification with patterns of general and mental health in a Spanish population. *International Journal of Epidemiology*, **32**, 950–8.

Muntaner, C., Lynch, J., and Oates, G.L. (1999). The social class determinants of income inequality and social cohesion. *International Journal of Health Services*, **20**, 699–732.

National Association of County and City Health Officials (NACCHO) (2002). *Creating Health Equity through Social Justice*. Draft Working paper. NACCHO, Washington.

Navarro, V. and Shi, L. (2001). The Political Context of Social Inequalities and Health. *International Journal of Health Services*, **31**, 1–21.

Popay, J. (2000). Social capital: the role of narrative and historical research. *Journal of Epidemiology and Community Health*, **54**, 401.

Poundstone, K.E., Strathdee, S.A., and Celentano, D.D. (2004). The social epidemiology of human immunodeficiency virus/acquired immunodeficiency syndrome. *Epidemiology Review*, **26**, 22–35.

Power, C. and Hertzman, C. (2004). Health and human development from life course research. In *Population Health:*

Policy dilemmas (eds. M. Barer, R. Evans, C. Hertzman and J. Heyman). Oxford University Press, Oxford.

Putnam, R. (2000). *Bowling alone: The collapse and revival of American community*. Simon & Schuster, New York.

Putnam, R. (2001). Foreword. In *Social capital and poor communities* (eds. S. Saegert, J.P. Thompson and M.R. Warren), pp. xv–xvi. Russell Sage Foundation, New York.

Raphael, D. (2006). Social determinants of health: Present status, unanswered questions, and future directions. *International Journal of Health Services*, **36**, 651–77.

Raphael, D. and Bryant, T. (2006). Maintaining population health in a period of welfare state decline: Political economy as the missing dimension in health promotion theory and practice. *Promotion & education*, **13**, 236–42.

Rose, G. (2001). Sick individuals and sick populations. *International Journal of Epidemiology*, **30**, 427–32.

Schwartz, S. (1994). The fallacy of the ecological fallacy: the potential misuse of a concept and the consequences. *American Journal of Public Health*, **84**, 819–24.

Sigerist, H. (1943). *Civilization and disease*. University of Chicago Press, Chicago.

Smith, G.D. and Egger, M. (1996). Commentary: understanding it all—health, meta-theories, and mortality trends. *British Medical Journal*, **313**, 1584–5.

Solar, O. and Irwin, A. (2007). *A conceptual framework for action on the social determinants of health*. Working paper of the WHO Department of Equity, Poverty and Social Determinants of Health and the Commission on Social Determinants of Health. WHO, Geneva.

Solar, O., Irwin, A., and Vega, J. (2004). Equity in health sector reform and reproductive health: Measurement issues and the health systems context. Unpublished working paper. WHO Health Equity Team, Geneva.

Susser, M., Watson, W., and Hopper, K. (1985). *Sociology in medicine*. Oxford University Press, New York.

Szreter, S. (2002). Rethinking McKeown: The relationship between public health and social change. *American Journal of Public Health*, **92**, 722–5.

Szreter, S. (2004). Industrialization and health. *British Medical Bulletin*, **69**, 75–86.

Szreter, S. and Woolcock, M. (2004). Health by association? Social capital, social theory, and the political economy of public health. *International Journal of Epidemiology*, **33**, 650–67.

Tajer, D. (2003). Latin American social medicine: Roots, development during the 1990s, and current challenges. *American Journal of Public Health*, **93**, 2023–7.

Tarlov, A. (1996). Social determinants of health: The sociobiological translation. In *Health and social organization* (eds. D. Blane, E. Brunner and R.Wilkinson), pp. 71–93. Routledge, London.

Virchow, R. (1985 [1848]). *Collected essays on public health and epidemiology*. Science History Publications, Cambridge.

Whitehead, M., Burström, B., and Diderichsen, F. (2000). Social policies and the pathways to inequalities in health: A comparative analysis of lone mothers in Britain and Sweden. *Social Science and Medicine*, **50**, 255–70.

WHO (2004). Glossary of equity, gender, human rights, poverty, social determinants and related issues in health. Unpublished working document. WHO Health Equity Team, Geneva.

WHO and UNICEF (1978). *Declaration of Alma Ata*. WHO, Geneva.

Wilkinson, R.G. (2000). Inequality and the social environment: A reply to Lynch *et al. Journal of Epidemiology and Community Health*, **54**, 411–3.

Wilkinson, R.G. and Pickett, K.E. (2006). Income inequality and population health: A review and explanation of the evidence. *Social Science and Medicine*, **62**, 1768–84.

2.3

Behavioural determinants of health and disease

Lawrence W. Green and Robert A. Hiatt

Introduction

That behaviour is associated with health and disease has never been in doubt. Indeed, the tendency to blame sinful, negligent, indulgent, ignorant, reckless, or selfish behaviour for health problems has too often placed undue emphasis on individual responsibility and culpability when the solution to health problems of populations demanded attention to the social and physical environment. But no matter how behaviour is framed or moralized in relation to its causes, it remains an inescapable variable in the pathway between ultimate upstream aetiologies and the incidence or prevalence of most diseases and health conditions downstream. Approaches to public health have sought throughout the history of civilization (1) to control or cajole the health-related behaviour of individuals, (2) to protect individuals from the behaviour of others, and (3) to mobilize the behaviour of groups to influence health-related social and physical environments.

This chapter reviews the ways in which behaviour relates to the spectrum of health and disease determinants, from environmental to genetic, in shaping health outcomes. It builds on the previous chapters in recognizing the powerful influence of socioeconomic factors, especially poverty, in influencing both behaviour and health. Many commentaries in the past two decades have attempted to correct the early overemphasis on behavioural determinants of health by discounting and sometimes disparaging any focus on individual behaviour in disease prevention and health promotion. This chapter seeks a middle ground, building on the growing understanding of the ecological context of the behaviour–health relationship. It seeks to integrate that knowledge in an approach to public health that acknowledges the reciprocal determinism of behavioural, environmental, and biologic determinants rather than minimizing the importance of behaviour in these complex interactions.

The shifting role of behaviour as a determinant of health and disease

Simple, discrete behaviours account for many of the infections and injuries of the past. Today's growing chronic disease burden relates more to complex behaviours. We use the term 'complex behaviour' to refer to combinations of interrelated practices and their environmental contexts, reflecting patterns of living influenced by the family and social history of individuals and communities, their environmental and socioeconomic circumstances, and their exposure to cultures and communications. We know that discrete behaviours can be influenced directly by health education targeted at individuals and groups. Complex behaviour changes more slowly and usually requires some combination of educational, organizational, economic, and environmental interventions in support of changes in both behaviour and conditions of living. This combination of strategies has defined health promotion and public health programmes addressing complex behaviour change (Green & Kreuter 2005; Smith *et al.* 2006).

Obesity and HIV/AIDS present the obvious contemporary examples of health-related conditions and diseases awaiting technological solutions, for which behaviour, in the meantime, is a necessary route of intervention and change. Virtually every public health breakthrough has had a behavioural change process that served the public until the technology was at hand. Then, behavioural change processes were needed to diffuse, adapt, and apply the new technology to varying cultural and social circumstances. Unless and until an obesity prevention vaccine or HIV vaccine is developed, society must depend on behavioural preventive measures to curb the spread of obesity and AIDS. These include, of course, policies, environmental changes, and health educational programmes that support behavioural changes.

Much of the early success in controlling HIV infections through change in sexual practices (especially use of condoms) among men in urban gay communities appear to have been in response to health education programmes (Petrow 1990). Reviews also show increases in the use of clean needles for at least 15 years among intravenous drug users (e.g. Wodak 2006), which has required a combination of policy and educational interventions to make clean needles accessible and more acceptable than the culture of needle-sharing. Evidence that health education leads to the regular use of condoms among sexually active adolescents, however, has not held up consistently (James *et al.* 2006; Koniak-Griffin & Stein 2006; Walker *et al.* 2006). The parallel lessons from the success of tobacco control programmes also point to the need for combined policy, regulatory, organizational, environmental, and educational interventions to influence population changes in tobacco consumption (Eriksen *et al.* 2007) and many of the same types of interventions are under consideration for obesity control (Mercer *et al.* 2005).

Specific behaviours and health—the causal links

Some behaviour clearly increases the risk of developing disease and can be considered a proximal cause of disease, such as hygienic practices that expose one to infections. Other behaviours correlate with and precede better health, increased longevity, and decreased disease risk, but their causal link is more tenuous, warranting their inclusion with more distal determinants, such as general dietary and physical activity patterns. Examining the relationships between specific behavioural patterns and indicators of health and disease status provides the foundation for assessing behavioural factors as population health determinants. Examining the covariation of these relationships with other characteristics of the populations and their environmental circumstances helps put behaviour into its ecological, social, and cultural context.

The causal link is relatively easy to establish for single-agent communicable or infectious diseases. Evidence from observational epidemiological studies, human experimental trials, and animal models, together with clear mechanisms of biological action, lead one to conclude that many behaviours are, in fact, contributing causes (causal risk factors) of specific diseases. Again, the easiest examples of clear causal linkages are those established for single-action behaviours such as ingesting a contaminated food, getting an immunization that confers lifetime immunity, or taking a one-dose medication that leads to rapidly improved symptoms, or even a cure. As the number of booster shots required for immunization or doses required for cure increase, the behaviour becomes more complex, requiring repetition or timing, and the causal linkage more difficult to unravel among the biomedical agent, the behaviour, and all the other events and circumstances that might have intervened and influenced the outcome along the way.

Complex behaviours and health—the causal pathways and synergies

More difficult still are causal attributions and allocations for long-term behavioural patterns that are not under medical supervision and relate to multiple-cause chronic diseases and conditions (Krieger 1984; Glass & McAtee 2006). We present three examples of evidence supporting causal links between behaviours and coronary heart disease: Smoking, diet, and physical activity. These three examples illustrate that even in the absence of direct experimental evidence in human beings, strong evidence of other types can be combined for the steps in a causal chain from behaviour through physiological effects to disease or health. In addition, the synergistic effects of two or more behaviours on health outcomes have been established.

A plausible biological model of the relationship between smoking behaviour and coronary heart disease has been available for decades (Dawber 1960). Observational epidemiological studies—including within- and between-population designs, case-control, and prospective designs—produced strong and consistent measures of association, the hypothesized temporal sequence, and dose–response relationships in subsequent decades (Stamler 1992). Additional randomized trials have included smoking cessation

programmes that provide experimental evidence for smoking as a cause of coronary heart disease. Although the overall results of the Multiple Risk Factor Intervention Trial (MRFIT) in the United States were disappointing, in both MRFIT (Okene *et al.* 1990) and the British trial on the effect of smoking reduction (Rose & Colwell 1992), cessation interventions showed decreases in coronary heart disease mortality respectively of 13 per cent after 20 years and 12 per cent after 10.5 years. In addition, when smokers at baseline from the experimental and control groups were pooled, quitters had a significant decrease in their risk of mortality from coronary heart disease compared with non-quitters (Okene *et al.* 1990).

On the dietary front, evidence that saturated fat and cholesterol consumption behaviour contributes to coronary heart disease came first from ecological studies showing a correlation between dietary patterns and serum cholesterol levels (Keys *et al.* 1958), and later dietary fat consumption levels, and the corresponding geographical coronary heart disease incidence rates and mortality (Keys 1970). A 30-year follow-up of the Framingham cohort samples showed that high levels of serum cholesterol predicted the risk of coronary heart disease development (Anderson *et al.* 1987). In a meta-analysis of 27 trials, Mensink and Katan (1992) found that changes in dietary saturated fat and cholesterol led to changes in serum cholesterol. In the Helsinki Heart Study, Frick *et al.* (1987) showed that interventions to lower serum cholesterol levels decreased the occurrence of coronary heart disease. A definitive demonstration of the diet–heart hypothesis by a true experimental study might never occur because of the large sample size required, the sustained differential changes needed between intervention and control groups, and the long-term follow-up required for such a trial. The strong evidence for each step in a causal chain from diet to coronary heart disease and mortality, however, led to major national and international recommendations that diet be a first-line approach to reduce blood cholesterol to prevent disease, and more urgently today in the face of the global obesity epidemic (e.g. Health Canada 2003; NHLBI 1993; US Department of Health and Human Services 2001; WHO 1990, 2000).

Physical inactivity as a risk factor for coronary heart disease is the third example. Evidence that physical inactivity contributes to coronary heart disease came from studies of the biological effects of exercise on cardiovascular physiology, observational epidemiological studies, and randomized controlled trials of physical activity and physiological coronary heart disease risk factors, such as high blood pressure, obesity, and diabetes. The biological effects of exercise training to enhance cardiovascular health were well established by the 1980s (McArdle *et al.* 1986). Epidemiological evidence continues to show consistent and relatively strong associations, the hypothesized temporal sequence, and a dose–response relationship between physical activity and coronary heart disease (Blair *et al.* 1993). Observational epidemiological and randomized controlled trials demonstrated the beneficial effects of physical activity on blood pressure (Arroll & Beaglehole 1992) and on blood lipids and lipoproteins (Lokey & Tran 1989), which have, in turn, been causally linked with subsequent coronary heart disease. The combination of these sources of evidence for each of the steps in a causal chain provides a plausible model for the sequence.

Some of the immediate causal risk factors are not themselves behaviours, but have determinants that are behaviours. In these cases, the behavioural determinants can be regarded as indirect risk factors that act earlier in the causal pathway. For example, a combination of overeating and sedentary behaviour produce high caloric intake and low energy output, which together mediate the behavioural determinants of obesity. Obesity, in turn, is a physiological risk factor for cardiovascular diseases and type 2 diabetes (Stern 1991).

Behaviour also contributes to the prognosis of diseases at each stage where the screening, diagnosis, or the compliance with prescribed regimens of treatment or self-care affects outcomes. For example, the prognosis of breast cancer depends on the stage of disease at which the woman obtains screening, diagnosis, and medical care. The prognosis for type 1 (insulin dependent) diabetes depends on the patient's compliance with his or her insulin prescriptions. Because behaviour is so central to disease outcomes, a large literature on patient education and patient compliance with medical regimens has been catalogued and subjected to meta-analyses with regularity (e.g. Mullen *et al.* 1985; D.G. Simons-Morton *et al.* 1992; Malik & Hu 2007).

Behavioural risk factors in population health

The causal pathways by which behaviour can influence health (or its negative manifestations) can be broadly classified as direct (as shown by arrow 1 in Fig. 2.3.1) and indirect, where the indirect pathways (arrows 2 and 3 in Fig. 2.3.1) are largely mediated through the environment or through healthcare organization and personnel. These three determinants of health—behaviour, environment, and healthcare organization—in addition to human biology, were cast as the 'Health Field Concept' as part of the Lalonde Report on the Health of Canadians (Canada 1974), which many credit with having launched the health promotion and population health movements in public health. The third indirect pathway could be drawn through genetics, the main pathway by which individuals can make some reproductive decisions independent of the medical care system, but such non-medically mediated decisions are largely mediated by the social environment. Figure 2.3.1 is hardly a full representation of the three sets of variables (behaviour, environment, healthcare organization), much less the genetic interactions, insofar as there is much reciprocal determinism between behaviour and each of the various environments, as well as with genetics. These environmental influences on behaviour will be examined in the next section, and behaviour's influence on the environment in a later section.

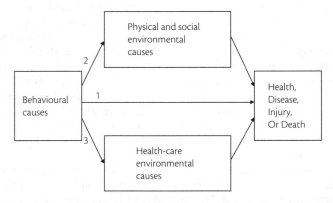

Fig. 2.3.1 Three pathways for behavioural influence on health, disease, injury, or death.

Behaviour itself as a risk factor for disease

The direct pathway suggested by Fig. 2.3.1 includes the broad array of actions people take, consciously or unconsciously, that can have an immediate or cumulative effect on their health status. The effect on health may be intended (health-directed) or unintended (health-related), but the behaviour is nevertheless direct in its effect. The most dramatic of these are the violent injury-causing actions people may take behind the wheel of an automobile, with weapons, or unintentionally with the careless use of tools or toxic substances or merely walking absent-mindlessly on a slippery or cluttered surface. Less dramatic, but no less lethal, are the cumulative little actions people take each time they light a cigarette, imbibe or inject an addictive or mind-altering substance, or abide by neglect of physical activity or healthful foods.

Table 2.3.1 lists the nine leading causes of death in most of the more developed countries, as reflected here by the United States, and relates those to the risk factors for each in column 2, which McGinnis and Foege (1993, 2004) and Mokdad *et al.* (2004) refer to as the 'actual causes of death'. Colditz (2001) has noted that more than half of all cancer is a consequence of behaviour, much of which is embedded in culture. Most of the risk factors in Table 2.3.1 are themselves behaviours. Those that are not behaviours themselves—such as high serum cholesterol, obesity, hypertension, and diabetes mellitus—are the consequence, in large part, of behaviours. The behavioural determinants of physiological risk factors in column 3 present some of the most challenging targets for public health intervention, because they require decreasing behaviours that are perceived as pleasurable (e.g. types of food, sedentary entertainment, spontaneous sexual encounters) and increasing behaviours perceived as boring, painful, or inconvenient (e.g. less sugary or salty foods, more strenuous or frequent physical activity, use of condoms). Their challenges are compounded by the fact that most of the instances of these behavioural determinants of risk can be carried out very privately with limited opportunity for monitoring or social influence.

Tobacco consumption alone accounts for a large proportion of deaths in developed countries, implicated as a direct risk factor in all five of the leading causes of death shown in Table 2.3.1. At least one of the three main behavioural risk factors—smoking, dietary practices, and alcohol use—is causally related to each of the 10 leading causes of death shown in Table 2.3.1. Active smoking has been established as a risk factor for coronary heart disease, diabetes, stroke, and adverse pregnancy outcomes, such as low birth weight, premature rupture of membranes, and abruption placentae (USDHHS 2004). As examples of how the behaviour of some individuals can influence the health of others, passive smoking (i.e. exposure to environmental tobacco smoke) has been related to lung cancer and other respiratory diseases, as an independent risk factor for coronary heart disease, and exposure to environmental tobacco smoke in the home has been associated with asthma, other respiratory conditions, and with ear infections in infants and children (US Department of Health and Human Services 2006). Although still controversial, the California Environmental Protection Agency (2005) has concluded from its reviews that passive smoking is also a risk factor for breast cancer.

As noted in previous chapters, the causes of death in developing countries differ markedly from the patterns reflected in Table 2.3.1, although the demographic profiles are converging. WHO estimates of the four leading causes of death for the developing countries have been respiratory diseases, infectious and parasitic diseases,

Table 2.3.1 The nine leading causes of death in the United States (2003), their generally accepted behavioural (in italics) and physiological risk factors, and the behavioural determinants of the physiological risk factors

Causes of death (age-adjusted death rates in the United States per 100 000 population)	Selected risk factors	Behavioural determinants of physiological risk factors
Diseases of the heart (232.3)	*Smoking* *Physical inactivity* High serum cholesterol Obesity Hypertension Diabetes mellitus	High-fat diet High-calorie diet, physical inactivity High-salt diet High-calorie diet (obesity)
Malignant neoplasms (190.1)	*Smoking* *High-fat diet* *Low-fibre diet* *Physical inactivity* Sexually transmitted diseases	*Sexual behaviours*
Cerebrovascular diseases (53.5)	Hypertension Atherosclerosis *Smoking*	*High-salt diet* *High-fat diet*
Chronic obstructive pulmonary disease (43.3)	*Smoking*	
Unintentional injuries (37.3)	*Alcohol abuse* *Unsafe driving* *Seat-belt non-use* *Smoking* *Drug use*	
Diabetes mellitus (25.3)	*Physical inactivity* Obesity	*High-calorie diet+*
Pneumonia and influenza (22.0)	*Drug use* Immunization Status Malnutrition	*Failure to receive immunization* Diet
Suicide (10.8)	*Alcohol use* *Hand gun use* *Drug use*	
Chronic liver disease and cirrhosis (9.3)	*Alcohol abuse*	

Source: Adapted from National Center for Health Statistics, CDC (2006), p. 179. Death: Final data from 2003. *National Vital Statistics Reports,* **54**, 1–120; Mokdad *et al.* (2004).

cardiovascular diseases, and perinatal mortality. As tobacco use has increased and problems of macro-nutrients have replaced some of the micro-nutrient problems in those countries, other chronic diseases, in addition to cardiovascular diseases, have increased. By 2020, according to WHO (1998) estimates, the tobacco epidemic is expected to kill more people than any single disease. Because it is a known probable determinant of at least 25 diseases, and the most important determinant of some of the leading causes of death, tobacco use will cause nearly 18 per cent of all deaths in developed countries and 11 per cent in developing countries. This alone warrants the concerted global attention to this behaviour that has been proposed by the Framework Convention on Tobacco Control.

Behaviour as a determinant of other risk factors

Besides the cumulative effect of behaviours on physiological risk factors, such as the energy balance mentioned earlier between calorie intake and physical activity producing weight gain, obesity, and hypertension, many of the health consequences of behaviour are secondary to their impact on the immediate environment. Individuals are not merely the passive victims of the environments they inhabit or traverse. They are agents of change in those environments, and their ability to alter or control environmental threats to their own health increases with technological innovations. The growing capacity of individuals and groups to alter their environments through technological means, such as transport, also produces negative consequences for their health. Hence, health promotion and health protection have emphasized mobilizing individuals and groups to undertake personal conservation behaviours and collective actions to support policy changes and regulatory initiatives in support of more healthful environments.

Among the most striking differences in health between the developed and the developing countries are the perinatal-juvenile mortality rates. In their analysis of 66 countries, Hertz *et al.* (1994) found the three most important predictors of infant mortality rates to be percentage of households with sanitation, total literacy rate, and the percentage of households without safe water. The major public health goals in developing nations have related to the provision of immunization, access to a sufficient supply of clean water, and the installation of proper sanitation facilities (WHO 1981). But the more recent Millennium Development Goals (MDG) aim to cut global poverty by half by the year 2015, with three goals focused directly on health, covering maternal mortality, infant mortality, HIV/AIDS, malaria, and tuberculosis.

These environmental and age-specific or disease-specific health measures, however, achieve their intended health goals only to the extent that an informed population accepts and uses them properly. A report by the World Bank (1993) suggested that the single most important public health policy for developing countries lies in the improvement of the education of young girls. Better educated women have fewer children, who tend to be healthier and, in turn, better educated and able to respond to the technological advances offered by such environmental measures. They also become a better informed electorate to demand and support healthful policies for the installation of such facilities. In short, behaviour remains a critical mediator of the relationships between environmental measures and health outcomes, as well as the relationship between the health needs and the political actions to create the environmental changes.

The behaviour–policy link in the causal chains becomes more important as the chronic diseases creep into the developing countries. Inspection of the recent trends in the richest of the developing countries provides evidence that improvement of the socioeconomic condition is accompanied by a shift in mortality towards the chronic diseases and their behavioural risk factors reviewed earlier. In Mexico, for example, as early as 1991, infectious and parasitic diseases were only the fourth leading cause of death, following diseases of the heart, malignant neoplasms, and accidents. Developing countries are now the primary target for market expansion for the multinational tobacco companies, with convenience food companies close behind them. Behaviour will be an issue both in personally resisting the temptations offered by these industries and in collective action to restrain their advertising, promotion, ingredients, and location.

Behaviour as a consequence of cognitions, environments, and genetics

Notwithstanding the implied simplicity of identifying a few behaviours that account for the majority of deaths in developed countries, those and other behaviours are highly complex, value-laden, and over-determined. Most behavioural risk factors and healthcare behaviours as well, are the product of a variety of component behaviours, tasks, or actions. For example, food consumption confronts most people with a chain of related behaviours that includes procuring and selecting food, planning menus or selecting from a menu, preparing or ordering foods, and eating with literally hundreds of food-related choices, including where to shop or eat, what to purchase or prepare, how to season food, and with whom to eat (B.G. Simons-Morton *et al.* 1986). One can identify similar chains of component behavioural choices for each of the other health behaviours identified in Table 2.3.1.

Not only are the behaviours complex, but each behaviour has numerous influences or determinants. Factors that influence behaviours can be grouped into three major categories (Green & Kreuter 2005, with adaptation from Andersen, 1969): Predisposing, enabling, and reinforcing, as shown in Fig. 2.3.2. Both positive and negative behaviours are predisposed, enabled, and reinforced by forces in the culture and the environment. This broad categorization has proved useful in public health programme planning (with more than 970 published applications, see www.lgreen.net for bibliography) because it groups the determinants of behaviour according to the major strategies used in public health to influence them. *Direct communications* through mass media, schools, worksites, other organizations, and through patient counselling in health clinics are used to influence the predisposing factors. *Indirect communications* through parents, teachers, clergy, community leaders, employers, peers, and others are used to strengthen the reinforcing factors with organizational rewards or social-normative influence. *Community organization, political activation, and training* strengthen the enabling factors by mobilizing and moving resources, policies, and building skills and capacities.

Predisposing factors

Predisposing factors reside in the individual and include attitudes, values, beliefs, and perceptions of need, but these are shaped over time by cultural and social exposures, which produce reinforcing factors (see below). Predisposing factors are those antecedents to behaviour that provide the rationale, motivation, or drive for an individual's or group's behaviour. They mostly fall in the psychological domain of determinants, though genetics and environment shape them across the life span. They include the cognitive and affective dimensions of knowing, feeling, believing, valuing, and having self-confidence or a sense of self-efficacy.

Because these determinants of behaviour reside in individuals, public health must seek to influence behaviour by assessing the prevalence and distribution of key predisposing factors and look

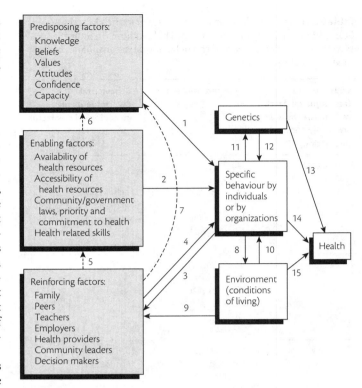

Fig. 2.3.2 This portion of the Precede–Proceed Model includes additional lines and arrows to outline a theory of causal relationships and order of causation and feedback loops for the three sets of factors influencing behaviour. In addition to the lines shown, an arrow from 'enabling factors' to 'environment' would elaborate the ecological aspect of factors that influence behaviour indirectly through changes in the environment. (Kreen & Kreater, 2005, p. 149, with permission.)

for opportunities to communicate differentially with various segments of the populations, according to an educational diagnosis or 'social marketing' assessment of their knowledge, attitudes, values, beliefs, and perceptions. The behavioural science literature, especially in health psychology, is replete with competing theories of the relative importance of particular predisposing factors and how they interact with each other (e.g. Glanz *et al.* 2002). Some of these theories, such as the Health Belief Model (Becker 1974), Social Cognitive Theory (Bandura 2004), and the Transtheoretical Model of Stages of Change (Prochaska *et al.* 2002), have become mainstays of the intervention literature on health education and behaviour change. These frequent uses of selected models have produced sufficient numbers of comparable studies or programme evaluations to permit meta-analyses of their applications across different health behaviours (e.g. Harrison *et al.* 1992; Netz *et al.* 2005; Spencer *et al.* 2005).

Enabling factors

Underplayed in most psychological studies of health behaviour, but critical to the role of public health as a complement to the roles of parents, schools, and mass media in the development of a healthy population, are the enabling factors influencing behaviour. These are often conditions of the environment that facilitate (or impede) the performance of a predisposition or motivated action by individuals or groups. Included are the availability, accessibility, and affordability of healthcare and community resources. Also included are conditions of living that act as facilitators or barriers to action, such as availability of transportation or child care to release a parent from that responsibility long enough to participate in a health programme, clinic, or service. It also includes features of the built environment, such as bicycle lanes, sidewalks, proximity of housing to workplaces, and other physical conditions of the environment that make physical activity more or less convenient and inviting (e.g. Taylor *et al.* 2007). Enabling factors also include new skills that a person needs—or new capacities that a group, organization, or community needs—to be able to accomplish health goals.

Public health addresses the enabling factors for behavioural change through policy changes and resource allocations at the national, regional, and local level, community organization for such policy and resource allocation at the local level when government programmes and services are insufficient or inappropriate to local perceptions of need. Training in the skills needed to take certain complicated actions is the other behavioural intervention used by public health to address the enabling factors.

In an era of constrained public health resources, many communities have resorted to more intensive community organization to build coalitions of multiple agencies including government and NGOs, and intersectoral collaboration between the health agencies and the community's schools, worksites, transportation, and other such sectors. Public–private collaboration on issues of enabling a more healthful food supply in school lunches, for example, or less accessibility of children to vending machines with cigarettes or 'junk food', have become increasingly common strategies for addressing the behaviour–environment interaction issues at the heart of most enabling factors.

Reinforcing factors

Before chronic diseases became the prevailing concern of public health in developed countries, behaviour was perceived as less important than today. The types of behaviour required to implement many of the most important public health interventions such as immunization and fluoridation were less complex. Immunizations, for example, could confer long-term immunity for an individual with a single act. Fluoridation or chlorination of water supplies could be implemented in many communities with no engagement of the public, although when fluoridation did become a local political issue requiring a local vote, the behaviour in question for most people was, again, a single action. As chronic diseases became more prevalent, the behaviours in question were largely ones that had to be repeated frequently, some for a lifetime, such as dietary practices, hypertension medication regimens, smoking cessation, and physical activity. For these behaviours, the predisposing and enabling factors remain important, but reinforcing factors take on increased importance because maintaining a behaviour requires reinforcement.

Reinforcing factors are those consequences of action that determine whether the actor receives positive (or negative) feedback and is supported socially or financially after it occurs. Reinforcing factors thus include social support, peer influences, and advice and feedback by healthcare providers, as well as a sense that the benefits of the action outweigh the costs. In consideration of the benefits (and costs), they also include physical consequences of behaviour, which may be separate from the social context. Examples include the feeling of well-being (or pain) caused by physical exercise and the alleviation of respiratory symptoms (or the experience of side effects) following the use of asthma medication, or gaining weight while quitting cigarettes.

Public health uses reinforcing factors such as denormalizing smoking in public places, social reinforcement with encouraging words in personal counselling, small-group health education sessions in which behaviour is publicly endorsed and praised, or mass media images of attractive role models with whom people wish to be associated by their own behaviour. No matter how effective these extrinsic reinforcements might be in the short term in strengthening a behavioural tendency, they must be internalized over time to become intrinsic motivation. Token rewards lead to token behaviour if the individuals do not replace them over time with the belief that the behaviour is intrinsically valuable because it accords with their own personal values (Green *et al.* 1986).

Table 2.3.2 gives examples of the more commonly identified influences on each of four most important behavioural risk factors. These behaviours interact with each other, such that changes in one influence predisposing, enabling, and reinforcing factors for others. Young women, for example, may take up smoking in the belief that it will help them control their appetite and thereby their weight. Other examples are athletes quitting smoking and limiting alcohol intake to improve their physical activity or sport performance; and contraceptive use leading to fewer, more spaced births, which lead in turn to women seeking other opportunities to improve their health and that of their families.

Public health strategies to influence determinants of behaviour

Another chapter in this volume will deal with the full range of health promotion and health education strategies (Kickbusch 2008). The focus of this section is specifically on how the aspects of the environment discussed above that shape health-related behaviour can be targeted for strategic intervention for public health purposes. Three types of strategies are used in public health to accomplish health promotion and disease prevention goals through behaviour change:

◆ *Educational strategies* inform and educate the public about issues of concern, such as the dangers of drug misuse, the benefits of automobile restraints, or the relationship of maternal alcohol consumption to foetal alcohol syndrome.

◆ *Automatic-protective strategies* are directed at controlling environmental variables, that minimize the need for individual decisions in structuring each behaviour, such as public health measures providing for milk pasteurization, fluoridation, infant immunizations, and the burning or chemical killing of marijuana crops, but these often involve individual and group decisions and actions about which policies to support, since they limit degrees of freedom in choice of behavioural options.

◆ *Coercive strategies* employ legal and other formal sanctions to control individual behaviour, such as required immunizations for school entry, mandatory tuberculosis testing of hospital employees, compulsory use of automobile restraints, and arrests for drug possession or use.

Table 2.3.2 Some known and suspected influences on four major behavioural risk factors

Cigarette smoking	Dietary practices	Alcohol use/abuse	Physical inactivity
Knowledge of adverse health effects of smoking	Personal food preferences	Expectations of alcohol effects	Beliefs in physical activity benefits
Attitudes about smoking	Cultural food preferences	Child of alcoholic	Attitudes toward physical activity
Skills in smoking cessation/prevention	Perceived social acceptance of foods	Alternatives to alcohol	Self-motivation
Cigarette cost	Social context of eating	Psychological stress	Self-efficacy
Availability of cigarettes	Availability and convenience of foods	Low self-esteem	Accessibility of exercise facilities
Cigarette advertising	Skills in menu planning	Early drinking experience	Skills in relapse prevention
Peer influences to smoke	Skills in food preparation	Heavy social drinking	Skills in goal setting
Social support for non-smoking	Skills in food selection	Parent and peer influences	Enjoyability of physical activity
	Food advertising	Alcohol advertising	Family support
		Cost of alcohol	Design of the built environment
		Availability of alcohol	
		Supervision of drinking	

Illustrative of successful public health measures reflecting this range of strategies directed at influencing health-related behaviours are the efforts to control tobacco consumption. Influencing tobacco-related knowledge and attitudes has been declared one of the great public health achievements of the twentieth century, at least in the United States (Centers for Disease Control 1999) and several other countries. Considering that these successes, as measured by the reductions in tobacco consumption behaviour, were achieved largely in the last third of the century, they represent both a remarkable turn-around of an epidemic of smoking behaviour that had increased inexorably through the first two-thirds of the century, and an inspiration for public health approaches to other health-related behaviours that now show similar epidemic trends. The application of the lessons from tobacco control to reversing, for example, the obesity epidemic through similar influences on dietary and physical activity behaviours has become a point of major public health debate in the early years of the new millennium (Eriksen *et al.* 2007; Green *et al.* 2006; Mercer *et al.* 2005).

Influences on smoking initiation and cessation are numerous, and many of them are also intertwined with diet, alcohol, and physical activity. Predisposing factors include attitudes about smoking and beliefs about and knowledge of the health effects of smoking. Enabling factors of access to tobacco products and price are influential. The price elasticity has been documented at a 3 per cent decrease in tobacco consumption for every 10 per cent increase in the price, and a greater relative decrease in youth, for whom disposable income is less (Jha & Chaloupka 2000; Ranson *et al.* 2002). The influence of raising taxes on cigarettes, then, has been a major public health strategy with known effects on consumption. With the dedication of part of the tax revenues to the funding of comprehensive tobacco control programmes, some jurisdictions have achieved a doubling and even tripling of the rate of decline in per capita consumption compared with other jurisdictions in the same country (Mercer *et al.* 2005). But more powerful still are the cumulative reinforcing factors of growing social support and pressure for smoke-free environments as smoking becomes denormalized with the decline in prevalence rates and the legal restrictions on smoking in public places (Eriksen *et al.* 2007).

Cigarette advertising and promotions by the tobacco industry have proved to be powerful negative predisposing and reinforcing influences on smoking behaviour that are highly adaptable to changing regulatory attempts to control their content and channels. Initial restrictions on US tobacco advertising in the broadcast media in the mid-1960s, for example, resulted in the tobacco industry voluntarily withdrawing from radio and television advertising, but adroitly using those resources from mass media to expand its advertising vastly on more targeted print media in magazines, billboards, and youth-oriented outlets. Sponsorship of sports and arts events and clubs, for example, provided a more targeted venue for reaching youth and other susceptible markets. Response of some jurisdictions in restricting these sponsorships has produced reductions in youth uptake of tobacco products (Hagmann 2002). Diversification of advertising to youth-oriented media and point-of-purchase settings such as stores near schools has resulted in increased restrictions in many jurisdictions. The results have been largely disappointing, which is attributed to the agility of the industry in finding loopholes and ways to circumvent the new legal restrictions.

Attempts to control the determinants of tobacco consumption also illustrate an essential public health lesson in the importance of comprehensive programmes to affect the complex behaviours associated with chronic diseases (CDC 1999). Comprehensive approaches have proved critical because:

♦ No single intervention reaches all segments of susceptible people in a population (Green & Glasgow 2006).

♦ No single intervention reaches different segments with the same degree of effectiveness (e.g. Contento *et al.* 1993).

♦ Different interventions are differentially effective in the different phases of change (Prochaska *et al.* 2002).

♦ Different interventions variously influence the predisposing, enabling, and reinforcing determinants of behaviour in a population (Green & Kreuter 2005).

This comprehensiveness lesson has been carried forward to public health efforts in diet, alcohol, and physical activity insofar as they have increasingly engaged multiple organizations in community coalitions and multiple sectors and national programmes to address the various determinants that extend beyond the purview of the medical and public health sectors at the local level.

The promotion of physical activity or active living illustrates the lessons of comprehensiveness and multi-sector involvement in public health strategies to influence a complex behaviour. The numerous influences on sedentary behaviour or physical activity include predisposing beliefs about the importance of physical activity and attitudes about physical activity, enabling accessibility of exercise facilities, walking lanes or paths, skills in relapse prevention and in goal setting, and reinforcing factors of discomfort or inconvenience of exercise, and family support (Frankish *et al.* 1998). Increasing attention has been given in recent years to the built environment, including the density of housing, mixed-use neighbourhoods, and sidewalks that encourage walking to and from home for shopping, work, and recreation; provision of mass transit that also supports walking the distance to and from transit stops rather than driving to work and other destinations (Frank 2000).

The recent growth of the active living field is an extension and integration of traditional public health approaches with more collaborative approaches involving sectors such as housing, parks and recreation, and transportation. It responds to the increasing recognition of the complexity of health-risk behaviours related to chronic diseases and their numerous determinants. The performance of each behaviour is interwoven with or ecologically embedded in other behaviours and their mutual genetic determinants and their social, cultural, and physical environments.

Behaviour as determinant of environmental and genetic predispositions

Population behavioural and educational diagnoses enable public health to intervene strategically on the behaviour of populations. But health problems have other determinants in the environment and in genetics. Behaviour also can play a role in influencing those determinants.

The reciprocal influence of individual behaviour on environments

A fundamental precept of human ecology is the reciprocal determinism of behaviour and the environment (Green *et al.* 1996). The literature on health promotion took a sharp turn away from behaviour in the 1980s to give attention to the policy and environmental determinants of health. This was partly in response to a period in which public health was perceived to have taken too much of a psychological approach to the determinants of health (Green 2006). As early as 1968, Edward S. Rogers had appealed to sociology for the assistance of public health needed from the social sciences to address the ecological issues (Rogers 1968). Psychologists, however, were more available, at least in the US, to step into the perceived social science void of public health and to take up the new professorships in public health. They brought an emphasis on testing theories of individual behavioural change. As the ecological imperative of multi-level interventions (individual, family, organizational, community, regional, national, and global) gained growing emphasis in public health (e.g. Green *et al.* 1996; Kickbusch 1989), a gradual turn to the study of behaviour-in-context gave reciprocal determinism a new lease on life in public health (Institute of

Medicine 2001, 2003; Stoto *et al.* 1997) in the decade bridging the millennium. One theory of behavioural change that gained particular public health prominence in this era was Albert Bandura's social cognitive theory, with its emphasis on self-efficacy and individual agency in changing one's environment at the same time that it gave prominence to the social environment in shaping behaviour (Bandura 2004).

Some of the environmental determinants of health beyond the behavioural control of individuals nevertheless lend themselves to group political behaviour or collective action through community intervention. Communities, neighbourhoods, or special-interest (self-help) groups can organize, vote, lobby, boycott, and otherwise support or prevent some environmental changes. To varying degrees, individuals can avoid or limit their exposure to environmental risks such as solar radiation, lead paint, and ambient smoke. In short, individual behaviour can be mobilized to influence the environment, so that individuals need not be seen only as passive objects of environmental influence.

The projected but still limited influence of behaviour on genetics

The Human Genome Project and the explosion of research on human genetics have raised very hopeful scenarios of 'personalized medicine', in which individuals could know more precisely their genetic risk of certain diseases or causes of death. The usual assumptions are that such information could be made readily available to individuals, and that having such information would be considerably more compelling in motivating behaviour than the usual statistical risk of groups of people without the personalized association with the individual in question.

The first assumption remains to be supported by true evidence of effectiveness. For example, in about 30 per cent of women with breast cancer, over-expression of a protein called HER2/neu is associated with a worse prognosis and in such women the drug trastuzumab is especially effective. The FDA approved the drug and a test for HER2/neu for use in women with metastatic breast cancer in 1998 and more recently for women with early stage breast cancer (Braga *et al.* 2006; Hortobagyi 2005; Piccart-Gebhart *et al.* 2005). The co-development and approval of the drug and test is considered one of the real successes of the application of genetics to modern medical practice and among the best examples of 'personalized medicine'. One might think the story is complete. However, although this information about the efficacy and availability of the test and the drug was published and promulgated by commercial backers, the behaviour of clinicians and their patients has been a more complicated matter. There is little known about how many women have access to testing and treatment. The costs of both are high and cost-effectiveness issues have not been resolved. Also how best to administer the test has not been resolved (e.g. timing) and there are reports of an increased risk of heart failure, the effect of which on acceptance is not known.

The second assumption, that having such information would motivate more concerted effort to change one's behaviour, is only partially supported by: (1) the logic and evidence from other areas of health counselling and communications that more personally tailored health information based on the individual's own family history or biological risk information adds motivational value to the experience with health advice that is based on more generic information (Kreuter & Wray 2003; Kreuter *et al.* 2003, 2004, 2005);

(2) limited direct evidence from the few instances in which such genetic information has been used to counsel individual behavioural choices of action. The latter is illustrated by the examples in the previous paragraph and those from prenatal testing and counselling for birth defects. However, a meta-analysis of 21 controlled trials showed that while genetic counselling improved knowledge of cancer genetics, it did not increase the level of perceived risk and few studies examined cancer surveillance behaviours (Braithwaite *et al.* 2006).

Public health faces two major limiting factors in pursuing this pathway of behaviour influencing health through genetic determinants: (1) the limited influence of the genes so far implicated in specific mortality or morbidity outcomes, and their interactions with the environment, (2) the ethics of offering such information to the individual with anything more than a cautionary note of possible relevance to their reproductive decisions or their behavioural choices. The first is a limit that could be partially overcome with further breakthroughs in the human genomics research. But apart from some prenatal tests for genetic defects in the fetus, most of the other genetic markers associated with predispositions to illnesses or premature mortality are highly interactive with other genes and the environment. Therefore, any course of action recommended to the individual remains probabilistic in its assurance of a health benefit. In combination with the other risk factors that can be more readily identified, the addition of personalized genetic information might raise the probabilities sufficiently to help the individual reach a tipping point in motivation to take action on complex health-related behaviours. But whether it really adds motivational value to what could be similarly known from a good family history has yet to be demonstrated.

The other limiting factors for this behaviour–genetic pathway as a public health consideration are the ethical complications that arise with the technology and the information. The concern, as in other screening technologies, with false-positive results can be multiplied in their ethical considerations for genetic information on individuals. The usual issues of protecting the privacy of such information and the potential discrimination in hiring, placement, retention, and promotion of individuals with known genetic predispositions will continue to be debated before the 'personalized medicine' potential of expanding the behaviour–genetic pathway can be pursued as public health policy. Meanwhile, private medicine is opening opportunities for individuals to explore this option in structuring their behavioural response to personal genetic information. Another chapter in this volume addresses human genetics more thoroughly.

The interaction of socioeconomic status (SES), environments, and behaviour

Of all the interactions in the association of behaviour and health, none is more pervasive, consistent, and robust than that of socioeconomic status. The relationship between SES and measures of health or mortality is shown in previous chapters to be a gradient rather than a threshold effect, though threshold effects are sometimes found beyond which income or other SES indicators have no further beneficial effects (e.g. Finch 2003). Those at the top of the SES hierarchy usually have better health and lower mortality rates than those just below them who are themselves better off than the others, and so on down to those in poverty at the very bottom.

The gradient adheres whether the SES measure is education, income, occupational status, or place of residence. The gradient globally is anchored at the lowest end by the poorest developing countries. Some one billion people globally live in extreme poverty on an income of just US$1 a day, of whom 70 per cent live in Asian and Pacific countries. Many of the poor lack access to basic health services and are at exaggerated risks for many of the leading causes of death in those countries.

The question here is how the mortality and morbidity gradients with socioeconomic status might operate through health-related behaviours and environments to suggest mechanisms by which the pervasive SES gradient influences health.

SES as a predisposing determinant of behaviour

The ecological perspective on SES as a determinant of behaviour related to health would suggest first that environments shape behaviour from early childhood onward. Shaping behaviour in the first instance (rather than enabling it in the second or reinforcing it in the third) qualifies this environmental influence as a predisposing factor. Homes, neighbourhoods, towns, cities, regions, and whole countries with their variable physical, social, economic, and cultural environments differ in relation to SES measured at individual, family, neighbourhood, and other geographic levels. Once the measures of SES and health or mortality are aggregated above the individual level, their relationships constitute ecological correlations. Studies have examined the ecological relationship between mortality rates and various indicators of social inequalities in geographical areas varying in size from metropolitan areas (Lynch *et al.* 1998) to whole countries (Wilkinson & Marmot 1998). These studies showed that those areas where inequalities between those at the top of the hierarchy and those at the bottom were the largest were also those in which the mortality gradient was the strongest (Wilkinson 1996). Similar findings were found with other indicators of social inequities such as differences in social capital (Kawachi *et al.* 1997). Health disparities between socioeconomic groups appear from Canadian data to increase with age across the lifespan, which supports the notion of a cumulative effect over time of the health- and mortality-SES gradient (e.g. Prus 2007).

One implication of this relative deprivation dimension of the SES-health gradient is that perception of one's status relative to others de-motivates or discourages one's efforts to take greater control over the behavioural and environmental determinants of one's health. Whether consciously discouraged or unconsciously conditioned by repeated confrontations with inequalities and inequities that conspire against one's efforts, the hypothesis is that disparities make those exposed to relative deprivation less predisposed or motivated to take preventive and healthcare actions. Two specific mechanisms have been suggested for this de-motivation or lack of predisposition to undertake behaviour. One is a chronic pessimism that has been found in adolescent children of lower SES parents, and that pessimism was associated with stress (Finkelstein *et al.* 2007). The other possibly related mechanism is the theoretical construct of 'self-efficacy', widely measured in association with social cognitive theory applications in health behaviour research (Bandura 2004).

SES as an enabling determinant of behaviour

Socioeconomic standing also confers capabilities and resources that enable the predisposed behaviours to be carried out, for better or for worse. With higher standing come more resources and the associated education and training that endow individuals, families, groups, and communities with enabling judgements, resources, and skills. No matter how motivated people may be by their predisposing factors, they may not have the income and other resources, including accessible and affordable services within reach of their residences or workplaces, to be able to carry out the behaviour without great sacrifice and inconvenience. But environmental variables of accessible fruit and vegetable outlets in local neighbourhoods, for example, only partially explain or mediate the relationship between SES and fruit or vegetable consumption (Ball *et al.* 2006).

The educational enabling influence of SES on behaviour

Among the SES indicators, education has for decades demonstrated the strongest association with most health-behaviour measures (Green 1970a,b; Metcalf *et al.* 2007). It also stands out among the indicators of inequities in confirming the relative deprivation hypothesis above (Kunst & Mackenbach 1994). Education can be viewed as a proxy for a variety of predisposing and enabling factors in explaining the causes of behavioural determinants as mediators of at least part of the SES-health gradient. Prominent among these are optimism (a predisposing factor) and education as an enabling or coping resource (Finkelstein *et al.* 2007), with the knowledge, attitudes, and skills that come with years of schooling.

The Canadian Health Promotion Survey (Adams 1993) showed that men and women with a higher level of education self-rated their health as excellent or good in a much higher proportion than individuals with lower education. The proportion of people in Canada who are smokers is double in people with elementary or lower education, compared with people with university degrees (Health and Welfare Canada *et al.* 1993). This spread in proportions of smokers was greater for the highest and lowest education categories than for the highest and lowest income or occupational status categories (Pederson 1993). Data from the major US community trials in cardiovascular disease prevention showed that the dramatic drop in smoking prevalence over the 1980s was more pronounced for people with higher education compared with peoples with less education (Winkleby *et al.* 1992 b; Luepker *et al.* 1993). The same trend was observed in Canada for the period 1985–1991 (Millar & Stephens 1993).

These historical associations between health behaviours and SES have been confounded in the more recent tracking of obesity, physical activity, and food consumption. The more sedentary work and modes of travel of a majority of white collar workers blurs the educational, income, and occupational correlations with physical activity (e.g. Canadian Institute for Health Information 2006; Tjepkema 2005). In Canada, for example, 'of the demographic variables examined, income, occupation, and employment status were unrelated to obesity, while education was negatively associated with the prevalence of obesity' (Raine 2004, p. 6.).

The cultural–environmental predisposing influence of SES

The strong relationships between education and smoking and other health behaviours are only slightly less so when adjusted for age, sex, and ethnicity (Winkleby *et al.* 1992; Shea *et al.* 1991). Culture and gender do appear to play important roles, but these are highly intertwined with education and acculturation. The early ecological studies remain some of the most compelling in establishing and

explaining the role of culture in health. The studies of Japanese men who had lived in Japan and emigrated to California showed clear dietary changes and increased heart disease and stroke rates only in their offspring, i.e. the second generation. Those who emigrated to Hawaii had intermediate rates of dietary change and coronary and stroke rates (Keys *et al.* 1970; Kato *et al.* 1973). As the Japanese became acculturated, they assumed both the dietary and cardiovascular patterns of their new country.

Another classic study providing evidence of the effects of culture on health was the series on the Roseto community. Early observations showed that this ethnically homogeneous Pennsylvania community experienced a significantly lower mortality from myocardial infarction than the nearby community of Bangor despite a higher prevalence of hypertension and obesity and a similar proportion of smokers (Lynn *et al.* 1967). These results were attributed to the apparent protective effect of a unique social, ethnic, and family cohesion in the community (Bruhn *et al.* 1982). More recent analyses show that Rosetans lost that relative protection over subsequent decades (Egolf *et al.* 1992). This loss was accompanied by an increase in the number of intermarriages of Rosetans with people of non-Italian decent, a decrease in social participation in Roseto, and an increase in the general wealth of the community, as the original Italian-born generation was gradually replaced by their ageing American-born offspring (Lasker *et al.* 1994).

In short, to the extent that minority cultures can remain sheltered from the pervasive influences of the majority culture, they can have powerful predisposing influences on health-related behaviour. With acculturation, however, comes the displacement of minority cultural influence with the majority culture. Culture, nevertheless, remains a conceptually useful construct for understanding both the minority and majority processes of socially transmitted beliefs and values that predispose people to one choice of behaviour over another.

SES as a reinforcing determinant of behaviour

A behaviour that is predisposed and enabled might still fail to persist beyond a trial stage of development if it fails to produce satisfying results. Satisfaction comes from various sources that can have the effect of reinforcing behaviour. SES can contribute to the availability of reinforcements by putting people into association with other people and environments that are more likely to produce satisfaction with behaviours. Two examples follow.

The 'status identity factor' and social norms

The social-normative theory underlying the notion of SES functioning like a reinforcing factor would predict that people will identify with a place in the social hierarchy that they can justify on the basis of their highest achievement. Unlike the usual measure of SES produced by averaging standardized or weighted measures of education, income, and occupation, one hypothesis derived from social reinforcement theory was that people will aspire to and adhere to that norm of a particular behaviour associated with their highest measure on the gradient of SES. For example, a person who is relatively high on education, but of moderate income and occupational status, would tend to adhere to the behavioural norms of the highest, rather than the average, of the three status scores. The hypothesis was tested in a California state-wide sample of mothers of children under 5, demonstrating that the immunization status of the children and five other measures of early childhood care followed a gradient with SES, but that the best predictor of the mother's behaviour on these five measures was her highest standardized SES among income, education, and occupation, not the average. This inferred 'status identity' of the mothers provided a basis for linking the psychological phenomena of identification and role modelling with the sociological concept of normative influence (Green 1970a).

Denormalizing behaviour

In retrospect, one of the most important elements of the tobacco control success of the last third of the twentieth century in the US and Canada was the 'denormalization' of smoking behaviour in public places (Eriksen et al. 2007). What had been a normative behaviour of smoking in the workplace and in restaurants, meeting rooms, and other public places became increasingly unacceptable, first by legal restrictions, then by social norms, by which the growing majority of non-smokers expected and even insisted on smoke-free environments. The combination of new smoke-free or 'clean air' ordinances and by-laws with mass media emphasizing the carcinogenic properties of second-hand smoke and the rights of non-smokers to be spared the exposure to this carcinogen resulted in a dramatic drop in this public behaviour. It was during this period of the 30-year decline in smoking that the rate of decline accelerated most dramatically. One reason for the importance of this element of the tobacco control campaigns was that the passage and enforcement of policies restricting a personal behaviour faced strong opposition as long as it was perceived by the public to be a matter of individual rights and the threat to be only to the person's own health. When the threat is seen to be to other people's health, especially to the health of children, the support of passage and enforcement of the laws and regulations grows. Other public health campaigns are attempting to model this experience, which builds on the social responsibility notions associated with communicable diseases of the past, but with most of the chronic disease-related behaviours, such as overeating and sedentary living, it has been more complicated to relate the normative behaviour of individuals to the health of others.

The interaction of socioeconomic status, gender, and behaviour

Men's and women's relative risk of disease or death in relation to specific behavioural risk factors such as smoking are generally similar (e.g. Oliveira et al. 2007), but their experiences with health differ markedly (Chapman Walsh et al. 1995). These differences cannot be attributed solely to biological determinants related to sexual differentiation (Krieger et al. 1993). The social construct of gender, as opposed to the biological categories of sex, was conceptualized to refer to cultural and social conventions, roles and behaviours assigned to men and women (Krieger 1996). These in turn shape the social, political, cultural, and economic circumstances experienced by men and women. Gender thus attempts to capture this differential experience that men and women have with their environment and the possibilities and constraints associated with these differences (Potvin & Frohlich 1998). A growing body of research is showing that some of these constraints and possibilities are interacting with the living conditions associated with SES to shape the health of people.

The correlation of SES with health appears stronger for men than for women; the SES-health gradient is steeper for men (Arber & Cooper 1999), except in their twenties and thirties when the gradients are similar (Matthews et al. 1999). The gender interactions with SES and health have been variously attributed to differential occupational experiences (e.g. Ross & Bird 1994), marital experiences (Koskinen & Martelin 1994), and degree of emancipation of women (Kawachi et al. 1999). These and other possible explanations generally require assumptions of behavioural mediators. Such mediators are more likely to be 'health-related' behaviour (e.g. sedentary living or food consumption patterns) rather than 'health-directed' behaviour (e.g. exercise or high-fibre diet). This distinction (Green & Kreuter 2005) recognizes the centrality of behaviour in the causal chains even when (perhaps especially when) it is not consciously health-*directed* behaviour.

Relationships among health-related behaviours

The interplay among habitual behavioural patterns and the socioeconomic and cultural conditions reviewed in the last half of this chapter leads one to put into a broader context the reductionist examinations, presented in the first half, of specific behaviours as they relate to health, disease, and mortality. The dynamic relationships among the specific measures creates a complex system of social, economic, cultural, and behavioural factors, interwoven with disease risk factors and health status, and influenced by the healthcare and physical environments.

Early studies of the relationships among health behaviours showed weak correlations, typically below $r=0.20$ (Green 1970b; Steele & McBroom, 1972). Those in subsequent studies that maintained correlations in the 0.20 range were smoking with alcohol use, alcohol use and exercise (Calnan 1989), and smoking and diet (Blaxter 1990). With the decline in smoking, less variation in smoking produces less co-variation with other behavioural variables. Given these low correlations, there is little evidence supporting a one-dimensional concept of health-related behaviours (Calnan 1994).

Conclusion

Behaviour is an inescapable link in the chain of causation between most environmental and genetic determinants and the health outcomes in which they are implicated. Some toxins and infectious environmental agents can affect health directly without behaviour as a mediator, but even these *can* be mediated by individual action to avoid exposures, and collective behaviour of groups or communities to protect themselves.

The *social* environment presents a further complexity in the mediating and moderating of behaviour and environment in their determination of population health. Most health-related behaviour occurs in the context of the social environment, so it involves the behaviour of other people as well as that of the person whose health is in question. The individuals are acting upon, and in reaction to, each other as their health outcomes are being shaped by their actions. This reciprocal determinism of behaviour and the social environment applies as well to the physical environment and the genetic determinants of health. These interactions make up the ecology of health, and call upon public health to take an ecological approach to the management of population health.

One way to structure the ecological approach to the planning of public health programmes in which behaviour change has a role is to examine the factors that influence behaviour in three categories of determinants: Predisposing factors, enabling factors, and reinforcing factors. These roughly correspond to strategies, respectively, that would use (1) direct communications to influence the knowledge, attitudes beliefs, and perceptions of the population concerning the behaviour–health relationship; (2) legal, engineering, financial, organizational levers and resource development that would enable or prohibit the behaviour; and (3) indirect communications through social organizations, parents, peers, employers, and others who control rewards and approval that would reinforce behaviour. By combining public health strategies directed at these three categories of determinants (predisposing, enabling, and reinforcing factors) the strategies will be comprehensive in their coverage and impact.

All of what has been understood as determinants of the health behaviour of individuals applies with some variation to the behaviour of health professionals, other practitioners and policy-makers who could serve as channels through which to reach individuals, groups, and whole populations to influence their health behaviour. The actions of all of these categories of individuals, as well as their organizations, can be analysed in relation to the factors that predispose, enable, and reinforce their actions, and these analyses can point, in turn, to the development of strategies to change those behaviours.

Acknowledgements

We are indebted to Denise Simons-Morton, MD, PhD, and Louise Potvin, PhD, co-authors of this chapter in the previous editions, for significant remnants of their earlier contributions that remain in this edition. We also thank Julie Miller for bibliographic assistance.

References

Adams, O. (1993). Health status. In *Health and welfare Canada. Canada's health promotion survey 1990: Technical report* (eds. T. Stephens and D. Fowler Graham), p. 23. Ministry of Supply and Services, Ottawa.

Adler, N.E., Boyce, T., Chesney, M.A. *et al.* (1994). Socioeconomic status and health: The challenge of gradient. *American Psychologist*, **49**, 15.

Andersen, R.M., Mullner, R.M., and Cornelius, L.J. (1987b). Black-white differences in health status: Method or substance. *Milbank Memorial Fund Quarterly*, **65** (Suppl 1), 71.

Anderson, K.M., Castelli, W.P., and Levy, D. (1987a). Cholesterol and mortality: 30 years of follow-up from the Framingham Study. *Journal of the American Medical Association*, **257**, 2176–80.

Anderson, P., Cremona, A., Paton, A. *et al.* (1993). The risk of alcohol. *Addiction*, **88**, 1493.

Anderson, R.M. (1969). *A behavioral model of families' use of health services.* University of Chicago Center for Health Administration Studies, Research Series No. 25, University of Chicago Press, Chicago.

Andersen, R.M., Mullner, R.M., and Cornelius, L.J. (1987). Black-white differences in health status: Method or substance. *Milbank Memorial Fund Quarterly*, **65** (Suppl 1), 71.

Antonovsky, A. (1967). Social class, life expectancy and overall mortality. *Milbank Memorial Fund Quarterly*, **45**, 31.

Arber, S. and Cooper, H. (1999). Gender differences in health in later life: The new paradox? *Social Science and Medicine*, **48**, 61.

Arroll, B. and Beaglehole, R. (1992). Does physical activity lower blood pressure: A critical review of the clinical trials. *Journal of Clinical Epidemiology*, **45**, 439–47.

Austoker, J. (1994a). Cancer prevention in primary care: Diet and cancer. *British Medical Journal*, **308**, 1610–14.

Austoker, J. (1994b). Cancer prevention in primary care: Reducing alcohol intake. *British Medical Journal*, **308**, 1549–52.

Ball, K., Crawford, D. and Mishra, G. (2006). Socio-economic inequalities in women's fruit and vegetable intakes: a multilevel study of individual, social and environmental mediators. *Public Health Nutrition*, **9**, 623–30.

Bartecchi, C.E., MacKenzie, T.D. and Schrier, R.W. (1994). The human cost of tobacco use, Part 1. *New England Journal of Medicine*, **330**, 907.

Basta, N.E. (2007). Community-level socio-economic status and cognitive and functional impairment in the older population. *European Journal of Public Health*, **18** (1): 48–54.

Becker, M.H. (1974). The Health Belief Model and personal health behaviour. *Health Education Monographs*, **2**, 324.

Berkman, L.F. and Syme, S.L. (1979). Social networks, host resistance, and mortality: A nine year follow-up of Alameda county residents. *American Journal of Epidemiology*, **109**, 186.

Berlin, J.A. and Colditz, G.A. (1990). A meta-analysis of physical activity in the prevention of coronary heart disease. *American Journal of Epidemiology*, **132**, 12–28.

Blair, S., Powell, K., Bazzarre, T. *et al.* (1993). Physical activity. American Heart Association Prevention Conference III: Behaviour change and compliance, keys to improving cardiovascular health. *Circulation*, **88**, 1402.

Blaxter, M. (1990). *Health and lifestyles*. Routledge, London.

Bor, W., Naiman, J.M., Anderson, M. *et al.* (1993). Socioeconomic disadvantage and child morbidity: An Australian longitudinal study. *Social Science and Medicine*, **36**, 1053.

Braga, S., dal Lago, L., Bernard, C. *et al.* (2006). Use of trastuzumab for the treatment of early stage breast cancer. *Expert Review of Anticancer Therapy*, **6**, 1153–64.

Braithwaite, D., Emery, J., Walter, F. *et al.* (2006). Psychological impact of genetic counseling for familial cancer: A systematic review and meta-analysis. *Familial Cancer*, **5**, 66–75.

Bruhn, J.G., Philips, B.U., and Wolf, S. (1982). Lessons from Roseto 20 years later: A community study of heart disease. *Southern Medical Journal*, **75**, 575.

Brunner, E. and Marmot, M. (1999). Social organization, stress and health. In *Social determinants of health* (eds. M. Marmot and R.G. Wilkinson), p. 17. Oxford University Press.

Bandura, A. (2004). Health promotion by social cognitive means. *Health Education and Behavior*, **31**, 143.

California Environmental Protection Agency (2005). *Proposed identification of environmental tobacco smoke as a toxic air contaminant*. California Environmental Protection Agency, Sacramento.

Calnan, M. (1989). Control over health and patterns of health-related behavior. *Social Science Medicine*, **26**, 435.

Calnan, M. (1994). Lifestyle and its social meaning. *Advances in Medical Sociology*, **4**, 69.

Canada (1974). *A new perspective on the health of Canadians (Lalonde Report)*. Department of National Health and Welfare, Ottawa.

Canadian Institute for Health Information (2006). *Improving the health of Canadians: Promoting healthy weights*. Canadian Institute for Health Information, Ottawa.

Carmelli, D., Swan, G.E., and Rosenman, R.H. (1986). The relationship between wives' social and psychologic status and their husbands' coronary heart disease. *American Journal of Epidemiology*, **122**, 90.

Cavelaars, A.E.J.M., Kunst, A.E., and Mackenbach, J.P. (1997). Socioeconomic differences in risk factors for morbidity and mortality in the European Community. *Journal of Health Psychology*, **2**, 90.

Centers for Disease Control and Prevention (1999). Achievements in public health 1900–1999: Tobacco use—United States, 1900–1999. *Morbidity and Mortality Weekly Reports*, **48**, 986–93.

Chapman Walsh, D., Sorensen, G., and Leanord, L. (1995). Gender, health and cigarette smoking. In *Society and health* (eds. B.C. Amick III, S. Levine, A.R. Tarlov, and D. Chapman Walsh), p. 131. Oxford University Press, New York.

Colditz, G.A. (2001). Cancer culture: epidemics, human behavior, and the dubious search for new risk factors. *American Journal of Public Health*, **91**, 357.

Colditz, G.A., Willett, W.C., Stampfer, M.J. *et al.* (1990). Weight as a risk factor for clinical diabetes in women. *American Journal of Epidemiology*, **132**, 501.

Connelly, S., O'Reilly, D., and Rosato, M. (2007). Increasing inequalities in health. Is it an artifact caused by the selective movement of people? *Social Science and Medicine*, **64**, 2008–15.

Contento, I.R., Basch, C., and Sheaa, S. (1993). Relationship of mothers' food choice criteria to food intake of preschool children: Identification of family subgroups. *Health Education Quarterly*, **20**, 227.

Corin, E. (1994). The social and cultural matrix of health and disease. In *Why are some people healthy and others not? The determinants of health populations* (eds. R.G. Evans, M.L. Barer, and T.R. Marmor), pp. 93–132. Aldine de Gruyter, New York.

Cotrell, L.S. (1976). The competent community. In *Further explorations in social psychiatry* (eds. B.H. Kaplan, R.N. Wilson, and A.H. Leighton), p. 195. Basic Books, New York.

Crawford, D., Ball, K., Mishra, G. *et al.* (2007). Which food-related behaviours are associated with healthier intakes of fruits and vegetables among women? *Public Health Nutrition*, **10**, 256–65. Erratum in *Public Health Nutrition*, **10**, 536.

Custer, S.J. and Doty, C.R. (1992). Assessment of self-motivation and selected physiological characteristics as predictors of adherence to exercise in a corporate setting. *Journal of Health Education*, **23**, 232.

Davis, N.J. and Robinson, R.V. (1988). Class identification of men and women in the 1970s and 1980s. *American Sociological Review*, **53**, 103.

Dawber, T.R. (1960). Summary of recent literature regarding cigarette smoking and coronary heart disease. *Circulation*, **22**, 164.

Egolf, B., Lasker, J., Wolf, S. *et al.* (1992). The Roseto effect: A 50-year comparison of mortality rates. *American Journal of Public Health*, **82**, 1089.

Emery, C.F. and Blumenthal, J.A. (1991). Effects of physical exercise on psychological and cognitive functioning of older adults. *Annals of Behavioral Medicine*, **13**, 99.

Epp, J. (1986). Achieving health for all: A framework for health promotion. *Health Promotion International*, **1**, 419.

Eriksen, M.P., Green, L.W., Husten, C.G. *et al.* (2007). Thank you for not smoking: The public response to tobacco-related mortality in the United States. In *Silent victories: The history and practice of public health in twentieth-century America.* (eds. J.W. Ward and C. Warren). New York: Oxford University Press.

Eriksen, M. P., Green, L. W., Huston, C. *et al.* (2007). Tobacco control in the United States: After the great public health triumphs of the Twentieth Century, what must we emphasize in the Twenty-First? In *A safer and healthier America: Public health in the 20th century* (eds. J.W. Ward and C.S. Warren), in press.

Ewart, C.K., Taylor, C.B., Reese, L.B. *et al.*(1983). The effects of early myocardial infarction exercise testing on self-perception and subsequent physical activity. *American Journal of Cardiology*, **51**, 1076.

Finch, B.K. (2003). Socioeconomic gradients and low birth-weight: Empirical and policy considerations. *Health Services Research*, **38**, 1819.

Finkelstein, D.M., Kubzansky, D.M., Capitman, J. *et al.*(2007). Socioeconomic differences in adolescent stress: The role of psychological resources. *Journal of Adolescent Health*, **40**, 127–34.

Fox, A.J., Goldblatt, P.O., and Jones, D.R. (1986). Social class mortality differentials: artifact, selection, or life circumstances. In *Class and health: Research and longitudinal data* (ed. R.G. Wilkinson), p. 35. Tavistock Publications, London.

Fox, S.H., Koepsell, T.D., and Daling, J.R. (1994). Birth weight and smoking during pregnancy – effect modification by maternal age. *American Journal of Epidemiology*, **139**, 1008.

Frank, L.D. (2000). Land use and transportation interaction: Implications on the public health and quality of life. *Journal of Planning Education and Research*, **20**, 6–22.

Frankish, C.J., Milligan, C.D., and Reid, C. (1998). A review of relationships between active living and determinants of health. *Social Sciences and Medicine*, **47**, 287–301.

Frick, M.H., Elo, M.O., Happa, K. *et al.* (1987). Helsinki Heart Study: Primary-prevention trial with gemfibrozil in middle-aged men with dyslipidemia. Safety of treatment, changes in risk factors, and incidence of coronary heart disease. *New England Journal of Medicine*, **137**, 1237–45.

Glanz, K., Rimer, B.K., and Lewis, F.M. (eds.) (2002). *Health behavior and health education: Theory, research, and practice*, 3rd edition. Jossey Bass, San Francisco.

Glass, T. A. and McAtee, M. J. (2006). Behavioral science at the crossroads in public health: Extending horizons, envisioning the future. *Social Science & Medicine*, **62**, 1650.

Goeppinger, J. and Baglioni, A.J., Jr (1985). Community competence: A positive approach to needs assessment. *American Journal of Community Psychology*, **13**, 507.

Gottlieb, N.H. and Green, L.W. (1987). Ethnicity and lifestyle health risk: Some possible mechanisms. *American Journal of Health Promotion*, **2**, 37.

Green, L.W. (1970a). Manual for scoring socioeconomic status for research on health behavior. *Public Health Reports* **85**, 185.

Green, L.W. (1970b). *Status identity and preventive health behaviour*. Pacific Health Education Reports, No. 1. University of California School of Public Health. Berkeley, CA.

Green, L.W. (1986). The theory of participation: A qualitative analysis of its expression in national and international policies. In *Advances in health education and promotion* (eds. W.B. Ward, Z.T. Salisbury, S.B. Kar, and J.G. Zapka), Vol. 1, Part A, p. 211. JAI Press, Greenwich, CT.

Green, L.W. (2006). Public health asks of systems science: To advance our evidence-based practice, can you help us get more practice-based evidence? *American Journal of Public Health*, **96**, 406.

Green, L.W. and Glasgow, R. (2006). Evaluating the relevance, generalization, and applicability of research: Issues in external validation and translation methodology. *Evaluation & the Health Professions*, **29**, 126.

Green, L.W. and Kreuter, M. (2005). *Health program planning: An educational and ecological approach*, 4th edition. New York, McGraw-Hill Higher Education.

Green, L.W. and McAlister, A.L. (1984). Macro-intervention to support health behavior: Some theoretical perspectives and practical reflections. *Health Education Quarterly*, **11**, 322.

Green, L.W., Orleans, C.T., Ottoson, J.M. *et al.* (2006). Inferring strategies for disseminating physical activity policies, programs, and practices from the successes of tobacco control. *American Journal of Preventive Medicine*, **31**(Suppl 4), S66.

Green, L.W., Richard, L., and Potvin, L. (1996). Ecological foundations of health promotion. *American Journal of Health Promotion*, **10**, 270.

Green, L.W., Wilson, A., and Lovato, C.Y. (1986). What changes can health promotion produce and how long will they last? Trade-offs between expediency and durability. *Preventive Medicine*, **15**, 508.

Haan, I., Kaplan, G.A., and Camacho, T. (1987). Poverty and health. Prospective evidence from the Alameda County Study. *American Journal of Epidemiology*, **125**, 989.

Hagmann, M. (2002). WHO attacks tobacco sponsorship of sports. *Bulletin of the World Health Organization*, **80**, 80.

Hancock, T. (1986). Lalonde and beyond: looking back at 'A new perspective on the health of Canadians'. *Health Promotion: An International Journal*, **1**, 93.

Harrison, J.A., Mullen, P.D., and Green, L.W. (1992). A meta-analysis of studies of the Health Belief Model. *Health Education Research*, **7**, 107.

Health and Welfare, Canada, Stephens, T., and Fowler Graham, D. (eds.) (1993). *Canada's health promotion survey 1990: Technical report*. Minister of Supply and Services, Ottawa.

Health Canada (2003). *Canadian Guidelines for Body Weight Classification in Adults*. Health Canada, Ottawa.

Hertz, E., Hebert, J.R., and Landon, J. (1994). Social and environmental factors and life expectancy, infant mortality, and maternal mortality rates: Results of a cross-national comparison. *Social Science and Medicine*, **39**, 105.

Hortobagyi, G.N. (2005). Trastuzumab in the treatment of breast cancer. *New England Journal of Medicine*, **353**, 1734.

House, J.S., Kessler, R.C., and Herzog, A.R. (1990). Age, socioeconomic status, and health. *Milbank Quarterly*, **68**, 383.

Hunninghake, D.B., Stein, E.A., Dujovne, C.A. *et al.* (1993). The efficacy of intensive therapy alone or combined with lovastatin in outpatients with hypercholesterolemia. *New England Journal of Medicine*, **328**, 1213.

Hunt, K. and Annandale, E. (1999). Relocating gender and morbidity: Examining men's and women's health in contemporary Western societies. Introduction to special issue on gender and health. *Social Science and Medicine*, **48**, 1.

Institute of Medicine (2001). *Health and behavior: The interplay of biological, behavioral, and societal influences*. National Academies Press, Washington, DC.

Institute of Medicine (2003). *The future of public health in the 21st century*. National Academies Press, Washington, DC.

James, S., Reddy, P., Ruiter, R. A. *et al.* (2006). The impact of an HIV and AIDS life skills program on secondary school students in Kaw Zulu-Natal, South Africa. *AIDS Education and Prevention*, **18**, 281.

Jha, P. and Chaloupka, F. J. (eds). (2000). *Tobacco control in developing countries*. Oxford University Press, New York.

Kaplan, R.M., Atkins, C.J., and Reinsch, S. (1984). Specify efficacy expectations medicate compliance in patients with COPD. *Health Psychology*, **3**, 223.

Kato, H., Tillotson, J., Nichaman, M.Z. *et al.* (1973). Epidemiological studies of coronary heart disease and stroke in Japanese men living in Japan, Hawaii, and California. Serum lipids and diet. *American Journal of Epidemiology*, **97**, 372.

Kawachi, I., Kennedy, B.P., Gupta, V. *et al.* (1999). Women's status and the health of women and men: A view from the States. *Social Science and Medicine*, **48**, 21.

Kawachi, I., Kennedy, B.P., Lochner, K. *et al.* (1997). Social capital, income inequality, and mortality. *American Journal of Public Health*, **87**, 1491.

Keil, J.E., Sutherland, S.E., Mapp, R.G. *et al.* (1992). Does equal socio-economic status in black and white mean equal risk of mortality. *American Journal of Public Health*, **82**, 1133–6.

Keys, A. (1970). Coronary heart disease in seven countries. *Circulation*, **41** (Suppl 1), 1.

Keys, A., Kimura, N., Kusukawa, A. *et al.* (1958). Lessons from serum cholesterol studies in Japan, Hawaii, and Los Angeles. *Annals of Internal Medicine*, **48**, 83.

Kickbusch, I. (1989). Approaches to an ecological base for public health. *Health Promotion*, **4**, 265–68.

Koniak-Griffin, D. and Stein, J. A. (2006). Predictors of sexual risk behaviours among adolescent mothers in a human immunodeficiency virus prevention program. *Journal of Adolescent Health*, **38**, 297.e111.

Koskinen, S. and Martelin, T. (1994). Why are socioeconomic mortality differences smaller among women than among men? *Social Science and Medicine*, **38**, 1385–96.

Kreuter, M.W. and Wray R.J. (2003). Tailored and targeted health communication: strategies for enhancing information relevance. *American Journal of Health Behavior*, **27** (Suppl 3), S227–32.

Kreuter M.W., Steger-May K., Bobra S. *et al.* (2003). Sociocultural characteristics and responses to cancer education materials among African American women. *Cancer Control*, **10** (5 Suppl), 69–80.

Kreuter, M.W., Skinner, C.S., Steger-May, K. *et al.* (2004). Responses to behaviorally vs culturally tailored cancer communication among African American women. *American Journal of Health Behavior*, **28**, 195–207.

Kreuter, M.W., Sugg-Skinner, C., Holt, C.L. *et al.* (2005). Cultural tailoring for mammography and fruit and vegetable intake among low-income African-American women in urban public health centers. *Preventive Medicine*, **41**, 53–62.

Krieger, N. (1984). Epidemiology and the web of causation. Has anyone seen the spider? *Social Science and Medicine*, **39**, 887.

Krieger, N. (1996). Inequality, diversity, and health: thoughts on 'race/ethnicity' and 'gender'. *Journal of American Medical Women's Association*, **51**, 133.

Krieger, N., Rowley, D.L., Herman, A.A. *et al.* (1993). Racism, sexism, and social class: Implications for study of health, disease, and well being. *American Journal of Preventive Medicine*, **9** (Suppl), 82.

Kuller, L.H., Ockene, J.K., Meilahn, E. *et al.* (1991). Cigarette smoking and mortality, MRFIT Research Group. *Preventive Medicine*, **29**, 638.

Kunst, A.E. and Mackenbach, J.P. (1994). The size of mortality differences associated with educational level in nine industrialized countries. *American Journal of Public Health*, **84**, 932.

Lahelma, E., Manderbaka, K., Rahkonen, O. *et al.* (1994). Comparison of inequalities in health: Evidence from national surveys in Finland, Norway, Sweden. *Social Science and Medicine*, **38**, 517.

Lahelma E., Martikainen, P., Rahkonen, O. *et al.* (1999). Gender differences in health in Finland: Patterns, magnitude and change. *Social Science and Medicine*, **48**, 7.

Lasker, J.N., Egolf, B.P., and Wolf, S. (1994). Community social change and mortality. *Social Science and Medicine*, **39**, 53.

Lokey, E.A. and Tran, Z.V. (1989). Effects of exercise training on serum lipid and lipoprotein concentrations in women: a meta-analysis. *International Journal of Sports Medicine*, **10**, 424.

Lorig, K. and Laurin, J. (1985). Some notions about assumptions underlying health education. *Health Education Quarterly*, **12**, 231.

Link, B.G. and Phelan, J. (1995). Social conditions as fundamental causes of disease. *Journal of Health and Social Behavior*, (special issue) 80.

Luepker, R.V., Rosamond, W.D., Murphy, R. *et al.* (1993). Socioeconomic status and coronary heart disease risk factor trends: The Minnesota Heart Health Survey. *Circulation*, **88**, 2172.

Lynch, J.W., Kaplan, G.A., Pamuk, E.R. *et al.* (1998). Income inequality and mortality in metropolitan areas of the United States. *American Journal of Public Health*, **88**, 1074.

Lynn, T.N., Duncan, R., Naughton, J.P. *et al.* (1967). Prevalence of evidence of prior myocardial infarction, hypertension, diabetes, and obesity in three neighboring communities in Pennsylvania. *American Journal of Medical Services*, **254**, 385.

McArdle, W.D., Katch, F.L., and Katch, V.L. (1986). *Exercise physiology: Energy, nutrition, and human performance*, 2nd edition. Lea and Febiger, Philadephia, PA.

McGinnis, J.M. and Foege, W.H. (1993). Actual causes of death in the United States. *Journal of the American Medical Association*, **270**, 2270.

McGinnis, J.M., and Foege, W. (2004). The immediate vs the important. *Journal of the American Medical Association*. **10**;291(10): 1263–4.

Macintyre, S. (1993). Gender differences in longevity and health in Eastern and Western Europe. In *Locating health: Sociological and historical explanations* (eds. S. Platt, T.H. Scott, and G. Williams), p. 57. Avebury UK, Aldershot.

Macintyre, S. (1997). The Black Report and beyond: What are the issues. *Social Science and Medicine*, **44**, 723.

Macintyre, S., Hunt, K., and Sweeting, H. (1996). Gender differences in health: Are things really as simple as they seem? *Social Science and Medicine*, **42**, 617.

Malik, V.S. and Hu, F.B. (2007). Popular weight-loss diets: from evidence to practice. *Nature, Clinical Practice, Cardiovascular Medicine*, **4**, 34–41.

Marmot, M.G., Rose, G., Shipley, M.J. *et al.* (1978). Employment grade and coronary heart disease in British civil servants. *Journal of Epidemiology and Community Health*, **32**, 244.

Marmot, M.G., Shipley, M.J., and Rose, G.A. (1984). Inequalities in death. Specific explanations of a general pattern? *Lancet*, **i**, 1003.

Marmot, M.G., Smith, G.D., Stansfeld, S. *et al.* (1991). Health inequalities among British civil servants: The Whitehall II study. *Lancet*, **337**, 1387.

Marmot, M.G., and Wilkinson, R.G. (eds.) (1999). *The social determinants of health*. Oxford University Press, Oxford.

Matthews, S., Manor, O., and Power, C. (1999). Social inequalities in health: Are there gender differences? *Social Science and Medicine*, **48**, 49.

McKinley, J.B. and Marceau, L.D. (2000). To boldly go . . . *American Journal of Public Health*, **90**, 25.

Mechanic, D. (1979). The stability of health and illness behavior: Results from a 16-year follow-up. *American Journal of Public Health*, **69**, 1142.

Mensink, R.P. and Katan, M.G. (1992). Effect of dietary fatty acids on serum lipids and lipoproteins: A meta-analysis of 27 trials. *Arteriosclerosis and Thrombosis*, **12**, 911.

Mercer, S. L. Kahn, L. K., Green, L.W. *et al.* (2005). Drawing possible lessons for obesity prevention and control from the tobacco control experience. Chapter 11 In *Obesity prevention and public health* (eds. D. Crawford and R.W. Jeffrey), pp. 231–64. New York and London: Oxford University Press, New York.

Metcalf, P., Scragg, R., and Davis, P. (2007). Relationship of different measures of socioeconomic status with cardiovascular disease risk factors and lifestyle in a New Zealand workforce survey. *New Zealand Medical Journal*, **120**(1248), U2392.

Millar, W.T. and Stephens, T. (1993). Social status and health risk in Canadian adults: 1985–1991. *Health Reports*, **5**, 143.

Mittendorf, R., Herschel, M. Williams, M.A. *et al.* (1994). Reducing the frequency of low birth weight in the United States. *Obstetrics and Gynecology*, **83**, 1056.

Mokdad, A.H., Marks, J.S., Stroup, D.F. *et al.*(2004). Actual causes of death in the United States, 2000. *Journal of the American Medical Association*, **291**, 1238. Erratum, *Journal of the American Medical Association*, **293**, 293.

Mullen, P.D., Green, L.W., and Persinger, G.S. (1985). Clinical trials of patient education for chronic conditions: A comparative meta-analysis of intervention types. *Preventive Medicine*, **14**, 753.

National Center for Health Statistics (2006). *Health, United States, 2006*. U.S. Department of Health and Human Services, Centers for Disease Control, p. 179, Hiattsville, MD.

Netz, Y., Wu, M.J., Becker, B.J. *et al.* (2005). Physical activity and psychological well-being in advanced age: A meta-analysis of intervention studies. *Psychology and Aging*, **20**, 272.

NHLBI (National Heart, Lung, and Blood Institute) (1993). *Detection, evaluation and treatment of high blood cholesterol in adults*, NIH Publication 93, p. 3095. National Institutes of Health, Bethesda, MD.

North, F, Syme, S.L., Feeney, A. *et al.* (1993). Explaining socioeconomic differences in sickness absence: The Whitehall II Study. *British Medical Journal*, **306**, 361.

Nuckolls, K.B., Cassels, J., and Kaplan, B.H. (1972). Psychosocial assets, life crisis and the prognosis of pregnancy. *American Journal of Epidemiology*, **95**, 431.

Ockene, J.K., Kuller, L.H., Svendsen, K.H., and Meilahn, E. (1990). The relationship of smoking cessation to coronary heart disease and lung cancer in the Multiple Risk Factor Intervention Trial (MRFIT). *American Journal of Public Health*, **80**, 954–8.

Office of Environmental Health Hazard Assessment (OEHHA), California Environmental Protection Agency (1997). *Health effects of exposure to environmental tobacco smoke*. Final report. Sacramento, CA.

Office of Health and Environmental Assessment (1992). *Respiratory, health effects of passive smoking: lung cancer and other disorders*. EPA/600/ (6-90/0006F), US Environmental Protection Agency, Cincinnati, OH.

Ogston, S.A. and Parry, G.J. (1992). EUROMAC. A European concerted action: maternal alcohol consumption and its relation to the outcome of pregnancy and child development at 18 months. Results-strategy of analysis and analysis of pregnancy outcome. *International Journal of Epidemiology*, **21** (Suppl 1), S45.

Oliveira, A., Buros, H., Maciel, M. J. *et al.* (2007). Tobacco smoking and acute myocardial infarction in young adults: A population-based case-control study. *Preventive Medicine*, **44**, 311.

Peck, M.N. (1994). The importance of childhood socio-economic group for adult health. *Social Science and Medicine*, **39**, 553–6.

Pederson, L. (1993). *Tobacco use. Canada's health promotion survey 1990: Technical report* (eds. Health and Welfare Canada, T. Stephens and D. Fowler Graham), pp. 97–108. Minister of Supply and Services Canada, Ottawa.

Petrow, S. (1990). *Ending the HIV epidemic*. Network Publications, Santa Cruz, CA.

Piccart-Gebhart, M.J., Procter, M., Leyland-Jones, B. *et al.* Herceptin Adjuvant (HERA) Trial Study Team (2005). Trastuzumab after adjuvant chemotherapy in HER2-positive breast cancer. *New England Journal of Medicine*, **353**, 1659–72.

Poland, B., Green, L.W., and Rootman, I.R. (2000). *Settings for health promotion: Linking theory and practice*. Sage, Thousand Oaks, CA.

Pooling Project Research Group (1978). Relationship of blood pressure, serum cholesterol, smoking habit, relative weight and ECG abnormalities to incidence of major coronary events: Final report of the Pooling Project. *Journal of Chronic Disease*, **31**, 201.

Potvin, L. and Frohlich, K.L. (1998). L'utilité de la notion de genre pour comprendre les inégalités de santé entre les homes et les femmes. *Ruptures, Revue Transdisciplinaire en Santé*, **5**, 142.

Prattala, R. Kaaristo, A., and Berg, M.A. (1994). Consistency and variation in unhealthy behaviour among Finnish men 1982–1990. *Social Science and Medicine*, **39**, 115.

Prochaska, J. O., Redding, C. A., and Evers, K. E. (2002). The Transtheoretical model and stages of change. In *Health behavior and health education: Theory, research, and practice*, 3rd edition (eds. K. Glanz, B. K. Rimer, and F. M. Lewis), pp. 99–120. Jossey-Bass, San Francisco.

Prus, S. G. (2007). Age, SES, and health: A population level analysis of health inequalities over the life course. *Sociology, Health and Illness*, **29**, 275–96.

Raine, K. D. (2004). *Overweight and obesity in Canada: A population health perspective*. Canadian Institute for Health Information, Ottawa.

Ranson, M.K., Jha, P., Chaloupka, F.J. *et al.* (2002). Global and regional estimates of the effectiveness and cost-effectiveness of price increases and other tobacco control policies. *Nicotine and Tobacco Research*, **4**, 311–19.

Richard, L., Potvin, L., Kishuck, N. *et al.* (1996). Assessment of the integration of the ecological approach in health promotion programs. *American Journal of Health Promotion*, **10**, 318.

Rimm, E.B., Manson, J.E., Stampfer, M.J. *et al.* (1993). Cigarette smoking and the risk of diabetes in women. *American Journal of Public Health*, **83**, 211.

Robbins, A.S. Manson, J.E., Lee, I.M. *et al.* (1994). Cigarette smoking and stroke in a cohort of US male physicians. *Annals of Internal Medicine*, **120**, 458.

Rogers, E.S. (1968). Public health asks of sociology . . . Can the health sciences resolve society's problems in the absence of a science of human values and goals. *Science*, **159**, 506.

Rose, G. and Colwell, L. (1992). Randomized controlled trial of anti-smoking advice: Final (20-year) results. *Journal of Epidemiology and Community Health*, **46**, 75.

Ross, C.E. and Bird, C.E. (1994). Sex stratification and health lifestyle: Consequences for men's and women's perceived health. *Journal of Health and Social Behavior*, **35**, 161.

Rozin, P. (1984). The acquisition of food habits and preferences. In *Behavior health: A handbook of health enhancements and disease prevention* (eds. J.D. Matarzzo, S.M. Weiss, J.A. Herd *et al.*), p. 590. Wiley, New York.

Rutten, A. (1995). The implementation of health promotion: A new structural perspective. *Social Science and Medicine*, **41**, 1627.

Shea, S., Stein, A.D., Basch, C.E. *et al.* (1991). Independent associations of educational attainment and ethnicity with behavioral risk factors for cardiovascular disease. *American Journal of Epidemiology*, **134**, 567.

Simons-Morton, B.G., O'Hara, N.M., and Simons-Morton, D.G. (1986). Promoting healthful diet and exercise behaviors in communities, schools, and families. *Family and Community Health*, **9**, 1.

Simons-Morton, B.G., Brink, S.G., Parcel, G.S. *et al.* (1990). *Preventing acute alcohol-related health problems in adolescents and young adults*. Centers for Disease Control, Atlanta, GA.

Simons-Morton, B.G., Greene, W.H., and Gottlieb, N.H. (1995). Social change. In *Introduction to health education and health promotion*, 2nd edition. p. 193. Waveland Press, Prospect Heights, IL.

Simons-Morton, D.G., Simons-Morton, B.G., Parcel, G.S. *et al.* (1988a). Influencing personal and environmental conditions for community health: A multilevel intervention model. *Family and Community Health*, **11**, 25.

Simons-Morton, D.G., Brink, S.G., Parcel, G.S. *et al.* (1988b). *Promoting physical activity among adults: A CDC community intervention handbook*. Center for Disease Control, Atlanta, GA.

Simons-Morton, D.G., Mullen, P.D., Mains, D.A. *et al.* (1992). Characteristics of controlled studies of patient education and counseling for prevention behaviors. *Patient Education and Counseling*, **19**, 175.

Smith, B.J., Tang, K. C., and Nutbeam, D. (2006). WHO Health Promotion Glossary: new terms. *Health Promotion International*, **21**, 340–5.

Spencer, L., Pagell, F., and Adams, T. (2005). Applying the transtheoretical model to cancer screening behavior. *American Journal of Health Behavior*, **29**, 36–56.

Stamler, J. (1992). Established major coronary risk factors. In *Coronary heart disease epidemiology: From aetiology to public health* (eds. M. Marmot and P. Elliott), pp. 35–66. Oxford University Press, Oxford.

Stamler, J., Wentworth, D., and Neaton, J.D., for MRFIT Research Group (1986). Is the relationship between serum cholesterol and risk of premature death from coronary heart disease continuous and graded. Findings in 356,222 primary screenees of the Multiple Risk Factor Intervention Trial (MRFIT). *Journal of American Medical Association*, **256**, 2823–8.

Steele, J. and McBroom, W. (1972). Conceptual and empirical dimensions of health behavior. *Journal of Health and Social Behavior*, **13**, 382.

Stern, M.P. (1991). Primary prevention of type II diabetes mellitus. *Diabetes Care*, **14**, 399.

Steuart, G.W. (1965). Health, behavior, and planned change. *Health Education Monographs*, **20**, 3.

Stoto, M. A., Green, L. W., and Bailey, L. A. (eds.) (1997). *Linking research and public health practice: A review of CDC's program of Centers for Research and Demonstration of Health Promotion and Disease Prevention*. National Academy Press, Washington, DC. http://books.nap.edu/catalog/5564.html

Stout, C., Morrow, J., Brandt, E.N. *et al.* (1964). Unusually low incidence of death from myocardial infarction in an Italian-American community in Pennsylvania. *Journal of American Medical Association*, **188**, 845.

Stronks, K., Van de Mheen, D., Loomanm C.W.N. *et al.* (1996). Behavioural and structural factors in the explanation of socio-economic inequalities in health: An empirical analysis. *Sociology of Health and Illness*, **18**, 653.

Taylor, W.C., Sallis, J.F., Lees, E. *et al.* (2007). Changing social and built environments to promote physical activity: Recommendations from low income, urban women. *Journal of Physical Activity and Health*, **4**, 54–65.

Tjepkema, M. (2005). *Nutrition: Findings from the Canadian Community Health Survey. Issue No. 1 measured obesity: Adult obesity in Canada*. Statistics Canada, Ottawa.

Townsend, P., Davison, N., and Whitehead, M. (1988). *Inequalities in health*. Penguin, Harmondsworth.

UNICEF (1993). *The state of the world's children 1993*. Oxford University Press, New York.

U.S. CDC (US Centers for Disease control). (1993). Cigarette smoking attributable mortality and years of potential life lost United States, 1990. *Morbidity and Mortality Weekly Reports*, **42**, 645.

U.S. Department of Health and Human Services (2001). *Healthy people 2001: National health promotion and disease prevention objectives*. UC Government Printing Office, Washington, DC.

U.S. Department of Health and Human Services (2004). *The health consequences of smoking: A report of the Surgeon General*. U.S. Department of Health and Human Services, Centers for Disease Control and Prevention, Coordinating Center for Health Promotion, National Center for Chronic Disease Prevention and Health Promotion, Office on Smoking and Health, Atlanta. US Government Printing Office, Washington, DC.

U.S. Department of Health and Human Services (2006). *The health consequences of involuntary exposure to tobacco smoke: A report of the Surgeon General—executive summary*. U.S. Department of Health and Human Services, Centers for Disease Control and Prevention, Coordinating Center for Health Promotion, National Center for Chronic Disease Prevention and Health Promotion, Office on Smoking and Health, Atlanta.

Verbrugge, L.M. (1989). The twain meet: Empirical explanations of sex differences in health and mortality. *Journal of Health and Social Behavior*, **30**, 282.

Villas, P., Cardenas, M., and Jameson, C. (1993). Instrument development using the PRECEDE model to distinguish users/triers from non-users of alcoholic beverages. *Wellness Perspectives: Research, Theory and Practice*, **10**, 46.

Walker, D., Gutierrez, J. P., Torres, P. *et al.* (2006). HIV prevention in Mexican schools: Prospective randomized evaluation of intervention. *British Medical Journal*, **332**, 1189.

Ward, J. W. and Warren, C. S. (eds.) (2007). *A safer and healthier America: Public health in the 20th century*. Oxford University Press, New York.

WHO (World Health Organization) (1981). *Global strategy for health for all by the year 2000*. WHO, Geneva.

WHO (World Health Organization) (1990). *Prevention in childhood and youth adult cardiovascular diseases: Time for action*. WHO technical report 792. WHO, Geneva.

WHO (World Health Organization) (1998). *Tobacco epidemic: Health dimensions*. Fact Sheet No. 154, revised. WHO, Geneva.

WHO (World Health Organization) (2000). *Obesity: Preventing and managing the global epidemic*. WHO technical report series no. 894. World Health Organization, Geneva.

Wilkinson, R.G. (1992a). Income distribution and life expectancy. *British Medical Journal*, **304**, 165.

Wilkinson, R.G. (1992b). National mortality rates: The impact of inequality. *American Journal of Public Health*, **82**, 1082.

Wilkinson, R.G. (1996). *Unhealthy society. The afflictions of inequality*. Routledge, London.

Wilkinson, R.G. (1999). Income inequality, social cohesion, and health: Clarifying the theory—A reply to Muntaner and Lynch. *International Journal of Health Services*, **29**, 525.

Wilkinson, R.G. and Marmot, M. (1998). *The solid facts*. World Health Organization, Geneva.

Wilkinson, R.G. and Pickett, K.E. (2008). Income inequality and socioeconomic gradients in mortality. *American Journal of Public Health*, **98**, 699–704.

Winkleby, M.A., Jatulis, D.E., Franck, E. *et al.* (1992a). Socio-economic status and health: how education, income, and occupation contribute to risk factors for cardiovascular disease. *American Journal of Public Health*, **82**, 816.

Winkleby, M.A., Fortman, S.P., and Rockhill, B. (1992*b*). Trends in cardiovascular risk factors by educational level: The Stanford Five City Project. *Preventive Medicine*, **21**, 592.

Wodak, A. (2006). Controlling HIV among injecting drug users: The current status of harm reduction. *HIV AIDS Policy and Law Review*, **11**, 77–80.

World Bank (1991). *World development report. Special population issues.* World Bank, Washington, DC.

World Bank (1993). *World development report 1993. Investing in health.* Oxford University Press, New York.

Genomics and public health

Alison Stewart, Wylie Burke,
Muin J. Khoury, and Ron Zimmerns

Introduction and historical perspectives

Public health has not traditionally been concerned with genomics. Practitioners of public health have regarded populations as essentially homogeneous, differing only in their exposures to environmental and social determinants of health such as poverty, poor housing, or toxic or infectious agents. Until recently, genomics and public health rarely came together except in the context of population screening programmes for certain genetic conditions. The first of these was newborn screening for the inherited metabolic disease phenylketonuria (PKU), for which biochemical screening and diagnostic tests became available during the 1960s (Botkin 2005). Although this genetic disease was rare, screening was recognized as a public health responsibility because early diagnosis and treatment of affected infants could prevent serious mental and physical disability in the population.

At around the same time, the speciality of medical genetics began to be recognized in some countries as a clinical discipline in its own right. As new interventions such as antenatal diagnosis for some genetic disorders were developed during the next few decades, geneticists and some public health professionals became involved in assessing population needs for services offering these interventions (Royal College of Physicians 1991) and, in countries such as the United Kingdom where public health has a role in healthcare service organization and delivery, in commissioning and allocating resources for them.

In some countries, enthusiasm for population screening broadened after the success of the early newborn screening programmes to include screening of sections of the adult population for some genetic conditions. In the United States, for example, mandatory screening of the African American population for sickle cell disease was introduced in the early 1970s. However the programme was ill-conceived: No clinical or public health benefits were identified, and there was evidence of stigmatization and discrimination against unaffected carriers of the condition (Markel 1997). Some other programmes met with more success, notably a carrier screening programme for Tay Sachs disease in the Ashkenazi Jewish community (Markel 1997) and screening for β-thalassaemia in Sardinia and Cyprus (Cao *et al.* 2002). Although newborn screening programmes continued, a general distrust of public health motives for population screening, together with the malign legacy of the eugenics movement of the early to mid-twentieth century, resulted during the late 1970s and 1980s in a general distancing of medical genetics from mainstream public health.

The impact of the 'new' genetics

In 1990, the Human Genome Project began. This ambitious enterprise aimed to sequence the entire 3 billion DNA base pairs of the human genome within a 15-year time frame, providing the raw material for discovering the sequences of the complete set of human genes and, eventually, finding out their functions and how they participate both in normal physiology and during the initiation and progression of disease. As it turned out, the sequencing project was finished ahead of schedule: A 'reference sequence' for the genome, including the almost complete sequences for its complement of around 25 000 genes, was published in 2003 (Collins *et al.* 2003).

The Human Genome Project accelerated progress in finding the genes that, when mutated, cause heritable diseases such as cystic fibrosis, Duchenne muscular dystrophy, and Huntington's disease. By the early years of the twenty-first century, the genes implicated in some 1800 of these genetic diseases (most of them very rare) had been identified and catalogued in the Online Mendelian Inheritance in Man database (http://www.ncbi.nlm.nih.gov/entrez/query.fcgi?db=OMIM). The availability of molecular diagnosis for many of these conditions began to transform the practice of medical genetics and spurred attempts to find better treatments.

During the same period, attention was also turning towards the subject of 'normal' human genetic variation and the opportunity of using the information and technology generated by the Human Genome Project to identify common genetic variants (or alleles) associated with disease in human populations (Willard *et al.* 2005). Many genetic epidemiology projects were initiated to search for gene–disease associations. In an effort to provide tools for such studies, the Human Genome Project consortia instigated first the single nucleotide polymorphism (SNP) project and then the HapMap project (Guttmacher & Collins 2005). The SNP and HapMap initiatives aimed to provide a map of common variation at the single-base level across the genome and to identify 'tagging' SNPs that characterized particular clusters of variants, or haplotypes, in different populations. These resources are beginning to bear fruit in successful whole-genome association studies, where markers distributed across the entire genome are scanned for possible association with a disease or other condition (Hirschhorn &

Daly 2005). These studies, often carried out by large international consortia and involving many thousands of study participants, have successfully identified common genomic variants associated with conditions including type II diabetes, coronary artery disease, and breast cancer (see, for example, The Wellcome Trust Case Control Consortium 2007).

The aim of all these studies is to achieve a better understanding of the molecular basis of human health and disease and to use this knowledge to develop a more accurate categorization of disease and susceptibility, together with new diagnostic technologies and more effective interventions, both preventive and therapeutic (Guttmacher *et al.* 2001; Collins & McKusick 2001). Alongside these aims is the hope of harnessing an understanding of human genomic variation to develop interventions that are targeted at those most likely to benefit.

Public health genomics

The population-level goals of the Human Genome Project, and the expectation that its achievements will in time bring profound changes both to clinical health services and to disease prevention, pose clear challenges and opportunities for public health practice (Khoury 1996). It may no longer be tenable for public health practitioners to regard populations as homogeneous, with 'one size fits all' answers to the problems posed by common, chronic conditions such as coronary heart disease, diabetes, or dementia. Genomic factors will also have to be incorporated into the assessment and control of important public health issues such as environmental health, nutrition, and infectious disease.

Nevertheless, doubts have been raised about the timing and occurrence of the widely touted 'genomics revolution' in medicine, and there are concerns that an over-emphasis on genomic contributors to disease may result in neglect of other factors such as environmental exposures, social structure, and lifestyle. Along with clear advances, genome-based research will almost certainly generate many promising ideas that do not ultimately yield health benefits.

As with other emerging technologies, the challenge is to devise an efficient strategy to distinguish between innovative advances and false leads. The potential benefits offered by the Human Genome Project need to be weighed against the resources required to implement them and against the potential harms.

The recognition of these challenges and opportunities and the need for a strategy to address them have led over the last decade to the emergence of the new field of public health genomics (Khoury 2003; Khoury *et al.* 2000; Stewart *et al.* 2007). The use of the term 'genomics' rather than 'genetics' signals that the subject matter is not confined to rare heritable diseases. The scientific basis for public health genomics is all the information stemming from the Human Genome Project and related '-omics' initiatives: Not only gene sequences and gene–disease associations, but also information about the spectrum of gene expression activity, gene products and metabolites in different tissue types, and in normal and disease states (functional genomics, proteomics, and metabolomics). Diagnostic and predictive biomarkers developed as a result of research in molecular and cell biology will increasingly be applied in clinical and preventive medicine, bringing opportunities to realize benefits for population health.

In this chapter, we will first outline the theoretical underpinnings of public health genomics: The recognition of genes as determinants of health, the importance of gene–environment interactions, and the relationships between genomic factors and disease. We will then look in more detail at some important areas where public health and genomics intersect: The use and evaluation of genetic and genomic tests, the criteria for population screening programmes involving genomic factors, and the use of genomics in disease prevention. This analysis will be followed by consideration of the ethical principles for the application of genomics in public health practice and, finally, by discussion of the challenges and prospects for public health genomics both immediately and in the coming decades.

We assume that readers have an understanding of the basic principles of genetics. For those needing background information or revision, there are many excellent Web-based tutorials such as *DNA from the Beginning*, produced by the Cold Spring Harbor Laboratory (http://www.dnaftb.org/dnaftb). A glossary of important terms and their definitions is provided in Box 2.4.1.

Genes as determinants of health

It has been known for many years that individuals differ in their susceptibility to environmental agents such as diet, housing, air and water quality, sanitation, and infectious agents. For example, in the nineteenth century when tuberculosis was rife in western European populations, physicians knew that individuals varied in their susceptibility to infection and attributed this variation to differences in individual 'constitution'. However, nothing was known about the 'constitutional' (essentially, genetic) factors involved, and so for all practical purposes they were ignored.

The new era of genomics mandates a change from this way of thinking, to one that explicitly recognizes genes as determinants of health (Fig. 2.4.1). An important feature of this model is that it emphasizes the interplay between genomic and environmental factors (an 'environmental' factor in this context is anything that is not genomic). Obesity presents a classic example. Genomic factors are known to influence an individual's appetite and sensation of satiation after a meal. Individuals with impaired mechanisms of appetite and satiation will seek more food and, if food is in abundant supply, will put on weight, sometimes to the point of obesity. Environmental factors can also influence genes: For example, ionizing radiation may cause DNA mutations that lead to cancer; if mutations affect germ-line cells, they may be transmitted to future generations.

Whether a disease appears to be primarily 'genetic' or 'environmental' depends on the relative prevalence of the causative factors. Once again, history provides an example. Vitamin D deficiency is known to cause the disease rickets, a discovery made during an era when the disease was relatively common due to the prevalence of childhood malnutrition. Today, however, childhood malnutrition is rare in the developed world, and the few cases of rickets that are seen are more likely to be caused by rare genetic disorders of vitamin D metabolism.

Rothman (1986) observed that any disease can be shown to be both 100 per cent inherited and 100 per cent environmental. The classic example is PKU. We refer to PKU as a genetic disease because the dietary factor, phenylalanine, is ubiquitous whereas the genetic

Box 2.4.1 Glossary of basic terms in genetics and genomics

Alleles	Variant forms of the same gene
Autosomes	Chromosomes that are not concerned with sex determination. Humans have 22 pairs of autosomes and two sex chromosomes
Biomarker	A factor used to indicate or measure a biological process (for example, a specific protein or genetic polymorphism)
Carrier	Usually refers to an individual who is heterozygous for a recessive disease-causing allele
Chromosomes	The structures within cells that carry the genetic information in the form of DNA
Dominant	A characteristic that is expressed even when the relevant gene is present in only one copy
Epigenetic	A factor or mechanism that changes the expression of a gene without affecting its DNA sequence, and is stably transmitted during cell division
Genome	The complete set of genetic information of an organism
Genotype	The specific genetic constitution of an individual
Germ-line	Relating to the sex cells, which transmit genetic information from one generation to the next
Haplotype	A specific set of alleles located on the same chromosome
Heterozygous	Carrying two different alleles of a gene
Homozygous	Carrying two identical alleles of a gene
Karyotype	A description of the number and structure of chromosomes in an individual
Locus	The location of a gene or DNA marker on a chromosome
Marker	A gene or other segment of DNA whose chromosomal position is known
Mendelian	Relating to the laws of inheritance discovered by Gregor Mendel
Meiosis	The specialized cell division that takes place when sex cells (sperm or eggs) are produced. The members of each chromosome pair separate so each sex cell receives only one copy of each gene
Mutation	A change in the sequence of DNA
Nucleotide	The molecular units that make up DNA and RNA. A nucleotide of DNA consists of a base (A, C, G, or T) linked to the sugar deoxyribose and a phosphate group
Penetrance	The likelihood that an individual carrying a specific genetic variant will show the characteristic determined by that variant
Phenotype	The observable traits of an organism
Polymorphism	A common genetic variant or allele (present in at least 1–2 per cent of the population)
Recessive	A characteristic that is only expressed when two copies of the relevant gene are present
SNP	Single nucleotide polymorphism: A DNA sequence variation that involves a change in a single nucleotide
Somatic	Relating to the cells of the body other than the germ-line (sex) cells and their precursors

defect is rare, occurring in around 1 in 10 000 births. If, in an alternative world, a population all had the genetic abnormality that we associate with PKU but phenylalanine was not found in the diet of that population, the few cases of PKU observed in that world would be deemed to be toxic or nutritional in origin.

It is clear, then, that the well-known 'nature versus nurture' debate in disease causation is meaningless, as are attempts to classify diseases as '*x* per cent genetic and *y* per cent environmental': All disease results from the combined effects of genes and environment. Box 2.4.2 presents some examples of effects of genetic and environmental exposures on disease risk.

The role of genes in disease

'Genetic' diseases

Although both genes and environment contribute to all diseases, in some cases a single alteration to the genetic code—a mutation—appears to be sufficient to cause disease. Examples of such classical 'genetic diseases' include cystic fibrosis, Huntington's disease, and sickle cell disease. Genetic diseases of this type are also sometimes known as Mendelian diseases because they show patterns of transmission from one generation to the next that conform to Mendel's laws of inheritance.

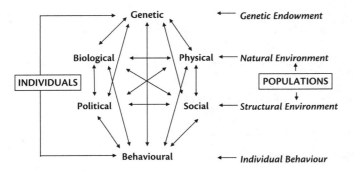

Fig. 2.4.1 Determinants of health.

Chromosomal disorders—caused by deletions, duplications, translocations, or inversions of whole chromosomes or chromosome segments—are also generally classed as genetic diseases because they are clearly correlated with an observable genetic lesion. An example of a chromosomal disorder is Down syndrome, which is caused by an extra copy of chromosome 21.

Although *potentially* heritable, genetic diseases are not always inherited. Almost all cases of Down syndrome arise as a result of a sporadic genetic lesion, usually during maternal meiosis. Some other genetic diseases show a similarly high proportion of sporadic cases. For example, approximately one-third of cases of the genetic disease tuberous sclerosis are inherited, whereas the remaining two-thirds arise from new mutations. In most cases, the cause of the new mutation is unknown.

In many countries of the developed world, specialist clinical genetics services care for individuals and families affected by genetic diseases. A recent book by Read and Donnai (2007) provides an excellent, practical background to all aspects of medical genetics and its clinical practice.

Mendelian diseases and chromosomal disorders are individually rare. However, collectively they represent a substantial burden of morbidity and mortality: Around 4000 Mendelian diseases have been recognized, with a combined birth frequency of approximately 1–2 per cent in populations in the developed world (Royal College of Physicians of London 1991).

The prevalence of genetic diseases may vary substantially in different populations, probably reflecting selective factors operating on the genes involved. For example, the birth prevalence of sickle cell disease, a recessive disorder, is very low in populations of Northern European origin, but as high as 1 in 80 in some black African populations (World Health Organization 1996). The reason is thought to be that, in the heterozygous state, sickle cell alleles confer resistance to malaria and so have been maintained by evolutionary pressures in populations exposed to malaria, despite the severe disadvantage they cause for homozygous individuals.

In some cases a 'founder effect' may be implicated: Particular alleles that arose in a small, isolated founder population may persist in the population through many generations if it remains relatively genetically isolated from other population groups. A probable example of a founder effect is the relatively high prevalence, in Ashkenazi Jews, of alleles causing the recessive disorder Tay Sachs disease.

The role of genes in common disease

Genes also play a role in susceptibility to the common diseases of later life such as coronary heart disease, type II diabetes, Alzheimer's dementia, and cancers. An indication that genomic factors are at work comes from the observation that in many cases such diseases show a tendency to 'run in families', though shared environment also contributes to familial effects. It is thought that genetic susceptibility to common disease is attributable to the combined action of many different common genomic variants that are individually of weak effect.

Box 2.4.2   Some patterns of relative risk in gene–environment interactions

The table shows three examples of different patterns of risk for three classical genetic diseases that have an environmental component, assuming dichotomous genetic susceptibility and environmental exposure.

In the first example, xeroderma pigmentosum (XP), exposure to ultraviolet light increases the risk of developing skin cancer in non-carriers of XP mutations, but the combination of these mutations and exposure to ultraviolet light vastly increases the risk. In theory, if individuals with XP mutations completely avoid ultraviolet light their risk of skin cancer becomes close to the background risk.

In the second example, phenylketonuria (PKU), only individuals with recessive mutations in the causative gene who are exposed to phenylalanine in the diet are susceptible to PKU.

In the third example, deficiency in the alpha-1-antitrypsin gene, both non-smokers who are at genetic risk and smokers who are not at genetic risk have an increased risk of developing emphysema, and the combination (smokers who are at genetic risk) is associated with the highest risk.

Gene variant	Environmental exposure	Relative risk (XP)	Relative risk (PKU)	Relative risk (emphysema)
Absent	Absent	1.0	1.0	1.0
Present	Absent	~1.0	1.0	Modest
Absent	Present	Modest	1.0	Modest
Present	Present	Very high	Very high	High

Reprinted with permission from Macmillan Publishers Ltd: Hunter, DJ. *Nature Reviews Genetics* **6**, 287–98, copyright 2005.

The genomic variants that affect susceptibility to common disease are so far mostly unknown. Many reported genotype–disease associations have not yet been independently validated though, as discussed previously, large-scale whole-genome association studies are now beginning to yield replicable associations. An example of an association that is supported by good evidence concerns alleles of the gene encoding the protein component of a blood lipoprotein, apolipoprotein E (APOE). Individuals with one copy of the APOE4 allele have a risk of Alzheimer's dementia that is 2.5–3 times the risk of individuals with two copies of the more common APOE3 allele. Homozygosity for the APOE4 allele increases the relative risk still further, to 10–15 times the risk of APOE3 homozygotes. Table 2.4.1 lists some other examples of validated gene–disease associations.

For some common diseases, including common cancers such as breast/ovarian cancer and colorectal cancer, there are families in which several family members are affected by the same disease, often at an early age, and the disease shows a Mendelian inheritance pattern through the family, suggesting the existence of a single mutation that confers a high risk of disease. In these Mendelian (single gene) subsets of common disease, genotype can be used with a fairly high degree of certainty to predict the development of disease.

An example is familial hypercholesterolaemia, a dominantly inherited condition that is characterized by a build-up of cholesterol and a high risk of premature cardiovascular disease. The disease is caused by mutations in a gene encoding a cell-surface receptor for a blood lipoprotein. About 1 in 500 people are thought to carry the mutant gene, and virtually all will develop symptoms of the disease at some stage of their life. In the population as a whole, only about 1 in 20 people who develop hypercholesterolaemia carry a strongly predisposing single-gene mutation; in general, single-gene subsets of common diseases account for a maximum of 5–10 per cent of the total burden of disease.

Complexities of gene–disease relationships

In Mendelian diseases and chromosomal disorders, a single genetic defect can be sufficient to cause disease. Such diseases are said to be completely or highly penetrant. The penetrance of a genotype is the probability that an individual with that genotype will be affected by the disease. Penetrance is always associated with a time frame; for example, lifetime penetrance, or penetrance by age 60, and so on. Cystic fibrosis is generally fully penetrant during early childhood, while Huntington's disease is fully penetrant by late middle age. Not all Mendelian diseases are fully penetrant, though in most cases penetrance is high; essentially, it is high penetrance that causes the disease to be recognized as Mendelian. For example, breast cancer associated with mutations in the BRCA1 gene has a lifetime penetrance of 40–85 per cent (Antoniou et al. 2003; the higher estimates come from families with multiple cases of the disease, and the lower estimates from population-based studies).

Incomplete penetrance is an indication that other factors are involved in determining whether an individual will be affected: These other factors may be other genes and/or environmental factors. Even for diseases whose penetrance is high, other genetic and/or environmental factors are likely to affect the expressivity of the disease: For example, characteristics such as the range and severity of symptoms, or the age of onset.

Complexity is also evident in the spectrum of mutations that may be associated with the 'same' disease. This phenomenon, known as genetic heterogeneity, is a complicating factor in the development and clinical application of genetic tests. Genetic heterogeneity may be allelic (different alleles of the same gene associated with the same disease) or non-allelic (alleles of different genes associated with the same disease; also called locus heterogeneity).

Genetic heterogeneity is extremely common. For example, more than 1000 different pathogenic mutations have been found in the CFTR gene associated with cystic fibrosis. Similarly, familial breast cancer may be caused by any of hundreds of different mutations in the BRCA1 or BRCA2 genes. Sometimes, particular mutations may be more common in a specific population. For example, in cystic fibrosis patients of Northern European origin the frequency of the ΔF508 mutation in the CFTR gene is about 70 per cent, whereas in African American cystic fibrosis patients it is only about 40 per cent. For this reason, clinical genetic testing protocols may need to be modified depending on the racial or ethnic origin of the person being tested.

DNA sequence variation is not the only source of variation in gene function. In multicellular organisms, different types of cells acquire their functional characteristics by expressing different subsets of their genome in a specific temporal pattern. Differential gene expression is associated with chemical modifications to the DNA (such as methylation) that do not change the primary DNA sequence and are termed epigenetic. As cells of a specific type multiply, they stably transmit these epigenetic modifications to the cells they give rise to. Epigenetic mechanisms are likely to play a role in mediating changes in gene expression in response to environmental signals (Jaenisch & Bird 2003). Disruption in epigenetic processes is known to play a role in some diseases, including cancer. Epigenetic changes are not generally thought to be heritable by the organism's offspring but there is some emerging evidence that trans-generational effects may occur (Richards 2006).

Because biological systems are so complex, it is almost always an over-simplification to speak in terms of a 'gene for' a particular characteristic or disease: No gene acts in isolation.

Table 2.4.1 Selected genetic associations validated through meta-analysis

Gene	Variant (contrast)	Disease	OR	95% CI
ACE	DD (DI/II)	Myocardial infarction	1.28	1.09–1.50
KCNJ11	E23K KK (EK/EE)	Diabetes type 2	1.92	1.29–2.97
TGFA	Taq1 (allele2 vs 1)	Nonsyndromic cleft lip	1.58	1.13–2.21
MTHFR	677 (TT vs CC/CT)	Neural tube defects	1.70	1.31–2.21
MAPT	Allele AD vs others	Parkinson disease	1.52	1.22–1.90
GSTM1	null/null vs others	Bladder cancer	1.54	1.27–1.86
F5	Leiden vs others	Preeclampsia	2.22	1.46–3.38
DRD2	Ser311Cys Cys vs ser	Schizophrenia	1.43	1.16–1.76

Noncomprehensive list from 50 genetic associations validated through meta-analysis as reported by Ioannidis et al. (2006).

Genetic and genomic tests

Virtually all medical tests are to some degree 'genetic', because genetic factors have played a part in the development of the characteristics (for example blood pressure, eyesight, or bone density) that are tested.

A US Task Force on Genetic Testing defined a genetic test as 'the analysis of human DNA, RNA, chromosomes, proteins, and certain metabolites in order to detect heritable disease-related genotypes, mutations, phenotypes, or karyotypes for clinical purposes' (Holtzman & Watson 1997). This definition implies that a genetic test is a test that enables a direct inference about the state of the germ-line genetic material. Any diagnostic test for a Mendelian disease or chromosomal disorder qualifies as a genetic test because it allows such an inference. For example, a renal ultrasound test for autosomal dominant polycystic kidney disease may be considered a genetic test because it enables the inference that there is or is not a lesion in one of the genes causally implicated in this disease. A biochemical analysis to detect haemoglobin variants causing sickle cell disease is also a genetic test. Any direct DNA test is a genetic test, whether it relates to a single-gene or chromosomal disorder, or to a low-penetrance genetic factor implicated in a common disease. However, a blood pressure test, for example, is not a genetic test by this definition because it does not enable any direct inference about the sequence or properties of a specific gene or genes.

The nature and implications of a genetic test can vary widely, depending largely on the penetrance of the condition or the genotype in question. It is important, when using the term genetic test, to be clear about whether it is being used to denote a test for a genetic (highly penetrant heritable) disease, or simply to mean a test of the genetic material (Zimmern 2001). A test for a genetic condition may have serious implications both for the person tested and for his or her blood relatives. In contrast, a test for a common DNA polymorphism associated with susceptibility to, say, coronary heart disease will probably have no more serious implications for health than analysis of blood lipids, and no greater consequences for other family members.

The US Task Force's definition specifically excludes somatic genetic tests, such as tests of the genetic material in tumour cells or gene expression profiles in different tissues or organs. However, the development, use, and evaluation of somatic genetic tests—perhaps better termed 'genomic tests'—also pose both opportunities and challenges for public health. Somatic genomic tests may also include tests for other complex genomic biomarkers such as proteomic or metabolomic profiles.

Uses of genetic and genomic tests

Genetic and genomic tests may be used in:

◆ Diagnosis of a disease.

◆ Prediction of risk for a disease.

◆ Prediction of response to a therapeutic or preventive intervention. The most familiar scenario is prediction of response to a therapeutic drug. This use of genetic test information is known as *pharmacogenetics*.

It has recently been suggested that this categorization in fact misses the point, and that diagnosis and prediction are only means to various ends. The ultimate purpose of carrying out a genetic test is (a) to reduce morbidity or mortality, (b) to provide salient health information that will benefit the clinical care of the patient, or (c) to enable reproductive choice; and the effectiveness of the test should be evaluated with regard to the stated purpose (Burke *et al.* 2007).

Diagnostic genetic tests

Diagnostic genetic tests may be used at any stage of life (preimplantation, prenatal, newborn, childhood, adolescence, or middle age) to detect a DNA or chromosomal variant (or variants) associated with a disease. At present they are only in routine clinical use for highly penetrant single-gene (Mendelian) diseases and chromosomal disorders (see Table 2.4.2 for some examples). In the future, DNA tests may be used to clarify the diagnosis of specific molecular subtypes of common disease.

Diagnostic DNA tests carried out before birth (preimplantation or prenatal genetic diagnosis) may be used by couples at risk of transmitting a specific genetic disease to determine whether the embryo or foetus is affected by the disease. The purpose of testing is to enable the couple to exercise reproductive choice by either preparing for the birth of an affected child or opting to terminate the pregnancy. In the case of preimplantation diagnosis, only unaffected embryos are used to establish a pregnancy.

Diagnostic genetic tests in the postnatal period may be used to provide a definitive diagnosis in cases where genetic disease is suspected. For example, in an infant affected by severe muscle wasting, a DNA test may confirm a diagnosis of Duchenne muscular dystrophy.

A special category of diagnostic test is a carrier test, which is used to detect a carrier of a Mendelian autosomal recessive or sex-linked disease. Individuals in families or populations affected by such diseases may wish to know whether they are carriers and therefore, although not themselves affected, at risk of transmitting the disease to their children.

Diagnostic genomic biomarkers

Genomic biomarkers such as gene expression, proteomic or metabolomic profiles convey information about the molecular-genetic characteristics of somatic cells that may be correlated with clinical parameters such as disease staging, prognosis, and response to therapy. Gene expression and proteomic profiling is an active area of clinical research, particularly in oncology. For example, gene expression profiling, using microarrays, has been used to distinguish different tumour subtypes in diffuse large B-cell lymphomas (Staudt & Dave 2005). Serum proteomic profiling has been investigated as a screening test for early diagnosis of ovarian cancer (Petricoin *et al.* 2002).

However, although one Phase III clinical trial of gene expression profiling in breast cancer is underway, and some commercial 'kits' for gene expression and proteomic profiling are available, these technologies are not yet ready for mainstream clinical implementation (Quackenbush 2006). Difficulties that need to be overcome include inadequate reproducibility, lack of standardization, failure to demonstrate improved outcomes as compared with current clinical practice, and poor positive predictive values, especially when used as screening tests in a population setting.

Predictive genetic tests

Because an individual's germ-line DNA remains largely unchanged throughout life, DNA testing can in some circumstances be used in

Table 2.4.2 Examples of molecular genetic tests

Condition	Genes	Reported uses of testing
Neurological		
Spinocerebellar ataxia	SCA1, SCA2, SCA3, SCA6, SCA7, SCA10, DRPLA	Diagnostic, predictive
Fragile X syndrome	FMR1	Diagnostic, antenatal
Huntington's disease	HD	Diagnostic, predictive, antenatal
Connective tissue		
Ehlers–Danos syndrome, vascular type	COL3A1	Diagnostic, antenatal
Marfan syndrome	FBN1	Diagnostic, antenatal
Oncological		
Familial adenomatous polyposis	APC	Diagnostic, predictive
Hereditary non-polyposis colorectal cancer	MLH1, MSH2, PMS2, MSH3, MSH6	Diagnostic, predictive
Familial breast/ovarian cancer	BRCA1, BRCA2	Diagnostic, predictive
Haematological		
Beta-thalassaemia	Beta-globin (HbB)	Carrier detection, antenatal
Haemophilia A	F8C	Prognostic, carrier detection, antenatal
Haemophilia B	F9C	Carrier detection, antenatal
Renal		
Polycystic kidney disease (autosomal dominant and autosomal recessive)	PKD1, PKD2, PKHD1	Predictive, antenatal
Multisystem		
Achondroplasia	FGFR3	Antenatal
Alpha1-antitrypsin deficiency	AAT	Diagnostic, predictive
Galactosaemia	GALT	Newborn screening, carrier detection, antenatal
Neurofibromatosis type 1	NF1	Antenatal
Neurofibromatosis type 2	NF2	Predictive, antenatal

Source: Adapted from Burke, W. *New England Journal of Medicine* **347**, 1867–75. Copyright 2002 Massachusetts Medical Society. All rights reserved.

an asymptomatic individual to predict the risk of a specific disease occurring in the future. The classic example is Huntington's disease, which may be predicted with almost 100 per cent certainty by a DNA test even before birth. A positive test result for a pathogenic mutation in the *APC* gene associated with familial adenomatous polyposis, an inherited form of bowel cancer, predicts future disease with 90–100 per cent certainty. In the context of highly penetrant Mendelian conditions, predictive testing is sometimes termed *presymptomatic testing*.

However, this high degree of predictive value is rare. Huntington's disease has a population prevalence of about 1 in 20 000–40 000, and fewer than 0.5 per cent of bowel cancer cases are thought to be due to inherited mutations in the *APC* gene. In relation to common disease, the predictive value of DNA test information is much lower; such tests may be better described as susceptibility or predispositional tests.

Pharmacogenetic tests

Heritable genetic factors are known to affect responses to many classes of therapeutic drugs. Variable responses may include increased or decreased sensitivity to the drug, as well as adverse or toxic drug reactions. For example, variants of genes encoding members of the cytochrome P450 family of enzymes affect dosage requirements for a wide range of drugs including warfarin, codeine, clozapine, and timolol (Wolf *et al.* 2000). Certain polymorphisms in the gene encoding the enzyme thiopurine *S*-methyltransferase (TPMT) are associated with serious adverse reactions to thiopurine immunosuppressive drugs, such as azathioprine, used in oncology and other fields of medicine (Gardiner & Begg 2006).

The concept underlying pharmacogenetics is that it may be possible to use DNA testing to tailor drug prescribing to an individual's genetic make-up, thereby optimizing response and minimizing adverse reactions. The path from discovery of a validated polymorphism influencing drug response to a clinically useful pharmacogenetic test is a complex one. The anti-coagulant drug warfarin provides an instructive example. Warfarin dose requirement is affected by variation in the *CYP2C9* gene (Sanderson *et al.* 2005). However, other factors such as age, sex, other genes, and drug interactions also affect warfarin response (and response to most other drugs); the predictive value of *CYP2C9* testing is not known accurately but may be only about 20 per cent (Sconce *et al.* 2005). It is not clear whether *CYP2C9* testing would offer appreciable advantages over current best practice in warfarin prescribing, which includes careful clinical evaluation of the patient and post-prescription monitoring.

Proposed pharmacogenetic tests need careful consideration on a case-by-case basis, including determination of sensitivity, specificity, positive and negative predictive values, and cost-effectiveness. The optimal parameters for a pharmacogenetic test will vary for different test indications.

Pharmacogenetic tests for heritable variants remain mostly at the research stage but some somatic pharmacogenetic tests are already in clinical use, particularly in oncology. An example is the typing of *HER2* gene expression in breast tumours to test for responsiveness to the drug Herceptin® (trastuzumab), an antibody drug that targets the HER2 protein on the surface of tumour cells.

Gene expression profiling is also under investigation as a tool to guide optimal treatment. For example, patients whose tumour gene expression profile, together with standard clinical criteria, indicates a good prognosis and a low probability of metastasis may be spared debilitating aggressive treatment with adjuvant chemotherapy. As discussed previously, gene expression profiling needs further evaluation before adoption for mainstream clinical use.

Evaluation of genetic and genomic tests

Public health professionals have a role in ensuring that any diagnostic, predictive, or pharmacogenetic tests used in clinical or public health practice are properly evaluated in order to protect patients and health services. A genetic test (or any other clinical test) encompasses more than a laboratory assay. Rather, it is a complex process that is part of an overall regime of disease prevention or management for a specific individual (Kroese *et al.* 2004). A test is best conceived of as the application of an assay for a particular disease, in a particular population, and for a particular purpose (Kroese *et al.* 2004). An assay may be deemed highly effective in one set of circumstances but not in another.

The first attempt to devise an evaluation framework for genetic tests was the ACCE project (Haddow & Palomaki 2004), using criteria originally proposed by the 1997 Task Force on Genetic Testing (Holtzman and Watson 1997). ACCE is an acronym standing for **A**nalytical validity, **C**linical validity, **C**linical utility, and **E**thical, legal, and social implications. Recently, it has been acknowledged that ethical, legal, and social implications such as potential discrimination, stigmatization, and psychosocial consequences form part of the assessment of the overall utility of a test (Grosse & Khoury 2006), and there has been a trend away from regarding them as a separable set of issues.

Analytical validity

The analytical validity is the means by which an assay is evaluated. It is defined as the assay's ability to measure accurately (in the case of a genetic test) the genotype of interest. It is important to define the genotype precisely. A test to detect 24 specific mutations in the *CFTR* gene is not the same test as one designed to detect only 4 mutations, for example. The test characteristics will differ in these two circumstances because the reference standard will be different. A distinction can also be made between open-ended assays such as karyotyping (microscopic examination of the chromosomes) or mutation scanning across a gene, in which any abnormality is sought, and closed assays, which specify in advance the spectrum of mutations or abnormalities the assay is designed to test (Burke & Zimmern 2007).

Clinical validity

Clinical validity is the ability of a test to diagnose or predict a specific phenotype (usually, a specific disease); here, the reference standard is a clinical one. The clinical validity of a test encompasses more than a demonstration of good epidemiological association between a test result (the presence of a genetic variant) and the disease. There must additionally be a formal evaluation of test performance in practice.

For closed assays, parameters such as sensitivity, specificity, positive and negative predictive values, likelihood ratios, and the receiver operating characteristic (ROC) curve can be measured. Even if there is a strong association between a genetic variant and a disease, as has been shown for the *TCF7L2* polymorphism and type II diabetes, a clinical test for this polymorphism may have very limited predictive value and thus poor clinical validity (Janssens *et al.* 2006).

Assessment of clinical validity is more difficult for open-ended assays. As a result, proxies must be used to estimate the clinical performance of an open-ended test. Microarray comparative genomic hybridization (CGH) offers an example (Subramonia-Iyer *et al.* 2007). CGH is a new technique for detecting submicroscopic chromosomal abnormalities, including some never detected before and some that are unlikely to be of clinical significance. In this setting, measures based on biological plausibility can be used to estimate the likelihood that a detected abnormality is clinically significant (e.g. nature and location of the abnormality; whether similar chromosomal abnormalities have been described in normal populations). With the use of these parameters, the test can be evaluated for its estimated diagnostic yield (proportion of those tested with a positive result) and false positive yield.

Clinical utility

Clinical utility refers to the likelihood that a test will lead to an improved health outcome, whether in terms of the clinical course of the disease by way of reduced mortality or morbidity, or in terms of reduced impact of the disease on the individual or his or her family. Factors that may be considered include the clinical risks and benefits of testing, such as the availability of an effective intervention and the risks associated with any interventions (Burke 2002; Burke *et al.* 2002), and health economic assessment.

Clinical utility may be poor if, for example, available interventions are not genotype-specific. Carriers of the Factor V Leiden or *G20210A* prothrombin variants have an increased risk for venous thromboembolism (VT). However, genetic testing of VT patients does not aid clinical management, as current evidence suggests that these genetic variants do not significantly increase the recurrence risk for VT.

Clinical utility has proved very difficult to assess in practice. Burke and Zimmern (2007), using criteria based on Donabedian's work on the quality of medical care, suggest that the main dimensions of clinical utility relate to the purpose for which a test is used (legitimacy, efficacy, effectiveness, and appropriateness), and the feasibility of test delivery (acceptability, efficiency, and the economic dimensions of optimality and equity) (Table 2.4.3).

The full evaluation of a genetic test is a complex process that requires significant resources. Because it is not possible to apply the full process to all tests, different levels of evaluation may be applied, depending on the nature of the test, its purpose, and the population in which it is to be carried out. For example, most tests for rare disorders require a less stringent programme of evaluation than tests for common disorders or population screening. This is because, when penetrance is high, the association between a positive test and ultimate outcome is more predictable, and the rarity of the condition means that the number of tests will be small.

In the United States, an ongoing model initiative of the Centers for Disease Control and Prevention, called the Evaluation of Genomic Applications in Practice and Prevention (EGAPP, http://www.egappreviews.org/default.htm), is attempting to integrate various models of genetic test evaluations including in-depth assessments and fast-track evaluation.

Genomics in disease prevention

All disease results from the combined effects of genetic and non-genetic factors. It follows that there may be opportunities to prevent disease by modifying either the genetic or the non-genetic component, or both. Juengst (1995) has distinguished these two theoretical modes of prevention as genotypic and phenotypic prevention, respectively.

Preventive strategies may be primary (preventing or delaying disease onset), secondary (encompassing early detection and treatment), or tertiary (delaying or preventing complications and deterioration).

Table 2.4.3 Key questions in genetic test evaluation

Domain	Questions
Assay	**How accurate is the assay?**
Analytical validity	What are the analytical sensitivity, specificity, PPV, and NPV of the assay, as compared to a gold standard?
Reliability and reproducibility	How reproducible are the test results under normal laboratory conditions?
Clinical validity	**What is the predictive value of the test in a defined population, for the specified disease?**
Gene–disease association	What is the strength of the association between genotype and disease?
	Is the genotype a minimally sufficient cause of disease?
	Is the genotype necessary for disease to occur?
Clinical test performance	What are the sensitivity, specificity, PPV, NPV, LR+, LR-, and ROC of the test, compared to a gold standard?
	If these measurements are not possible, what is the basis for proposing clinical validity for the test?
Clinical utility	
Test purpose	**What is the purpose of the test?**
Legitimacy	Is the proposed test in keeping with societal values, norms, and ethical principles?
	Is test delivery in compliance with laws and regulations?
Efficacy	Can the test and associated services achieve the intended purpose under ideal circumstances?
Appropriateness	What are the benefits and negative consequences of testing?
	Do the benefits sufficiently outweigh the negative consequences?
Feasibility of test delivery	**Can the test and associated services be delivered equitably, and in an acceptable manner, for a reasonable cost?**
Acceptability	Is the test delivered in conformity to the wishes, desires, and expectations of patients and their families?
Efficiency	Can the cost of the test and associated services be lowered without diminishing benefits? If there is an alternative for achieving the same purpose, is the test more or less efficient?
Optimality	What are the costs of the test relative to the benefits? Is a formal analysis of cost-effectiveness needed?
Equity	Can the test and associated services be provided equitably among different members of the population?

Source: Burke and Zimmern (2007).

Genotypic prevention

Genotypic prevention is a mode of primary genetic prevention. Examples include the use of antenatal genetic diagnosis and termination of pregnancy by couples wishing to avoid the birth of a child affected by a serious genetic disease. Genotypic prevention must always be a matter for personal choice by the individuals concerned, not a public health goal. Couples who know they are at risk of transmitting a genetic disease to their child should receive specialist advice and counselling by clinical genetics professionals before they make their choice.

Preimplantation genetic diagnosis (PGD) is considered by some to be a more acceptable form of genotypic prevention as it involves embryo selection rather than abortion, but there may still be ethical objections on the grounds that those embryos that are not selected for implantation are destroyed. Purchasers and commissioners of health services may also place restrictions on the use of PGD because of the high costs of the procedure, which involves *in vitro* fertilization as well as complex processes of embryo biopsy and molecular genetic testing.

In some countries, there are explicit programmes of antenatal genetic screening for some genetic diseases. Under such programmes, a whole population or population subgroup, who may not be aware that they are at risk, is offered a screening test to determine if the risk of their having an affected child is sufficiently high for them to be offered a definitive diagnostic test for the condition in question. For example, the United Kingdom has a national antenatal screening programme for Down syndrome (National Collaborating Centre for Women's and Children's Health 2003) and antenatal carrier screening programmes for sickle cell disease and the thalassaemias (NHS Sickle Cell and Thalassaemia Screening Programme). All pregnant women are offered screening as part of routine antenatal care. In countries such as the United Kingdom (but not in all countries) such programmes are considered ethically acceptable as long as informed choice by individuals determines who takes up the offer of screening.

Using genomics in secondary prevention: Newborn screening

Unfortunately most highly penetrant genetic diseases are incurable, but clinical management of many of these conditions has improved in recent years, and for some conditions life expectancy has increased significantly. In some cases, early detection of the disease, and early initiation of treatment, can significantly reduce mortality and morbidity. The classic example is the disease PKU, which is caused by deficiency of the enzyme phenylalanine hydroxylase (Kaye *et al.* 2006). If the disease is untreated, build-up of phenylalanine causes irreversible brain damage soon after birth. Early detection and initiation of a phenylalanine-free diet enables near-normal development. Sickle cell disease and cystic fibrosis also respond to early diagnosis and initiation of treatment in the newborn period, though the benefits are less dramatic than for PKU (Kaye *et al.* 2006). Newborn screening programmes may have other less direct benefits, such as in sparing parents of an affected child the often prolonged process of obtaining a diagnosis and in counselling parents about the risk to subsequent pregnancies.

Newborn screening programmes for various conditions are in place in many western countries (see Table 2.4.4 for examples). In some jurisdictions, including the United States, newborn screening programmes are state-mandated. In others, for example the United Kingdom, parental consent is sought.

The apparent success of newborn screening for PKU, the development of new diagnostic technologies such as tandem mass spectrometry, and powerful advocacy by some patient groups have led to pressure for widening newborn-screening programmes to include an increasing number of conditions [see, for example, the recent recommendations of the American College of Medical Genetics (Watson *et al.* 2006)].

However, serious concerns have been expressed about pressure to expand newborn screening panels (Botkin *et al.* 2006; Grosse *et al.* 2006). A major criticism is that many of the additional conditions depart from the key criteria identified by Wilson and Jungner (1968) for ensuring that population screening programmes deliver public health benefits. These criteria include the need to demonstrate that the natural history of the disorder is understood, that the characteristics of the screening test have been thoroughly

evaluated, that an effective preventive intervention is available, and that screening is necessary to prevent death or serious disability.

For many of the conditions represented in the American College of Medical Genetics screening recommendations, evidence is not available to fulfil these criteria. Moreover, screening has the potential to cause harm (Grosse *et al.* 2006). Problems may include unnecessary or even harmful therapies given either to children who are incorrectly identified as having a disease or to children with mild or asymptomatic disease. False positive results may cause acute parental anxiety and damage family well-being. Insufficient thought has been given to the implications of identifying unaffected carriers of recessive conditions. Screening programmes have resource implications and opportunity costs that have not been sufficiently considered.

A further consideration is the need to ensure that health-service capacity, structures, and resources are in place to enable effective long-term follow-up of individuals identified by newborn screening programmes, so that the health benefits of early identification are not subsequently lost. There is evidence for a lack of effective long-term management of some individuals identified by newborn screening programmes for PKU and sickle cell disease (Botkin *et al.* 2006). For all these reasons, it has been suggested that new screening programmes should initially be introduced only within a research paradigm, so that their risks and benefits can be carefully assessed before widespread implementation (Botkin 2005).

Table 2.4.4 Examples of genetic disorders included in newborn screening programmes

Disorder	Screening method	US states offering screening	Offered in the UK?	Treatment
Phenylketonuria	Guthrie bacterial inhibition assay Fluorescence assay Amino-acid analyser Tandem mass spectrometry	All	Yes	Diet restricting phenylalanine
Congenital hypothyroidism	Measurement of thyroxine and thyrotropin	All	Yes	Oral levothyroxine
Sickle cell disease	Haemoglobin electrophoresis Isoelectric focusing High-performance liquid chromatography Follow-up DNA analysis	All	Yes	Prophylactic antibiotics Immunization against *Diplococcus pneumoniae* and *Haemophilus influenzae*
Galactosaemia	Beutler test Paigen test	All	No	Galactose-free diet
Maple syrup urine disease	Guthrie bacterial inhibition assay	Most	No	Diet restricting intake of branched-chain amino acids
Congenital adrenal hyperplasia	Radioimmunoassay	Most	No	Glucocorticoids Mineralocorticoids Salt
Cystic fibrosis	Immunoreactive trypsinogen followed by DNA testing	Some	Yes	Improved nutrition Management of pulmonary symptoms
Medium-chain acyl CoA dehydrogenase deficiency (MCADD)	Tandem mass spectrometry	Most	Planned	Avoidance of fasting Aggressive medical management during illness

The approach to the assessment of potential population screening programmes varies in different countries. In the United Kingdom, a National Screening Committee considers the evidence base for all proposed screening programmes, including those for genetic conditions. The Health Technology Assessment programme has carried out reviews of newborn screening for some conditions (see, for example, Pandor *et al.* 2004), and most proposed programmes are piloted on a regional basis before being rolled out nationally. For example, a national newborn screening programme for medium chain acyl CoA dehydrogenase deficiency (MCADD) is being introduced following a successful pilot study (National Screening Committee 2007). Critics of this cautious approach claim that lives are lost and children harmed by long delays before programmes are introduced. Ideally, research and clinical trials of new screening technologies should be funded promptly and adequately so that evidence to inform decisions about proposed screening programmes can be obtained as efficiently as possible.

Using genomics in primary phenotypic prevention of disease

The Holy Grail for those wishing to apply genomics in public health would be the ability to use genotypic information to identify individuals who are at increased risk of disease and who could be offered opportunities to reduce their risk by means of interventions aimed at modifiable environmental factors such as diet. However, this is by no means a simple goal to attain.

The predictive value of genotypic information

The first problem in using genotypic information for prevention is the low penetrance of most of the alleles implicated in susceptibility to common disease. Individually, such alleles are typically associated with odds ratios of around 1.1–2, though rarer alleles may confer higher risks (see Table 2.4.1 and Janssens *et al.* 2004). For this reason, the positive and negative predictive values of tests for single alleles are likely to be low (see Fig. 2.4.2): Most individuals who tested positive would gain no benefit from a preventive intervention because they would not have developed the disease in any case. Those who tested negative might be falsely reassured.

Some applications of the use of genotypic information in prevention have already been suggested. For example, since the discovery of the *HFE* gene, which is mutated in the iron-overload disease hereditary haemochromatosis, population screening for hereditary haemochromatosis has been proposed, based on *HFE* genotype. The rationale is that serious disease (liver cirrhosis, fibrosis, or diabetes) may be prevented by the simple procedure of frequent phlebotomy. However, although about 25–50 per cent of people with a predisposing *HFE* genotype have evidence of iron overload, it is not known how many of these people would, if untreated, progress to symptomatic disease; the penetrance of overt liver disease may be as low as 1–10 per cent. Public health has played an important role in the evidence-based evaluation of population screening for hereditary haemochromatosis. (Box 2.4.3)

It has been suggested that the predictive power of genotypic information would be increased if more alleles were considered together. This approach is sometimes called genomic profiling (Yang *et al.* 2003). Although individuals who carry multiple risk alleles will have a very high risk of disease, these individuals constitute a very small percentage of the population (Janssens *et al.* 2004). For the bulk of the population, genomic profiling will be extremely complex, depending on the number of risk genotypes tested for, the spectrum of risk alleles an individual carries, and the odds ratios associated with each of them (Janssens & Khoury 2006).

Pleiotropic effects of susceptibility genes must also be taken into account. For example, the *APOE4* variant increases risk for both Alzheimer's dementia and coronary heart disease but reduces risk for macular degeneration. Interventions aimed at preventing the negative effects of a gene variant might increase risk for another disease.

Behavioural responses to genomic risk information

A second question is whether risk information based on genetic factors is likely be effective in motivating the sustained behavioural change that would be needed to achieve health benefits. Current evidence on this issue is limited and more research is needed. Research to date suggests that risk information alone plays only a small part in people's ability to change their behaviour (Marteau & Lerman 2001). The availability of an effective intervention is important, as is the individual's assessment of his or her ability to achieve behavioural change; this assessment, in turn, is strongly dependent on the person's familial and social environment.

There is some evidence that reactions to genetic risk information may differ from those to other types of risk information. For example, one study compared attitudes about risk-reducing interventions in people with a clinical diagnosis of familial hypercholesterolaemia, with and without a mutation-positive DNA test result (Marteau *et al.* 2004). Although there was no difference in people's belief that cholesterol-lowering interventions were important for their health, those with a DNA-based diagnosis were less likely to believe that dietary intervention would be effective and more likely to believe that cholesterol-lowering medication would be required. This reaction suggests some degree of fatalism in attitudes about genetic information and the need to present genetic risk information in such a way that it does not undermine the individual's belief in the efficacy of behavioural change.

There could also be a danger that information indicating an average or reduced genetic risk might be falsely reassuring, leading people to underestimate their risk and ignore advice about a healthy lifestyle. To date there is little evidence that false reassurance is a significant concern, though some more subtle effects of negative genetic test results have been observed. For example, among people with a family history of Alzheimer's disease (and therefore at increased risk), those whose risk estimate included a negative test result for the *APOE4* polymorphism perceived their risk as lower than those with the same risk estimate based only on family history information (LaRusse *et al.* 2005).

A further relevant factor is the likelihood that people will take up an offer of genetic testing to indicate their risk. The public health impact of genetic susceptibility testing is likely to be low if few are motivated to take advantage of it. Those who have poor motivation to improve their health through behavioural and lifestyle change, or perceive a test result as a threat to their well-being rather than an opportunity to improve their health, are unlikely to perceive benefits from genetic susceptibility testing.

High-risk versus population approaches to prevention

The fundamental rationale for using genomics in the primary prevention of common diseases with environmental causes has also been questioned (see, for example, Merikangas & Risch 2003).

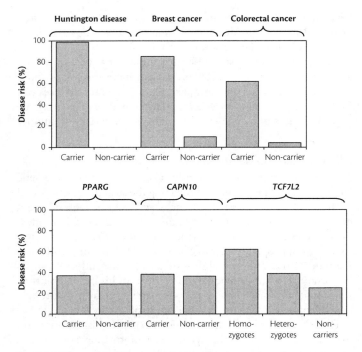

Fig. 2.4.2 Disease risks of carriers and non-carriers in genetic testing. In monogenic (Mendelian) disorders (top panel), carriers have a substantially increased risk of disease; non-carriers have a disease risk that approximates the population average. In the case of common disease (bottom panel), because risk alleles are generally common (population frequency >1 per cent), carriers and non-carriers have disease risks that are only slightly higher or slightly lower, respectively, than the population average. Reproduced from Janssens and Khoury (2006).

One argument is based on Rose's (1985) observation that a greater reduction in overall disease incidence can be achieved by a small reduction in disease risk over a whole population, whereas targeting an intervention at a high-risk group results in a larger absolute reduction in risk for those individuals. However, the example of obesity, discussed at the beginning of this chapter, suggests that population-level interventions may not be successful if they fail to take individual differences into account: Advice about healthy and moderate eating may have little effect on individuals whose genomic make-up predisposes them to a constant craving for high-calorie food. Moreover, Rose also pointed out that the population and high-risk approaches to prevention are complementary: Both have a role to play in prevention.

A further issue is the need for caution in applying population-derived risk estimates to decisions about individual patients (Rockhill *et al.* 2000). For example, Elmore and Fletcher (2006) have calculated that, although the Gail model for breast cancer risk prediction performs well at a population level, with a concordance of 0.96 between the expected and actual number of women in a population who develop breast cancer, at an individual level the concordance is only about 0.6. This problem is, of course, not unique to risk estimates based on genetics. Population-based risk estimates may best be used to stratify risk (so that, for example, an individual falls into a specific quintile) rather than to attempt to pinpoint individual risk. Population-based data will generate hypotheses about preventive action but these hypotheses must be tested rigorously in prospective outcome studies.

In summary, there is currently insufficient evidence to support the use of genetic testing or genomic profiling in the primary prevention of common diseases (Haga *et al.* 2003). In the future,

---

Box 2.4.3 Public health action to evaluate a proposed population screening programme: Hereditary haemochromatosis

With discovery of the *HFE* gene in 1996 and the identification of *HFE* mutations as the primary cause of hereditary haemochromatosis, many experts identified *HFE* mutation testing as a model for genetic screening of adult populations. Public health leadership has played an important role in evaluating this potential intervention.

1997   Meeting convened in the United States by National Human Genome Research Institute (NHGRI) and Centers for Disease Control and Prevention (CDC) to evaluate state of knowledge about *HFE* and hereditary haemochromatosis, resulting in:

     ◆ Consensus statement calling for more research on *HFE* mutation penetrance before screening

     ◆ Series of articles defining current knowledge and practice standards

1999   International jury convened to develop evidence-based recommendations regarding screening for haemochromatosis, under auspices of CDC and European Association for the Study of the Liver

     ◆ Jury recommended against population screening in absence of research documenting outcome benefit

     ◆ Jury recommended that diagnosis of hereditary haemochromatosis be reserved for symptomatic patients (as opposed to asymptomatic patients identified by biochemical or DNA-based testing)

2000–04 Population-based study of screening for hereditary haemochromatosis in 100 000 subjects funded by National Heart Lung and Blood Institute and NHGRI

     ◆ Penetrance of HFE mutations low (consistent with smaller studies from USA, Australia, and Europe)

     ◆ Symptomatic hereditary haemochromatosis rare

2004   Launch of CDC Web site (http://www.cdc.gov/genomics/training/perspectives/hemo.htm) providing education about hereditary haemochromatosis for healthcare providers and the general public.
        Emphasis on identification of early symptoms of hereditary haemochromatosis by healthcare providers and a family tracing approach rather than population-based screening.

scientifically validated genotypic risk information may be best used to enhance the predictive value of a 'package' of risk information that also incorporates measures of lifestyle and behavioural factors as well as relevant phenotypic biomarkers. Further research is needed to determine the best way to communicate genetic risk information in order to achieve beneficial health outcomes.

Using family history in disease prevention

It is likely to be many years, perhaps decades, before it will be possible to use genotypic information routinely in the assessment of risk for common chronic diseases. It has been suggested that, in the meantime, family history information represents a useful surrogate that could be used more effectively and systematically in preventive healthcare than is currently the case (Yoon *et al.* 2002).

Family history is a risk factor for almost all diseases of public health significance, including most chronic diseases. Family history reflects the consequences of shared genetic variation at multiple loci (first-degree relatives such as siblings share 50 per cent of their genes), shared exposures to environmental factors, and shared behaviours.

Methods have been proposed for quantifying the risk associated with family history based on the number of family members affected, the degree of closeness of their biological relationship to the individual under consideration, and their ages at onset of disease (Yoon *et al.* 2002). From this information about their relatives, it is suggested that people can be stratified into average risk, moderate risk, and high risk groups and given appropriate preventive advice (Khoury *et al.* 2005). Those at average risk would be encouraged to adhere to standard public health prevention recommendations. Those at moderate or high risk would be given personalized recommendations including, for example, assessment and modification of risk factors, lifestyle changes, alternative early detection strategies, and perhaps chemoprevention. Those at high risk would also be referred to the specialist clinical genetics service to investigate the possibility of a high-penetrance genetic disorder. Although only a few people are expected to fall into the high risk group, a much larger number will be assessed as being at moderate risk, offering the possibility of augmenting and improving the standard population approach to prevention.

Risk stratification based on family history is already in clinical practice as a form of triage for individuals concerned about a family history of some common cancers, such as breast/ovarian and colorectal cancer [see, for example, guidelines of the United Kingdom's National Institute for Health and Clinical Excellence (2006) for management of women with a family history of breast cancer]. This approach is not, however, used proactively as a screening programme.

The added value of the proactive use of family history risk-stratification as an adjunct to population-level prevention activities needs rigorous evaluation (Khoury *et al.* 2005). Issues that must be addressed include the degree of accuracy of family history reporting, the optimum algorithm for stratifying risk, and the value of family history as a motivator for behavioural change. Particularly rigorous evaluation will be needed if a positive family history is used as an indication for any preventive intervention that carries risk, such as chemoprevention. Health service providers, particularly family practitioners, will need education and training in taking and assessing family histories, and provision must be in place for effective follow-up of individuals who fall into higher-risk groups. Health economic analysis should also form part of the overall assessment of the family history approach.

Genomics and public health ethics

The combination of genetics and public health has had an uneasy history, largely because of the legacy of the eugenics movement. Even today, there are still concerns about the potential tension between the population-level objectives of public health and the sensitive and personal nature of genomic information. It is important to allay these fears, which in many cases arise from an exaggerated perception of the 'power' of genomic information and from a misunderstanding of the motives of public health professionals who become involved with genomics.

The legacy of eugenics

The term 'eugenics', literally meaning 'well born', was coined by Francis Galton in 1883. Its central philosophy was that the human gene pool could be 'improved' by selective breeding (Kevles 1995). Individuals judged to have a 'good' genetic constitution would be encouraged to have children, while those with 'poor' genes would be discouraged. The idea gained ground both in a number of European countries (including the United Kingdom and Sweden) and in the United States. Some eugenic programmes involved the involuntary sterilization of large numbers of people deemed genetically 'unfit' because they were poor, homeless, or 'morally degenerate'. In Nazi Germany, eugenic principles were invoked to justify the murder of millions of people.

The application of eugenics to humans is problematic on two key counts: First, that eugenic programmes violate human rights; and second, that 'good' and 'poor' human characteristics are complex traits that have no objective definition and result from multiple genetic, environmental, and social influences. Even if 'good' and 'bad' traits could be defined, it would be impossible to select simultaneously for multiple 'good' traits and against multiple 'bad' traits. The eugenics movement has been rightly condemned, and repudiated in most countries of the world.

Use of genomic information: Balancing the rights of individuals and society

Revulsion against eugenics has led to an insistence that genomic information is the property of the individual and his or her family. Individual autonomy, informed consent, and the privacy and confidentiality of genomic information have been paramount concerns. Numerous authors have warned about the dangers of stigmatization and discrimination against individuals on the basis of genetic characteristics.

Recently there have been attempts to re-balance the ethical debate and to move away from the concept that genetic information necessarily has a power and significance beyond that of other types of personal medical information—a concept known as 'genetic exceptionalism' (Murray 1997). The serious issues faced by families affected by highly penetrant genetic diseases do not generally apply to the luckier majority whose genetic risk of disease is much lower (Janssens & Khoury 2006).

The focus of public health is the population rather than the individual. The development of applications for genomics in population health will depend on the willingness of individuals to allow their genomic information to be used in population-based research projects designed to investigate low-penetrance genomic variants and gene–environment interactions that affect disease susceptibility.

Concerns have been raised about the privacy and confidentiality of the genetic information of individuals participating in such projects. For example, full anonymization of samples and data may not be possible because the research may depend on the ability to link data to individuals. Moreover, the prospective nature of some epidemiological projects can mean that informed consent is difficult to implement fully: Individuals may be asked to consent now to future uses of their samples and data that are currently unknown.

However, the ethical problems of large population studies may have been over-played. Population-based research involving genetics will have meaningful public health implications but these studies will not generally reveal clinically relevant information about individual participants and consequently will entail few physical, psychological, or social risks for those individuals or their families (Beskow et al. 2001). Although individual rights must be upheld, and genetic information must be protected just like any other personal data, community-centred ethical values such solidarity, altruism, and citizenry must also be given due weight (Knoppers & Chadwick 2005). In this view, biobanks and population genomic research are seen as global public goods to be used for the benefit of current society and future generations (Knoppers 2005).

These arguments do not deny the importance of high ethical standards for population-based projects and biobanking initiatives, in order to maintain the degree of public confidence that will be essential for the success of these long-term projects. Iceland's deCODE project attracted criticism as a result of the Icelandic Government's decision to assume that every individual in the country would be a participant in the project unless they specifically opted out, and to grant a commercial monopoly on any results from the project to the deCODE company. Other large-scale population biobanking projects (see Table 2.4.5, later in this chapter) have been more careful to avoid ethical controversy, for example by establishing mechanisms for independent ethical oversight, paying careful regard to procedures for seeking informed consent from participants, and carrying out public consultations on project plans. Such measures appear to command broad approval although some disquiet persists, for example over issues such as feedback of results to individuals, and terms for commercial access to samples and data. The international Public Population Project in Genomics (P3G) (http://www.p3gconsortium.org) is providing a platform for sharing best practice in ethical standards for biobanking initiatives.

Integrating genomics into public health practice

We are moving from an era in which genetics has been a small specialist clinical service dealing with patients and families affected by rare heritable diseases, to one in which genomic information and technologies may become a normal part of mainstream clinical and public health practice (Guttmacher et al. 2001). During the past 10 years, public health professionals have begun to realize that this transformation must be rationally managed and to put in place organizations and strategies for achieving this aim.

The emergence of public health genomics

During the 1990s, some public health professionals in the United States and the United Kingdom began to realize that public health practice must take account of developments in genomics. In the United States, the report of a Task Force on Genetics and Disease Prevention convened by the Centers for Disease Control and Prevention (CDC) led to the establishment of the Office of Genetics and Disease Prevention (now the National Office of Public Health Genomics, NOPHG, http://www.cdc.gov/genomics) at CDC in Atlanta in 1997 (Centers for Disease Control and Prevention 1997). At around the same time, the idea of public health genomics as a new subdiscipline of public health began to emerge and multidisciplinary academic programmes in public health genomics were developed at the Universities of Michigan and Washington (Austin et al. 2000).

In the United Kingdom, two reports to Government by expert advisory groups signalled the first awareness, on the part of the country's National Health Service, that genomics would in time evolve beyond the confines of a small specialized service for rare genetic disorders (NHS Central Research and Development Committee 1995, 1996). The first public health organization with an explicit interest in genomics was the Public Health Genetics Unit (now the Foundation for Genomics and Population Health, http://www.phgfoundation.org), established in Cambridge in 1997.

In the decade since 1997, public health genomics has increased in strength and influence. A growing body of academic literature has established the intellectual foundations of the discipline. Projects and activities undertaken at the NOPHG, the Foundation for Genomics and Population Health and elsewhere have made important contributions in areas such as genetic test evaluation, human genome epidemiology, and public policy for the use of human tissue and genomic information. Other groups focused on public health genomics have been set up within both government organizations (for example, the Office of Population Health Genomics in the Western Australian Department of Health) and academia (for example, Centers of Genomics and Public Health at the Universities of Washington and Michigan).

The Bellagio model for public health genomics

In 2005, a multidisciplinary workshop attended by 18 experts from the United States, United Kingdom, France, Germany, and Canada was convened in Bellagio, Italy, with the aim of seeking a consensus on the definition, scope, and goals of public health genomics (Bellagio group 2005; Burke et al. 2006). The group arrived at the following definition:

Public health genomics is the responsible and effective translation of genome-based knowledge and technologies for the benefit of population health.

Building on this consensus definition, the workshop developed a visual representation of the 'enterprise' of public health genomics (Fig. 2.4.3). The functions and activities shown in dark grey define the scope of the field. Several key features emerge from this representation:

1. The input to the enterprise is knowledge generated by genome-based science and technology, together with knowledge derived from academic research in the population sciences, as well as the humanities and social sciences.

2. The driving force of public health genomics is knowledge integration. This term encompasses the activity of selecting, storing, collating, analysing, integrating, and disseminating knowledge,

both within and across disciplines. It is the means by which information is transformed into knowledge.

3. The integrated and interdisciplinary knowledge base is used to underpin four core sets of activities:

(a) Communication and stakeholder engagement (including, for example, public dialogue and involvement, and engagement with industry)

(b) Informing public policy (including applied legal and policy analysis, engagement in the policy-making process, seeking international comparisons, and working with government)

(c) Developing and evaluating health services (including strategic planning, manpower planning, and capacity building; service review and evaluation; and development of new programmes and services)

(d) Education and training (including programmes of genetic literacy for health professionals and generally within society, specific training for public health genomics specialists, and development of courses and materials).

4. The mode of working of public health genomics is described by the cycle of analysis—strategy—action—evaluation, which is a widely recognized representation of public health practice. .

5. Public health genomics does include a research component, shown at the bottom of the diagram. This component is not generally basic research; rather, it is programmes of applied and translational research that contribute directly to the goal of improving population health and also identify gaps in the knowledge base that need to be addressed by further basic research.

6. Public health genomics does not operate in a vacuum. It is embedded within a social and political context and is informed by societal priorities.

7. Double-headed arrows throughout the diagram indicate the dynamic and interactive nature of the enterprise: It generates knowledge as well as using it, and it is modulated by the effects of its own outputs and activities.

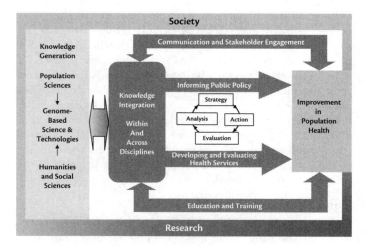

Fig. 2.4.3 The 'enterprise' of public health genomics. The scope of public health genomics is defined by the areas shown in dark grey.

An international network, the Genome-based Research and Population Health International Network (GRaPH *Int*, http://www.graphint.org) has been established to support the development of public health genomics and the sharing of resources worldwide (Stewart *et al.* 2006). The administrative hub of the network is based in Montreal and funded by the Public Health Agency of Canada.

Challenges and prospects for public health genomics

Integrating genomics into public health and behavioural research

Research is needed to strengthen the evidence base for applications of genomics in public health, particularly with respect to major public health problems such as obesity, outbreaks of infectious disease, or effects of exposure to environmental toxins and pollutants (Khoury *et al.* 2004, 2005).

Toxicogenomics and nutrigenomics

Toxicogenomics (sometimes referred to as 'ecogenomics') and nutrigenomics are important evolving areas of research that are attempting to unravel interactions between genomic variants and responses to toxic environmental agents and dietary constituents, respectively. There is good evidence that genomic variants do affect responses to these exposures but, as with alleles associated with susceptibility to common disease, the predictive value of the individual risk alleles is generally low. For example, a polymorphism in the *DPB1* gene (part of the major histocompatibility complex, which encodes components of the immune system) increases risk of sensitization to inhaled beryllium dust, encountered by workers in the nuclear industry. However, although the relative risk conferred by the sensitizing *DPB1* allele is high (odds ratio ~10), the specificity of the *DPB1* marker is low, thus limiting its utility.

Many reported associations and gene–environment interactions in toxicogenomics and nutrigenomics have not been independently confirmed. For example, different studies have found opposite effects of the Pro12Ala variant of the PPAR-γ gene on the association between the dietary P:S (polyunsaturated:saturated fat) ratio and body mass index. Although non-replication can be due to poor study design, under-powered studies, and type 1 errors, these differences could also reflect true differences between the populations studied, as well as the known biological complexity of the role of PPAR-γ.

The fields of toxicogenomics and nutrigenomics are in their infancy, and it is likely that many years of research will be needed before validated evidence will be available to inform public health action. It is also important to ensure that this evidence, when it does become available, is used responsibly. Genetic effects on responses to environmental toxins or dietary components may identify some individuals or populations at high risk for whom specific preventive advice may be appropriate. Toxicogenomic and nutrigenomic research will also reveal important aspects of the biological mechanisms of interaction between environmental exposures and the human body. Such information could lead, for example, to better definition of the lowest tolerable dose for a toxin, based on the most susceptible genotype.

In terms of prevention, however, genomics is unlikely to supersede the value of standard public health advice for the bulk of the population. Public health practitioners must ensure that the benefits and risks of any proposed interventions or programmes based on toxicogenomics or nutrigenomics are carefully weighed, and that people are not misled by unsupported claims made by companies selling direct-to-consumer genetic test kits.

Infectious disease

The complete genomes of many important human pathogens have been sequenced, including those of the organisms implicated in tuberculosis, malaria, plague, leprosy, diphtheria, cholera, and typhoid. Genomic information is being used to develop new diagnostics, vaccines, and drug treatments. For example, genomic technology has improved diagnosis of leishmaniasis and dengue fever in some Latin American countries (Singer & Daar 2001). Research on the genome of the malaria parasite *Plasmodium falciparum* identified an unusual biochemical pathway for steroid synthesis and suggested that a drug known to inhibit a crucial step in a similar pathway operating in bacteria and plants might be useful in treating malaria. The drug, fosmidomycin, has shown promise in several clinical studies.

The process of infection involves not just the pathogen genome but also that of the host organism. The genomes of human populations have co-evolved with those of the pathogens that infect them, and resistance or susceptibility to infection has been a strong selective pressure in human evolution. A wide range of human genes, including the highly polymorphic genes of the immune system, are involved in human responses to pathogens. In some cases a single genetic variant appears to be significantly associated with susceptibility or resistance to a disease. For example, a specific polymorphism in the gene encoding the cell-surface receptor molecule CCR5 is associated with resistance to infection by human immunodeficiency virus (HIV). This gene was chosen for analysis because the receptor was known to be involved in entry of the virus into specific cells of the immune system. Analysis of genomic variants in resistant individuals may suggest new mechanisms and targets for drug development, or strategies for enhancing protective immunity in exposed populations.

Behavioural research

Public health programmes of disease prevention depend to a large extent on promoting behavioural change, but genomics has so far had little impact on behavioural research. As discussed earlier in this chapter, there is a need for better understanding of the effect of genotypic risk information on human behaviour (Marteau & Lerman 2001). It is particularly important, for example, that individuals who believe genetic testing has revealed they are at reduced risk from, for example, bladder cancer due to smoking, or coronary heart disease due to a high-fat diet, do not interpret 'reduced risk' as 'no risk'.

In addition, the role of genomic factors in health-related behaviours must be more fully explored. For example, genomic factors are known to affect the likelihood that smokers will develop lung cancer, but the picture is incomplete without an understanding of the genomic factors that affect risk-taking behaviour and nicotine addiction. A fuller understanding of the role of genomics in human behaviour may suggest new strategies to promote public health and prevent avoidable death and disease.

The impact of genomics on epidemiology

Genomics offers new opportunities for epidemiological research. In time, the familiar 2×2 table correlating disease status (for example, in a case-control study) with the presence or absence of an exposure or risk factor may routinely be replaced by a 2×4 table in which the underlying genotype at a particular locus or groups of loci will be measured and evidence sought for interaction with the risk factor.

New tools and resources are being developed for epidemiological studies involving genomics. For example, as mentioned earlier in this chapter, genomics is inspiring the establishment of large population cohorts and 'biobanks' to provide resources for the discovery and characterization of genes associated with common diseases (Table 2.4.5). In addition to promoting gene discovery, biobanks will help epidemiologists to quantify the occurrence of diseases in different populations and to understand their natural histories and risk factors, including gene–environment interactions. Large cohorts may also be used for nested case-control studies or case-only studies as an initial screening method. These studies will produce a large amount of data on disease risk factors, lifestyles, and environmental exposures, and they will provide opportunities for data standardization, data sharing, and joint analyses (Khoury *et al.* 2004; Davey Smith *et al.* 2005).

Genomic research may also help to identify unknown environmental risk factors for disease or confirm suspected environmental risk factors, through the approach of Mendelian randomization (Davey Smith *et al.* 2005). The reasoning behind this approach is that if a genetic polymorphism affects the level of a biological intermediate in a way that mirrors the effect of an environmental exposure on the same intermediate, and if the biological intermediate in turn affects disease risk, then an association between the polymorphism and disease risk can act as a proxy for the relationship between the environmental exposure and disease risk. Mendel's law of random assortment of traits during transmission from parents to offspring means that this proxy relationship can be viewed as protected from the various confounding factors that affect observational studies of exposures.

The concept of Mendelian randomization can be illustrated by the example of the *C677T* polymorphism of the methylenetetrahydrofolate reductase (*MTHFR*) gene, which is needed for conversion of homocysteine to methionine (Khoury *et al.* 2005). The *C677T* polymorphism reduces MTHFR enzyme activity and increases levels of homocysteine, thereby mimicking the effects of low dietary folate intake. Thus a confirmed association between the *C677T* polymorphism and neural tube defects enhances causal inferences about the role of folate in neural tube defects. Although Mendelian randomization can potentially help epidemiologists derive better causal inferences about environmental exposures and disease, its application is currently limited by the paucity of confirmed genotype-disease associations, and incomplete understanding of the gene functions and biological pathways involved in the pathogenesis of common diseases.

Human genome epidemiology

Although thousands of gene–disease associations have been reported, only a small fraction of these have been independently replicated and fewer still can be considered fully validated (Khoury *et al.* 2007). Problems include publication bias, confounding by

Table 2.4.5 Examples of large population-based research biobanks (planned and current)

	Sample size (*n*)	Participating countries	Recruitment	Age at recruitment	URL
Cohort studies					
EPIC Europe	>500 000	Ten European countries	1993–97	45–74	http://www.iarc.fr/epic/Sup-default.html
CARTaGENE	50 000 (in two phases)	Quebec	2007–09 (Phase 1)	25–69	http://www.cartagene.qc.ca
Generation Scotland	50 000 family members	Scotland	Ongoing	35–55	http://129.215.140.49/gs/
UK Biobank	500 000	England	Ongoing	40–69	http://www.ukbiobank.ac.uk
Twin cohorts					
GenomEUtwin	>600 000 twin pairs	Six European countries	Varies among the eight different twin cohorts	Various	http://www.genomeutwin.org
Total populations					
DeCode Genetics	>100 000	Iceland	Ongoing	Various	http://www.decode.com
Esonian Genome Project	>100 000	Estonia	Ongoing	Various	http://www.geenivaramu.ee
Western Australian Genome Project	~2 000 000	Western Australia	Awaits funding	Various	http://www.genepi.org.au

Source: Adapted (and updated) from Davey Smith Ebrahim, S. Lewis, S. (2005). *Lancet* **366**, 1484–98.

population stratification, faulty selection of control subjects, genotyping errors, deviations from Hardy–Weinberg equilibrium, linkage disequilibrium issues, misclassification of exposures and outcomes, inadequate statistical power, and type 1 errors (false positive associations). These problems point to a need for systematic evaluation and meta-analysis of studies to identify validated associations, question unsubstantiated claims, and flag promising candidates for further investigation.

The Human Genome Epidemiology Network, HuGENet, is a global collaboration of individuals and organizations that develops methods and guidance for integrating and disseminating knowledge on the prevalence of genomic variants in different populations, genotype–disease associations, gene–gene and gene–environment interactions, as well as evaluating genetic tests for screening and prevention (Khoury 1999; Little *et al.* 2003).

HuGENet's Web-accessible knowledge base captures ongoing publications in human genome epidemiology and is searchable by disease, gene, and disease risk factors. In collaboration with several journals, HuGENet also sponsors systematic reviews of the evidence on genotype–disease associations, using specific published guidelines for this work (the HuGENet handbook) as well as applying quantitative methods for evidence synthesis. Over 50 HuGENet reviews have been published on various diseases ranging from single-gene conditions to common complex diseases.

In 2005, HuGENet formed a network of investigator networks; these are mostly disease-specific research consortia that share knowledge, experience, and resources for human genome epidemiology investigations. The HuGENet Network of Networks has published a 'road map' for using consortia-driven pooled data and meta-analyses to augment the knowledge base on gene–disease associations (Ioannidis *et al.* 2006) and guidelines on the assessment of cumulative evidence on genetic associations (Ioannidis *et al.* 2008). HuGENet is also working on ways of integrating genetic

epidemiological evidence on gene–disease associations with biological evidence.

Genomics in the developing world

Genomics and genomic technology will not replace traditional public health measures such as combatting malnutrition, providing clean water and access to sanitation, alleviating poverty, and promoting sexual health. However, genomics offers potential benefits to the developing world, for example in more rapid and accurate diagnosis of infectious disease (as discussed earlier in this chapter), enhancing the nutritional value of staple foods, bioremediation to reverse environmental degradation, and prevention of widespread human suffering by better recognition and management of genetic disease (Daar *et al.* 2002; Genomics Working Group of the Science and Technology Task Force of the United Nations Millennium Project 2004).

It will be appropriate for different countries to adopt different strategies depending on the nature of their health problems, their economic situation, their social and political climate, their clinical and public health infrastructure, and the availability of trained medical and public health personnel. It is important to ensure that applications of genetics and genomic technology are thoroughly evaluated in pilot studies; that local expertise is fully engaged at all stages of the research, development and implementation pathway; and that international aid is focused appropriately on developing local capacity, networks, and partnerships to cascade expertise and promote best practice.

Management and prevention of genetic disease

As mentioned earlier in this chapter, the developing world carries the heaviest burden of genetic disease, contributing to a birth defects prevalence that is 50–100 per cent higher than in the developed world (Christianson *et al.* 2006). The most prevalent genetic disorders in the developing world are the haemoglobin disorders (sickle cell disease and thalassaemia) and glucose-6-phosphate deficiency. Approximately 7 per cent of the world's population are carriers of a haemoglobin disorder, and 300 000–400 000 babies with severe forms of these diseases are born every year, mostly in tropical regions (Weatherall & Clegg 2001). The public health impact of haemoglobin disorders is substantial and in some regions is increasing, as falling rates of childhood mortality due to malnutrition and infection mean that more individuals survive to present for diagnosis and treatment. Demographic changes such as migration are also increasing the prevalence of haemoglobin disorders in the developed world.

Chromosomal disorders and multifactorial conditions with a strong genetic component also have a significant impact on the developing world. For example, lack of effective family planning, leading to high birth rates for older mothers, contributes to a significant birth prevalence for Down syndrome. Congenital heart defects and neural tube defects make a substantial contribution to childhood mortality and morbidity. High rates of consanguineous marriages in some societies may increase the birth frequency of rare recessive diseases.

As a first step towards improving management and prevention of genetic conditions, both low-income and middle-income countries should seek to educate their communities and health professionals about these conditions, promote family planning, improve maternal health and nutrition, and establish child health services (Christianson *et al.* 2006). If economic and political circumstances allow, it may be possible to establish a medical genetics service, including training appropriate health professionals in clinical diagnosis of genetic conditions and basic genetic counselling, and considering implementation of appropriate neonatal and antenatal screening programmes.

Cultural, religious, and economic factors dictate different strategies in different countries, but all countries with a significant prevalence of haemoglobin disorders need good diagnostic facilities and provision for treatment. For sickle cell disease, the most cost-effective approach is likely to be the development of national centres with expertise in screening, DNA diagnosis, education, counselling, and management of the conditions (World Health Organization Advisory Committee on Health Research 2002). Ideally, such centres would support and train personnel for a network of peripheral screening clinics focusing on neonatal screening and administration of oral antibiotic prophylaxis in childhood, and taking the lead in programmes of public education.

The thalassaemias present a different range of problems. Simple and cheap diagnostic techniques are available to diagnose the condition and detect carriers. However, disease management is more complex and costly than for sickle cell disease because the severe forms require lifelong blood transfusion (using blood that has been screened to prevent transmission of pathogens) and expensive drug treatment to remove the excess iron introduced by multiple transfusions. In some countries, programmes of antenatal carrier screening are considered acceptable to reduce the birth prevalence of disease. Once again, the model of centralized diagnostic laboratories and a network of peripheral screening clinics (in this case, for antenatal screening) may be appropriate. Antenatal carrier screening programmes have been in operation for many

years in some Mediterranean countries, where as a result the birth frequency of β thalassaemia has fallen by over 80 per cent (Cao *et al.* 2002).

In some middle-income, developing countries, such as the countries of Southeast Asia, changing lifestyles are leading to an increasing burden of disease from multifactorial conditions such as heart disease and diabetes, which may before long overtake communicable diseases as the major public health scourge in these countries. Although, as in the developed world, preventive strategies will be aimed at altering diet and lifestyle, some of the genetic variants underlying susceptibility to these conditions are likely to be population-specific. Genomic research in developing-world populations will be needed for a full understanding of the aetiology of disease and may point to a need for therapies and preventive interventions that are tailored for different population groups.

Genomic technologies in the developing world

In the wider sphere of genomic biotechnology, too, different strategies are appropriate for different countries (Genomics Working Group of the Science and Technology Task Force of the United Nations Millennium Project 2004). For some of the poorest countries, cheap genomics-based diagnostics may be cost-effective in programmes of infectious disease monitoring and control. International collaborations between the developed and developing world can help scientists in developing countries to gain access to appropriate technology, and to adapt this technology to a low-resource setting and a specific set of local conditions. Ongoing evaluation of any applications is also essential.

Some middle-income countries such as Cuba, Brazil, and Thailand are in a position to be able to develop their own biotechnology capacity. Governments in such countries need to create a favourable policy environment for genomic technology by investing in appropriate research, instituting transparent legal and regulatory frameworks and protection for intellectual property rights, stimulating their own biotechnology and pharmaceutical industries, and fostering public–private partnerships that are accountable to the public interest (World Health Organization Advisory Committee on Health Research, 2002). Policies for applications of genomics and genetics must be sensitive to the ethical and cultural values of the country.

Training partnerships between industrialized and developing countries can help to develop human resources, and in some cases joint academic or clinical appointments can prevent the 'brain drain' of highly trained scientists and clinicians to more lucrative jobs in the developed world. Innovative industrial partnerships between the developed and developing world can, if carefully managed, help to provide both resources and expertise for the development of local industry.

Education and training

In both the developed and the developing world, public health professionals must be prepared for the impact genomics will have on their practice (Austin *et al.* 2000; Burton 2003). As well as a working knowledge of basic genetics, they will need an understanding of human genome epidemiology and the criteria for evaluation of genetic tests, and an appreciation of the ethical, legal, psychosocial, and policy dimensions of applications of genomics and genomic technologies.

A set of competencies in genomics for the US public health workforce has been developed by the US National Office of Public Health Genomics (2001). Competencies are documented for the workforce as a whole and for specific groups including leaders/administrators, clinicians, epidemiologists, health educationalists, laboratory staff, and environmental health workers.

In addition, some individuals will require an in-depth knowledge of public health genomics, for example, those involved in screening and other preventive programmes, health service development and evaluation, public health education, and policy analysis and development. Educational programmes in public health genomics are already underway at some centres.

Conclusion

The full benefits of genomics for clinical medicine and public health are likely to take many years to materialize; public health genomics must play a long game (Halliday *et al.* 2004; Davey Smith *et al.* 2005). However, there is a need now to establish capacity and infrastructure for the decades ahead. Leadership, sharing of resources (Box 2.4.4), and knowledge through international networks such as GRaPH *Int* and the Public Health Genomics European Network (PHGEN, http://www.phgen.nrw.de/typo3/index.php), programmes of professional education and training, and engagement with public policy development for genomics will all contribute to timely progress.

Several challenges must be addressed. A concerted interdisciplinary effort will be required to understand interactions between genetic, environmental, and social contributors to health. Genome-based technologies and interventions need to be critically evaluated through prospective study of health outcomes. Effective implementation of genome-based advances will require new policy and educational initiatives.

Genomic research offers great promise for population health benefit. However, potential uses of genomic information must be critically scrutinized. Some seemingly promising technologies or interventions may yield little benefit or pose unexpected harms; others may provide unique opportunities to improve health.

Box 2.4.4 Examples of some current initiatives in public health genomics

Centres

National Office of Public Health Genomics, US Centers for Disease Control and Prevention

http://www.cdc.gov/genomics
Carries out research on how human genomic discoveries can be used to improve health and prevent disease. Established and coordinates the HuGE Net (Human Genome Epidemiology Network) initiative.

Foundation for Genomics and Population Health (formerly the Public Health Genetics Unit)

http://www.phgfoundation.org
Multidisciplinary group that assesses advances in genetic science and their impact on health services and healthcare policy.

Centers for Genomics and Public Health

http://www.sph.umich.edu/genomics/
http://depts.washington.edu/cgph/
Established by collaboration between the US Centers for Disease Control and Prevention and the Association of Schools of Public Health, and located at the Universities of Michigan and Washington. The Centers contribute to the knowledge base, provide technical assistance to local, state, and regional public health organizations and develop and deliver training to the public health work force.

Genomics, Health, and Society

http://genopole-toulouse.prd.fr/index.php?id=57
A multidisciplinary research centre located at the Toulouse Genopole, University of Toulouse, France, and including biologists, clinicians, geneticists, lawyers, sociologists, and economists.

Office of Population Health Genomics, Western Australian Department of Health

http://www.genomics.health.wa.gov.au/home/index.cfm
Aims to facilitate the integration of genomics into all aspects of public health, policy, and programmes.

Resources

HumGen

http://www.humgen.umontreal.ca
An international database on the legal, ethical, and social aspects of human genetics, developed as a collaboration between academia, government, and industry by the Centre de recherche en droit public at the University of Montreal.

Box 2.4.4   Examples of some current initiatives in public health genomics *(Continued)*

GDPinfo

http://apps.nccd.cdc.gov/genomics/GDPQueryTool/default.asp

   A searchable database of all the documents available on the Office of Genomics and Disease Prevention Website, including the HuGE Net database.

PHGU Genomics Policy Database

http://www.phgfoundation.org/policydb

   A searchable web-based database of literature on policy development for genomics in health services and healthcare.

Projects

Evaluation of Genomic Applications in Practice and Prevention (EGAPP)

http://www.cdc.gov/genomics/gtesting/egapp.htm

   The project aims to develop a coordinate process for evaluating genetic tests and other genomic applications that are in transition from research to clinical and public health practice.

P3G Consortium—Public Population Project in Genomics

http://www.p3gconsortium.org/

   An international consortium to provide the international population genomics community with the resources, tools, and know-how to facilitate data management for improved methods of knowledge transfer and sharing.

Canadian Programme on Genomics and Global Health

http://www.utoronto.ca/jcb/genomics/index.html

   Promotes the use of genomics and biotechnologies to improve health in developing countries.

HuGE Net

http://www.cdc.gov/genomics/hugenet/default.htm

   A global collaboration of individuals and organizations committed to the assessment of the impact of human genome variation on population health and how genetic information can be used to improve health and prevent disease.

Cross-disciplinary partnerships, research infrastructures, and effective communication among stakeholders will promote an efficient and beneficial translation process.

References

Antoniou, A. *et al*. (2003). Average risks of breast and ovarian cancer associated with BRCA1 or BRCA2 mutations detected in case series unselected for family history: A combined analysis of 22 studies. *American Journal of Human Genetics*, **72**, 1117–30.

Austin, M.A., Peyser, P.J., and Khoury, M.J. (2000). The interface of genetics and public health: Research and educational challenges. *Annual Review of Public Health*, **21**, 81–9.

Bellagio group (2005). *Genome-based research and population health*. Report of an international workshop held at the Rockefeller Foundation Study and Conference Center, Bellagio, Italy, 14–20 April 2005. http://www.graphint.org/docs/BellagioReport230106.pdf.

Beskow, L.M. *et al*. (2001). Informed consent for population-based research involving genetics. *JAMA*, **286**, 2315–21.

Botkin, J.R. (2005). Research for newborn screening: Developing a national framework. *Pediatrics*, **116**, 862–71.

Botkin, J. *et al*. (2006). Newborn screening technology: Proceed with caution. *Pediatrics*, **117**, 1800–5.

Burke, W. (2002). Genetic testing. *New England Journal of Medicine*, **347**, 1867–75.

Burke, W. and Zimmern, R. (2007). *Moving beyond ACCE: An expanded framework for genetic test evaluation*. Paper prepared for the UK Genetic Testing Network.

Burke, W. *et al*. (2002). Genetic test evaluation: information needs of clinicians, policy makers, and the public. *American Journal of Epidemiology*, **256**, 311–8.

Burke, W., Khoury, M.J., Stewart, A. *et al*. for the Bellagio group (2006). The path from genome-based research to population health: Development of an international public health genomics network. *Genetics in Medicine*, **8**, 451–8.

Burke, W., Zimmern, R.L., and Kroese, M. (2007). Defining purpose: A key step in genetic test evaluation. *Genetics in Medicine*, **9**, 675–81.

Burton, H. (2003). *Addressing genetics, delivering health*. Public Health Genetics Unit, Cambridge, UK.

Cao, A., Rosatelli, M.C., Monni, G. *et al*. (2002). Screening for thalassaemia: A model of success. *Obstetrics and Gynecology Clinics of North America*, **29**, 305–28.

Centers for Disease Control and Prevention (1997). *Translating advances in human genetics into public health: A strategic plan*. http://www.cdc.gov/genomics/about/strategic.htm

Christianson, A., Howson, C.P., and Modell, B. (2006). *March of Dimes global report on birth defects. The hidden toll of dying and disabled children*. March of Dimes Birth Defects Foundation. White Plains, New York.

Collins, F.S. and McKusick, V.A. (2001). Implications of the human genome project for medical science. *JAMA*, **285**, 540–4.

Collins, F.S., Morgan, M., and Patrinos, A. (2003). The human genome project: Lessons from large-scale biology. *Science*, **300**, 286–90.

Daar, A., Thorsteindottir, H., Martin, D.K. *et al*. (2002). Top ten biotechnologies for improving health in developing countries. *Nature Genetics*, **32**, 229–32.

Davey Smith, G., Ebrahim, S., Lewis, S. *et al*. (2005). Genetic epidemiology and public health: Hope, hype, and future prospects. *Lancet*, **366**, 1484–98.

Elmore, J.G. and Fletcher, S.W. (2006). The risk of cancer risk prediction: "What is my risk of getting breast cancer?" *Journal of the National Cancer Institute*, **98**, 1673–5.

Gardiner, S.H. and Begg, E.J. (2006). Pharmacogenetics, drug metabolising enzymes and clinical practice. *Pharmacological Reviews*, **58**, 529–90.

Genomics Working Group of the Science and Technology Task Force of the United Nations Millennium Project (2004). *Genomics and global health*. University of Toronto Joint Centre for Bioethics, Toronto.

Grosse, S.D. and Khoury, M.J. (2006). What is the clinical utility of genetic testing? *Genetics in Medicine*, **8**, 448–50.

Grosse, S.D., Boyle, C.A., Kenneson, A. *et al*. (2006). From public health emergency to public health service: The implications of evolving criteria for newborn screening panels. *Pediatrics*, **117**, 923–9.

Guttmacher, A.E. and Collins, F.S. (2005). Realizing the promise of genomics in biomedical research. *JAMA*, **294**, 1399–402.

Guttmacher, A.E., Jenkins, J., and Uhlmann, W.R. (2001). Genomic medicine: Who will practice it? A call to open arms. *American Journal of Medical Genetics*, **106**, 216–22.

Haddow, J. and Palomaki, G. (2004). ACCE: A model process for evaluating data on emerging genetic tests. In *Human genome epidemiology* (eds. M. Khoury, J. Little, and W. Burke), pp. 217–33. Oxford University Press, Oxford.

Haga, S.B., Khoury, M.J., and Burke, W. (2003). Genomic profiling to promote a healthy lifestyle: Not ready for prime time. *Nature Genetics*, **34**, 347–50.

Halliday, J.L., Collins, V.R., Aitken, M.A. *et al*. (2004). Genetics and public health – evolution, or revolution? *Journal of Epidemiology and Community Health*, **58**, 894–9.

Hirschhorn, J.N. and Daly, M.J. (2005). Genome-wide association studies for common diseases and complex traits. *Nature Reviews Genetics*, **6**, 95–107.

Holtzman, N.A. and Watson, M.S. (eds.) (1997). *Promoting safe and effective genetic testing in the United States*. Final report of the Task Force on Genetic Testing. http://www.genome.gov/10001733

Hunter, D.J. (2005). Gene-environment interactions in human disease. *Nature Reviews Genetics*, **6**, 287–97.

Ioannidis, J.P.A., Trikalinos, T.A., and Khoury, M.J. (2006). Implications of small effect sizes of individual genetic variants on the design and interpretation of genetic association studies of complex diseases. *American Journal of Epidemiology*, **164**, 609–14.

Ioannidis, J.P.A. *et al*. (2006). A road map for efficient and reliable human genome epidemiology. *Nature Genetics*, **38**, 3–5.

Ioannidis, J.P.A. *et al*. (2008). Assessment of cumulative evidence on genetic associations: interim guidelines. *International Journal of Epidemiology* **37**, 120–32.

Jaenisch, R. and Bird, A. (2003). Epigenetic regulation of gene expression: How the genome integrates intrinsic and environmental signals. *Nature Genetics*, **33**(Suppl.), 245–54.

Janssens, A.C.J.W. and Khoury, M.J. (2006). Predictive value of testing for multiple genetic variants in multifactorial diseases: Implications for the discourse on ethical, legal and social issues. *Italian Journal of Public Health*, **4**, 35–41.

Janssens, A.C., Gwinn, M., Valdez, R. *et al*. (2006). Predictive genetic testing for type 2 diabetes. *BMJ*, **333**, 509–10.

Janssens, A.C.J.W., Pardo, M.C., Steyerberg, E.W. *et al*. (2004). Revisiting the clinical validity of multiplex genetic testing in complex disease. *American Journal of Human Genetics*, **74**, 585–8.

Juengst, E.T. (1995). 'Prevention' and the goals of genetic medicine. *Human Gene Therapy*, **6**, 1595–605.

Kaye, C.I. *et al*. (2006). Newborn screening fact sheets. *Pediatrics* **118**, e934–63.

Kevles, D.J. (1995). *In the name of eugenics: Genetics and the uses of human heredity*. Harvard University Press, Cambridge, USA.

Khoury, M.J. (1996). From genes to public health: The applications of genetic technology in disease prevention. *American Journal of Public Health*, **86**, 1717–22.

Khoury, M.J. (1999). Human genome epidemiology (HuGE): Translating advances in human genetics into population-based data for medicine and public health. *Genetics in Medicine*, **1**, 71–3.

Khoury, M.J. (2003). Genetics and genomics in practice: The continuum from genetic disease to genetic information in health and disease. *Genetics in Medicine*, **5**, 261–8.

Khoury, M.J., Burke, W., and Thomson, E.J. (2000). *Genetics and public health in the 21st century*. Oxford University Press, New York.

Khoury, M.J., Davis, R., Gwinn, M. *et al*. (2005). Do we need genomic research for the prevention of common diseases with environmental causes? *American Journal of Epidemiology*, **161**, 799–805.

Khoury, M.J., Little, J., Gwinn, M. *et al*. (2007). On the synthesis and interpretation of consistent but weak gene-disease associations in the era of genome-wide association studies. *International Journal of Epidemiology*, **36**, 439–45.

Khoury, M.J., McCabe, L.L., and McCabe, E.R.B. (2003). Population screening in the age of genomic medicine. *New England Journal of Medicine*, **348**, 50–8.

Khoury, M.J., Millikan, R., Little, J. *et al*. (2004). The emergence of epidemiology in the genomics age. *International Journal of Epidemiology*, **33**, 936–44.

Knoppers, B.M. (2005). Of genomics and public health: Building public 'goods'. *Canadian Medical Association Journal*, **173**, 1185–6.

Knoppers, B.M. and Chadwick, R. (2005). Human genetic research: Emerging trends in ethics. *Nature Reviews Genetics*, **6**, 75–9.

Kroese, M., Zimmern, R.L., and Sanderson, S. (2004). Genetic tests and their evaluation: Can we answer the key questions? *Genetics in Medicine*, **6**, 475–80.

LaRusse, S. *et al*. (2005). Genetic susceptibility testing versus family history-based risk assessment: Impact on perceived risk of Alzheimer disease. *Genetics in Medicine*, **7**, 48–53.

Little, J. *et al*. (2003). The human genome project is complete. How do we develop a handle for the pump? *American Journal of Epidemiology*, **157**, 667–73.

Markel, H. (1997). Scientific advances and social risks: Historical perspectives of genetic screening programs for sickle cell disease, Tay Sachs Disease, neural tube defects and Down Syndrome, 1970–1997. Appendix 6 in *Promoting safe and effective genetic testing in the United States. Final report of the Task Force on Genetic Testing* (eds. N.A. Holtzman and M.S. Watson). http://www.genome.gov/10001733

Marteau, T. and Lerman, C. (2001). Genetic risk and behavioural change. *BMJ*, **322**, 105–6.

Marteau, T. *et al*. (2004). Psychological impact of genetic testing for familial hypercholesterolaemia within a previously aware population: A randomized controlled trial. *American Journal of Medical Genetics*, **128**, 285–93.

Merikangas, K.R. and Risch, N. (2003). Genomic priorities and public health. *Science*, **302**, 599–601.

Murray, T. (1997). Genetic exceptionalism and 'future diaries': Is genetic information different from other medical information? In *Genetic secrets: Protecting privacy and confidentiality in the genetic era* (ed. M.A. Rothstein), pp. 60–73. Yale University Press, New Haven.

National Collaborating Centre for Women's and Children's Health (2003). *Antenatal care: Routine care for the healthy pregnant woman*. http://www.rcog.org.uk/resources/Public/pdf/Antenatal_Care.pdf

National Institute for Health and Clinical Excellence (2006). *Familial breast cancer: The classification and care of women at risk of familial breast cancer in primary, secondary and tertiary care*. http://www.nice.org.uk/guidance/CG41

National Office of Public Health Genomics (2001). *Genomic competencies for the public health workforce*. http://www.cdc.gov/genomics/training/competencies/default.htm

National Screening Committee (2007). *National Screening Committee policy – medium chain acyl CoA dehydrogenase deficiency screening*. http://www.library.nhs.uk/guidelinesfinder/ViewResource.aspx?resID=57173

NHS Central Research and Development Committee (1995). *Genetics of common disease*. Department of Health, London.

NHS Central Research and Development Committee (1995). *Report of the Genetics Research Advisory Group*. Department of Health, London.

NHS Sickle Cell and Thalassaemia Screening Programme. *Policy framework for antenatal screening programme for England*. http://www.kcl-phs.org.uk/haemscreening/Documents/AnScreenPolicy.pdf

Pandor, A., Eastham, J., Beverley, C. *et al.* (2004). Clinical effectiveness and cost effectiveness of neonatal screening for inborn errors of metabolism using tandem mass spectrometry. *Health Technology Assessment*, **8** (12).

Petricoin, E.F. *et al.* (2002). Use of proteomic patterns in serum to identify ovarian cancer. *Lancet*, **16**, 572–7.

Quackenbush, J. (2006). Microarray analysis and tumour classification. *New England Journal of Medicine*, **354**, 2463–72.

Read, A. and Donnai, D. (2007). *New clinical genetics*. Scion, Bloxham.

Richards, E.J. (2006). Inherited epigenetic variation – revisiting soft inheritance. *Nature Reviews Genetics*, **7**, 395–401.

Rockhill, B., Kawachi, I., and Colditz, G.A. (2000). Individual risk prediction and population-wide disease prevention. *Epidemiological Reviews*, **22**, 176–80.

Rose, G. (1985). Sick individuals and sick populations. *International Journal of Epidemiology*, **14**, 32–8.

Rothman, K.J. (1986). *Modern epidemiology*. Little, Brown and Company, Boston.

Royal College of Physicians of London (1991). *Purchasers' guide to genetic services in the NHS*. Royal College of Physicians, London.

Sanderson, S., Emery, J., and Higgins, J. (2005). CYP2C9 variants, drug dose, and bleeding risk in warfarin-treated patients: A HuGENet systematic review and meta-analysis. *Genetics in Medicine*, **7**, 97–104.

Sconce, E.A. *et al.* (2005). The impact of *CYP2C9* and *VKORC1* genetic polymorphism and patient characteristics upon warfarin dose requirements: Proposal for a new dosing regimen. *Blood*, **106**, 2329–33.

Singer, P.A. and Daar, A.S. (2001). Harnessing genomics and biotechnology to improve global health equity. *Science*, **294**, 87–9.

Staudt, L.M. and Dave, S. (2005). The biology of human lymphoid malignancies revealed by gene expression profiling. *Advances in Immunology*, **87**, 163–208.

Stewart, A., Brice, P., Burton, H. *et al.* (2007). *Genetics, health care and public policy*. Cambridge University Press, Cambridge.

Stewart, A., Karmali, M., and Zimmern, R. (2006). GRaPH Int: An international network for public health genomics. In *Genomics and public health. Legal and socio-economic perspectives* (ed. B.M. Knoppers), pp. 257–71. Martinus Nijhoff Publishers, The Netherlands.

Subramonia-Iyer, S. *et al.* (2007). Array-based comparative genomic hybridization for investigating chromosomal abnormalities in patients with learning disability: Systematic review and meta-analysis of diagnostic and false-positive yield. *Genetics in Medicine*, **9**, 74–9.

The Wellcome Trust Case Control Consortium (2007). Genome-wide association study of 14,000 cases of seven common diseases and 3,000 shared controls. *Nature*, **447**, 661–78.

Watson, M.S. *et al.* (eds.) (2006). Newborn screening: Toward a uniform screening panel and system. Executive summary. *Genetics in Medicine*, **8** (Suppl), 1S–11S.

Weatherall, D.J. and Clegg, J.B. (2001). Inherited haemoglobin disorders: An increasing global health problem. *Bulletin of the World Health Organization*, **79**, 704–12.

Willard, H.F., Angrist, M., and Ginsburg, G.S. (2005). Genomic medicine: Genetic variation and its impact on the future of health care. *Philosophical Transactions of the Royal Society Series B*, **360**, 1543–50.

Wilson, J.M.G. and Jungner, G. (1968). *Principles and practice of screening for disease*. Public health paper no. 34. World Health Organization, Geneva.

Wolf, C.R., Smith, G., and Smith, R.L. (2000). Science, medicine and the future: Pharmacogenetics. *BMJ*, **320**, 987–90.

World Health Organization (1996). *Control of hereditary diseases*. WHO, Geneva. http://whqlibdoc.who.int/trs/WHO_TRS_865.pdf

World Health Organization Advisory Committee on Health Research (2002). *Genomics and world health*. World Health Organization, Geneva.

Yang, Q. *et al.* (2003). Improving the prediction of complex diseases by testing for multiple disease susceptibility genes. *American Journal of Human Genetics*, **72**, 636–49.

Yoon, P.W., Scheuner, M.T., Peterson-Oehlke, K.L. *et al.* (2002). Can family history be used as a tool for public health and preventive medicine? *Genetics in Medicine*, **4**, 304–10.

Zimmern, R. (2001). What is genetic information: Whose hands on your genes? *Genetics Law Monitor*, **1**, 9–13.

2.5

Water and sanitation

Thomas Clasen and Steven Sugden

Abstract

The lack of safe drinking water and basic sanitation impose a heavy health burden, especially on young children and the poor; it also aggravates poverty, poor school attendance, and overall development. Unlike many of the other challenges in public health, the water and sanitation solutions are well-known. However, despite strong evidence of the effectiveness and cost-effectiveness of improved water and sanitation against diarrhoea and certain other diseases and support for the intervention at the highest international levels, coverage still lags behind the MDG targets, especially for sanitation. This chapter describes the aetiological agents of the leading water- and sanitation-related diseases, presents the evidence concerning the effectiveness of water and sanitation interventions to prevent such diseases, and summarizes the economic implications of such interventions and some of the other non-health benefits associated therewith. Recent and emerging developments in water, sanitation, and health are discussed, including new methods for assessing and measuring the risks associated with unsafe water and sanitation, technologies, programmatic approaches, and implementation strategies. The chapter closes with a discussion of some of the continuing challenges in water and sanitation, including efforts to scale up interventions among the most vulnerable populations in an effort to secure the benefits of water and sanitation for all.

Introduction

Background

Safe drinking water and sanitary waste disposal are among the most fundamental of public health interventions. When readers of the *British Medical Journal* were asked in 2006 to name the 'greatest medical advance' since 1840, their top choice was clean drinking water and waste disposal, beating antibiotics, anaesthesia, vaccines, and germ theory (Ferriman 2007). Deaths from diarrhoeal diseases and typhoid fever showed dramatic declines in Europe and North America when cities and towns began filtering and chlorinating their water and safely disposing of human and animal excreta (Cutler & Miller 2005). The field of epidemiology arguably has its origins in John Snow's nineteenth century mapping of cholera cases and the eventual intervention at London's Broad Street pump that demonstrated waterborne transmission of the disease.

While diseases associated with poor water and sanitation are now comparatively unknown in higher income countries, they still impose a heavy burden elsewhere, especially among young children, the poor, the immuno-compromised, and the displaced. Diarrhoeal diseases alone kill an estimated 1.7 million people each year, and account for 17 per cent of deaths in children under five in developing countries (WHO 2005). According to the World Health Organization (WHO), 94 per cent of such deaths could be averted by improvements in water, sanitation, and hygiene (Prüss-Üstün & Corvalán 2007). Because they interfere with normal adsorption of nutrients, the diseases associated with poor water and sanitation are also a major cause of malnutrition, a separate source of significant morbidity and mortality (Fewtrell *et al.* 2007).

Water and sanitation are not only a matter of public health, but also of poverty, equity, and justice (UNDP 2006). Because they are less likely to have access to safe water and sanitation, the poor bear most of the burden of water-related diseases, driving them further into poverty through lost productivity and expenditure on treatment (Blakley *et al.* 2006). Time spent in collecting water from distant sources and the inability to procure sufficient quantities of water for irrigating crops, watering animals, and carrying out other productive activities aggravates poverty. Inadequate water and sanitation are also associated with poor school attendance (Hutton *et al.* 2007). For these and other reasons, water and sanitation have been recognized as a fundamental human right (UNICEF 1999; United Nations 2002).

Nevertheless, basic water security and sanitation still elude much of the world's population living in low-income countries. An estimated 1.1 billion people lack improved access to water supplies; 2.6 billion people—40 per cent of the world's population—lack access to improved sanitation. Coverage is lowest in developing regions, where people are most vulnerable to infection and disease. In Africa, improved water and sanitation coverage is just 56 per cent and 37 per cent, respectively (WHO/UNICEF 2005). Rural areas also lag behind their urban counterparts, with three times as many rural dwellers lacking improved sanitation as urban dwellers; improved water reaches less than 50 per cent of rural populations in 27 developing countries. If current trends continue, more than half of the rural population will still be without sanitation coverage in 2015, and more than 700 million mainly poor rural dwellers will still lack improved water (WHO/UNICEF 2006).

The shortfall in water and sanitation coverage is not the result of a failure to recognize the need or declare goals at the highest international levels. The 1977 Mar del Plata Declaration by the United Nations expressed the goal of providing safe water and sanitation for all by 1990, launching the Water and Sanitation Decade (1981–1990) (Cairncross 1992). In 1990, the UN renewed the call and extended the deadline to the end of the century. The United Nations Millennium Development Goals (MDGs) call for halving, by 2015, the portion of the population without sustainable access to safe drinking water or basic sanitation (United Nations 2000). As the research described in this chapter suggests, such coverage would not only advance the environmental security targets under MDG Goal 7, but also make contributions to reducing poverty (Goal 1), increasing primary education (Goal 2), promoting gender equality (Goal 3), reducing child mortality (Goal 4), and combating major diseases (Goal 6). In a further effort to attract attention to this deficit and additional priority to the sector, the United Nations General Assembly declared 2005–15 as the Decade for Action, Water for Life (WHO/UNICEF 2005), and 2008 as the International Year of Sanitation.

Traditionally, much of the work in water and sanitation has been undertaken by engineers and has consisted of infrastructural improvements. Low-cost community- and household-based interventions, such as protected wells, boreholes, and communal stand pipes for improved water supplies, and various types of latrines, septic tanks, and composting systems for improved sanitation, have been largely conceived by and constructed with the assistance of engineers. There are numerous books, manuals, and other resources that describe these systems in detail, including Cairncross and Feachem (1993), DFID (1998), Davis and Lambert (2002), the quarterly *Waterlines*, and the World Bank Water and Sanitation Programme (WSP) *Field Notes* (www.wps.org). Readers are encouraged to refer to such sources for details on the design, installation, and operation of such systems, technology innovations, and the programmatic challenges associated with achieving widespread use on a sustained basis.

This chapter focuses solely on the public health issues concerning water and sanitation. After introducing some basic terminology, it begins by describing the diseases associated with inadequate water and sanitation and their contribution to the overall burden of disease. It then presents evidence of the effectiveness of water and sanitation interventions to prevent such diseases, the economic implications (especially cost-effectiveness and cost–benefits) of such interventions, and some of the other non-health benefits associated therewith. Recent and emerging developments in water, sanitation, and health are then discussed, along with some issues relevant to designing water and sanitation interventions. The chapter closes with a discussion of some of the continuing challenges in water and sanitation, including efforts to scale up interventions among the most vulnerable populations in an effort to secure the benefits of water and sanitation for all.

Terminology

At the outset, it is useful to understand some of the terminology used in describing the diseases, transmission routes, and interventions associated with the water and sanitation sectors. Water-related diseases are sometimes classified according to their disease transmission routes as *waterborne* (ingested in drinking water),

water-washed (associated with inadequate supplies of water for proper personal hygiene), *water-based* (transmitted through an aquatic invertebrate host), or linked to a *water-related vector* (involving an insect vector breeding in or near water) (White *et al.* 1972). Most waterborne organisms that are human pathogens colonize the gut of humans and certain other mammals and are transmitted through the *faecal–oral* route. The transmission of common waterborne diseases can thus be interrupted by improvements in sanitation (*excreta disposal*), personal hygiene (especially *hand washing*), and microbiological *water quality*, while those that are water-washed are impacted by improvements in *water supplies* (quantity and access) for personal hygiene. Improving water supplies can also help prevent water-based diseases (such as schistosomiasis and dracunculiasis) by reducing the need to enter infected water bodies.

The term 'sanitation' is vague with multiple meanings. Within the sanitation sector two definitions are used. Under the broader definition, sanitation extends to the process whereby people demand, effect, and sustain a hygienic and healthy environment for themselves. This definition could include safe food production, solid waste management, industrial waste, hygiene behaviour change, hand washing, control of chemicals, environmental pollution, storm water drainage, wastewater disposal, human settlements, prevention and control of communicable diseases, HIV/AIDS, vector and vermin control, occupational health and safety, mining and quarrying, port health, and disposal of the dead. A second definition is more specific, extending only to the process of separating humans from their excreta. This chapter uses this second, more specific definition and regards sanitation as a system in which excreta is (i) collected safely and with dignity, (ii) transported to a suitable location, (iii) treated or contained for some period of time, and (iv) reused and/or discharged to the environment.

The MDG targets for water and sanitation are expressed in terms of *sustainable access to safe drinking water* and of *basic sanitation*. The water target has been interpreted as 'sufficient drinking water of acceptable quality as well as sufficient quantity of water for hygienic purposes' (UN Millennium Project 2005). Basic sanitation, in turn, has been defined as 'the lowest-cost option for securing sustainable access to safe, hygienic, and convenient facilities and services for excreta and sewage disposal that provide privacy and dignity, while at the same time ensuring a clean and healthy living environment both at home and in the neighbourhood of users' (UN Millennium Project 2005). Progress toward the MDGs, however, is measured with reference to the Joint Monitoring Programme (JMP) which adopts an indicator approach based on facilities or level of service. For water supplies, the JMP distinguishes only between *improved water supplies* (piped-in tap water, public tap/standpipe, borehole/tubewell, protected well/spring, rainwater harvesting), and *unimproved water supplies* (surface water, unprotected well/spring, tankered water, bottled water). *Improved sanitation* includes a private flush or pour-flush toilet or latrine connected to a piped sewer system or septic system, simple pit latrine with slab, ventilated improved pit (VIP) latrine, or composting toilet; *unimproved sanitation* includes any other flush or pour-flush latrine, open pit latrine, bucket latrine, hanging latrine, any public or shared facility, or open defecation (WHO/UNICEF 2002).

Burden of disease

General

Poor water and sanitation are associated with a variety of infectious diseases transmitted through various pathways by helminths, protozoa, bacteria, and viruses. Table 2.5.1 summarizes the most important of these diseases, their transmission routes, aetiological agents, and epidemiological significance. Further details are provided in Sections 'General' *et seq.* Some of these diseases also contribute to malnutrition, a separate cause of substantial morbidity and mortality that is not reflected in the direct burden of disease figures cited below (Black *et al.* 2003).

Certain diseases associated with water are not addressed in this chapter. First, in addition to microbial agents, water is a medium for the transmission of chemical pathogens, including arsenic and other metals, fluoride, nitrates, and volatile organic compounds (including pesticides and herbicides). Accordingly, WHO guidelines and many national water standards establish maximum allowable limits for such chemicals (WHO 2004). However, except for arsenicosis and fluoridosis, which are especially serious in focal areas in Asia and parts of Africa, most of these contaminants represent hazards to health only over the longer term. Second, although improvements in water supplies (to discourage contact with water) and point-of-use water treatment (with filters) are important interventions in preventing dracunculiasis (Cairncross *et al.* 2002), efforts to control Guinea worm infection have been largely successful and the disease is now of public health interest in limited areas. Finally, this chapter does not address a variety of diseases associated with waterborne pathogens, such as poliomyelitis and hepatitis A & E, which are controlled mainly by vaccines and other non-environmental measures (Leclerc *et al.* 2002).

Diarrhoeal diseases

Diarrhoeal diseases kill an estimated 1.8 million people each year (WHO 2005). Among infectious diseases, diarrhoea ranks as the third leading cause of both mortality and morbidity (after respiratory infections and HIV/AIDS), placing it above tuberculosis and malaria. Young children are especially vulnerable, bearing 68 per cent

Table 2.5.1 Principal infectious diseases, disease agents, transmission routes, and annual morbidity and mortality related to poor water and sanitation

Disease	Aetiological agent	Transmission	Morbidity*	Mortality*
Diarrhoea (dysentery, cholera)	**Viruses** *Rotavirus*	Faecal–oral	4 billion (annual)	1.8 million
	Bacteria *E.coli (ETEC)* *Shiguella* sp. *Salmonella* sp. *Vibrio* sp. *Campylobacter* sp.	Faecal–oral		
	Protozoa *Giardia lambia* *Cryptosporidium parvum* *Emtamoeba histolytic*	Faecal–oral		
Schistosomiasis	*S. haematobium* *S. mansoni* *S. japonicum*	Penetration through skin exposed to contaminated freshwater	187 million	27 000–280 000
Ascariasis	*Ascaris lumbricoides*	Faecal–oral	1.2 billion	
Trichuriasis	*Trichuris trichuria*	Faecal–oral	795 million	
Hookworm infection	*Necator americanus*	Penetration through skin exposed to faecally-contaminated soil	740 million	
	Ancylostoma duodenale	Faecal–oral		
Typhoid and paratyphoid fever	*Salmonella* sp.	Faecal–oral	26 million	216 000
Trachoma	*Chlamydia trachomatis*	Fingers Clothing Eye-seeking flies (*M. sorbens*) Coughing/sneezing	6 million blind 150 million with active trachoma	

*Estimates vary according to method. Morbidity and mortality estimates for diarrhoeal disease are from WHO (2005); those for soil-transmitted helminth infections (STH) (ascariasis, trichuriasis, hookworm) and schistosomiasis are from deSilva *et al.* (2003) and Hotez *et al.* (2006). Mortality estimates for STH and schistosomiasis vary significantly, depending on the method used for estimation (Hotez *et al.* 2006). Typhoid and paratyphoid estimates are from Crump *et al.* (2004). Trachoma figures are from Kumaresan and Mecaskey (2003).

of the total burden of diarrhoeal disease (Bartram 2003). Among children younger than 5 years, diarrhoea accounts for 17 per cent of all deaths (United Nations 2005). For those infected with the human immunodeficiency virus (HIV) or who have developed acquired immunodeficiency syndrome (AIDS), diarrhoea can be prolonged, severe, and life-threatening (Hayes *et al.* 2003).

Diarrhoea is characterized by stools of decreased consistency and increased number. The clinical symptoms and course of the disease vary greatly with the age, nutritional and immune status, and the pathogen (Black & Lanata 1995). Most cases resolve within a week, though a small percentage continue for 2 weeks or more and are characterized as 'persistent' diarrhoea. Dysentery is a diarrhoeal disease defined by the presence of blood in the liquid stools. Though epidemic diarrhoea such as cholera and shigellosis (bacillary dysentery) are well-known risks, particularly in emergency settings, their global health significance is small compared to endemic diarrhoea (Hunter 1997).

The immediate threat from diarrhoea is dehydration, a loss of fluids and electrolytes. Thus, the widespread promotion of oral rehydration therapy (ORT) has significantly reduced the case-fatality rate associated with the disease. Such improvements in case management, however, have not reduced morbidity, which is estimated at four billion cases annually (Kosek *et al.* 2003). And since diarrhoeal diseases inhibit normal ingestion of foods and adsorption of nutrients, continued high morbidity is an important cause of malnutrition, leading to impaired physical growth and cognitive function, reduced resistance to infection, and potentially long-term gastrointestinal disorders.

The infectious agents associated with diarrhoeal disease are transmitted chiefly through the faecal–oral route (Leclerc *et al.* 2001). Safe excreta disposal thus represents a primary barrier that should contribute to the prevention of indirect transmission via food, water, hands, fomites, and mechanical vectors (flies) (Fig. 2.5.1). A wide variety of bacterial, viral, and protozoan pathogens excreted in the faeces of humans and animals are known to cause diarrhoea. The importance of individual pathogens varies among settings, seasons, and conditions. Although diarrhoea is also associated with the ingestion of metals, nitrates, organics, and other chemicals, the burden of disease arising from such exposure is small relative to infectious diarrhoea (Hunter 1997).

Schistosomiasis

Schistosomiasis affects 187 million people all over the world, with *S. haematobium* and *S. mansoni* being the most common species. The schistosomiasis life cycle involves contamination of freshwater by eggs-carrying excreta and urine and an intermediate host, a freshwater snail. Larvae released in the water infect humans by penetrating through the skin. Parasites develop and migrate to the intestines and bladder where thousands of eggs are produced. Like other intestinal helminths, schistosomes are associated with impaired physical and mental development and anaemia. Furthermore, schistosomiasis may cause serious damage to the bladder and intestine walls as a result of parasite egg entrapment within tissues. Chronic infection with *S. haematobium* has been associated with increased risk of bladder cancer in adulthood (Gryssels *et al.* 2006).

Soil-transmitted helminth infection

More than two billion of the world's population, mostly in developing countries, are infected with soil-transmitted helminths. About 300 million people suffer from heavy worm load and related severe morbidity (deSilva *et al.* 2003). *Ascaris lumbricoides, Trichuris trichuria*, and hookworm (*Ancylostoma duodenale* and *Necator americanus*) are the most prevalent intestinal helminths. Transmission occurs via ingestion of eggs present in faecally-contaminated soil, or via penetration of the larvae through the skin. Children are particularly vulnerable to chronic and heavy infections which result in malnutrition, stunted growth, reduced physical fitness, and impaired cognitive development (Stephenson *et al.* 2000). Hookworm infection is an important cause of anaemia, not only in children, but also among women of reproductive age and pregnant women leading to premature birth and low birth-weight (Hotez *et al.* 2004).

Typhoid and paratyphoid fevers

While enteric fevers such as typhoid and paratyphoid were leading causes of waterborne disease in previous centuries, morbidity and mortality diminished dramatically with the provisions of disinfected water supplies and improved sanitary facilities (Cutler & Miller 2005). The aetiological agents for typhoid and paratyphoid fevers

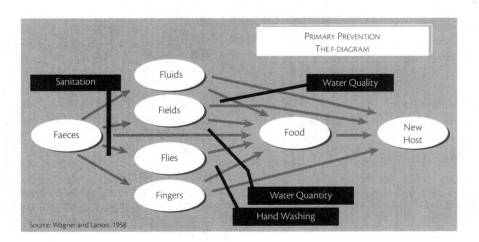

Fig. 2.5.1 The F-diagram (from Wagner & Lanois 1958).

are *Salmonella typhi* and *Salmonella paratyphi*; a proposed new nomenclature would change the *S. typhi* to *S. enterica* serovar Typhi and *S. paratyphi* to *S. enterica* serovar Paratyphi A and B. A recent review estimates 21 million cases of typhoid annually, causing 216 000 deaths (Crump *et al.* 2004). The milder paratyphoid accounts for an additional 5 million cases each year.

Trachoma

Trachoma accounts for 15 per cent of world blindness, with 6 million people affected and 150 million at risk of visual impairment (Kumaresan & Mecaskey 2003). Trachoma is caused by repeated eye infection with *Chlamydia trachomatis*. Children are the main reservoir for infection, with high prevalence of active trachoma (Mabey *et al.* 2003). Repeated infections result in deformation of the upper eye lid, abrasion of the cornea, and progressive loss of vision in later life. *C. trachomatis* is transmitted from the discharge of an infected eye via contaminated fingers, clothing, and eye-seeking flies (*M. sorbens.*) Although the role of flies in the transmission of infection remains unclear, studies have shown that *M. sorbens* breed mainly in solid human faeces present in the environment and not in latrines (Emerson *et al.* 2000). Thus, safe excreta disposal may play an important role in reducing trachoma transmission. Improving water supplies and sanitationis part of the WHO-backed SAFE (surgery, antibiotics, facial hygiene, environmental improvement) strategy for controlling and preventing the disease.

Effectiveness of water and sanitation in preventing disease

Barriers to transmission of faecal–oral diseases

As illustrated by the so-called 'F-diagram' (Fig. 2.5.1), the safe disposal of human faeces is the primary barrier in preventing faecal–oral transmitted diseases. Without removing excreta from potential contact with humans, animals, and insects, pathogens may be carried on unwashed hands, in contaminated water or food, or via flies and other insects on to further human hosts. Whether or not sanitation is adequate, hands can become contaminated with faeces, especially during anal cleansing following defecation or in cleaning a child after defecation. This may result in further transmission, either directly or indirectly through food, water, or other beverages, or fomites. Accordingly, hand washing is an important secondary barrier to faecal–oral disease transmission (Curtis & Cairncross 2003). Other secondary barriers include (i) water quality interventions to prevent contamination (e.g. safe distribution and storage or use of a residual disinfectant to prevent recontamination), (ii) water supply interventions to increase the quantity and availability of water for personal and domestic hygiene, (iii) proper cooking and food handling, and (iv) control of mechanical vectors such as flies.

Rigorously assessing the impact of water and sanitation interventions on human health presents a number of methodological problems (Blum & Feachem 1983; Esrey *et al.* 1986). Blinded, randomized, controlled trials (RCTs), the gold standard of epidemiological evidence (Chapter 6.8), are impossible for most water and sanitation interventions, as it is impractical or politically inexpedient to randomly deliver the intervention to large numbers of a study population while leaving others as controls, and often impossible to blind

infrastructural interventions. Studies that purport to achieve sufficient sample size by randomly allocating the intervention to the population of one village while using a second village serve as controls are, in fact, a one-to-one comparison, yielding a sample size of just two and limiting the statistical significance of any observed differences (Blum & Feachem 1983). Most interventional studies of water and sanitation follow a quasi-randomized (quasi-experimental) design where the intervention has not been allocated randomly, but the investigators otherwise treat as a controlled trial. Blinded RCTs have been used to assess certain water quality interventions of household-based interventions (Colford *et al.* 2002). Recent studies of sanitation interventions have followed cluster-randomized (Emerson *et al.* 2004) and step-wedge approaches (Smith & Morrow 1996) to address some of the challenges of RCTs to assess water and sanitation interventions.

Most studies of the water and sanitation thus follow observational designs (cross-sectional, case-control, and cohort studies). While these studies can yield valuable information in developing hypotheses and seeking associations between the intervention and outcome of interest, they must measure and control for numerous known confounders. Age is particularly important: Diarrhoeal disease morbidity and mortality is highest among children after weaning and before development of immune systems; other enteric infections also tend to follow demographic patterns consistent with their exposure. Faecal–oral diseases such as diarrhoea are characterized by significant seasonal variations that make it difficult to make before–after comparisons (as opposed to comparisons with a contemporaneous control group) and challenging to estimate sample sizes (Schmidt *et al.* 2007). Other important confounders include quantity and quality of water available, distance and other barriers to access, collection and storage practices, sanitation facilities, and use, and hygiene practices. Households who take special steps to improve their water supplies or build latrines are self-selected and, as they also tend to be wealthier, better educated, and more conscious of hygiene, are more likely to adopt other behaviour that protect their families from faecal–oral disease.

Regardless of the study design, there are significant challenges in assessing the effectiveness of water and sanitation interventions to prevent diarrhoeal disease. First, there are different ways of defining the disease itself. While many studies use the standard WHO definition for diarrhoea (3 or more loose stools in 24 h) (WHO 1993), others use local definitions (Moy *et al.* 1991). Although some studies use clinical assays or serology to confirm infection, most assessments of diarrhoeal diseases rely on self-reporting which can be biased by recall errors (especially for periods longer than the previous 48 h) and potential reporting since diarrhoea is private or embarrassing and often regarded as more of an annoyance than a disease. Comparing results between studies is also complicated by different measures of disease frequency (incidence, period prevalence, longitudinal prevalence) and measures of effect of the intervention (risk ratios, rate ratios, odds ratios, longitudinal prevalence ratios). While collecting information on incidence may be necessary for assessing risk, longitudinal prevalence may be a more efficient means of measuring the effectiveness of an intervention while minimizing Hawthorne effect and courtesy bias and the challenge of distinguishing separate episodes of diarrhoea (Morris *et al.* 1996; Schmidt *et al.* 2007). Another common error in the analysis of results is the failure to adjust the data for lack of independent observations (e.g. repeated observations of the same subject and for intra-cluster correlations, such as among subjects living within the same household). Owing to the challenges of measuring actual use of a latrine or improved water supply, many studies fail to report on compliance with the intervention even though this has been shown to be an important aspect of the effectiveness of the intervention.

It is important for those engaged in research involving water and sanitation interventions to consider these methodological issues when designing studies and assessments. These issues should also be borne in mind in evaluating the evidence of the effectiveness of water and sanitation interventions described in the next section.

Evidence of effectiveness

Scores of studies have been conducted and published on the effectiveness of water, sanitation, and hygiene interventions to prevent infection and disease. By one estimate, more than 285 studies were published between 1980 and 2003 solely on water quality interventions to prevent diarrhoea (Clasen *et al.* 2006). Systematic reviews (Chapter 6.14) are a means of identifying, summarizing, synthesizing, explaining, and assessing the methodological quality of evidence of the effectiveness of health interventions with a variety of studies relating to a particular health intervention. In some cases, such reviews also employ meta-analysis or other statistical methods to estimate the pooled effect of the intervention across the studies included in the review. A number of such reviews have examined the evidence of effectiveness of water, sanitation, and hygiene interventions to prevent disease and infection.

Diarrhoeal diseases

Table 2.5.2 summarizes the results of five different systematic reviews of water and sanitation interventions to prevent diarrhoeal diseases published over the last 25 years. They demonstrate that

improvements in water quantity, water quantity and quality, water quality and availability, and sanitation all make substantial contributions to the prevention of diarrhoeal diseases.

In the past, Esrey's conclusions have been oversimplified to suggest that improving water quantity and sanitation may be more effective in preventing diarrhoea than improving water quality. An analysis of the actual review, however, suggests that only when the water supply is delivered on plot are the health gains realized (Cairncross & Valdmanis 2006). This is consistent with the more recent reviews. Clasen *et al.* (2006) suggest that household-based interventions are about twice as effective in preventing diarrhoeal diseases than conventional interventions at the source or point of distribution (e.g. protected wells, boreholes, and communal tap stands), and are roughly comparable to the impact of hand washing and sanitation. The biological basis for the added protection offered from point-of-use interventions has been shown in dozens of studies that demonstrate how water that is safe at the source becomes contaminated during collection, storage, and use in the home (Wright *et al.* 2004). Among household-based interventions, filtration was associated with the largest reductions in diarrhoeal disease, perhaps because it also improves water aesthetics which may increase use (compliance) with the intervention.

Recent reviews also challenge three other widely-held notions in public health engineering. First, the evidence does not suggest that an improved supply of water is essential for water quality interventions to prevent diarrhoea (Clasen *et al.* 2006). This finding confirms the WHO's recent strategy to pursue household water treatment and safe storage as a means of accelerating the health gains of safe drinking water, even though it may not reduce the 1.1 billion currently without access to improved water supplies. Second, water quality interventions appear to be effective in preventing diarrhoea regardless of whether they are deployed in settings where sanitation

Table 2.5.2 Estimate of effect* (and number of studies) of systematic reviews of water and sanitation interventions to prevent diarrhoeal diseases

Intervention (Improvement)	Esrey *et al.* (1985) (range)	Esrey *et al.* (1991)	Fewtrell *et al.* (2005) (95% CI)	Clasen *et al.* (2006) (95% CI)	Clasen *et al.* (2008) (95% CI)
Water quantity	25% (0–100%) (17)	27% (7)			
Water quality			0.69 (0.53–0.89) (15)	0.57 (0.46–0.70) (38)	
Source	16% (0–90%) (9)	17% (7)	0.89 (0.42–1.90) (3)	0.73 (0.53–1.01) (6)	
Household			0.65 (0.48–0.88) (12)	0.53 (0.39–0.73) (32)	
Chlorination				0.63 (0.52–0.75) (16)	
Filtration				0.37 (0.28–0.49) (6)	
Solar disinfection				0.69 (0.63–0.74) (2)	
Floc-disinfection				0.69 (0.58–0.82) (6)	
Water quality and availability	37% (0–82%) (8)	16% (22)	0.75 (0.62–0.91) (6)		
Water and sanitation		20% (7)			
Sanitation	22% (0–48%) (10)	22% (11)	0.68 (0.53–0.87) (2)		0.67 (0.50–0.82) (7)

*For studies by Esrey and colleages, estimate of effect is the median reduction in diarrhoeal disease from the reported studies; for other studies, estimate of effect is the pooled risk ratio from meta-analysis using random effects model. To compare results, the percentage reduction is 1−RR (e.g. RR of 0.69 implies a 31% reduction in risk).

is improved or unimproved (Clasen *et al.* 2006). This is in contrast to conclusions that interventions to improve water quality are effective only where sanitation has already been addressed (Esrey 1986; VanDerslice & Briscoe 1995). Finally, contrary to conventional wisdom and results from disease-transmission modelling (Eisenberg *et al.* 2007), sub-group analysis does not demonstrate that the effectiveness of a water quality intervention to prevent diarrhoea is enhanced by adding hygiene instruction, a separate vessel to treat or store water, or by improving sanitation or water supply (Fewtrell *et al.* 2005; Clasen *et al.* 2006). This is consistent with the finding that the effectiveness of a water quality intervention does not depend on the baseline conditions in regard to other environmental parameters that are associated with diarrhoea. At the same time, it implies that the cost and effort of combining the water quality intervention with improved hygiene, water storage, water supply, or sanitation may not be justified on the basis of an incremental effect on diarrhoeal disease.

With respect to sanitation interventions, Esrey and colleagues reported median reductions in diarrhoea of 22 per cent (range of 0–48 per cent) from 10 studies of interventions that included excreta disposal (Esrey *et al.* 1985). A subsequent review that also included sanitation interventions reported a medium reduction in diarrhoea morbidity of 22 per cent from 11 studies (36 per cent from five studies the investigators deemed rigorous) (Esrey *et al.* 1991). An update of the Esrey reviews which was limited to interventional research designs identified just four such studies of improved sanitation, only two of which provided data that they could use in a meta-analysis (Fewtrell *et al.* 2005). Fewtrell and colleagues reported the interventions to be protective, with a pooled relative risk of 0.68 (95 per cen CI: 0.53–0.87)—a 32 per cent reduction in diarrhoea that would appear consistent with Esrey's findings. More recently, Clasen and colleagues reported a pool risk ratio from seven randomized and quasi-randomized controlled studies of 0.67 (95 per cent CI: 0.50–0.88), corresponding to a 33 per cent reduction in risk (Clasen *et al.* 2008). All of the interventional studies included in the Fewtrell and Clasen reviews combined the sanitation intervention with a water supply (and in some cases, hygiene) intervention, making it impossible to tease out the effect attributable solely to the improvement in excreta disposal facilities. Nevertheless, the consistency of results among these reviews and the underlying studies does provide some confidence that sanitation interventions are protective against diarrhoeal disease. And observational studies—such as a recent cohort study in Brazil in which increased sewer connections was associated with a 26 per cent reduction in diarrhoea (95 per cent CI: 15–37 per cent) (Barretto 2007)—provide additional support.

Soil-transmitted helminth infection

Esrey and colleagues (1991) reported a 4 per cent median reduction in hookworm (*Ancylostoma*) infection from nine studies of combined sanitation and water interventions; the reduction was also 4 per cent in the only included study they deemed rigorous. Esrey also reported a 4 per cent reduction in hookworm in the single study reporting on a sanitation intervention alone. Combined improvements in water supplies and sanitation were associated with a 28 per cent reduction in ascariasis morbidity from 11 studies (29 per cent from four rigorous studies).

In their review of randomized and quasi-randomized controlled trials of interventions to improve excreta disposal, Clasen and colleagues (2008) found consistent evidence that the interventions

were protective, even though the limited number of clusters in each study made it impossible to calculate confidence intervals around the point estimates or to pool estimates using meta-analysis. The three studies that reported *Ascaris* infection as an outcome found the intervention group had reductions of 34 per cent (Chandler *et al.* 1954), 73 per cent (Messou *et al.* 1997), and 39 per cent (Zhang *et al.* 2000) compared to controls. The two studies that reported hookworm infection also found the intervention to be protective, with reductions of 87 per cent (Messou *et al.* 1997) and 66 per cent (Chandler *et al.* 1954). Two studies also reported the intervention to be effective against intestinal parasites that they did not specify: Chen *et al.* (2004) recorded a 77 per cent reduction in the intervention group compared with controls, while Zhang *et al.* (2005) found a 56 per cent reduction.

Schistosomiasis

Esrey and colleagues (1991) reported a median reduction in the prevalence of schistosomiasis of 73 per cent (range 59–87 per cent) from four water and sanitation interventions; the reduction was 77 per cent among the three studies they deemed rigorous. Piped-in water supplies and community washing and bathing facilities that reduced contact with surface waters were especially protective, leading to reductions in both prevalence and severity (Esrey *et al.* 1991). The reviewers noted that in Kenya, the installation of boreholes without laundry or shower facilities failed to reduce infection.

Two recent quasi-randomized, controlled interventional studies from China also suggest that improved excreta disposal is protective against schistosomiasis. In a 3-year quasi-RCT, Chen *et al.* (2004) recorded a 43 per cent reduction from combined water, sanitation, and hygiene interventions that also included a snail control component. Zhang *et al.* (2005) reported a 45 per cent reduction in a 2-year quasi-RCT that included water, sanitation, and hygiene. Once again, these trials did not include sufficient clusters to reliably calculate confidence intervals around the point estimates of effect.

Typhoid and paratyphoid

No studies of water or sanitation interventions to prevent typhoid or paratyphoid have been reported. Nevertheless, there is evidence suggesting the effectiveness of water quality interventions. Cutler and Miller (2005) have shown the historical evidence on reductions in mortality associated with the introduction of clean water and sanitation in the United States. Recent case-control studies do suggest that the diseases are still associated with unsafe water and sanitation. In a recent study in Uzbekistan where typhoid remains endemic, cases were more likely to drink unboiled surface water outside the home (OR 3.0, 95 per cent CI: 1.1–8.20) (Srikantiah *et al.* 2007). In a similar case-control study in Bangladesh, drinking unboiled water at home was a significant risk factor (OR 12.1, 95 per cent CI: 2.2–65.6) (Ram *et al.* 2007). Among the risk factors for typhoid and paratyphoid in an urban setting in Indonesia were lack of a toilet in the household (OR 2.20, 95 per cent CI: 1.06–4.55) and use of ice cubes (OR 2.27; 95 per cent CI: 1.31–3.93).

Trachoma

The evidence of the effectiveness of environmental interventions (including water and sanitation) alone to prevent active trachoma is not clear (Rabiu *et al.* 2007). Reviews of the WHO-backed SAFE strategy for trachoma control conclude that there is comparatively weak evidence of the effectiveness of the 'F' (facial cleanliness) and

'E' (environmental improvement) components that encompass improved access to water and better sanitation (Emerson *et al.* 2000a; Kuper *et al.* 2003). In a 6-month cluster RCT of 21 villages in the Gambia, Emerson and colleagues (2004) reported a reduction in fly catches among study clusters receiving latrines. However, the prevalence of active trachoma associated with the intervention was not statistically lower than among seven control clusters (RR 0.81, 95 per cent CI: 0.54–1.22). While trachoma is a water-washed disease that may be impacted by increased access to water, there is also a paucity of evidence that face washing alone is protective against active trachoma (Ejere *et al.* 2004) despite consistent evidence that improved facial hygiene was associated with lower prevalence of disease (Emerson 2000).

Economic implications of water and sanitation interventions

Economic evaluation

Although the evidence suggests that water and sanitation interventions are effective in preventing diarrhoea and certain other faecal–oral diseases, the extent to which interventions are ultimately deployed will not be determined on their effectiveness alone. With limited resources, particularly in developing countries, governments are forced to allocate health expenditures to an array of public health challenges. While public sector decisions on health expenditures are often based on political commitments or other expediencies, economic efficiency, by definition, requires that resources be directed to their most productive use. In the health context, such allocative efficiency means identifying and focusing on the intervention that will produce the greatest health gains for a given investment of resources (Witter *et al.* 2000). This implies more than cost; the lowest cost intervention is seldom the most effective. Economic evaluation is normally a function of both the cost of the intervention and the return on that cost, measured either in terms of overall economic benefits (a *cost–benefit analysis* or CBA) or in the realization of a social objective, such as the prevention of disease (a *cost-effectiveness analysis* or CEA). In a CBA, all of the outcomes of the investment are valued in economic terms, and the output is expressed as a return on the investment or the cost–benefit ratio. The output of a CEA is a ratio (the cost-effectiveness ratio) between the cost of the intervention and an operational outcome measured in its own units. For health interventions, a common unit of measurement is disability adjusted life years (DALYs) averted as a result of the intervention.

Cost-effectiveness analysis

In its *2002 World Health Report*, the WHO assessed the cost-effectiveness of interventions to increase coverage of water and sanitation services in accordance with the MDGs (WHO 2002). It concluded that achieving the MDG for improved water supplies would be the least costly to implement in each region, at a global cost of approximately I\$37.5 billion over 10 years. It estimated health gains of approximately 30 million DALYs worldwide. A more recent CEA of water quality interventions to prevent diarrhoeal disease reached a similar conclusion when comparing source-based improvements to household-based interventions (Clasen *et al.* 2007). Among household-based interventions, point-of-use chlorination

using sodium hypochlorite was the most cost-effective; additional health gains could be achieved at higher costs with household-based filters. In the lowest-income parts of Africa, for example, the cost per DALY averted was US\$53 for household chlorination, US\$61 for household solar disinfection, US\$123 for source-based interventions, and US\$142 for household filters. Direct cost saving, even if limited to the WHO estimates of those corresponding to health-related expenditures, more than offset the costs of implementing most water quality interventions. This means that governments, who are chiefly incurring such costs, would reduce their overall outlays by investing in the implementation of such interventions rather than in the treatment of cases of diarrhoeal disease.

In a recent CEA of improvements in water supplies and sanitation that included the value of time savings from improving the access as well as health benefits, Cairncross and Valdmanis (2006) reported a cost-effectiveness ratio of US\$94 per DALY averted for installation of hand pumps or standposts, US\$223 for household connections, US\$47 for water sector regulation and advocacy, more than US\$270 for latrine construction and promotion, and US\$11 for promotion of basic sanitation.

Cost–benefit analysis

In another WHO-funded study, Hutton and colleagues (2007) assessed the cost–benefit ratios in 17 WHO epidemiological sub-regions of five categories of water and sanitation interventions based on the MDG water and sanitation targets and additional steps to minimize environmental exposure. The interventions included (1) improvements required to meet the MDGs for water supply, (2) interventions to meet the water and sanitation MDG, (3) increasing access to improved water and sanitation for everyone, (4) providing disinfection at point-of-use over and above increasing access to improved water supply and sanitation, and (5) providing regulated piped water supply in house and sewage connection with partial sewerage for everyone. Costs of the interventions were based on WHO estimates and included the full economic cost of construction and maintenance. Predicted reductions in the incidence of diarrhoeal disease were calculated for each intervention based on the expected population receiving these interventions. Benefits were based on such reductions in disease, and included time savings associated with better access to water and sanitation facilities, the gain in productive time due to less time spent ill, health sector and patient costs saved due to less treatment of diarrhoeal diseases, and the value of prevented deaths.

The analysis yielded a vast amount of valuable data on the cost of each intervention and on each of the categories of benefits. Table 2.5.3 summarizes the results of the analysis for the epidemiological sub-regions that comprise the continent of Africa. Significantly, most of the overall economic benefit is derived from time savings from improved access to water and sanitation. The cost–benefit ratio in Africa is 11, meaning a return of US\$11 for every dollar invested in water and sanitation. In all regions and for all five interventions, the cost–benefit ratio is greater than 1, with values in developing regions of between 5 and 28 for Intervention 1, between 3 and 34 for Intervention 2, between 6 and 42 for Intervention 3, and between 5 and 60 for Intervention 4; returns were lowest (between 1.27 and 4.84) for Intervention 5. Significantly, the main contributor to benefits was the saving of time associated with better access to water supply and sanitation services; health benefits were a

Table 2.5.3 Economic benefits from investments in improved water and sanitation in Africa (based on Hutton 2007)

	Meeting MDG target	Full coverage of safe water and basic sanitation
Cases of diarrhoea avoided annually	173 million cases	245 million cases
Productive days gained annually	456 million	647 million
Value of productive days gained annually	US$116 million	US$168 million
Health sector treatment costs averted annually	US$1695 million	US$2410 million
Value of time saved	US$15 877 million	US$33 972 million
School days gained annually	99 million	140 million
Cost of interventions per year	US$2020 million	US$4040 million
Total economic benefits per year	US$22 910 million	US$44 040 million
Dollar benefits return per dollar invested (Cost Benefit Ratio)	11	11

comparatively minor part of the overall. While the authors review possible sources of financing- based benefits, they conclude that the health sector budget, which is often meagre anyway, cannot and should not be expected to fund improvements in water and sanitation.

Providing services and allocating costs

Cost-effectiveness analyses and cost–benefit analyses suggest that improvements in water and sanitation yield both health and other valuable benefits, not only to those who receive the intervention but also to the public sector. Inadequate water and sanitation services also have significant externalities (costs imposed on others), such as the costs of over-extraction from water supplies, pollution of water sources, and environmental degradation. Even those who promote water as a basic right accept that some value must be attached to water to reduce waste, encourage conservation and promote higher value uses. Infrastructural improvements in water and sanitation often fail to be initiated or sustained because of a reluctance to charge fully for the cost of delivering the services, inefficiency in collecting such charges or diversion of the fees away from operation and maintenance. Understanding who benefits from improvements in water and sanitation can help justify the allocation of costs and secure financing.

While water and sanitation services are traditionally provided by the public sector, private entrepreneurs, ranging from individual water vendors to large-scale concessionaires of water supply and sewer systems, also play a role. Studies that assess willingness to pay and ability to pay regularly show that people of even modest means can and will contribute to the cost of improving water and sanitation services in many cases (Whittington and Briscoe 1990; Whittington *et al.* 2002). For water, interventions that increase the convenience, reliability, quantity, and quality of water are especially attractive. Urban sanitation is particularly well-suited to the service sector, though even rural latrines are often constructed by specialized masons. Careful planning to assess and match the demand for improvements with the target population's willingness-to-pay help

guide decisions on the appropriate level of services and ensure their financial sustainability.

Other benefits of water and sanitation interventions

Improving water availability (quantity and access)

As the Section 'Evidence of effectiveness' makes clear, improving water availability—even without a corresponding improvement in water quality—is associated with reductions of diseases transmitted through waterborne, water-washed, and water-based routes. This is partly due to the well-established relationship between the amount of water that people use and the time required to collect it (Cairncross & Feachem 1993). Figure 2.5.2 shows the plateau-shaped curve that characterizes water consumption patterns based on service levels. While significant quantities of water are used if delivered directly to the home, the quantity used is fairly constant when the collection time is 5–30 min and further diminishes for longer collection times. In lower-income settings, average daily per capita consumption is about 150 l for those with household

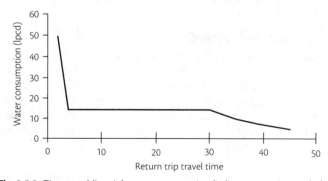

Fig. 2.5.2 Time travel (in min) versus consumption (in litres per capita per day) (from Cairncross & Feachem 1993).

connections, 50 l for yard taps, and just 15 l for communal sources such as stand posts, wells, and springs. Thus, assessments of water availability are expressed in terms of distance: Normally 1 km or round trip collection time (normally 30 min) (WHO/UNICEF 2000) but 0.5 km in disaster response (Sphere Project 2004).

Examining the evidence, a recent WHO report concludes that a minimum quantity of water for basic health protection is 20 l/person/day (Hutton & Bartram 2003). Of this, 7.5 l is for consumption (hydration and food preparation) and therefore must be of a quality to present minimal health risk; the balance is for basic personal and domestic hygiene. The report recognizes, however, that in addition to the direct health benefits associated with improving water supplies, there are indirect health and other benefits. Indirect health benefits may accrue from reducing the amount of time collecting water which can then be used more effectively at home caring for children or engaging in other productive activities (Cairncross 1987). Services at clinics, medical posts, and other healthcare facilities also benefit from improved water supplies. Sufficient water for irrigating gardens and crops can improve nutrition and generate income (Thompson *et al.* 2001). Vending water and making and selling beverages can also impact poverty. Finally, to the extent that people are paying for water, improved water supplies may result in savings that can be used for food and other necessities that may impact health outcomes.

Ecological sanitation

Within the sanitation sector there is an active group of advocates who promote the use of ecological sanitation (Winblad & Simpson-Hébert 2004). Ecological sanitation (EcoSan) works on the principle that urine and faeces are not just waste products, but assets that if properly managed, can contribute to better health and food production and reduce pollution. Managing such assets includes reducing pathogen loading to a safe level which is achieved by a combination of drying the faeces, increasing the pH, and storage for at least 12 months. Without good latrine management, pathogens can survive and create a risk to public health. The pathogen which causes greatest concern is *Ascarisis,* which has a long persistence in the environment and a low infective dose (Cairncross & Feachem 1993). Public health risks need to be balanced against the potential benefits. In areas where land fertility is low, artificial fertilizer is expensive, and livelihoods are dependent on subsistence farming, the benefits of using excreta as a fertilizer/soil improver could be considerable. Even when potential benefits can be demonstrated, local beliefs and taboos may limit acceptability or prevent adoption of the practice (Jackson 2005).

Improved school attendance

Improved water and sanitary facilities has been shown to result in increased attendance for a variety of reasons. Reduced incidence of disease results in fewer days of school missed as a result of illness. In Africa alone, Hutton and colleagues (2007) estimated that meeting the MDGs for water and sanitation would increase school attendance by 99 million days annually; full access to basic water and sanitation for all would increase school attendance by 140 million days each year. The sanitary needs of girls and the negative impact that lack of sanitation adversely impact their attendance levels. A UNICEF sanitation project in Bangladesh led to an 11 per cent increase in female enrolment by building appropriate school sanitation (UNICEF 1999). In Uganda, 94 per cent of girls reported problems at school during menstruation and 61 per cent reported staying away from school (IRC 2006). Cultural and religious constraints in many settings make menstruation a taboo. If menstruation lasts over a week, there is a tendency for girls to skip the entire school year (Bharadwaj & Patkar 2004). Sanitation pays an important role in improving educational access for children with disabilities, through the improvement of paths, latrine floors, and installation of handrails (Bannister *et al.* 2005).

Security and gender equality

Improved sanitation and water supplies improve security and gender equality for women and girls. Household sanitation can increase their safety by avoiding the dangers of sexual assault and harassment faced when practising open defecation or using latrines away from their homes. Safe, private, and proximate latrines are a particular issue for women in emergencies and conflicts (Sphere Project 2004). Research in Kenya revealed that women would defecate into plastic bags and throw them into streets ('flying toilets') because they feared being raped when using latrines shared with men (Maili Saba 2005). They were also afraid of being seen to be using latrines too regularly and preferred to bathe within their own homes after dark where they felt safer. Young children often prefer open defecation due to fear of falling into pits in poorly-designed or unsuitably-adapted latrines.

Advancing the fight against HIV/AIDS

It is well known that access to safe drinking water and sanitation prolongs the lives of people living with HIV/AIDS (PLWHA) by reducing the risk of opportunistic infections, including diarrhoeal diseases (Hayes 2003). Household-based water treatment has been shown to be an effective intervention in preventing mortality and morbidity in a population with one or more persons infected with HIV (Colford *et al.* 2005; Lule *et al.* 2006). Point-of-use water treatment products are now included in health kits for PLWHA (Colindres *et al.* 2007). Efforts are also underway to ensure that mothers infected with HIV have safe drinking water (or point-of-use water treatment products) to prepare infant formula for use as an alternative to breastfeeding in order to minimize mother–child transmission.

Recent and emerging developments in water and sanitation

Water safety plans and microbial risk assessment

Traditionally, the water sector relied on compliance with end-product standards to ensure the safety of drinking water. Most drinking water standards are based on WHO guidelines that establish maximum limits for known or suspected microbial and chemical pathogens as well as physical/aesthetic characteristics. Under this approach, drinking water is to be free of pathogens at the point of delivery as demonstrated by the absence of a prescribed indicator of faecal contamination, such as *E. coli* or thermotolerant coliforms (TTC). However, in the third edition of the WHO *Guidelines for Drinking-Water Quality* (GDWQ), the WHO adopted a risk assessment and risk management approach for improving drinking water quality (WHO 2004). The approach calls on water providers to develop and implement water safety plans similar to the hazard assessment critical control point (HACCP) approach used in the food industry to identify and control potential threats to safety.

This latest rolling revision to the GDWQ also encourages greater surveillance to verify compliance.

This risk-based approach uses health-based targets for water quality. This is based on quantitative microbial risk assessment (QMRA), an approach developed for calculating the burden of disease from potential pathogens. QMRA sets pathogen limits based on the evidence concerning exposure assessment, dose–response analysis, and risk characterization (Haas *et al.* 1999). Risk assessment and acceptable levels of risk are expressed in terms of DALYs. Reference pathogens are defined for each category of microbes. Significantly, these do not necessarily coincide with long-standing indicator organisms and may require capacity building in new laboratory techniques. Limited country-specific data and other resources may also delay full implementation of this approach in many countries.

Wastewater reuse

QMRA is also used in the recently-published second edition of the WHO's *Guidelines for the Safe Use of Wastewater, Excreta and Greywater* for agriculture and aquaculture (WHO 2006). As an estimated 70 per cent of water withdrawals from surface and sub-surface sources are used for agricultural purposes (WRI 2007), the agricultural sector is particularly eager to develop safe, economical, and effective water sources for crop irrigation. Wastewater can be high in plant nutrients (nitrogen, phosphorus, and potassium), minimizing the need for chemical fertilizers and producing higher incomes for farmers (Ensink & van der Hoek 2007). As municipalities in lower-income settings struggle to treat even drinking water, however, few are able to remove potential pathogens from wastewater, leaving an estimated 80 per cent of sewage untreated. The WHO *Guidelines* attempt to balance the benefits of wastewater reuse with the need for food security. As treated wastewater is also being increasingly viewed as a potential source of drinking water in water stressed regions, additional guidance based on public health evidence will be necessary.

Household-based water treatment

For the hundreds of millions who lack household water connections that provide drinking water on a 24–7 basis, water is often collected and stored in the home until needed. It is well known that even water that is safe at the point of collection undergoes frequent and extensive re-contamination during collection (or compromised distribution), storage, and use in the home (Wright *et al.* 2004). While providing safe, piped in, disinfected water to each household is an important goal, even meeting the MDG targets for 50 per cent coverage would entail an investment of tens of billions of dollars each year to connect households at the rate of 300 000 per day (WHO/UNICEF 2005). Accordingly, the WHO and others have called for other approaches that will accelerate the heath and economic gains associated with safe water while progress is made in improving infrastructure.

Interventions to treat and maintain the microbial quality of water at the point of use are among the most promising of these alternatives (Sobsey 2002). In many settings, both rural and urban, populations have access to sufficient quantities of water, but that water is unsafe. Because point-of-use interventions ensure the microbiological integrity of the water at the point of ingestion, they are more likely to deliver health benefits. Recent systematic reviews have shown household-based interventions (home-based boiling, chlorination, filtration, solar disinfection, and flocculation/disinfection) to be significantly more effective than traditional, non-reticulated source-based interventions (protected wells and springs, boreholes, communal tap stands) in improving microbiological water quality and reducing diarrhoeal disease (Fewtrell *et al.* 2005; Clasen *et al.* 2006). The up-front cost of treating such water at the point-of-use can be dramatically less than the cost of conventional water treatment and distribution systems. Point-of-use water treatment, such as household-based chlorination, is the most cost-effective intervention to prevent diarrhoeal disease across a wide range of countries and settings (WHO 2002; Clasen *et al.* 2007). It is also among the most cost-beneficial (Hutton *et al.* 2007). In 2003, the WHO helped organize the International Network for the Promotion of Safe Household Water Treatment and Storage, a global collaboration of UN and bilateral agencies, NGOs, research institutions, and the private sector committed to improved household water management as a component in water, sanitation, and hygiene programmes. The Network's Website contains a considerable amount of information on household water management (http://www.who.int/household_water/en).

Technologic and programmatic innovations

Efforts to improve water supplies and sanitation, particularly in rural and remote locations, have proved especially challenging. Despite concerted efforts over past decades, the situation for many has not improved dramatically (Thompson *et al.* 2001). While a variety of communal and household-level options have been promoted as alternatives to customary approaches in order to improve water quality, quantity, and proximity, some of these have been found wanting in terms of technological suitability, cost, and sustainability. New challenges include natural or man-made chemical contamination, saline intrusion, increasing urbanization, falling water tables, threats associated with climate change, and increasing demand for agricultural and industrial uses of water (Chapter 2.10). High upfront costs, lack of financing, uncertain land tenure, inadequate skilled masons for construction, pit-emptying, longer-term waste disposal, and urbanization are major challenges in sanitation.

Public health professionals, programme implementers, social entrepreneurs, and the private sector have responded to these challenges by developing and promoting a variety of technological and programmatic innovations for improving water supplies and sanitation, especially among low-income populations. In water, these include developments in rainwater harvesting, water locating, borehole drilling, well digging, locally-fabricated pumps and other water lifting devices, self-supply strategies, chemical filters, and adsorption technologies. In sanitation, communal private latrines have been promoted widely in India and elsewhere, and technologies include cheaper, lightweight squatting slabs, composting toilets, digestion chemicals, multi-chamber pits, pit-emptying, and improved separation of liquid and solid excreta. Many of these innovations are accompanied by entrepreneurial initiatives, microfinance, and base-of-the-pyramid (BOP) marketing. While some of these innovations appear promising, lessons from the past suggest that understanding and responding to the particular circumstances present in a given setting—and especially what the target population itself wants and is willing to pay for—are especially important in achieving large-scale sustainable improvements that will also impact public health.

Water and wastewater testing and microbiology

American Public Health Association (APHA), the American Water Works Association (AWWA), and the Water Environment Federation (WEF) jointly publish *Standard Methods for the Examination of Water and Wastewater*, the definitive guide for water quality testing. The twenty-first edition published in 2005 contains methods for assessing physical properties, metals, inorganic non-metallic constituents, aggregate organic constituents, individual organic compounds, radioactivity, toxicity, microbiological examination, and biological examination (APHA *et al.* 2005). Nevertheless, there are continuing debates about even fundamental issues, such as the use of indicators of faecal contamination such as coliforms, thermotolerant coliforms (TTC), and *Escherichia coli* (Gleeson & Gray 1997). The International Water Association's Health Related Water Microbiology Specialist Group is a rich source of research and new developments in the microbiology of water and waste, including water and wastewater treatment and its effects on health and the environment (including chlorinated by-products), methods in microbiology, microbe tracking and behaviour in water systems and the environment, rapid testing and monitoring, issues presented by bioterrorism, epidemiology and microbial risk assessment, and treatment processes.

Total sanitation

First developed in Bangladesh in 1999 and now expanding elsewhere, Community-Led Total Sanitation (CLTS) is an approach that empowers local communities to stop open defecation and to build and use latrines without the support of external hardware subsidies. Through the use of participatory techniques, community members analyse their own sanitation situation, including the extent of open defecation and the possibilities of faecal–oral contamination. This is designed to ignite a personal sense of disgust and shame that translates into collective action to reduce the impact of open defecation (Kar 2003). By triggering collective behaviour change, CLTS places the community, rather than the household, at the centre of the decision-making process. Peer pressure and civic pride are important motivating factors. The particular design of a latrine is secondary to the emphasis on 100 per cent coverage. The results can be impressive, with whole communities changing from open defecation to latrine use in a matter of months (Kar 2003). The approach has since been rolled out in Africa and Asia, and there is some evidence of its sustainability (Kar & Bongartz 2006).

Sanitation marketing

Sanitation marketing uses a commercial approach to the production and delivery of sanitation technologies and engages the private sector for production and delivery in a financially and institutionally sustainable manner (Jenkins & Sugden 2006). Such a marketing approach has been recommended over typical public-sector promotion of sanitation since it helps ensure that people choose to receive what they want and are willing to pay for, is financially sustainable, is cost-effective, and can be taken to scale (Cairncross 2004). Sanitation marketing adopts a consumer perspective, starting with an understanding of which products and services the target population wants, will pay for, will maintain, and are appropriate to the local context. It seeks to develop a sustainable sanitation industry which is not dependent on external donors for hardware subsidies or long-term support for its continuation. It recognizes the household as the key decision maker regarding their defecation practice and the importance of effective public private partnerships. The extent to which the approach is capable of reaching the base of the economic pyramid has not yet been shown.

Scaling up sanitation; subsidies

Recent research has begun to explore the drivers and constraints toward latrine adoption (Jenkins & Curtis 2005; Jenkins & Scott 2007). Results demonstrate that while public health and economic benefits are the main societal reasons for investing in sanitation, householders have different reasons for wanting a latrine (Table 2.5.4). Research has shown that the rate of uptake of sanitation interventions increases as information spreads from one household to another, much like the adoption curves that characterize many new innovations (Cairncross 2004; Jenkins and Curtis 2004). Householder-perceived advantages of using a latrine become apparent as housing density starts to increase and when the need for privacy, convenience, and maintaining dignity become more important.

Subsidizing latrine construction is a controversial issue within the sanitation sector. Public incentives to private individuals are justified in an economic sense when there are externalities—social benefits that go beyond the private benefits associated with a given private action (Gregersen 1984; Pardo 1990). As the public health benefits of limiting open defecation are greater than the private benefits an individual gains by choosing use of latrines over open defecation, sanitation may constitute a public good, thus justifying subsidies. However, for scaling up of sanitation to be successful, subsidies must be used to encourage householders to build and use latrines and help them overcome the constraints rather than to cover the actual costs of construction. Moreover, the public service priority needs to focus on safely and efficiently managing excreta within the larger community, especially in dense urban slums, after it has left the private domain of households (Methra & Knapp 2005; Evans *et al.* 2004). Inappropriately-applied subsidies also have the negative effects of creating dependency, distorting the behaviour of the private supply market, and perhaps most importantly, not reaching the poor.

Challenges in water and sanitation

Failure to treat diarrhoea as a serious disease

One of the threshold constraints to scaling up water and sanitation is the belief that diarrhoea—the main health threat associated with poor water and sanitation coverage—is not a disease. Figueroa and Kinkaid (2008) cite numerous studies from various countries in which participants reported diarrhoea to be a natural and even desirable condition, especially in young children, not worthy of special preventative measures. Although health benefits often lack significant motivational impetus for driving preventative measures, the fact that diarrhoea is not even considered a disease by many of the most vulnerable populations further limits this strategy. Among policy makers and health officials faced with a variety of life-threatening diseases, diarrhoea may not receive the commitment of resources that its status as the third leading cause of morbidity and mortality from infectious disease would suggest it deserves.

Despite UN and other initiatives to draw attention to the need to expand water and sanitation coverage, there is no corresponding

WATER AND SANITATION 171

Table 2.5.4 Inventory of stated benefits of improved sanitation from the private vs. public perspectives

Household perspective *	Society-public perspective **
◆ Increased comfort	◆ Reduced excreta-related disease burden (morbidity and mortality) leading to:
◆ Increased privacy	◇ Reduced public healthcare costs
◆ Increased convenience	◇ Increased economic productivity
◆ Increased safety, for women, especially at night, and for children	◆ Increased attendance by girls at school (for school sanitation) leading to broad development gains associated with female education
◆ Dignity and social status	◆ Reduced contamination of ground water and surface water resources
◆ Being modern or more urbanized	◆ Reduced environmental damage to ecosystems
◆ Cleanliness	◆ Increased safety of agricultural and food products leading to more exports
◆ Lack of smell and flies	◆ Increased nutrient recovery and reduced waste generation and disposal costs (for ecological sanitation)
◆ Less embarrassment with visitors	◆ Cleaner neighbourhoods
◆ Reduced illness and accidents	◆ Less smell and flies in public places
◆ Reduced conflict with neighbours	◆ More tourism
◆ Good health in a very broad cultural sense, often linked to disgust and avoidance of faeces	◆ National or community pride
◆ Increased property value	
◆ Increased rental income	
◆ Eased restricted mobility due to illness, old age	
◆ Reduced fertilizer costs (ecological sanitation)	
◆ Manure for crop production (ecological sanitation)	

*Compiled from the following case studies and project reports based on household interviews, surveys, and group discussions in many different settings: Jenkins (1999, 2004); Jenkins and Curtis (2005); Obika *et al.* (2002); Mukherjee (2000); Allen (2003); Ellmendorf and Buckles (1980); D'Souza (2005); WSP-EAP (2002); WSP (2004).
** Reasons for public action stated in studies and documents but rarely quantified or ranked (Evans *et al.* (2004); Jenkins and Sugden (2006)).

source of funds to meet the challenge. Roll Back Malaria, the Global Fund to Fight HIV/AIDS, Tuberculosis and Malaria, and the Presidents Emergency Plan for AIDS Relief (PEPFAR) are examples of high profile, well-financed, international campaigns against important infectious diseases. Though diarrhoea accounts for more mortality and morbidity than tuberculosis or malaria, there is no global fund or presidential initiative to address it even though it is largely preventable as evidenced by the minimal disease in middle- and high-income countries. Unless and until diarrhoea is recognized as a significant health threat rather than an embarrassing annoyance, it is not likely to attract its share of health resources.

Lack of public-sector coordination

In most countries, a variety of agencies and authorities are responsible for some part of water and sanitation. These typically include the ministries of water, health, water resources, environment, local government, rural development, and education. In many cases, there are also federal, regional, district, and local levels of government. Rarely do any of these ministries take full responsibility for all aspects of water or of sanitation. The result is often a patchwork effort that lacks funding and coordination. There are important examples of successful coordinated public sector efforts. In South Africa, strides in sanitation are occurring because of a national decision and plan which set out targets, clear strategies, significant resources, and accountability (Muller 2002). Ethiopia has also achieved considerable success in improving water and sanitation coverage, particularly in the Southern Nations, Nationalities and

Peoples Region, where a commitment at the senior levels translated into coordinated and sustained action (Bibby & Knapp 2007).

Bias toward large, infrastructural solutions

Public-sector advocacy, funding, and support has been shown to be an important factor in the successful scaling up of oral rehydration salts, insecticide-treated nets, and other interventions directed at environmental health. To date, however, governmental support for community and household-based water and sanitation interventions programmes has not been extensive in most countries. This is due in part to the engineering orientation of the applicable ministries, and their emphasis on larger-scale, infrastructural improvements, especially in urban and peri-urban settings. Nearly all populations who do not enjoy piped-in water on a 24–7 basis express priority for increasing the quantity and access to water over improving its quality. Governments respond accordingly, aware not only of the political value from these popular projects (and the particularly photogenic value of water emerging from massive new pipes), but also the economic gains that are available from reducing the time people spend collecting and transporting water to their homes and from the productive use of water in agricultural activities. Multilateral and bilateral funding also tends to focus on such infrastructural water projects, despite compelling evidence that HWTS is more cost beneficial and highly cost-effective (Hutton *et al.* 2007; Clasen *et al.* 2007).

The term 'sanitation' is not only vague; it is often used interchangeably with the term 'sewerage'. Sewerage refers to a system of sewers that convey wastewater to a treatment plant and as such is depended on the provision, operation, and maintenance of an infrastructure of pipes, pumps, and screens. If working correctly, sewerage systems separate humans from their faeces, and is therefore a form of sanitation. But sewers are not the only form, and arguably not the most important with regard to increasing sanitation coverage in Africa. In Dar es Salaam, Kampala, and other African cities, 70 per cent of the population are served by pit latrines and only 10–12 per cent by the sewer system, despite heavy investment in the latter. This proportion is unlikely to increase over the coming years as cities are rapidly growing and sewerage systems are very expensive. Even so, Ministries of Water are often mainly interested in sewer systems and ignore on-site solutions. As the poor often cannot afford to connect to sewer systems, and the households served by the rehabilitated sewers already had access to sanitation, the net impact of the investment on the MDGs, health, and poverty reduction is limited. The funding allocated to low-cost, low-technology excreta management solutions used by the vast majority of the world's poor is comparatively low. The consequence of the bias towards sewer solutions is to direct resources away from the poor.

Uncertainty about the role of the private sector

Water and sanitation have traditionally been supplied by the public sector, particularly in Europe and North America where coverage, service levels, and costs are optimal. As governments, particularly in lower-income settings, have been unable to deliver services such as power, transportation, and even health and education to much of the population, they are increasingly relying on the private sector to provide such services. There are some apparent success stories where the private sector, through concessions, public–private partnerships, or other vehicles, enhance the coverage and service level of water and sanitation though increased investment and improved management of fee collection and delivery. At the same time, there are at least some notorious cases, such as Cochabamba, Bolivia, where a concession was opposed due to the perception at least that the private sector partners were putting profits ahead of performance. There is certainly a need for regulation, as these services are usually a natural monopoly and market forces, if left unchecked, will favour delivery to higher-density and higher income areas where paybacks are faster and costs/risks lower. The United Nations Development Programme (UNDP), World Bank, and others have examined the constructive role that the private sector can play in helping scale up the delivery of water and sanitation services (UNDP 2007). Balancing the potential contribution of the private sector against the needs of the target population will continue to represent a significant challenge for policy makers.

Decoupling sanitation from water

Since the 1990s, there has been an effort to always integrate water supply, sanitation, and hygiene promotion in developing countries within the same project. As a result, sanitation and hygiene have piggy backed on the political and community demand for improved water supplies. However, many effective interventions to improve excreta disposal do not require improvements in water supplies. While the water supply sector is dominated by engineers who lean towards technical solutions, sanitation and hygiene promotion rely more heavily on understanding and changing behaviour, a different set of skills. As a result, staff in integrated projects naturally

concentrate on water supplies, whilst excreta disposal fails to receive the resources it requires. The sanitation element is usually built around the process of providing the water supply; in fact, sanitation differs in that it requires a household rather than a community decision, requires more time, and is more complex from a behaviour change perspective. By decoupling sanitation from water, it may be possible to increase coverage more rapidly, particularly in remote areas in which water interventions are unlikely to reach in the near future.

Excreta disposal in urban unplanned areas

While urban areas generally have higher rates of sanitation than rural areas, the rapid growth of informal settlements and urban slums presents a particular challenge for sanitation (WHO/UNICEF 2006). The lack of planning controls can result in ever increasing housing densities as plots are divided and subdivided either to house expanding extended families or to increase rental income. Eventually the area becomes saturated. This complicates excreta management in two ways: (i) streets and passages become very narrow making it impassable for latrine- and septic-emptying vehicles, and (ii) the space available in each compound is insufficient to build initial or replacement latrines.

Another important and sensitive question with urban sanitation is the divide between public and private responsibility. Public funds are used to install, manage, and maintain public sewers and tariffs or taxation used to recover costs. No such publicly funded services are provided for the poor living in the unplanned high density areas, and excreta disposal is regarded as being the sole responsibility of the household. It is arguable that the public health benefits from providing an appropriate pit emptying service could be so great that it warrants total public funding and provided free of charge to the poor.

Conflicting objectives in sanitation

Sanitation projects usually aim for a combination of four often-conflicting objectives. The first is to build a large number of latrines in a relatively short time, driven in part by the MDGs or national targets. In such cases, projects often use a supply-driven approach that coerces, entices, or persuades householders to build latrines by providing a generous subsidy, normally in the form of free hardware and/or labour. But when funding ends, the delivery and support mechanisms dissolve and the community members are left, as they started, with a lack of latrine component supply chains and nowhere to turn to for support. The second objective is to develop a sustainable sanitation industry that can continue providing latrines for many generations to come. This requires a good understanding of demand, the motivations and constraints of households in building and using latrines and the use of marketing techniques to develop, promote and supply better latrine components. This is a longer-term process which will not result in large number of latrines being built in a short period of time and is therefore not attractive to politicians, donors, government officials, and implementers wanting instant MDG-driven solutions and to be seen to be doing something. The third objective driving sanitation is to enhance sustainable livelihoods and environmental improvements. This can be achieved by taking an ecological sanitation approach to latrine building which ensures that the nutrients in the excreta are reused to grow crops. The fourth objective is organizational insistence that their work must be targeted at the poorest of the poor. These are the most risk adverse, hardest to reach, price sensitive members of the population who are also likely to be the least well educated and socially or politically connected. This makes them the least likely people to benefit from either a supply- or a demand-driven approach. While a targeted, sustainable, demand-driven, livelihood-enhancing latrine building programme that builds a large number of latrines in a short period of time is the ideal, decision makers need to understand the weaknesses of each approach and prioritize their expectations accordingly.

Conclusion

Unlike many of the other challenges in public health, the solutions for eliminating most of the disease burden associated with poor water and sanitation are well known. All but the poor have enjoyed the health, economic, and other benefits associated with safe drinking water and basic sanitation for decades. The fact that hundreds of millions still lack access to these fundamental resources is a scandal that generations have allowed to persist simply as a matter of misguided priorities. And as the 'haves' continue to make rapid gains, they are not only increasing the gap over the 'have-nots' but also using up larger amounts of the world's limited water supplies and capacity for waste disposal, making it more difficult and costly for others to join their privileged club.

The need to extend water and sanitation coverage is acknowledged at the highest international levels, and progress is being made. Whether these efforts will be any more successful than those expressed in previous international declarations and goals is not yet clear. As the poor continue to wait for the piped-in water supplies and sanitary disposal that they deserve, however, it is incumbent on the public health community to develop, assess, and promote effective, low-cost, and sustainable alternatives and creative delivery strategies in order to accelerate access to the health gains associated with safe drinking water and basic sanitation.

Key points

- While safe drinking water and sanitation are widely recognized as fundamental public health interventions, more than a sixth of the world's population still lack improved water supplies and 40 per cent lack basic sanitation.

- The infectious diseases associated with unsafe drinking water and poor sanitation impose a heavy burden, especially on the poor, the very young and the immuno-compromised; they also aggravate poverty, education, and economic development.

- There is strong evidence that interventions to improve water supplies or sanitation can be effective in preventing diarrhoea, soil-transmitted helminth infections, schistosomiasis, and typhoid fevers.

- Water and sanitation interventions have also been shown to be cost-effective and cost-beneficial, with significant savings to the public sector from reduced healthcare costs; there is also evidence of other economic and developmental benefits from improved access to water and sanitation.

- A variety of recent and emerging developments, including new methods for assessing and monitoring the risk of diseases associated with water and sanitation as well as alternative technologies, programmatic approaches, and implementation strategies, may contribute to improved targeting, coverage, uptake, and sustainability.

- Nevertheless, significant political, social, economic, and developmental challenges must be addressed in order to successfully scale up some of these interventions on a sustainable basis and thus provide the most vulnerable populations with the health and other benefits of safe drinking water and sanitation.

References

Allan, S.C. (2003). *The WaterAid Bangladesh / VERC 100% sanitation approach: Bangladesh*. IDS Working Paper 194. Institute of Development Studies, Brighton, Sussex.

APHA (2005). *Standard methods for the examination of water and wastewater*, 21st edition. American Public Health Association, the American Water Works Association (AWWA) and the Water Environment Federation (WEF), Washington, DC.

Bannister, M., Hannan, M.D., Jones, H. *et al.* (2005). *Water and sanitation for all: Practical ways to improve accessibility for disabled people*. 31st WEDC Conference, Maximising the benefits from water and environmental sanitation. Kampala, Uganda.

Barreto, M.L., Genser, B., Strina, A. *et al.* (2007). Effect of city-wide sanitation programme on reduction in rate of childhood diarrhoea in northeast Brazil: Assessment by two cohort studies. Lancet, **370**(9599), 1622–8.

Bartram, J. (2003). New water forum will repeat old message. *Bulletin of the World Health Organization*, **83**, 158.

Bharadwaj, S. and Patkar, A. (2004). *Menstrual hygiene and management in developing countries: Taking stock*. Junction Social, Social Development Consultants.

Bibby, S. and Knapp, A. (2007). *From burden to communal responsibility: A sanitation success story from southern region in Ethiopia*. Field Note. Washington: World Bank Water and Sanitation Programme.

Black, R.E. and Lanata, C.F. (1995). Epidemiology of diarrhoeal diseases in developing countries. In (eds. M.J. Blaser, P.D. Smith, J.I. Ravdin, H.B. Greenberg, and R.L. Guerrant) *Infections of the gastrointestinal tract*. Raven Press, New York.

Black, R.E., Morris, S.S. and Bryce, J. (2003). Where and why are 10 million children dying every year? *Lancet*, **361**, 2226–34.

Blakely, T., Hales, S., Kieft, C. *et al.* (2005). The global distribution of risk factors by poverty level. *Bulletin of the World Health Organization*, **83**, 118–126.

Blum, D. and Feachem, R.G. (1983). Measuring the impact of water supply and sanitation investments on diarrhoeal diseases: Problems in methodology. *International Journal of Epidemiology*, **12**, 357–65.

Cairncross, S. (1987). The benefits of water supply, In (ed. J. Pickford) *Developing world water*. Grosvenor Press, London.

Cairncross, S. (1992). *Sanitation and water supply: Practical lessons from the decade*. The World Bank, Washington DC.

Cairncross, S. (2004). *The case for marketing sanitation*. Field Note. Nairobi: Water and Sanitation Programme Africa.

Cairncross, S. and Feachem, R. (1993). *Environmental health engineering in the tropics: An introductory text*, 2nd edition). John Wiley & Sons Ltd., Chichester, West Sussex.

Cairncross, S., Muller, R., and Zagaria, N. (2002). Dracunculiasis (Guinea Worm Disease) and the eradication initiative. *Clinical Microbiology Reviews*, **15**, 223–46.

Cairncross, S. and Valdmanis, V. (2006). Water supply, sanitation and hygiene promotion. In (eds. D.T. Jamison, J.G. Breman, A.R. Measham *et al.*) *Disease control priorities in developing countries*, pp. 771–92, The World Bank, Washington DC.

Chandler (1954). A comparison of helminthic and protozoan infections in two Egyptian villages two years after the installation of sanitary improvements in one of them. *The American Journal of Tropical Medicine and Hygiene*, **3**, 59–73.

Chen, G., Wang, M.H.S., Ou, N. *et al.* (2004). Observation on the effect of the comprehensive measures of replacing cattle with machine and reconstructing water supply and lavatory to control the transmission of schistosomiasis. *Journal of Tropical Disease & Parasitology*, **2**, 219–22.

Clasen, T., Bostoen, K., Boisson, S. *et al.* (2008). *Improved excreta disposal for the prevention of diarrhoea, helminth infections and trachoma: A systematic review* (submitted).

Clasen, T., Do Hoang, T., Boisson, S. *et al.* (2008). Lessons in household water treatment from a cross-sectional study in rural Vietnam. *Environmental science & technology* (in press).

Clasen. T., Haller, L., Walker, D. *et al.* (2007). Cost-effectiveness analysis of water quality interventions for preventing diarrhoeal disease in developing countries. *Journal of Water and Health*, **5** (4), 599–608.

Clasen, T., Roberts, I., Rabie, T. *et al.* (2006). *Interventions to improve water quality for preventing diarrhoea (Cochrane Review)*. In The Cochrane Library, Issue 3, 2006. Update Software, Oxford.

Colford, J.M. Jr, Saha, S.R., Wade, T.J. *et al.* (2005). A pilot randomized, controlled trial of an in-home drinking water intervention among HIV + persons. *Journal of Water and Health*, **3** (2), 173–84.

Colford, J.M., Rees, J.R., Wade, T.J. *et al.* (2002). Participant blinding and gastrointestinal illness in a randomized, controlled trial of an in-home drinking water intervention. *Emerging Infectious Diseases*, **8**, 29–36.

Colindres, R., Mermin, J., Ezati, E. *et al.* (2007). Utilization of a basic care and prevention package by HIV-infected persons in Uganda. *AIDS Care*, **24**, 1–7.

Crump, J.A., Luby, S.P., and Mintz, E.D. (2004). The global burden of typhoid fever. *Bulletin of the World Health Organization*, **82**, 346–53.

Curtis, V. and Cairncross, S. (2003). Effect of washing hands with soap on diarrhoea risk in the community: A systematic review. The *Lancet Infectious Diseases*, **3**, 275–81.

Cutler, D. and Miller, G. (2005). The role of public health improvements in health advances: The twentieth-century United States. *Demography*, **42** (1), 1–22.

Davis, J. and Lambert, R. (2002). *Engineering in emergencies*. Intermediate Technology Publications, Ltd., London.

DFID (1998). *Guidance manual on water supply and sanitation programmes*. UK Department of International Development, London.

deSilva, N.R., Brooker, S., Hotez, P.J. *et al.* (2003). Soil-transmitted helminth infections: Updating the global picture. *Trends in Parasitology*, **19**, 547–51.

Eisenberg, J.N., Scott, J.C., and Porco, T. (2007). Integrating disease control strategies: Balancing water sanitation and hygiene interventions to reduce diarrheal disease burden. *American journal of Public Health*, **97** (5), 846–52.

Ejere, H., Alhassan, M.B., and Rabiu, M. (2004). *Face washing promotion for preventing active trachoma*. The Cochrane Database of System Reviews 2004, Issue 3.

Emerson, P.M., Bailey, R.L., and Mahdi, O.S. (2000). Transmission ecology of the fly *Musoca sorbens*, a putative vector of trachoma. *Transactions of the Royal Society of Tropical Medicine and Hygiene*, **94**, 1–5.

Emerson, P.M., Cairncross, S., Bailey, R.L. *et al.* (2000a). Review of the eidenc ebase fo the 'F' and 'E' component of the SAFE strategy for trachoma control. *Tropical medicine & international health*, **5** (8), 515–27.

Emerson, P.M., Lindsay, S.W., Alexander, N. *et al.* (2004). Role of flies and provision of latrines in trachoma control: Cluster-randomised controlled trial. *Lancet*, **363** (9415), 1093–8.

Ensink, J.H. and van der Hoek, W. (2007). New international guidelines for wastewater use in agriculture. *Tropical Medicine & International Health*, **12** (5), 575–7.

Esrey, S.A. and Habicht, J-P. (1986). Epidemiologic evidence for health benefits from improved water and sanitation in developing countries. *Epidemiologic Reviews*, **8**, 117–28.

Esrey, S.A., Feachem, R.G., and Hughes, J.M. (1985). Interventions for the control of diarrhoeal diseases among young children: Improving water supplies and excreta disposal facilities. *Bulletin of the World Health Organization*, **64**, 776–72.

Esrey, S.A., Potash, J.B., Roberts, L. *et al.* (1991). Effects of improved water supply and sanitation on ascariasis, diarrhoea, dracunculiasis, hookworm infection, schistosomiasis, and tracoma. *Bulletin of the World Health Organization*, **69**, 609–21.

Evans, B., Hutton, G., and Haller, L. (2004). *Closing the sanitation gap—the case for better public funding of sanitation and hygiene*. Commission on Sustainable Development, Oslo.

Ferriman, A. (2007). BMJ readers choose the "sanitary revolution" as greatest medical advance since 1840. *British Medical Journal*, **334**, 111.

Fewtrell, L., Kaufmann, R., Kay, D. *et al.* (2005). Water, sanitation, and hygiene interventions to reduce diarrhoea in less developed countries: a systematic review and meta-analysis. *The Lancet Infectious Diseases*, **5**, 42–52.

Fewtrell, L., Pruss-Ustun, A. Bos, R. *et al.* (2007). *Water, sanitation and hygiene—quantifying the health impact at national and local levels in countries with incomplete water supply and sanitation coverage*. Environmental Burden of Disease series No. 15. World Health Organization, Geneva.

Figueroa, M.E. and Kincaid, D.L. (2008). Social, cultural and behavioral correlates of household water treatment and storage. World Health Organisation Geneva (in press).

Gleeson, C. and Gray, N. (1997). *The Coliform Index and waterborne disease*. E & FN Spon, London.

Gryssels, B., Polman, K., Clerinx, J. *et al.* (2006). Human schistosomiasis. *Lancet*, **368**, 1106–18.

Guerrant, D.I., Moore, S.R., Lima, A.A.M. *et al.* (1999). Association of early childhood diarrhoea and cryptosporidiosis with impaired physical fitness and cognitive function four-seven years later in a poor urban community in Northeast Brazil. *The American Journal of Tropical Medicine and Hygiene*, **61**, 707–13.

Gundry, S., Wright, J., and Conroy, R. (2003). A systematic review of the health outcomes related to household water quality in developing countries. *Journal of Water and Health*, **2** (1), 1–13.

Haas, C.N., Rose, J.B., and Gerba, C.P. (1999). *Quantitative microbial risk assessment*. John Wiley & Sons, New York.

Hayes, C., Elliot, E., Krales, E. *et al.* (2003). Food and water safety for persons infected with human immunodeficiency virus. *Clinical Infectious Diseases*, **36**(Suppl 2), S106–9.

Hotez, P., Brooker, S., Bethony, J. *et al.* (2004). Hookworm infection. *The New England Journal of Medicine*, **351**, 799–807.

Hotez, P.J., Bundy, D.A.P., Beegle, K. *et al.* (2006). Helminth infections: Soil-transmitted helminth infections and schistosomiasis. In (eds. B.D.T. Jamison, A.R. Measham, C *et al.*) *Disease control priorities in developing countries*, 2nd edition, pp. 467–97. Oxford University Press.

Hunter, P.R. (1997). *Waterborne disease epidemiology and ecology*. John Wiley & Sons, Chichester.

Hutton, G. and Bartram, J. (2003). *Domestic water quantity, service level and health*. World Health Organization, Geneva.

Hutton, G., Haller, L., and Bartram, J. (2007). Global cost-benefit analysis of water supply and sanitation interventions. *Journal of Water and Health*, **5** (4), 481–502.

IRC Water and Sanitation Centre (2006). Girl friendly toilets for school girls. (downloaded from http://www.schools.watsan.net/page/319).

Jackson, B. (2005). *A review of EcoSan experience in Eastern and Southern Africa*. Field Note. Washington: World Bank Water and Sanitation Programme.

Jenkins, M.W. and Curtis, V. (2005). Achieving the "good life"; why some people want latrines in rural Benin. *Social Science & Medicine,* **61,** 2446–59.

Jenkins, M.W. and Scott, B. (2007). Behavioral indicators of household decision-making and demand for sanitation and potential gains from social marketing in Ghana. *Social Science & Medicine,* **64** (12), 2427–42.

Jenkins, M.W. and Sugden, S. (2006). *Rethinking sanitation—Lessons and innovation for sustainability and success in the New Millennium.* UNDP HDR2006, Sanitation Thematic Paper, London School of Hygiene and Tropical Medicine.

Kosek, M., Bern, C., and Guerrant, R.L. (2003). The global burden of diarrhoeal disease, as estimated from studies published between 1992 and 2000. *Bulletin of the World Health Organization,* **81,** 197–204.

Kar, K. (2003). *Subsidy or self-respect? Participatory total community sanitation in Bangladesh.* IDS Working Paper 194. Institute of Development Studies, Brighton, Sussex, UK.

Kar, K. and Bongartz, J. (2006). Update on some recent developments in community-led total sanitation. Institute of Development Studies, Brighton, Sussex, UK.

Kuper, H., Solomon, A.W., Buchan, J. *et al.* (2003). A critical review of the SAFE strategy for the prevention of blinding trachoma. *The Lancet Infectious Diseases,* **3**(6), 372–81.

Kumaresan, J. and Mecaskey, J. (2003). The global elimination of blinding trachoma: Progress and promise. *The American Journal of Tropical Medicine and Hygiene,* **69,** 24–28.

Leclerc, H., Schwartzbrod, L., and Dei-Cas, E. (2002). Microbial agents associated with waterborne diseases. *Critical Reviews in Microbiology,* **28** (4), 371–409.

Lule, J.R., Mermin, J., Ekwaru, J.P. *et al.* (2005). Effect of home-based chlorination and safe storage on diarrhea among person with HIV in Uganda. *Tropical Medicine and International Health,* **73,** 926–33.

Mabey, D.C., Solomon, A.W., and Foster, A. (2003). Trachoma. *Lancet,* **362**(9379), 223–9.

Mackenbach, J. (2007). Sanitation: Pragmatism works. *British Medical Journal,* **6334** (Suppl 1), s17.

Maili Saba Research Report (2005). Livelihood and gender in sanitation and hygiene water services among urban poor.

Maybe, D., Solomon, A.W., and Foster, A. (2003). Trachoma. *Lancet,* **362,** 223–9.

Methra, M. and Knapp, A. (2005). *The challenge of financing sanitation for meeting the millennium development goals.* Commissioned by the Norwegien Ministry of the Environment for the Commission on Sustainable Development. Water and Sanitation Program—Africa. The World Bank, Nairobi, Kenya.

Messou, E., Sangare, S.V., Josseran, R. *et al.* (1997). Effect of hygiene measures, water sanitation and oral rehydration therapy on diarrhea in children less than five years old in the south of Ivory Coast. *Bulletin de la Société de pathologie exotique,* **90** (1), 44–7.

Morris, S.S., Cousens, S.N., Kirkwood, B.R. *et al.* (1996). Is prevalence of diarrhoea a better predictor of subsequent mortality and weight gain than diarrhea incidence? *American Journal of Epidemiology,* **144,** 582–8.

Moy, R.J.D., Booth, I.W., McNeish, A.S. *et al.* (1991). Definitions of diarrhoea. *Journal of Diarrhoeal Diseases,* **9** (4), 335.

Mukherjee, N. (2000). *Myth vs. reality in sanitation and hygiene promotion.* Field Note, Jakarta: World Bank Water and Sanitation Programme—East Asia and the Pacific.

Muller, M. (2002). *The National Water and Sanitation Programme in South Africa.* Field Note, Water and Sanitation Program—Africa: The World Bank, Nairobi, Kenya.

Obika, A., Jenkins, M., Howard, G. *et al.* (2002). *Social marketing for urban sanitation, Inception Report.* DFID KAR Project R7982. WEDC, Loughborough, UK.

Prüss-Üstün, A. and Corvalán, C. (2007). *Preventing disease through healthy environments: Towards an estimate of the environmental burden of disease.* World Health Organization, Geneva.

Rabiu, M., Alhassan, M., and Ejere, H. (2007). *Environmental sanitary interventions for preventing active trachoma.* Cochrane Database of Systematic Reviews 2007, Issue 4.

Ram, P.K., Naheed, A., Brooks, W.A. *et al.* (2007). Risk factors for typhoid fever in a slum in Dhaka, Bangladesh. *Epidemiology and Infection,* **135** (3), 458–65.

Rubenstein, A., Boyle, J., Odoroff, C.L. *et al.* (1969). "Effect of improved sanitary facilities on infant diarrhea in a Hopi village." *Public Health Reports,* **84** (12), 1093–7.

Schmidt, W.P., Luby, S.P., Genser, B. *et al.* (2007). Estimating the longitudinal prevalence of diarrhea and other episodic diseases: continuous versus intermittent surveillance. *Epidemiology,* **18** (5), 537–43.

Smith, P.G. and Morrow, R.H. (1996). *Field trials of health interventions in developing dountries: A Toolbox.* (2nd edition) Macmillan Education Ltd., London.

Sobsey, M.D. (2002). *Managing water in the home: Accelerated health gains from improved water supply.* The World Health Organization (WHO/SDE/WSH/02.07), Geneva.

Sphere Project (2004). *Humanitarian Charter and minimum standards in disaster response.* The Sphere Project, Geneva.

Srikantiah, P., Vafokulov, S., Luby, S.P. *et al.* (2007). Epidemiology and risk factors for endemic typhoid fever in Uzbekistan. *Tropical Medicine and International Health,* **12** (7), 838–47.

Stephenson, L.S., Latham, M.S., and Ottensen, E.A. (2000). Malnutrition and parasitic helminth infections. *Parasitology,* **121,** S23–38.

Thompson, J., Porras, I.T., Tumwine, J.K. *et al.* (2001). *Drawers of Water II: 30 years of change in domestic water use and environmental health in East Africa.* IIED, London.

Thylefors, B., Negrel, A.D., and Dadzie, K.Y. (1995). Global data on blindness. *Bulletin of the World Health Organization,* **73,** 115–21.

UN Millennium Project (2005). *UN millennium project task force on water and sanitation—Health, dignity and development: what will it take?* Earthscan, London.

UNDP (2007). *Beyond scarcity: Power, poverty and the global water crisis.* United Nations Development Programme: Human Development Report 2006.

United Nations (2000). United Nations Millennial Declaration. General Assembly Res. 55/2 (18 September 2000).

United Nations (2002). United Nations Committee on Economic, Cultural and Social Rights, General Comment 15, 27 November 2002.

Van Derslice, J. and Briscoe, J. (1995). Environmental interventions in developing countries: Interactions and their implications. *American Journal of Epidemiology,* **141,** 135–44.

Wagner, E.G. and Lanois, J.N.(1958). *Excreta disposal for rural areas and small communities.* WHO monograph series NO.39. WHO, Geneva.

White, G.F., Bradley, D.J., and White, A.U. (1972). *Drawers of water: Domestic water use in East Africa.* University of Chicago Press, Chicago.

Whittington, D. and Briscoe, J. (1990). Estimating the willingness to pay for water services in developing countries: A case study of the use of contingent valuation surveys in Southern Haiti. *Economic Development. & Cultural Change,* **38** (2), 293–311.

Whittington, D., Pattanayak, S., Yang, J-C. *et al.* (2002). Household demand for improved piped water services in Kathmandu, Nepal. *Water Policy.* **4** (6), 531–56.

WHO (1993). *The management and prevention of diarrhoea: Practical guidelines,* 3rd edition. World Health Organization, Geneva.

WHO (2004). *Guidelines for drinking-water quality,* Vol. 1, 3rd edition. World Health Organization, Geneva.

WHO (2005). *Progress towards the millennium development goals, 1990–2005.* World Health Organization, Geneva.

WHO (2006). *Guidelines for the safe use of wastewater, excreta and greywater,* Vols. 1–4. World Health Organization, Geneva.

WHO/UNICEF (2002). *Global water supply and sanitation assessment.* The World Health Organization and the United Nations Children's Fund, Geneva.

WHO/UNICEF (2005). *Water for life: Decade for action 2005–2015.* World Health Organization and United Nations Children's Fund Joint Monitoring Program, Geneva.

WHO/UNICEF (2006). *Meeting the MDG drinking water and sanitation target: The urban and rural challenge of the decade.* The World Health Organization and the United Nations Children's Fund, Geneva.

Winblad, U. and Simpson-Hébert, M. (eds.), (2004): *Ecological sanitation.* Stockholm Environmental Institute.

Witter, S., Ensor, T., Jowett, M. *et al.* (2000). *Health economics for developing countries.* Macmillan Education Ltd., London.

WRI (2007). Water Resources Institute. EarthTrends Environmental Resource Portal (downloaded from http://earthtrends.wri.org/text/water-resources/variable-10.html).

Wright, J., Gundry, S., Conroy (2003). Household drinking water in developing countries: A systematic review of microbiological contamination between source and point-of-use. *Tropical Medicine and International Health,* **9** (1), 106–17.

WSP-EAP (2002). *Selling sanitation in Vietnam: What works?* Jakarta: World Bank Water and Sanitation Program—East Asia and the Pacific.

Zhang, S-Q, Wang, T-P, Tao, C-G *et al.* (2005). Observation on comprehensive measures of safe treatment of night-soil and water supply, replacement of bovine with machine for schistosomiasis control. *Zhongguo Xue Xi Chong Bing Fang Ji Za Zhi* [*Chinese Journal of Schistosomiasis Control*], **17** (6), 437–42.

Zhang, W-P, Liu, M-X., Yin, W-H. *et al.* (2000). Evaluation of a long-term effect on improving drinking water and lavatories in rural areas for prevention of diseases. *Ji Bing Kong Ji Za Zhi* [*Chinese Journal of Disease Control & Prevention*], **4** (1), 76–8.

2.6

Food and nutrition

Prakash S. Shetty

Introduction

Food and nutrition are important determinants of a wide range of diseases of public health importance worldwide. Nutrition is a broad and complex subject which includes nutrient–gene interactions and the induction of such diseases as diabetes mellitus, coronary heart disease, and cancer and to conditions like impaired brain development. Nutrition also deals with the social, economic, and cultural issues related to making the right food choices, purchasing and eating the 'correct' types of food and in the 'appropriate' quantities as well as the factors that determine daily human activity and behaviour related to food. Thus, just as our gradual acquisition of the knowledge of microbiology influenced our understanding of infectious diseases, which in turn led to preventive measures for the population, so the historical advances in the field of nutrition have led to a more coherent understanding of the patterns of and the prevention of diet-related diseases of public health importance throughout the world.

Fluctuations in disease rates depend on environmental factors which include food and nutrition as one of the primary determinants. In the developing world, numerous deficiency diseases persist, which are the result of nutrient deficiencies in the daily diet. These now coexist with the increasing incidence of diet-related chronic diseases, which are typical of industrialized and economically developed countries. Thus developing societies now bear the 'double burden' of malnutrition with the emergence of the so called 'diseases of affluence' amidst persisting under-nutrition in their populations.

Significant changes in the patterns of disease and the causes of premature death within a population have little to do with advances in curative medicine and therapeutics. The changes in health depend largely on the environmental changes which include changes in social and economic conditions, the implementation of immunization programmes, improvements in women's social and educational status within the society, and changes in agriculture and food systems and in the availability of food. These changes have, in turn, been influenced in recent times by globalization and the increasing global trade and the social and cultural interactions that affect agricultural practices, the food systems, and the industrial and manufacturing sector and affect individual diets and lifestyles. National policies that seek to promote principally economic activity and international trade to boost foreign exchange earnings ignore the impact of these measures on the health of the populations.

Most of the beneficial environmental influences on the other hand, operate through changes in the provision and access to hygienic and nutritious food; the availability of potable water, clean housing, sanitary surroundings, and lack of exposure to environmental toxins. Economic development is normally accompanied by improvements in the quantity and quality of a nation's food supply and improvements in the immediate environment and living standards of the community. These changes contribute to a nutritionally mediated improvement in the body's resistance to infections and the mutual interdependence of the immune and nutritional state of the population probably explains at least some of the gains in public health in Britain in the last century (McKeown 1976).

The quantitative and qualitative changes in our food patterns that lead to such dramatic changes in life expectancy also result in the problems of diet-related chronic diseases, but these are not inevitable. Diet-related chronic diseases occur typically in middle and later adult life and can by increasing the incidence of premature mortality undermine the gains in life expectancy. More importantly they lead to morbidity and the resultant disability adjusted life years lost as well as contributing to economic losses and reducing the quality of life. These diet-related chronic diseases are traditionally regarded as manifestations of overconsumption and self-indulgence in an affluent society. In practice, some of these chronic diseases may be compounded by relatively deficient intakes of some nutrients thus emphasizing the need for a diversified and balanced daily diet for good health.

Nutrition has re-emerged as of fundamental importance in public health. Nutritional issues were seen in industrialized and developed societies as relating to deficiency diseases which were conquered in the early part of the twentieth century while continuing to persist in the relatively poor, developing countries. Now, however, food and nutrition are recognized as one of the principal environmental determinants of a wide range of diseases of public health importance throughout the world. These diseases reflect the cumulative impact of a variety of pathophysiological processes over a lifetime and the interactions are often seen as reflecting individual genetic susceptibility, but the different disease patterns of groups living on different diets being manifestly a societal reflection of the impact of dietary factors. The display of nutrient–gene interactions is evident, for example, in obesity, alcoholism, cardiovascular disease, non-insulin dependent diabetes mellitus, many gastrointestinal disorders, neural tube defects, and the most prevalent cancers.

As molecular epidemiology unravels the basis for genetic susceptibility to these disorders, physicians interested in metabolic medicine eventually look for the gene inducers or repressors which then prove to be of dietary or environmental origin. Societal features which determine human behaviour and economic well-being as well as climate, tradition, culture, and the role of women, all affect food patterns and dietary practices. These are the features which need to be recognized when considering public health rather than simply the epidemiological aspects of dietary disease. This chapter seeks to take a global view of food and nutrition in public health terms and so nutritional deficiency disorders as well as other diet related diseases of public health importance would be considered. This is particularly important because deficiency diseases are widespread in several parts of the world and yet coexist in the same country with chronic adult diseases usually found in affluent, developed societies. Vitamin deficiencies, both clinical and subclinical continue to manifest in poor communities as well as in apparently healthy populations. Threat of hunger and starvation and severe dietary inadequacy resulting in malnutrition often emerges during conflict and other man-made emergencies. The chapter is structured in such a way that it deals with both sides of the 'mal' nutrition in humans.

Hunger and malnutrition

The pre-eminent determinant of hunger or household food insecurity is poverty in societies. The recognition that poverty and hunger go hand in hand is manifest in the UN's Millennium Development Goal 1 (MDG 1), which specifies targets for the reduction of both global poverty and hunger by the year 2015. Improving household food security is one of the stated objectives of all democratic societies and constitutes an important element of the human right to adequate food. *Food security* is defined as the access by all people at all times to the food they need for an active and healthy life. The inclusion of the term household ensures that the dietary needs of all the members of the household are met throughout the year. The achievement of household food security requires an adequate supply of food to all members of the household, ensuring stability of supply all year round, and the access, both physical and economic, which underlines the importance of the entitlement to produce and procure food. Food insecurity exists when individuals lack access to sufficient amounts of safe and nutritious food and, therefore, are not consuming enough for an active and healthy life. This situation may be a result of the unavailability of food, inadequate purchasing power, or inappropriate utilization of food at the household or individual level. Thus food security at the household level is a complex phenomenon attributable to a range of factors that vary in importance across regions, countries, and social groups, as well as over time (Shetty 2006). It is described in terms of the availability and stability of good quality, safe and nutritious food supplies, and the access to, and utilization of, this food. All these criteria must be met for the consumption of a healthy diet and the achievement of nutritional well-being.

Availability relates to the adequacy of a varied and nutritious food supply and is influenced principally by factors that promote agricultural production and trade. Issues that influence these factors include policies and incentives, access to natural resources, and the availability of agricultural inputs, skills, and technologies including biotechnology. Stability of the level and types of foods available for

consumption is subject to seasonality and by the sustainability of the production and farming systems in practice. These factors, in turn, depend on the efficiency of market systems, including pricing mechanisms and infrastructure such as transport and warehousing, which influences the distribution and flow of food. While reduction of food losses through improvements in food storage and processing also affect stability, the nature of the farming system adopted and its effect on the environment and on sustainability is also a key determinant of the stability of food supplies in the medium- to long term.

Access that a community, household, or individual has to food is a reflection of the ability to either grow and retain the food grown for consumption, to purchase the food from the market, or to acquire it by a combination of strategies that Amartya Sen (1981) has described as representing 'entitlements' to food. This system depends on a range of factors such as: Access to resources such as land, water, agricultural inputs, and improved technologies; the nature of the food marketing system and the infrastructure to support it; purchasing power and food prices; consumer perceptions, behaviour, and preferences. Utilization is more concerned with the biological availability of the food after it has been ingested. While age, body size, and physical activity levels influence food utilization, the absence of disease and parasitic infestations also influences the utilization of nutrients by the body. As a consequence, utilization of food is largely influenced by factors such as health, clean water, and good sanitation.

The causes of malnutrition on the other hand are multi-dimensional and its determinants include both food and non-food related factors, which often interact to form a complex web of biological, socioeconomic, cultural, and environmental deprivations. Although establishing a relationship between these variables, and the indicators of malnutrition do not necessarily imply causality, they do demonstrate that in addition to food availability many social, cultural, health, and environmental factors influence the prevalence of malnutrition. Although, in general, people suffering from inadequacy of food are poor, not all the poor are undernourished. Even in households that are food secure, some members may be undernourished. Income fluctuations, seasonal disparities in food availability, and demand for high levels of physical activity, and proximity and access to marketing facilities may singly or in combination influence the nutritional status of an individual or a household. For example, the transition from subsistence farming to commercial agriculture and cash crops may help improve nutrition in the long run, however, they may result in negative impacts over the short term unless accompanied by improvements in access to health services, environmental sanitation, and other social investments. Rapid urbanization and rural to urban migration may lead to nutritional deprivation of segments of society. Cultural attitudes reflected in food preferences and food preparation practices, and women's time constraints including that available for child-rearing practices, influence the nutrition of the most vulnerable in societies. Inadequate housing and overcrowding, poor sanitation, and lack of access to a protected water supply, through their links with infectious diseases and infestations, are potent environmental factors that influence biological food utilization and nutrition. Inadequate access to food, limited access to healthcare, and a clean environment and insufficient access to educational opportunities are in turn determined by the economic and institutional structures as well as the political and ideological superstructures within society. The links between food security and malnutrition are evident as nutritional status is the outcome indicator. The presence of undernutrition is not only causally related to food insecurity at the household or individual level, but is also determined by other health-related factors such as access to safe water, good sanitation, and healthcare as well as the care practices that include proper breastfeeding and complementary feeding and ensuring fair and appropriate intra-household food distribution.

Poor nutritional status of populations affects physical growth, intelligence, behaviour, and learning abilities of children and adolescents. It impacts on their physical and work performance and has been linked to impaired economic work productivity during adulthood. Inadequate nutrition predisposes them to infections and contributes to the negative downward spiral of malnutrition and infection. Good nutritional status, on the other hand, promotes optimal growth and development of children and adolescents. It contributes to better physiological work performance, enhances adult economic productivity, increases levels of socially desirable activities, and promotes better maternal birth outcomes. Good nutrition of a population manifested in the nutritional status of the individual in the community contributes to an upward positive spiral and reflects the improvement in the resources and human capital of society.

Low birth weight

Intrauterine growth retardation resulting in low birth weights constitutes a major public health problem in developing countries. A WHO Technical Report (1995) recommended that the 10th percentile of a sex-specific, birth-weight-for-gestational-age distribution be designated for the classification of small-for-gestational-age infants. It is difficult to establish with certainty in all cases whether the reduced weight at birth is the result of *in utero* growth restriction. However, in populations in developing countries with high incidence of small for gestational age infants, the likelihood is that this is largely the result of intra-uterine growth retardation. The definition of intra-uterine growth retardation (IUGR) is an infant born at term (i.e. >37 weeks of gestation) with a low birth weight (i.e. <2500 g). The causes of IUGR are multiple and involve many different factors. The most important determinant of infant weight at birth is the maternal environment of which nutrition is the single most important factor. Poor maternal nutritional status at conception and inadequate maternal nutrition during pregnancy can result in IUGR. Short maternal stature, low maternal body weight and body mass index at conception, and inadequate weight gain during pregnancy are factors that are associated with IUGR. In developing countries IUGR is closely related to conditions of poverty and chronic undernutrition of economically disadvantaged mothers.

More than 96 per cent of low-birth-weight infants are born in the developing world and 20 million children are born each year weighing <2500 g, accounting for 16 per cent of all births in the developing world—a rate more than double the level in the developed world (7 per cent) (UNICEF 2007). The incidence of low birth weight varies across regions, but South Asia has the highest incidence, at 31 per cent with India being home to 40 per cent of all low-birth-weight babies in the developing world.

Low birth weights due to IUGR are associated with increased morbidity and mortality in infancy. It is estimated that term infants weighing less than 2500 g at birth have a four-times increased risk of neonatal death as compared to infants weighing between 2500 and 3000 g and 10 times higher than those weighing between 3000 and 3500 g. The risk of morbidity and mortality in later infancy is also considerably high in these low-birth-weight infants. In developing countries this is largely due to increased risk of diarrhoeal disease and respiratory infections. Barker's studies have consistently demonstrated a relationship between low birth and later adult disease and provide an important aetiological role for foetal undernutrition in amplifying the effect of risk factors in later life in the development of chronic diseases like heart disease and diabetes mellitus in adult life (Barker 2004).

Childhood undernutrition

The clinical conditions of childhood undernutrition or malnutrition are widely recognized as kwashiorkor, marasmus, and the mixed condition of marasmic kwashiorkor. These severe forms of malnutrition are, however, the tip of an iceberg of widespread mild and moderate childhood undernutrition within the community. It is this form of undernutrition in infants and children that is relevant from a public health nutrition perspective.

Poor diet and nutrition are not the only causes of childhood undernutrition. The determinants of child undernutrition can be considered as operating at three levels of causality: Immediate, underlying, and basic (Smith & Haddad 2000). The immediate determinants are dietary intakes and health status which are in turn influenced by three underlying determinants—household food insecurity, the concept of care for children and their mothers, and the health environment which includes access to safe water and to sanitation. Care encompasses such variables as breast-feeding and proper complementary feeding practices, the education of women—the caregiver, their status, their autonomy, and their access to resources. A poor health environment can result in frequent episodes of infection such as diarrhoeal diseases and even respiratory infections. A vicious cycle may be established with an intestinal infection in a young child leading to anorexia, intestinal damage with malabsorption, and secretory diarrhoea which then does not remit because the poor nutritional state of the child maintains the immunological deficit and this impairs the recovery of the intestine. Traditionally children in poor communities, fail to thrive once they have succumbed to an infectious disease and they then languish, responding poorly to standard therapy and failing to grow even when presented with apparently adequate amounts of food.

Undernutrition in childhood is characterized by growth failure, resulting in a body weight that is less than ideal for the child's age. Hence, in children, assessment of growth has been the single most important measurement that best defines their health and nutritional status. Measures of height and weight are therefore the commonly used indicators of the nutritional status of the child. Classification of childhood malnutrition based on height, weight, and age continues to be the backbone of nutritional assessment methods for both population and individual assessments (WHO 1995). Hitherto the standard reference for comparison has been the National Center for Health Statistics and WHO international reference population; however WHO has recently developed international growth standards for children, which will replace them (WHO 2006).

Children throughout the world when well fed and free of infection tend to grow at similar rates whatever their ethnic or racial origin and healthy children everywhere can, when fed appropriately, be expected to grow on average along the 50th centile of a reference population's weight and height for age. By expressing both height and weight as standard deviations or Z-scores from the median reference value for the child's age the normal range will correspond to the 3rd and 97th centile (i.e. ±2 SDs or ±2 Z-scores). By expressing data in this way, it is possible to express the weight and height data for all children across a wide age range in similar Z-score units and thereby produce a readily understandable comparison of the extent of growth retardation at different ages and in different countries.

A deficit in height is referred to as 'stunting', whereas a deficit in weight-for-height is considered as 'wasting'. These two measures are subsumed in the original designation of a child's failure to grow in terms of weight-for-age. Clearly this measure includes both the wasting and stunting features but fails to distinguish the important differences between the two. Wasting can occur on a short-term basis in response to illness with anorexia or malabsorption or because the child goes hungry for several weeks. Changes in weight-for-height therefore reflect the impact of short-term changes in nutritional status. Growth in height, however, is much more a cumulative index of long-term health because growth in length or height stops when a child develops an infection and the subsequent growth may be slow during the recovery period. Children normally grow in spurts and intermittently. Energy intake is not a crucial determinant of height and the energy cost of growth and weight gain is only 2–5 per cent of total energy intake once the child is 1 year of age. Impairment or slowing of growth in height occurs in many communities at the time of weaning and up to about 2 years of age and affects a fair proportion of children in many developing countries. Once the children have failed to maintain their proper growth trajectory for stature they tend to remain on the lower centiles and 'track' at this low level for many years.

Global estimates of the main forms of child undernutrition *viz* underweight and stunting as well as their prevalence in individual countries is compiled on a regular basis by WHO (de Onis *et al.* 2004) and the most recent available data is summarized in Table 2.6.1. Comparisons from earlier estimates indicate that the prevalence of underweight and stunting remain high despite substantial progress in most regions in the 1990s. In most parts of Africa the numbers of underweight and stunting increased during this period while the dramatic progress in Asia is outweighed by the persisting high prevalence and numbers of children affected. Stunting is a serious problem in both these regions and reflects poor nutrition during the early growth period; often the result of frequent infectious episodes during this period. Physical stunting is associated with poor mental development and socioeconomic deprivation resulting from reduced physical abilities and employment opportunities in adult life. Stunting in South Asia seems also to be related to the high incidence in low birth weight in this region.

Underweight in children is being used as an indicator for monitoring progress towards the Millennium Development Goals (MDG). Overall current analyses demonstrates some progress in reducing child undernutrition; but is uneven and in some countries has even deteriorated. To achieve the MDG more concerted effort is needed, especially in those regions with stagnating or increasing trends in child undernutrition. Well-nourished children have a better chance of surviving and growing into healthy adults. Improving child nutrition requires attention to all three components, i.e. access to adequate and safe food, freedom from illness, and appropriate care. Ensuring optimal child health and growth can contribute to a healthy adult population and accelerate economic growth of countries.

Table 2.6.1 Current estimates and progress since 1990 in the prevalence and numbers of child undernutrition globally and in developing countries of Africa, Asia, and Latin America

	Underweight		Stunting	
	1990	2005	1990	2005
Global				
Prevalence (%)	26.5	20.6	33.5	24.1
Numbers (× 10⁶)	163.4	127.2	206.5	149.1
Africa				
Prevalence (%)	23.6	24.5	36.9	34.5
Numbers (× 10⁶)	25.3	34.5	39.6	48.5
Asia				
Prevalence (%)	35.1	24.8	41.1	25.7
Numbers (× 10⁶)	131.9	89.2	154.6	92.4
Latin America				
Prevalence (%)	8.7	5.0	18.3	11.8
Numbers (× 10⁶)	4.8	2.8	10.0	6.5

Prevalence expressed as percentage below -2 SD of NCHS/WHO international reference value.
Global estimates are predominantly developing countries in the three regions.
Latin America includes the Caribbean.
Estimates reported by de Onis *et al.* (2004).

Adult undernutrition

For the last 50 years, nutritionists have focused on vulnerable groups in society, i.e. children, pregnant and nursing mothers, and the elderly, because they were considered to be particularly susceptible to nutritional deficiencies. It is now becoming apparent that undernutrition among the young adults has been neglected and this may have profound significance for the economic growth of developing countries. One simple measure of undernutrition in adults is adult weight in relation to height and *body mass index* (BMI) (i.e. body weight in kilograms divided by the square of the height in metres) is considered the most suitable index for both under- and overnutrition in adults (Shetty & James 1994). The choice of BMI for the assessment of nutritional status of adults was based on the observation that BMI was consistently highly correlated with body weight (a proxy for the available energy stores within the body) and was relatively independent of the stature of the individual. Adults with a BMI <18.5 are considered to be chronically undernourished while those with BMI >25 and >30 are considered overweight and obese, respectively (WHO 2000); and the same BMI cut-offs apply to both males and females. BMI is not only a sensitive index of adult undernutrition but also allows variations in relation to socioeconomic status, and seasonal fluctuations in the availability of food in the community to be detected. Undernourished adults show considerable impairment of physical well-being and exercise capacity and susceptibility to illness. The ability to promote and sustain effective agricultural productivity, particularly in rural societies, may therefore be limited by the vigour and well-being of the adults on whom the vulnerable in society depend. Thus, it is important to consider adult undernutrition alongside other vulnerable segments in a community.

Anthropometric measures of adult undernutrition provides an opportunity for objective estimates of the prevalence of undernutrition worldwide, hitherto dependent on estimates of food availability in countries and the numbers of people food insecure. In practice, children and adults may adapt to a shortage of food by reducing their physical activity without changing their body weight. Thus, measures of the prevalence of low weight-for-height provide only a limited index of food insecurity as physical activity is fundamental to children's play and exploration and therefore to their mental development. Similarly, in adults physical activity is desirable not only for physiological well-being and for limiting the development of chronic disease but also to allow societies to prosper through physically demanding economic activity and those sound developments which rely on an energetic and enterprising population.

For many years, the Food and Agriculture Organization of the UN (FAO) has attempted to assess the global prevalence of undernutrition by relating complex measures of food supply and its variable distribution between households with estimates of the population's energy needs (Naiken 2003). The number of undernourished estimated most recently by FAO, based on their method, is 854 million, of which 820 million are in developing countries (FAO 2006). Since reducing by half the proportion of the hungry or food insecure by 2015 is one of the targets set in MDG1, monitoring progress using this method has considerable importance. It is apparent that there has been progress in this direction although it has been recognized that progress has been slow in the last decade as compared to the previous decade. While the prospect of meeting the MDG1 target are good, progress has been variable with some regions such as Central Africa and East Asia having shown a worsening of the situation with increase in numbers of undernourished. Reliable global estimates of adult undernutrition based on BMI are not available since nutritional surveys rarely include adult men and the issue of adult undernutrition has also largely been ignored. With awareness of the increasing problem of overweight and obesity, it is likely that more information based on anthropometric surveys of adults will be generated which will also provide for data on adult undernutrition.

Public health initiatives that deal with this problem worldwide have to recognize that the basic causes of malnutrition are clearly political and socioeconomic. Agricultural revolutions such as the green revolution have increased food availability and helped meet the food needs of the population. Agricultural productivity has increased worldwide and developing countries are increasingly producing more food even when expressed on a per capita basis. Food prices for most commodities, particularly for cereals, have also fallen and been at their lowest until recently. However, poverty is often the basis of a failure to have access to food even when it is available and even when the prices are low as they are currently. Accelerated food production will alleviate hunger only to the extent that the resources used in the process reduce poverty more than they would if used in other ways. Thus food entitlement decline is a more important force in sustaining poverty and undernutrition than a decline in the availability of food in developing societies.

Micronutrient malnutrition

Micronutrient malnutrition, also referred to as 'hidden hunger' is caused by lack of adequate micronutrients such as vitamins and minerals in the habitual diet. Diets deficient in micronutrients are characterized by high intakes of staple food and cereal crops, but low consumption of foods rich in bioavailable micronutrients such as fruits, vegetables, and animal and marine products.

Micronutrient deficiencies are important from a public health perspective as they affect several billion people worldwide (Table 2.6.2) and can impair cognitive development and lower resistance to disease in children and adults. They increase the risk to both mothers and infants during childbirth and impair the physical ability and economic productivity of men. The costs of these deficiencies in terms of lives lost and reduced quality of life are enormous not to mention the economic costs to society. Strategies to combat micronutrient deficiencies in communities have included: (i) *Supplementation* of specific nutrients to meet the immediate deficits. (ii) *Fortification* of staple food items in the daily diet—another successful strategy that has been adopted to deal with specific nutrient deficiencies—a good example is the fortification of common salt with iodine to tackle iodine deficiency and goitres. (iii) *Food-based approaches* which include promoting kitchen gardens to enable families to produce and consume a diversified diet rich in vitamins and improve the nutrition of households—promoted extensively to reduce vitamin A deficiency in developing countries. (iv) A potential strategy under investigation is to improve the nutrient quality of commonly consumed staples by agricultural biotechnology such as genetically modified crops—a process referred to as *biofortification*. The micronutrient deficiencies that will be addressed below in this chapter include only the significant ones from a public health viewpoint.

Iron deficiency

Iron deficiency is probably the most common nutritional deficiency disorder in the world and affects over 2 billion people with anaemia. Hence it is a major public health problem with adverse consequences especially for women of reproductive age and for young children. The predominant cause of iron deficiency worldwide is

Table 2.6.2 Estimated global impact of micronutrient malnutrition

Micronutrient malnutrition	Estimated impact
Vitamin A deficiency	140 million pre-school children affected with VAD[1]
	Contributes to 1.15 million deaths in children every year[2]
	4.4 million children suffer from xeropthalmia[1]
	6.2 million women suffer from xerophthalmia[1]
Iron deficiency	2.0 billion women (96 million of them pregnant)[2]
	67 500 maternal deaths per year from severe anaemia[2]
Iodine deficiency	1.98 billion at risk with insufficient or low iodine intakes[3]
	15.8% of population worldwide have goitre[3]
	17.6 million infants born mentally impaired every year[2]
Folate deficiency	Responsible for 200 000 severe birth defects every year[2]

[1] SCN (2004) *Fifth report on the world nutrition situation: Nutrition for improved development*
[2] UNICEF/Micronutrient Initiative (2004) *Vitamin and mineral deficiency: A World progress report*
[3] WHO (2004) *Iodine status worldwide*

nutritional, the diet failing to provide for the body's requirements of iron. In tropical countries, intestinal parasitosis exacerbates iron deficiency by increasing the loss of blood from the gastrointestinal tract. The increase in malaria in these countries also contributes to the anaemia. A low intake of iron and/or its poor absorption then fails to meet the enhanced demands for iron and anaemia results.

The consequences of iron deficiency are numerous as iron plays a central role in the transport of oxygen in the body and is also essential in many enzyme systems. Iron deficiency leads to changes in behaviour, such as attention, memory, and learning in infants and small children, and also negatively influences the normal defence systems against infection. T-lymphocyte function, phagocytosis, and the killing of bacteria by neutrophilic leucocytes are affected. In pregnant women iron deficiency contributes to maternal morbidity and mortality, and increases risk of foetal morbidity, mortality, and low birth weight (Viteri 1997). Iron deficiency results in a reduction in physical working capacity and productivity of adults both in agricultural and industrial work situations. These functional impairments are economically important as it is estimated that median value of productivity losses is about 0.9 per cent GDP and the economic impact of iron deficiency can vary from 2 per cent GDP in the case of Honduras to 7.9 per cent in Bangladesh (Horton & Ross 2003).

Iron deficiency disorders encompass a range of body iron depletion states. The least severe is *diminished iron stores* diagnosed by decreased serum ferritin levels and not usually associated with adverse physiological consequences. The intermediate, *iron deficiency without anaemia* on the other hand, is severe enough to affect production of haemoglobin without haemoglobin levels falling below clinical criteria indicative of anaemia and is characterized by decreased transferrin saturation levels and increased erythrocyte protoporphyrin. The severe form with clinical manifestation is *Iron Deficiency Anaemia*.

Iron deficiency anaemia (IDA) is a serious problem worldwide and the dominant cause in all cases is nutritional iron deficiency (Table 2.6.3). The highest prevalence figures for IDA are seen in developing countries: In infants and pre-school children (39 per cent), school-age children aged 5–14 years (48.1 per cent), and women

aged between 15 and 59 years (52 per cent) (WHO 2001). Even in industrialized, developed countries the prevalence of IDA is significant and the estimated prevalence is 20.1 per cent among infants and pre-school children aged 0–4 years, 22.7 per cent among pregnant women, and 12 per cent in the elderly aged 60+ years. Based on the estimates of IDA as a risk factor for mortality, the total attributed global burden is estimated at 841 000 deaths and over 35 million DALYs (Stolzfus *et al.* 2004).

In Africa, Asia, and South America, the availability of iron in the diets has been deteriorating and IDA continues to be a massive public health problem. The availability of iron in the diet for absorption is affected by both the forms of iron and the nature of foods concurrently ingested. Iron exists in the diet in two forms: (i) as 'haem iron' it is found only in animal sources and is readily available for absorption and is not influenced by other constituents of the diet; and (ii) as 'inorganic iron' it is not readily available and is strongly influenced by factors present in foods ingested at the same time. Both animal foods and ascorbic acid (vitamin C) promote the absorption of inorganic iron. Diets, which are primarily cereal and legume-based, may contain much iron but, in the absence of co-factors such as ascorbic acid or presence of phytates, they provide only low levels of bioavailable iron. Concern about iron deficiency is an important nutritional reason for recommending the consumption of at least some meat as well as foods with ascorbic acid for populations who rely predominantly on a cereal-based diet.

The strategies to combat iron deficiency include: (1) iron *supplementation*; (2) iron *fortification* of certain foods; (3) *dietary modification* to improve the bioavailability of dietary iron by modifying the composition of meals; and (4) *parasitic disease control*. Iron and folate supplementation programmes for pregnant women are currently widely implemented in several countries; many countries have a universal preventive supplementation policy during pregnancy. Iron supplementations aimed at pre-school or school-aged children are being carried out in several countries. Fortification of foods with iron is a preventive measure aimed at improving and sustaining adequate iron nutrition over a longer term. Many industrialized countries like Canada and the United States have fortified foods with iron and studies in developing countries have demonstrated the

Table 2.6.3 Numbers of people (in millions) affected with iron deficiency anaemia based on blood haemoglobin concentration in different regions of the world

	Children		Women (15–49 years)		Men
	0–4 years	**5–14 years**	**Pregnant**	**All women**	**(15–59 years)**
	(millions)	(millions)	(millions)	(millions)	(millions)
WHO Regions					
Africa	45.2	85.2	10.8	57.8	41.9
Americas	14.2	40.6	4.5	53.8	19.4
Southeast Asia	111.4	207.8	24.8	215.0	184.8
Europe	12.5	12.9	2.4	27.1	13.3
Eastern Mediterranean	33.3	37.9	7.7	60.2	41.5
Western Pacific	29.8	156.8	9.7	158.7	174.4
Total All Regions	**246.4**	**541.2**	**59.9**	**572.6**	**475.3**

Source: Compiled from WHO (2001): *Iron Deficiency Anemia: Assessment, prevention and control.*

effectiveness of iron fortification of foods provided these programmes are based on careful planning and follow well-established guidelines (Viteri 1997). Improvement in the supply, consumption, and the bioavailability of iron in food is an important strategy to improve iron status of populations. The bioavailability of iron in foods is influenced by the composition of the meal and food preparation methods. The consumption of ascorbate-rich foods enhances iron absorption while limiting the content of phytate which inhibits iron absorption, will improve iron bioavailability. Malaria and intestinal parasites (especially hookworm) are important contributors to IDA in endemic areas. In populations where hookworm is prevalent, effective treatment of this helminth infection has reduced IDA in school-aged children (Stoltzfus *et al.* 1997). Thus, strategies that address iron nutrition, whether food based, or by supplementation or fortification, must be integrated with programmes such as malaria prophylaxis, helminth control, environmental health, and control of other micronutrient deficiencies to maximize effectiveness (WHO 2001).

Iodine deficiency

The term 'iodine deficiency disorder' (IDD) refers to a complex of effects arising from deficient intakes of iodine. The mountainous areas of the world are likely to be iodine deficient because the rain leaches the iodine from the rocks and soils. The most severely deficient areas are the Himalayas, the Andes, the European Alps, and the vast mountainous regions of China, i.e. elevated regions subject to glaciation and high rainfall which run off into rivers. It also occurs in flooded river valleys of Eastern India, Bangladesh, and Burma. The Great Lake basins of North America are also iodine deficient. Excessive intakes of goitrogens in food, (due to the excessive consumption of *cassava* or the *brassica* group of vegetables) and in water (water-borne goitrogens in Latin America) as well as the deficiency of certain trace elements in the soil or food chain (such as selenium) may interfere with the uptake and metabolism of iodine in the body and can thus cause or amplify the effects of iodine deficiency.

The prevalence of manifest IDD in the form of goitre varies globally and at present is confined to developing countries, largely because public health initiatives such as iodization of salt have been introduced in the developed world, and most have mandated or permitted salt iodization. Iodine deficiency and goitre is still prevalent in Central and Eastern Europe. According to recent estimates the goitre prevalence in developing countries is 15.8 per cent (WHO 2004). However, this figure masks the enormous numbers who are at risk of IDD based on urinary iodine status which reflects the insufficiency of iodine intake in the diet (Table 2.6.4). Iodine deficiency is also responsible for over 200 000 severe birth defects worldwide while also contributing to lower the intellectual capacity of almost all nations reviewed, by as much as 10–15 percentage points (UNICEF/Micronutrient Initiative 2004).

IDD in humans is predominantly the result of a primary deficiency of iodine in the diet. Both water and foods are sources of iodine, with marine fish being the richest source of iodine. Milk and meat are also rich sources of iodine. Fruits, legumes, vegetables, and fresh water fish are also important additional sources. Plant foods are likely to show a reduced content of iodine if the iodine content of the soils in which they are grown is low. Goitrogens in the diet are of secondary importance as aetiological factors in IDD. It has been shown that staple foods consumed largely by poor rural populations, such as cassava, maize, sweet potatoes, lima beans contain cyanogenic glucosides which release a goitrogen thiocyanate. Cassava is now implicated as an important contributor to the endemic goitre and cretinism in non-mountainous Zaire and in Sarawak in Malaysia. Selenium deficiency in the soil can result in manifestations of IDD in the presence of modest iodine deficiency since selenium is essential for thyroid metabolism. Selenium deficiency is now recognized as an aetiologic factor in the IDD in several regions of China.

Iodine is readily absorbed from the diet and forms a very important element in the synthesis of thyroid hormones in the body. Thyroid hormones are essential for normal growth and development. Just prior to birth, the levels of the biologically active triiodothyronine (T_3) increase and prepare the organism for the transition from intra-uterine to extra-uterine life. Failure to synthesize sufficient T_3 as a result of iodine deficiency may be a factor in the stillbirths that occur as a part of the spectrum of IDD. Thyroid hormone deficiency leads to severe retardation of growth and maturation of all organs. The brain is particularly susceptible to damage during the foetal and early postnatal periods. It is now confirmed that the thyroidal control of neonatal brain development is more important than foetal brain development since early and optimal thyroid hormone treatment after birth can lead to substantial improvement in thyroid function. The spectrum of IDDs in humans, from the foetus to the adult, have been outlined by Hetzel (1987).

Table 2.6.4 Proportion of population and number of individuals with insufficient iodine intake in school-age children (6–12 years) and the general population and total goitre prevalence in the same UN regions

UN Region	Insufficient iodine intake (urinary iodine <100 µg/l)		Total goitre prevalence
	School age children	General population	
Africa	42.7% (59.7 million)	43.0% (324.2 million)	26.8%
Asia	38.3% (187.0 million)	35.6% (1239.3 million)	14.5%
Europe	53.1% (26.7 million)	52.7% (330.8 million)	16.3%
Latin America and the Caribbean	10.3% (7.1 million)	10.0% (47.4 million)	4.7%
North America	9.5% (2.1 million)	64.5% (19.2 million)	–
Oceania	59.4% (2.1 million)	64.5% (19.2 million)	12.9%
Total	**36.5% (285.4 million)**	**35.2% (1988.7 million)**	**15.8%**

Summarized from *Iodine Status Worldwide*; WHO (2004).
Figures in parenthesis are numbers of individuals at risk estimated from UN population estimates for 2002.

The public health initiatives for correcting iodine deficiency require the provision of adequate iodine to the individual. This has been achieved by one of several methods: *Iodization* of salt has been the most favoured method and has greatly reduced the prevalence of IDDs in Switzerland, the United States, and New Zealand. Since its first successful introduction in the 1920s in Switzerland (Burgi *et al.* 1990) successful programmes have been reported in Central and South America, in Europe (Finland), and in Asia (China and Taiwan). However, several developing countries have encountered problems with their salt iodization programmes because it is difficult to produce and maintain enough high-quality iodized salt for large populations such as in India and Bangladesh. The extra costs of iodized salt and its availability and distribution in remote regions can also be a problem. These issues may be compounded by cultural prejudices about the use of iodized salt and the loss of iodine with cooking if salt is not added after cooking. *Iodized oil* injections have been used to prevent goitre and cretinism in New Guinea (Pharoah & Connolly 1987). Iodized oil is suitable for mass programmes and can be carried out alongside mass immunization programmes. These methods have been successful in China, Indonesia, and Nepal. The major problems with iodized oil are the cost, the initial discomfort, and the likely potential disadvantage associated with the transmission of Hepatitis B and HIV with the use of needles. The need for a primary healthcare team to inject the iodized oil can be a further disadvantage. Iodized oil by mouth may be an alternative and primarily health centres can readily administer this scheme. Oral iodized oil has been shown to be as effective in a single oral dose as an intramuscular injection (Phillips *et al.* 1988). However, the effects of oral iodized oil seem to last for only half as long as a similar dose of injected iodized oil. They do not, however, suffer from the disadvantages of iodized oil injections so it is a preferred method for use in remote areas. The IDDs are excellent examples of nutritional deficiency disorders of public health importance which can readily be abolished if mass community programmes are undertaken.

Vitamin A deficiency

Vitamin A deficiency leads to night blindness and xerosis (dryness) of the conjunctiva and cornea and disrupts the integrity of their surface and causes corneal clouding and ulceration and may lead to blindness in children. Xerophthalmia continues to be a major cause of childhood blindness despite the intensive prevention programmes of the last two decades. It is a widespread problem and the parts of the world most seriously affected include South and Southeast Asia, and many countries in Africa, Central America, and the Near East. Extrapolations from the best available data suggest that 140 million children under 5 and more than 7 million pregnant women suffer from vitamin A deficiency every year (SCN 2004). This report also states that another 4.4 million children and 6.2 million women suffer from xerophthalmia. Nearly half of the cases of VAD and xerophthalmia occur in South and Southeast Asia.

An additional 20–40 million suffer from mild or sub-clinical deficiency of vitamin A, which we now recognize as having serious consequences for survival since vitamin A deficiency (VAD) is now known to decrease the child's resistance to infections and increase mortality. Even before eye signs of VAD are detectable, changes in the surface linings of the gastrointestinal and respiratory tracts occur along with changes in cell-mediated immunity and these can increase the risk of morbidity and even mortality associated with infections in children. Recent evidence suggests that VAD may be associated with increased maternal morbidity and even mortality. The estimates are that between 1.2 and 3 million children and significant numbers of mothers die associated with vitamin A deficiency. Vitamin A is also now known to be involved in foetal development, haematopiesis, spermatogenesis, appetite, and physical growth.

Vitamin A is the parent of a class of compounds called retinoids. Pro-vitamin A carotenoids, chiefly β-carotene, is also included in the vitamin A family. Preformed vitamin A is chiefly found in dairy products such as milk, butter, cheese, egg yolk, in some fatty fish, and in the livers of farm animals and fish. Carotenes are generally abundant in yellow fruits (papayas, mangoes, apricots, peaches) and vegetables (carrots). Absorption of vitamin A is about 80 per cent complete in the presence of an adequate fat intake, while the absorption of carotenoids is highly bile salt dependent. Vitamin A (retinol and retinoic acid) plays a very important role in the body in cellular development and differentiation. Retinol also has a vital role in normal vision, particularly by the rods in the retina. Thus, one of the earliest manifestations of vitamin A deficiency is night blindness.

There is now increasing evidence that vitamin A supplements in deficient populations can reduce morbidity, mortality, and blindness. Xerophthalmia has become less prevalent in recent years in hyperendemic areas such as Indonesia and India. Intervention strategies that may have contributed to this include periodic megadose vitamin A supplementation either in the form of capsules, syrup, or as an injected dose. It is now the practice to provide vitamin supplements along with immunization programmes in many countries with the objective of providing at least one dose of vitamin A per year for all children aged 6 months to 5 years. The fortification of dietary items which are universally consumed, e.g. sugar, in Central America (Arroyave *et al.* 1981) and monosodium glutamate in Indonesia (Muhilal *et al.* 1988) have had a favourable impact on the vitamin A status of the whole population. Following on the success of sugar fortification in Central America it has been successfully tried in Zambia and South Africa and the Philippines have successfully implemented fortification of cereals (wheat and maize flour) with vitamin A (UNICEF/Micronutrient Initiative 2004). The problems with food fortification are essentially logistical and technological and many developing countries are beginning the process of fortifying staple foods and condiments with vitamins (and minerals) including margarine, cooking oil, and soya sauce. Food supplies from different regions of the world show limited vitamin A availability, but the problem is exacerbated by a tendency to withhold vegetables and fruits from children and from pregnant and lactating women for cultural and other reasons in some parts of the world. Nutrition education is the only answer when vitamin A deficiency develops despite fruit and vegetable sources of the vitamin being in plentiful supply. These foods are not incorporated into the diets of young children and mothers, due either to lack of knowledge or cultural biases. Nutrition education together with practical advice and help with growing cheap, nutritious vegetables in home kitchen gardens may help eradicate vitamin A deficiency. Horticultural approaches are increasingly recognized for their effectiveness and potential sustainability in improving not only vitamin A status, but also micronutrient status generally. The importance of combining increased vitamin A levels in the food supply with nutrition education and appropriate social marketing that promotes consumption by vulnerable groups within populations cannot be underestimated. Economic development and poverty reduction programmes are likely to improve the socioeconomic status and may indirectly contribute to reducing the problem of VAD.

Folate deficiency

Folate enables cell division and tissue growth. Adequate folate in the diet helps prevent malformations that affect the neural tube and spinal cord such as anencephaly and spina bifida as well as other birth defects like cleft lip and palate. Without adequate folate in the diet, 2 in every 1000 pregnancies may end up with a serious birth defect. Folate deficiency is also associated with increased risk of pre-term delivery and low birth weight (Scholl & Johnson 2000) and may also contribute to anaemia especially in pregnant and lactating mothers (Dugdale 2001). It may thus contribute indirectly to increased maternal illness and mortality. With the increasing awareness of the role folate plays in reducing the risk of heart disease and stroke, a case is being made for folate fortification of flour, a strategy already adopted in the United States and Canada.

It is important to acknowledge the contribution of several Non Government Organizations (NGOs), many of them specialized in addressing specific micronutrient deficiencies (e.g. International Council for the Control of Iodine Deficiency Disorders (ICCIDD) with the objective of the sustainable elimination of IDD) while many others such as Micronutrient Initiative (MI) tackle all major micronutrient deficiencies of public health significance. It would be futile to mention all of them, apart from emphasizing the important role they play in numerous ways to deal with the problem of 'hidden hunger' worldwide. They closely work in partnership with governments, AID agencies, and with the UN agencies and the community to further this laudable objective.

This section has hitherto dealt with only some of the more important nutritionally determined deficiency disorders of public health importance. It is important to recognize that segments of populations in the world suffer from other nutritional disorders such as those due to the deficiency of fluoride, zinc, selenium, B group vitamins, and ascorbic acid. Some of these seem to occur during seasonal deficiencies in their availability and accompany famine and conflict situations when they are seen in refugee camps. It is important to recognize that in all regions of the world there are still some populations affected by one or more of these deficiencies despite the significant advances that have been made in controlling nutritional deficiency disorders. In some regions of the world, largely the result of increasing population size, the numbers of undernourished are increasing even if the population prevalence is declining. In many there is shift in the severity of the deficiency diseases with decreasing numbers with severe deficiency and increasing numbers with mild to moderate deficiencies. For a majority of these countries there is still the need to pursue vigorous policies and targeted action to combat the various nutritional deficiency disorders as a part of the comprehensive health-oriented national food and nutrition policies.

Consequences of undernutrition and micronutrient deficiencies

An issue that deserves attention is to ask the question whether humanitarian considerations apart, does widespread undernutrition and micronutrient malnutrition matter? And is there a case for investing in better nutrition? According to UNICEF, approximately half the economic growth achieved by developed countries of Western Europe since 1790 until 1980 can be attributed to better nutrition and improved health and sanitation (UNICEF 1997). The social and economic costs, apart from costs to the individual due to poor nutrition, are huge. Improving nutrition of communities reduces healthcare costs. More than half of child mortality in developing countries is attributable to underweight and the consequent increased risk of infectious diseases. Underweight is the leading risk factor in the global burden of disease and, among developing countries with high mortality, it contributes to nearly 15 per cent of the attributable disability adjusted life years (DALYs) (WHO 2002). Preventing low birth weight and stunting also reduces childhood mortality and morbidity. The intimate links between undernutrition in early life including low birth weight and the increasing risk of chronic disease in later adult life is well established. Diagnosis and treatment of chronic diseases like heart disease, diabetes, and cancer is expensive and will distort the limited public health budgets of developing countries.

Undernourished children become smaller adults and demonstrate lower physiological performance and reduced physical and work capacity. Employment prospects and productivity of short-statured and undernourished individuals is impaired (Spurr 1987). It shortens productive lives and increases absence due to illness; impacting in turn on economic productivity of countries. Micronutrient deficiencies such as iron deficiency in adults also impairs physical capacity and work productivity and contributes to economic losses.

Poor nutrition impairs cognitive development and learning in undernourished children in developing societies. Grantham-McGregor (1995) has demonstrated that children who are stunted and live in deprived circumstances have major deficits in intellectual and cognitive development and social behaviour. Children's scholastic ability in their teens can be strongly influenced by interventions in the second and third year of life. Iodine deficiency and the syndrome of cretinism is another example of the role of nutrition in brain development and function. Even postnatal iodine deficiency can lead to slowing of mental processing that results in permanent impairment of mental development because of the need for adequate nutrition during critical periods of brain development. Similarly, Pollitt (1991a,b) has demonstrated that iron deficiency anaemia can permanently handicap children at a crucial time in their development even though iron deficiency per se is not enough to produce demonstrable clinical deficiency. Grantham-McGregor's (1995) studies show that food that stimulates longitudinal bone growth also stimulates brain development, thus implying a more generic demand for a range of nutrients if mental function is to improve. All of these have significant relevance to the fact that childrens' education is the cornerstone to social and economic development of nations and is now an important component of the MDGs (MDG2). The benefits of sustained mental and physical development from childhood into adult life ensures that healthy adults with the physical capacity to maintain high work outputs and with the intellectual ability to flexibly adapt to new technologies in this rapidly globalizing world will be a national asset. The importance of food and nutrition in the development of human capital in developing societies can never be underestimated.

Strategies to address the problem of undernutrition in developing societies

Reduction of poverty and hunger are high up among the MDG since achieving MDG 1—halving poverty and hunger by 2015 is central to achieving the other health-related MDGs. Economic growth and development should reduce the burden of undernutrition, but the reduction is slow and many people continue to suffer needlessly. There is thus a need for well-conceived policies for sustainable economic growth and social development that will benefit the poor and the undernourished. Given the complexity of factors that determine malnutrition of all forms, it is important that appropriate food and agricultural policies are developed to ensure household food security and that nutritional objectives are incorporated into development policies and programmes at national and local levels in developing countries. The deleterious consequences of rapid growth and development need to be guarded against and policies need to be in place to prevent one problem of malnutrition replacing another in these societies.

The pre-eminent determinant of household food insecurity is poverty in societies. Several policy measures undertaken by governments in developing countries are aimed at ensuring food supply and household food security. These include:

◆ Macroeconomic policies and economic development strategies that ensure both public-sector and private-sector investment in agriculture and food production.

◆ Appropriate policies to promote expansion and diversification of food availability and agricultural production in a stable and sustainable manner, and to regulate the import or export of foods and agricultural products to ensure food security.

◆ Policies that help create adequate employment opportunities for the rural poor and improving market efficiencies and opportunities.

◆ Policies that improve distribution and access to land, and to other resources such as credit, as well as other agricultural inputs.

◆ Legislating for policies that deter discrimination and ensure equal status for women, and ensuring their effective implementation.

◆ Identification of good and culturally appropriate caring practices and policies that protect, support, and promote good care and nutrition practices for children.

◆ Policies that enable public health measures to reduce the burden of infectious diseases and to ensure access to primary healthcare.

It is hoped that with good governance and democracy and with well-targeted aid from developed countries the implementation of these policies and the relevant programmes will reduce the burden of hunger and undernutrition in developing countries of the world.

Diet, nutrition, and chronic non-communicable diseases

The evidence relating food and nutrition to chronic non-communicable diseases such as non-insulin-dependent diabetes mellitus, and cancers comes from population-based epidemiological investigations and from controlled trials. Descriptive population-based epidemiological investigations yield valuable data which lead to important hypotheses, but they cannot be used alone to establish the causal links between diet and disease. The most consistent correlation between diet and chronic diseases has emerged from comparisons of populations or segments of population with substantially different dietary habits. Analytical epidemiological studies, such as cohort studies and case control studies that compare information from groups of individuals within a population usually provide more accurate estimates of such associations. It is important to recognize when examining population-based epidemiological data relating diet to disease that every population consists of individuals who vary in their susceptibility to each disease. Part of this difference in susceptibility is genetic. As the diet within a population changes in the direction that measures the risk of the specific disease, an increasing proportion of individuals, particularly those most susceptible to the risk, develop the disease. As a result of this inter-individual variability in the interaction of diet with an individual's genetic make-up and therefore the individual's susceptibility to disease, some diet–disease relationships are difficult to identify within a single population. In experimental clinical studies and randomized and controlled trials, long exposures may be required for the effect of the diet as a risk factor to be manifest. Strict inclusion criteria for participants need to be adopted to show the effect with small numbers in a reasonable length of time. These in turn may restrict the study to homogenous samples and thus limit the applicability of results to the population at large. Despite these limitations, when carefully designed studies show consistent findings of an association between specific dietary factors and a chronic disease, they generally indicate a cause and effect relationship.

Diet, nutrition, and cardiovascular diseases

The commonest cardiovascular diseases that are diet-related are coronary heart disease and hypertension.

Coronary heart disease (CHD)

CHD emerged as a burgeoning public health problem in Europe and North America after World War II and by the end of the 1950s had become the single major cause of adult death. The rates of CHD show marked international differences with overall rates being higher among men than women. Mortality rates are seven-fold higher in some Eastern European countries while three-fold differences are evident between Scotland and Spain or Portugal. Migration can contribute to either an increase as in the case of Japanese moving to the United States or decrease when Finns move to Sweden—migrants tending to approach the rates in their host countries. In the case of migrants from South Asia to the United Kingdom, however the rates exceed the hosts implying some genetic susceptibility increasing risk in the host environment.

Several prospective studies have documented the relationship between habitual diets and the risk of CHD in a given population. These longitudinal studies have shown that several foods and nutrients in the diet are protective and reduce risk of CHD—they include whole grain cereals, fish, fruits and vegetables, nuts, and moderate intakes of red wine while others such as dietary cholesterol, trans fatty acids, and increased consumption of coffee may increase the risk of CHD.

The nearly five-fold difference in CHD rates among different countries and the intra-population variations in rates, by socioeconomic class, ethnicity, and geographical location, have brought to our attention the dietary basis of CHD. The marked changes in CHD rates in migrant populations that moved across a geographical gradient in CHD risk provided further evidence of the environmental nature of the causative factor. The WHO Expert Committee on Prevention of CHD (1982) concluded, after reviewing the data on the relationship between blood cholesterol and the risk of CHD, that the relationship of lipids in the diet and blood met the criteria for an epidemiological association to be termed causal. These data were backed by several intervention trials in volunteers, clinical studies, and a wide range of animal experiments demonstrating the effects of diet on coronary artery atherosclerosis.

This relationship between dietary factors and CHD was supported by the results of the Seven Country Study (Keys 1980). The *saturated fat intake* varied between 3 per cent total energy in Japan and 22 per cent in Eastern Finland while the 15-year CHD incidence rates varied between 144 per 10 000 in Japan and 1202 per 10 000 in Eastern Finland. The annual incidence of CHD among 40–59-year-old men initially free of CHD was 15 per 100 000 in Japan and 198 per 100 000 in Finland. Measurement of food consumption by the people in 16 well-defined cohorts in seven countries and its correlation to 10-year incidence rate of CHD deaths provided further support for this causal association. The strongest correlation was noted between CHD and percentage of energy derived from saturated fat, while total fat was not significantly correlated with CHD.

In the Seven Country Study, the *serum total cholesterol* values were 165 mg dl in Japan and 270 mg dl in Eastern Finland, and suggested that the variation in serum total cholesterol levels between populations could be largely explained by differences in saturated fat intake and CHD incidence. On a population basis, the risk of CHD seems to rise progressively within the same population with increases in plasma total cholesterol. Observational studies suggest that one population with an average total cholesterol level 10 per cent lower than another will have one-third less CHD and a 30 per cent difference in total cholesterol predicts a four-fold difference in CHD (WHO 1990). The Seven Country Study showed a strong positive relationship between saturated fat intake and total cholesterol level; populations with an average saturated fat intake between 3 and 10 per cent of the energy intake were characterized by serum total cholesterol levels below 200 mg dl and by low mortality rates from CHD. As saturated fat intakes increased to greater than 10 per cent of energy intake a marked and progressive increase in CHD mortality was noticed. Saturated fats raise total and *low-density lipoprotein* (LDL) cholesterol; and of these fatty acids myristic and palmitic acids abundant in diets rich in dairy and meat products have the greatest effects (Table 2.6.5).

Several prospective studies have shown an inverse relation between *high-density lipoprotein* (HDL) cholesterol and CHD incidence. However, HDL cholesterol levels are influenced by several non-dietary factors and HDL levels do not contribute to explain differences in CHD mortality between populations. HDL levels are increased by alcohol, weight loss, and by physical activity. Populations who have high intakes of mono-unsaturated fatty acids (from olive oil) or have diets rich in n-3 polyunsaturates of marine origin (like Eskimos) also have low CHD rates. Both *mono-unsaturated* and n-3 and n-6 *polyunsaturated fatty acids* (PUFAs) lower plasma total and LDL cholesterol; PUFAs more effective than mono-unsaturates (Kris-Etherton 1999; Mori & Beilin 2001). There is good evidence that some isomers of fatty acids, such as *trans fatty acids* increase the incidence of CHD by increasing LDL cholesterol levels and decreasing the HDL levels, by interfering with essential fatty acid metabolism, and by enhancing the concentrations

Table 2.6.5 Summary of strength of evidence of dietary and lifestyle factors and risk of developing cardiovascular disease

Evidence	Decreased risk	No relationship	Increased risk
Convincing	Regular physical activity	Vitamin E supplements	Myristic and palmitic acids
	Linoleic acid		Trans fatty acids
	Fish and fish oils[1]		High sodium intake
	Vegetables and fruits		Overweight
	Potassium		High alcohol intake[4]
	Alcohol intake (low to moderate)[2]		
Probable	α Linolenic acid	Stearic acid	Dietary cholesterol
	Oleic acid		Unfiltered boiled coffee
	NSP[3]		
	Whole grain cereals		
	Nuts (unsalted)		
	Plant sterols/stanols		
	Folate		

Adapted from WHO/FAO (2003) *Diet, nutrition and the prevention of chronic diseases*
[1] Eicosapentaenoic acid and docosapentaenoic acid
[2] For CHD risk
[3] NSP= non starch polysaccharide
[4] For risk of stroke

of the lipoprotein Lp(a) which, in genetically susceptible people, seems to be an additional risk factor through mechanisms which include an anti-plasminogen effect to limit fibrinolysis.

Other dietary components, e.g. *dietary fibre or complex carbohydrates* in the diet seem to influence serum cholesterol levels and the incidence of CHD. Population sub-groups consuming diets rich in plant foods with a high content of complex carbohydrates have lower rates of CHD; vegetarians have a 30 per cent lower rate of CHD mortality than non-vegetarians and their serum cholesterol levels are significantly lower than that of lacto-ovo-vegetarians and non-vegetarians. *Alcohol* consumption also reduces the incidence of CHD. A number of observational studies suggest that light-to-moderate drinkers have a slightly lower risk of CHD than abstainers. However, the relationship between alcohol intake and CHD is complicated by changes in blood pressure and also the nature of the alcoholic drink. The presence of phenolic compounds in red wine may contribute to the benefits of drinking red wine as compared to alcohol consumption *per se* in reducing the incidence of CHD.

The risk of CHD in individuals is dominated by three major factors: (i) High serum total cholesterol, (ii) high blood pressure, and (iii) cigarette smoking (WHO 1982). There is also a synergism between risk factors, with the Japanese notable for their high smoking rates and hypertension but very low cholesterol levels: Smoking and hypertension are particularly harmful to individuals with high cholesterol levels. Body weight changes induced by diet and levels of physical activity, are strongly related to changes in serum total cholesterol, blood pressure, and obesity. Obesity in turn, particularly when associated with high waist circumference or waist/hip ratio, is strongly related to diabetes mellitus, both of which are risk factors for CHD.

Hypertension and stroke

The risk of CHD and that of cerebrovascular disease presenting clinically as stroke, increases progressively throughout the observed range of blood pressure, in a number of different countries (MacMohan *et al.* 1990). From the combined data it appears that there is a five-fold difference in CHD and a ten-fold risk of stroke over a range of diastolic blood pressure of only 40 mm Hg. Analysis indicates that a sustained difference of only 7.5 mm Hg in diastolic blood pressure confers a 28 per cent difference in risk of CHD and a 44 per cent difference in risk of stroke.

Nutritional determinants of hypertension are contributory factors and are causally linked to stroke. Obesity and alcohol intake are related to hypertension since weight reduction and restricting alcohol intake can lower blood pressures. The dietary factors that are implicated (in addition to alcohol and caffeine intakes) are excessive sodium and saturated fat intake and low potassium and calcium intake. The role of dietary sodium in hypertension has been a subject of considerable debate. A critical review concluded that there was the relationship between intakes of salt and the prevalence of hypertension (Glieberman 1973). However, in a majority of the studies the methods for assessing both dietary sodium and blood pressure were inadequate. The Intersalt Study (1988) compared standardized blood pressure measurements with 24 h urinary sodium excretion in 10 000 individuals aged 20–59 years in 32 countries and showed that populations with very low sodium excretion (implying low sodium intakes) had low median blood pressures, a low prevalence of hypertension, and no increase in blood pressure with age. Although sodium intake was related to blood pressure levels and also influenced the extent to which blood pressures increased with age, the overall association between sodium, median blood pressure, and the prevalence of hypertension was less than significant.

A number of explanations have been put forward to explain why meticulous studies such as the Intersalt Study underestimate the relationship between dietary sodium and blood pressure. These include among others: Unreliability of assessing dietary intake of sodium accurately; genetic variability; and the contribution of other factors such as obesity or alcohol intake. Recent meta-analysis has correlated blood pressure recordings in individuals with measurements of their 24 h sodium intake (Law *et al.* 1991); an association which increases with age and with the initial blood pressure. The results of intervention trials of sodium restriction support this relationship. Aggregation of the results of 68 cross-over trials and 10 randomized control trials of dietary salt reduction have shown that moderate dietary salt reduction over a few weeks lowers systolic and diastolic blood pressure in those individuals with high blood pressure (Law *et al.* 1991). It was estimated that such reductions in salt intake by population would reduce the incidence of stroke by 26 per cent and that of CHD by 15 per cent in Western countries. Reduction of salt in processed food would lower blood pressure even further and would prevent as many as 70 000 deaths per year in the United Kingdom. Results of therapeutic trials of drug therapy also support the fact that the incidence of stroke can be reduced if blood pressure is lowered, although the beneficial effect of lowering the incidence of CHD is lower than expected.

The other dietary component that has been investigated by the Intersalt Study (1988) is potassium. Urinary potassium excretion, an assumed indicator of intake, was negatively related to blood pressure as was the urinary sodium/potassium concentration ratio. It has also been observed that potassium supplementation reduces blood pressure in both normotensive and hypertensive subjects (Cappucio & MacGregor 1991). Some, but not all, cross-sectional and intervention studies suggest a beneficial effect of calcium intake on blood pressure. Epidemiological studies also consistently suggest lower blood pressures among vegetarians than non-vegetarians independent of age and body weight. These studies may also support the role of other dietary components because vegetarian diets rich in complex carbohydrates are also rich in potassium and other minerals.

Nutritional intervention is likely to reduce the occurrence of hypertension and the consequent complications of stroke and CHD in the community, as demonstrated in Finland where the average blood pressure has fallen by nearly 10 mm Hg and the prevalence of hypertension is only a quarter of what it was prior to the intervention. Along with the falls in average cholesterol levels, CHD and stroke rates in Finland have fallen dramatically as the population's diet was transformed to change its fat content and to more than double the average vegetable and fruit intakes. The decline in CHD and stroke rates was predominantly dependent on the fall in cholesterol and blood pressure levels respectively and these changes occurred despite increasing obesity rates (Puska *et al.* 1995).

A summary of the strength of evidence (convincing and probable) on diet and lifestyle factors and risk of developing cardiovascular diseases (CHD and stroke) based on the recent Joint WHO/FAO Expert Consultation is provided in Table 2.6.5 (WHO/FAO 2003). There is now general agreement on the population strategies that need to be adopted to reduce both the frequency and extent of the risk factors of cardiovascular disease based on this report. The nutritional approach including increasing physical activity is aimed at reducing obesity, lowering blood pressure, lowering total and LDL cholesterol and increasing HDL cholesterol, and lowering sodium intakes. Current recommendations take into consideration both the entire spectrum of cardiovascular risks including effects on thrombosis as well as providing a holistic approach to recommending a healthy diet which will reduce all chronic non-communicable diseases including cancers. These recommendations include lowering total fat intake to between 30 and 35 per cent of total calories, restricting saturated fat intake to a maximum of 10 per cent of total calories, increasing contribution from monounsaturated and polyunsaturated fatty acids (n-3 and n-6 PUFAs), and to increase intakes of complex carbohydrates or dietary fibre. Translated into food components this would mean reducing in particular intake from animal fat, hydrogenated and hardened vegetable oils, and increasing the consumption of cereals, vegetables, and fruits.

Diet, nutrition, and cancers

It is now widely accepted that one-third of human cancers could relate directly to some dietary component (Doll & Peto 1981) and it is probable that diet plays an important role in influencing the permissive role of carcinogens on the development of many cancers. Thus up to 80 per cent of all cancers may have a link with nutrition.

Evidence that diet is a determinant of cancer risk comes from several sources. These include correlation between national and regional food consumption data and the incidence of cancers in the population. Studies on the changing rates of cancer in populations as they migrate from a region or country of one dietary culture to another have contributed to many important hypotheses. Case control studies of the dietary habits of individuals with and without a cancer and prospective studies as well as intervention trials have provided evidence for the effects of diet on cancer. The section below discusses only those human cancers where the role of diet or a nutrient is reasonably well established (summarized in Table 2.6.6). Many other cancers in which aspects of the diet may have a possible role have not been discussed since the aim is not to make this section exhaustive and all inclusive.

Cancers of the gastrointestinal tract may be influenced by the diet. The intake of alcohol appears to be an independent risk factor for oral, laryngeal, and pharyngeal cancers as well as for oesophagus, liver, and breast cancers. Consumption of salted fish (Cantonese style), preserved and fermented foods containing nitrosamines as weaning foods or from early childhood may introduce a substantial risk of *nasopharyngeal cancer. Stomach cancer* is also associated with diets comprising large amounts of salted and salty foods and low levels of fresh fruit and vegetables which may contain nutrients that possibly inhibit the formation of nitrosamines. Non-starchy vegetables, allium vegetables (onion, garlic, etc.), and fruits probably decrease risk of stomach cancer.

Cancers of the colon and rectum are the third commonest form of cancer and the incidence rates are high in Western Europe and North America while they are low in sub-Saharan Africa (Boyle *et al.* 1985). Almost all the specific risk factors of colon cancer are of dietary origin. International comparisons indicate that diets low in dietary fibre or complex carbohydrates and high in animal fat and animal protein increase the risk of colon cancer. The epidemiological data relating foods containing dietary fibre to colorectal cancer generally support the existence of an inverse relationship between the intake of foods which are rich in dietary fibre and colon cancer risk and meta analysis indicates a 10 per cent decreased risk per 10 g fibre per day. Diets rich in fibre are also rich sources of nutrients such as antioxidant vitamins and minerals with potential cancer inhibiting properties. Vegetarian diets seem to provide a protective effect from the risk of colon cancer. There is now convincing evidence that red meat and processed meat in the diet increases the risk of colon and colorectal cancers while physical activity decreases risk. Alcohol intake in men and women as well as obesity and abdominal fatness increase risk of this cancer (WCRF/AICR 2007).

Primary *liver cancers* have been correlated with mycotoxin (aflatoxin) contamination of foodstuffs. The primary causal factor for *lung cancer*, a leading cause of death among men, is cigarette smoking. Several studies have shown an interactive effect between cigarette smoking and low frequency of intake of green and yellow vegetables rich in β-carotene. In prospective studies, the frequency of the consumption of foods rich in β-carotene has been inversely associated with lung cancer risk. However, high intakes of β-carotene as supplements increases risk significantly; and so does arsenic in drinking water.

Breast cancer is a common cause of death among women both in the United States and in the United Kingdom. The most convincing evidence is that lactation protects against risk of breast cancer in both pre- and post-menopausal women. Physical activity probably also decreases risk while increase in body fatness after menopause increases risk. While other nutritional factors related to life events such as greater birth weight, attained adult stature, and weight gain increase risk, consumption of alcoholic drinks also convincingly increases risk of breast cancer both pre- and post-menopause.

Dietary factors thus seem to be important in the causation of cancers of many sites and dietary modifications may reduce cancer risk. In general diets high in plant foods, especially vegetables and fruits, are strongly associated with a lower incidence of a wide range of cancers. Such diets tend to be low in saturated fat, high in complex carbohydrate and fibre, and rich in several antioxidant vitamins. Sustained and consistent intake of alcohol, physical inactivity, and obesity and body fatness are also associated with several cancers. On the basis of the evidence, a recent report (WCRF/AICR 2007) makes the following recommendations: (i) be as lean as possible within the normal range of body weight for height and be physically active. (ii) Eat mostly foods of plant origin and limit intake of red meat and avoid processed meat. (iii) Limit consumption of energy dense foods and avoid sugary drinks. (iv) Limit alcohol intake. (v) Limit consumption of salt, and avoid mouldy food. (vi) Mothers must be encouraged and supported to breast-feed their children.

Table 2.6.6 Associations between nutritional factors and some common cancers

Cancer	Decreasing risk of cancer	Increasing risk of cancer
Breast	Lactation	Alcohol
	Physical activity	Obesity
Colorectal	Physical activity	Processed red meat
	NSP/dietary fibre	Alcohol
	Milk, calcium	Obesity
Endometrium and kidney	Physical activity	Obesity
Liver		Aflatoxin
		Alcohol
Lung	Fruits	High-dose supplements of β-carotene
	Physical activity	
Mouth, larynx, pharynx	Vegetables and fruits	Alcohol
Nasopharynx		Salted fish*
Oesophagus	Fruits and vegetables	Alcohol
		Obesity
Pancreas	Folate rich foods	Obesity
Prostate	Lycopene and selenium-rich foods	High-calcium diets
Stomach	Fruits and vegetables	High salt intake

Compiled from WCRF/AICR, (2007): *Food, nutrition, physical activity and the prevention of cancer: A global perspective.*
Both convincing and probable evidence for decreasing and increasing risk combined
NSP= non starch polysaccharide/dietary fibre
* Specifically Cantonese style salted fish

Diet, lifestyles, and obesity

Obesity is one of the most important public health problems and the prevalence of obesity is increasing in the developed, industrialized world. Even in developing countries, relatively affluent and urbanized communities in countries undergoing rapid economic growth and transition are showing an increasing prevalence of obesity among adults and children.

Overweight and obesity is normally assumed to indicate an excess of body fat. Like adult undernutrition, body mass index (BMI) is used as an indicator of choice to diagnose obesity in adults and Table 2.6.7 outlines the diagnostic criteria for overweight and obesity in infants and children, adolescents, and adults (WHO 1995; WHO 2000). Recent recommendations include the suggestion that a BMI of between 18.5 and 24.9 in adults be considered appropriate weight for height. A BMI between 25 and 29.9 is indicative of overweight and possibly a pre-obese state, while obesity is diagnosed at a BMI >30. The main health risk of obesity is premature death due to heart disease and hypertension and other chronic diseases. In the presence of other risk factors, (both dietary and non-dietary), obesity increases the risk of CHD, hypertension, and stroke. In women, obesity seems to be one of the best predictors of cardiovascular disease. Longitudinal studies have demonstrated that weight gain, both in men and women, is significantly related to increases in cardiovascular risk factors. Weight gain was strongly associated with increased blood pressure, elevated plasma cholesterol, and triglycerides and hyperglycaemia (fasting and post-prandial). The distribution of fat in the body in obesity may also contribute to increased risk; high waist–hip ratios (i.e. fat predominantly in abdomen and not subcutaneous) increase the risk of heart disease and type 2 diabetes. The coexistence of diabetes is also an important contributor to morbidity and mortality in obese individuals. Obesity also carries increased risk of gall bladder stones, breast and uterine cancer in females, and possibly of prostate and renal cancer in males as well as osteoarthritis of weight bearing joints and obstructive sleep apnoea. While obesity contributes to social problems such as low self-esteem and reduced employability it is also associated with increasing mortality both in smokers and non-smokers.

Several environmental factors, both dietary and lifestyle related, contribute to increase in obesity in communities. Social and environmental factors that either increase energy intake and/or reduce physical activity are of primary interest. Changes in the environment that affect the levels of physical activity among children and adults and changes both in the food consumed and in the patterns of eating behaviour may contribute to increase energy intakes beyond one's requirement, thus causing obesity. Increased intake of dietary fat as energy dense food may result in poor regulation of appetite and food intake while fibre-rich complex carbohydrates tend to bulk the meal and limit intakes. International comparisons reveal that obesity increases as the fat percentage of calories in the diet increases (Lissner & Heitmann 1995). Patterns of eating, particularly snacking between meals, may contribute to increased intakes. However, evidence supports the view that much of the energy imbalance which is responsible for the epidemic of obesity in modern societies is largely the result of dramatic reductions in physical activity levels (both occupational and leisure time) when food availability is more than adequate.

Tackling overweight and obesity that is approaching epidemic proportions worldwide is of crucial importance since it is associated

Table 2.6.7 Diagnostic criteria for overweight and obesity in infants and children, adolescents, and adults

Infants and children		
(all ages)	Weight-for-height	>+2 Z scores
Adolescents		
Overweight	BMI-for-age	>85th percentile
Obese	BMI-for-age	>85th percentile of BMI plus
	Triceps-for-age	>90th percentile of TSkf
	Subscapular-for-age	>90th percentile of SSSkf
Adults		
Normal weight range	BMI	18.5–24.9
Overweight or pre-obese	BMI	25–29.9
Obese-Grade I	BMI	30–39.9
Grade II	BMI	35–39.9
Grade III	BMI	>40

Adapted from WHO (1995). *Physical status: the use and interpretation of anthropometry* and WHO (2000). *Obesity: Preventing and managing the global epidemic.*

with several co-morbidities and the consequent increased healthcare costs. It has been estimated that the direct costs of obesity for healthcare in the United States in 1995 was US$70 billion and that of physical inactivity another US$24 billion (Colditz 1999). These are enormous costs and a huge drain on healthcare budgets of countries.

Preventive measures to tackle the increasing obesity worldwide are reliant on the strength of evidence related to the factors that increase or reduce the risk of weight gain. The WHO report (WHO 2003) provides a summary of the evidence, but a more recent and critical review of the evidence is provided in Table 2.6.8 (WCRF/AICR 2007). Preventive measures have to start very early and primary prevention may have to be aimed at young children. This includes nutrition education of children and parents and dealing with problems of school meals, snacking, levels of physical activity, and other related issues. Public health initiatives need to address all social and environmental issues that contribute to the increasing energy and fat intakes and reduce physical activity levels. Since the issues are complex, attempts have to be made to interact with a wide range of stakeholders related to agriculture and trade, education, sport, transportation, etc., and address issues relevant to work sites, schools, supermarkets and deal with marketing, advertising, and promoting activity, etc., and not merely expect the health sector to provide solutions. A recent high-level exercise in the United Kingdom is a good example of such an integrated approach to the problem (Foresight 2007).

Non-insulin dependent diabetes mellitus (NIDDM)

NIDDM is a chronic metabolic disorder which occurs in middle adulthood and is strongly associated with an increased risk of CHD. NIDDM has to be distinguished from insulin dependent diabetes as well as from gestational diabetes of pregnancy. Obesity is a major risk factor for the occurrence of NIDDM; the risk being related both to the duration and the degree of obesity. The occurrence of

Table 2.6.8 Summary of factors that decrease risk (i.e. promote appropriate energy intake relative to energy expenditure) and those that increase risk (i.e. promote excess energy intake relative to energy expenditure) of weight gain and obesity

Evidence	Decreased risk	Increased risk
Convincing	Physical activity	Sedentary living
Probable	Low-energy-dense foods	Energy-dense foods
	Being breastfed	Sugary drinks
		'Fast foods'
		Television viewing

Source: Adapted from WCRF/AICR (2007): *Food, nutrition, physical activity and the prevention of cancer: A global perspective.*
1. Low-energy-dense food whole grain cereals, cereal products, non-starchy vegetables, and dietary fibre.
2. Energy-dense foods are mostly from animal fat and fast foods.
3. Sugary drinks have sucrose or high-fructose corn syrup.

NIDDM in a community appears to be triggered by a number of environmental factors such as sedentary lifestyle, dietary factors, stress, urbanization, and socioeconomic factors. Certain ethnic or racial groups seem to have a higher incidence of NIDDM, these include Pima Indians, Nauruans, and South Asians (i.e. Indians, Pakistanis, and Bangladeshis). NIDDM also seems to occur when the food ecosystem rapidly changes, e.g. urbanization of Australian aborigines or adoption of Western dietary patterns by Pima Indians.

The cause of NIDDM is unclear, but it seems to involve both an impaired pancreatic secretion of insulin and the development of tissue resistance to insulin. Overweight and obesity, particularly the central or truncal distribution of fat accompanied by a high waist/hip ratio and a high waist circumference seems to be invariably present with NIDDM. Hence the most rational approach to preventing NIDDM is to prevent obesity. Weight control and increasing physical activity levels is fundamental both as a population strategy for the primary prevention of this disorder and also to tackle high-risk individuals. Physical activity improves glucose tolerance by weight reduction and by its beneficial effects on insulin resistance. Diets high in plant foods are associated with a lower incidence of NIDDM, and vegetarians have a lower risk than non-vegetarians.

Expert groups have provided dietary recommendations for both the primary prevention of NIDDM, the management of diabetes, and the reduction of secondary complications which include CHD risk and the renal, ocular, and neurological complications of diabetes. Prevention of weight gain and reduction of obesity is the key, as is increasing levels of physical activity. The specific dietary recommendations include providing diets with carbohydrates providing 55–60 per cent of energy, maximizing content of complex carbohydrates and dietary fibre (non starch polysaccharide intake of 20 g per day) and reduction of simple sugar intakes. In addition the general recommendations for fat (saturated fat to <10 per cent of calories) is emphasized due to the associated high risk of CHD. Maintaining a desirable body weight and preventing weight gain is most important.

Diet and osteoporosis

The increase in numbers of elderly in the developed world has seen an increase in health problems of the elderly, which affects their quality of life. Fracture of the hip is an important health problem, particularly among post-menopausal women. Fractures occur in the elderly following what appears as relatively trivial falls when there is osteoporosis and the density of the bone is reduced. Bone density increases in childhood and adolescence and reaches a peak at about 20 years of age. Bone density falls from menopause in women and from about the age of 55 years in men. The variation in bone density between individuals and different racial groups is large and of the order of ±20 per cent. Since bone density declines with increasing age, those that attain high levels of peak bone mass at the end of adolescence and retain higher levels of bone density during adulthood become osteoporotic with advancing age much more slowly than those with lower bone densities to start with. Hence the range of factors that influence the attainment of peak bone density may play a crucial role in the development of osteoporosis and the occurrence of fractures as age advances.

Several factors determine the onset of osteoporosis and include the lack of oestrogen in post-menopausal women, degree of mobility, smoking, and alcohol intake. Calcium intake is a likely dietary determinant that may contribute to the onset and degree of osteoporosis. Evidence from some countries tends to indicate that the osteoporosis may be diet related since the fracture rate is halved among individuals in the higher calcium intake range compared to those on low calcium diets. However, there are regions where the lower rates of fracture due to osteoporosis are associated with lower calcium intakes. For example, the rates are lower in Singapore as compared with the United States, although the calcium intakes are lower than in the United States. The traditional emphasis on calcium intakes possibly reflects the recognition of its importance in contributing to the density of bone during growth and the need for attaining dense bones at the peak of adult life. High-protein and high-salt diets are known to increase bone loss while calcium supplements, well above what may be considered physiological, in post-menopausal women, may help to reduce the rate of bone loss and slow down the development of osteoporosis. Adequate levels of vitamin D either from the diet or by synthesis in the skin on exposure to sunlight are important factors that diminish risk of osteoporosis. Poor vitamin D status in the elderly have been linked with age-related bone loss and osteoporotic fractures. Many other nutrients may be important for long-term bone health and the prevention of osteoporosis. High intakes of alcohol increase risk of osteoporosis. Above all, the evidence is convincing that physical activity is an important determinant of good bone health.

It is generally believed that populations in developing countries are at less risk of developing osteoporosis in spite of low calcium intakes. This may be related to the fact that they do more physical work, smoke less, drink less alcohol, and have diets which are generally not high in protein or salt content. However, osteoporosis is seen in developing countries in regions where low intakes of dietary calcium are associated with high fluoride intakes. No osteoporosis occurs if high intakes of fluoride are accompanied by dietary intakes of calcium which are also high.

Diet and dental caries

Dental caries is a common disease of the teeth, which results in decay of the tooth surface, usually beginning in the enamel.

An essential feature in the causation of dental caries is dental plaque which is largely made up of microorganisms. Dietary sugars diffuse into the dental plaque where they are metabolized by the microorganisms to acids which can dissolve the mineral phase of the enamel causing dental decay. The process is, however, much more complex and is related to the quantity and quality of saliva produced in the mouth among other factors.

The evidence relating diet to dental caries is vast and has been well reviewed (Rugg-Gunn 1993). The overwhelming evidence indicates that sugars are cariogenic. There is good correlation between the sugar supply (in g per person per day) and the occurrence of dental caries in children and adults (WHO/FAO 2003). The consumption of refined sugar is a recent phenomenon in many parts of the world and seems to have been accompanied by an increase in dental caries in communities which were hitherto free of the problem. Cross-sectional studies correlating an individual's sugar consumption with the incidence of dental caries has demonstrated significant correlations between the two, particularly among young children. It also appears that the consumption of sugars between meals is associated with a marked increase in caries while consumption of sugars with meals is associated only with a small increase. Sucrose seems to be the predominant dietary agent that is cariogenic, although the current emphasis is on the consumption of all free sugars, particularly between meals. Despite suggestions that starch is also cariogenic, careful analysis of epidemiological data from several countries suggests that a much closer relationship exists between dental caries and free sugars than between caries and starchy cereal foods. Fresh fruit, although it contains intrinsic sugars, has a lower cariogenic potential while fruit juices are cariogenic, which may be related to the added sugars in fruit juices or from the lack of adequate salivary stimulation. Food may also contain protective factors that may prevent the occurrence of dental caries. This includes a sufficient daily ingestion of fluoride. Inorganic phosphates in the diet also seem to protect against dental caries.

Prevention of dental caries can be achieved by health education aimed at the individual beginning in infancy. Avoidance of the addition of free sugars to bottle feeds and milk and fruit drinks are a must. An adequate intake of fluoride is desirable quite early in life. During childhood and adolescence, the restriction of the three major sources that contribute to two-thirds of our intake of sugars, i.e. confectionery, table sugar, and soft drinks, will help reduce the increment of caries in childhood. At local and national level, the main interventions should include fluoridation of water supply, labelling of foods, and possible changes in policies that promote the production and marketing of free sugars.

Population nutrient intake goals in the prevention of chronic diseases

The distribution and determinants of risk factors in a population have direct implications for population-based prevention strategies. The foremost attribute that needs recognition is that risk typically increases across the spectrum of the risk factor and is a continuum. Thus those individuals at increased risk are not a distinct group or deviant minority, but a part of the risk continuum. Hence, population-based strategies must seek to shift the whole distribution of risk factors downwards and thus help reduce population incidence of the disease.

Population nutrient intake goals represents the mean population intake of the nutrient that is judged to be consistent with the maintenance of good health; health in this context implies a low prevalence of diet-related diseases in the population. There is usually no single best value and the safe range of intakes that constitute the nutrient goals would be consistent with maintenance of health. If the existing population averages move outside the recommended ranges, health concerns are likely to arise. Thus population nutrient intake goals are useful signposts for population-based strategies to help shift the risk distribution in a population downwards and thus reduce risk of the disease within the population. The recommended population nutrient goals based on critical examination of the available evidence from a recent Expert Consultation (WHO/FAO 2003) are summarized in Table 2.6.9.

Emerging food and nutrition issues of public health concern

Over the last decade several issues of public health concern related to food and nutrition have emerged both in the developed, industrialized countries, and in developing societies of the world. These include the problems related to the microbiological safety of foods, the frightening prospect of an epidemic of spongiform encephalopathies, concerns related to genetically modified foods, issues related to labelling of processed foods, and the emerging epidemic of diet-related chronic diseases and obesity in developing societies. Some of these issues will be dealt with briefly under this section.

Food safety

Food safety refers to whether food is safe for human consumption and hence lacking in biological and chemical contaminants that have the potential to cause illness. The increasing concern over the safety of foods in the developed world is a paradox in that the epidemiological evidence on the safety of foods is quite contrary to

Table 2.6.9 Ranges of the population nutrient intake goals

Dietary factor/nutrient	PNI goal*
Total fat	15–30%
Saturated fat	<10%
Polyunsaturated fatty acids (PUFAs)	6–10%
n-6 PUFAs	5–8%
n-3 PUFAs	1–2%
Trans fatty acids	<1%
Monounsaturated fats (MUFAs)	By difference
Total carbohydrate	55–75%
Free sugars	<10%
Protein	10–15%
Cholesterol	<300 mg per day
Sodium chloride	<5 g per day
Fruits and vegetables	>400 g per day

Source: Summarized from WHO/FAO (2003)
* Expressed as per cent of energy

the perceptions of the public and the media that the food available now is less safe than it used to be. The improvements in public health have virtually eradicated primarily food-borne infections that were until recently associated with considerable morbidity and mortality. The common food-borne diseases currently encountered are usually associated with mild self-limiting gastroenteritis. Studies of risk perception suggest that the public becomes alarmed by health threats which are disproportionate to the actual risk associated with the disease and that this public concern is fuelled by the media which make health issues into media health scares depending on the newsworthiness of the incidents.

There have been several food-borne epidemics in the developed world that have raised concerns about food safety in recent years. These include for instance the *Salmonella enteritidis pt4 (Se4)* epidemic. This was attributed to the ability of *Se4* to invade the oviduct of poultry and get deposited in the albumin of the egg. At the consumer level the outbreak of the infection was linked to the use of raw egg in recipes or cross-contamination from raw to cooked foods. *Campylobacter* infection is the commonest food-borne disease in the United Kingdom and the increase in its incidence may partly be explained by the better ascertainment and reporting of cases associated with this infection. The more recent food scare was the emergence of *E. coli 0157* in Scotland. The emergence of this food-borne infection which caused several deaths include changes in husbandry and the movement of livestock as well as the rapid growth of the fast food industry and poor food hygiene in these environments. *Listeria* is another cause of food-borne disease which is a good example of the role of international trade and globalization in the spread of food-borne diseases.

In the developing world the issues of food safety are related to microbiological agents that contaminate food and water and spread disease rapidly in the warm humid environments of these countries aided by the improper or poor food hygiene practices, poor environmental sanitation, and inadequate regulation of food-related commerce. The safety of foods in the developing world is also compromised by the presence of toxins such as aflatoxins which result from contamination with mycotoxins due to poor food storage practices or due to cyanogens in the diet due to inadequate preparation of staple foods such as cassava. In addition, the food chain in these poor countries is contaminated by pesticide and chemical residues thus compromising the safety of the food consumed by the populations in these countries.

Genetically modified (GM) foods

Another issue that has emerged over recent years and has created a considerable degree of controversy is the use of biotechnology to produce genetically modified foods. Genetic modification of food crops can be used to reduce food losses by increasing resistance to drought, frost, diseases and pests, and help control weeds and reduce post-harvest losses. Biotechnology can improve the nutritional value of foods, for example by increasing protein or micronutrient content or by reducing saturated fat content. They could help slow down ripening so that foods retain their quality much longer. Biotechnology can increase both the yield and the quality of crops grown on existing farmland and thereby reduce pressure on wildlife habitats. In the developed world, particularly in the United Kingdom and Europe, the opposition to GM foods is based largely on ecological arguments that raise concerns regarding the ecological

damage that may follow large-scale use of GM crops. In the poor, developing countries the concerns are more related to the use of the 'terminator gene' technology and the dependence on the large multinationals for seeds and chemicals that the small farmers will inherit. At the heart of this controversy and the raging debate is the gulf between plant breeders, seed and agrochemical industries who promote biotechnology, and the campaigners who argue that GM technology may have hazardous consequences on the environment. This is a debate replete with numerous paradoxes and the climate of mistrust, some of it associated with the not too recent BSE and nvCJD scare, is obscuring the real issues and clouding objective decisions from being made with regard to the production and consumption of GM foods (Dixon 1999). Agricultural biotechnology is essential to increase food production to an increasing global population that is increasingly diverting food from human use to biofuels and animal feed; the latter the consequence of increased meat consumption with economic growth, as seen in China. It has the potential to improve the quality of the food to address both nutritional needs as well as consumer demands. It is interesting to note that the perception and acceptance of GM foods in developing societies, once the terminator gene threat has passed, is widely at variance to the concerns in developed countries (FAO 2004).

Food labelling

An important source of information for the consumer about the food on the supermarket shelf is the label on a food product. Food labels provide information that may be of interest to the consumer, especially with regard to the added chemicals (additives, pesticide residues, colouring and flavouring agents, and preservatives), fats, sugars, and energy content. Although, about two-thirds of shoppers claim to read the information on the labels of new or unfamiliar food products to check their contents, this interest in labels does not mean that consumers always understand the information in the labels. Consumers are even more confused by the nutrition information panel which appears on many food labels.

Food label information is usually designed by experts. A prototype label is produced by the *Codex Alimentarius Commission* of the FAO and WHO which is the Organization charged with advising on international food standards, and this prototype is followed by Food Standards Committees around the world. According to this prototype the nutrients—energy, carbohydrate, protein, and fats are listed according to their amounts per serving and per 100 g. Most consumers however, have hardly any idea of what a 100 g serving is, or for that matter what a normal or average serving is. A further problem is that these labels designed by experts is also beset with problems with terminology. One example is the term 'carbohydrate', which covers a wide range of compounds including sugars and starches, which have quite different health-related properties. Health benefits or nutritional claims are also not meant to be part of the food labels and they also do not provide information to cover ecological and ethical issues which may be of concern for some consumers. More recently the need to highlight the source or origin of foods and in particular the labelling of GM sources of the food product has been a serious concern of consumers. In January 2007, the Food Standards Agency in the United Kingdom agreed on the nutritional criteria for a 'traffic light' labelling of food products to identify products high in fat, sugar, and salt. While consumer organizations supported this move some of the major food companies and super markets have opposed the scheme. Food labelling is an important issue of public health concern and despite the considerable progress made so far there is much to be achieved.

Functional foods

New food products are being marketed as health-enhancing or illness-preventing foods. These are called functional foods or otherwise as 'pharmafoods' or 'nutriceuticals' or novel foods. Functional foods are generally defined as food products that deliver a health benefit beyond providing nutrients. The health benefits of functional foods may be conferred by a variety of production and processing techniques which include: Fortification of certain food products with specific nutrients, using phytochemicals and active microorganisms, and by genetic modification of foods. The topic of functional foods is complex and controversial. An assumption implicit in the functional foods and health benefit claims is that the food supply needs to be fixed or doctored (or medicalized) on public health grounds. The assumption therefore is that the current food supply is in some way deficient, that the habitual diets are inadequate and a technological fix will solve the problem. Thus the emerging debate viewed from the perspective of the proponents of functional foods is that these novel foods may reduce healthcare expenditure by promoting good health and that functional foods are a legitimate nutrition education tool, which will help inform consumers of the health benefits of certain food products. The opponents on the other hand rightly state that it is the total diet that is important for health. They believe that the functional foods are a 'magic bullet' approach which enables manufacturers to indulge in marketing hyperbole, exploit consumer anxiety, and essentially blur the distinction between food and drugs. Ironically the production and marketing of functional foods is on the rise in most developed countries.

Emerging epidemic of obesity and diet-related chronic diseases and the 'double burden' of malnutrition in developing societies

A critical examination of the principal causes of mortality and morbidity worldwide indicates that malnutrition and infectious diseases continue to be significant contributors to the health burden in the developing world. Although reductions in the prevalence of undernutrition is evident in most parts of the developing world, the numbers of individuals affected remain much the same or have even increased, largely the result of increases in the population in these countries. What is striking, however, is that the health burden due to non-communicable diseases (NCDs) such as heart disease and cancer is dramatically increasing in some of these developing countries with modest per capita GNPs, particularly among those that are in some stage of rapid developmental transition. Even the modest increases in prosperity that accompany economic development seems to be associated with marked increases in the mortality and morbidity attributable to these diet-related NCDs. These transitions in the disease burden of the population are mediated by changes in the dietary patterns and lifestyles which typify the acquisition of urbanized lifestyles.

Most developing countries, particularly those in rapid developmental transition, are in the midst of a demographic and epidemiologic transition. Economic development, industrialization, and globalization are accompanied by rapid urbanization. These developmental forces are bringing about changes in the social capital of these societies as well as increasing availability of food and changing lifestyles. The changes in food and nutrition are both quantitative and qualitative; there is not only access to more than adequate food among some sections of the population, but also a qualitative change in the habitual diet. Lifestyle changes contribute to a reduction in physical activity levels (occupational and leisure time) which promote obesity. The essence of these changes is captured by the term 'nutrition transition' (Popkin 1994), which accompanies the demographic and epidemiologic transition in these countries. The poor consumer resistance and inadequate regulation compromises food safety and increases contaminants in the food chain. In addition the deterioration of the physical environment, particularly the increase in levels of environmental pollution, contributes to the health burden. These developing societies suffer a 'double burden'—an unfinished agenda of pre-existing widespread undernutrition superimposed by the emerging burden of obesity and chronic diseases.

Food and nutrition in the prevention of diseases of public health importance

The public health approach to the prevention of nutrition and diet-related diseases requires the adoption of health-oriented nutrition and food policies for the whole population. In most developing countries, the first priority must be ensuring the production or procurement of adequate food supply and its equitable distribution and availability to the whole population along with the elimination of the various forms of nutritional deficiencies which include protein-energy malnutrition, vitamin, mineral, and trace element deficiencies. Efforts must also be made to improve the quality of the food which includes ensuring food safety while reducing spoilage and contamination of foods as well as diversifying the availability and use of foods. In agrarian societies, consideration must be given to the short- and long-term effects of agricultural policies that affect the income and buying power of the small producers. Particular attention needs to be paid to the impact the promotion of cash and export crops has on the availability and ability to procure the principal staples in the diet. Special attention needs to be paid to the feasibility of fortification of foods to deal with localized or widespread deficiencies of iodine, iron, and vitamin A as a mass intervention measure.

In developed countries, the burgeoning costs of tertiary healthcare related to the diagnosis and management of the increasing burden of obesity and diet-related NCDs has had an impact. There is increasing recognition of the need for prevention-oriented health and nutrition policies, and changes in behaviour and lifestyle to reduce the occurrence of these diseases. Some developed countries have been active in the field of public education using national dietary guidelines as a major stimulus. It is important to remember that nutrition education of the public operates in the area where advice is given on a balance of probabilities, rather than irrefutable evidence or any degree of certainty. There is bound to be information that does not fit in with the consensus view since the consensus is based on the balance of the available evidence. It is important to recognize that the causes of these chronic diseases are complex and dietary factors are only a part of the explanation. Individuals differ in their susceptibility to the adverse health effects of specific dietary factors or deficiencies of others. Within the context of public health the focus is the health of the whole population and interventions are aimed at lowering the average level of risk to the health of the whole population.

Changes in consumer preferences have emerged, initially among the upper socioeconomic and educated masses. The media attention, along with the behavioural changes in food preferences and food choices are in turn influencing the industry to modify the systems for food production and processing. However, progress in changing consumer behaviour and preferences is by its nature intrinsically rather slow and has until recently largely occurred without support from public policies in any but the health sector. The process of changing unsatisfactory dietary practices and thus promoting health is not easy to achieve both socially and politically. Despite these limitations the occurrence of and mortality associated with some diet-related NCDs such as heart disease have declined reflecting possible changes in lifestyles of the population.

The dynamic relationship between changes in a population's diet and changes in its health is reflected well in two critical situations. One is the changes in disease and mortality profiles of migrant populations moving from a low risk to a high risk environment. An example of this is the change in disease pattern of the Japanese migrants to the United States. The other is the rapid change seen within a country as rural to urban migration occurs or more frequently as a developing country undergoes rapid industrialization and economic development, and in the process acquires a dietary change and the consequent morbidity and premature mortality profile characteristic of a developed country. Several developing countries have urban pockets of affluent diet and lifestyles and related disease burdens in the midst of problems typical of a poor, developing country. Such countries in transition, like India and Brazil, bear the dual burdens of diseases of affluence and the widespread health problems of a poor country. Developing countries can hence benefit by learning from the experience of dietary change and adverse health effects of the developed world and the aim should be to avoid the diseases and premature deaths related to the changes in diets and lifestyles. By recognizing this problem, governments of developing countries can gain for their people the health benefits of avoiding nutritional deficiencies without encouraging at the same time the development of diet-related NCDs that invariably accompany economic and technological development.

It is thus possible for a country to achieve a reduction in infant and childhood mortality and an increase in life expectancy by the pursuance of health and nutrition policies that aim to provide adequate and equitable access to safe and nutritious food and to minimize at the same time the occurrence of diet-related chronic diseases. This in turn will help avoid the social and economic costs of morbidity and premature death in middle age—a period of highest economic activity and productivity to the nation and to society at large. If such a socially and economically desirable goal is to be achieved, then national governments in both developing and developed countries must aim towards achieving a population-based dietary change (WHO 1990). In the pursuance of this objective, FAO and WHO jointly established the scientific basis for developing and using Food-Based Dietary Guidelines (FAO/WHO 1996).

The development of Food-Based Dietary Guidelines (FBDGs)

FBDGs are developed and used in order to improve the food consumption patterns and nutritional well-being of individuals and populations. Guidelines would be needed by all countries given the important role that food and dietary practices play in nutrition-related disorders; both due to deficiencies or excesses. FBDGs can address specific health issues without the need to fully understand the biological mechanisms that may link constituents of food and diet with disease. However, FBDGs do take into account the considerable epidemiological data linking specific food consumption patterns with a low or high incidence of certain diet-related diseases.

Disseminating information and educating the public through the FBDGs is a 'user friendly' approach since consumers think in terms of foods rather than nutrients. They provide a means for nutrition education mostly as foods for the public. They are intended for use by individual members of the general public, are written in ordinary language, and as far as possible avoid the use of technical terms in nutritional science. FBDGs will vary with the population group and has to take into account the local or regional dietary patterns, practices, and culture. It is important to recognize that more than one dietary pattern is consistent with good health. This will enable the development of food-based strategies that are appropriate for the local region and take into consideration the local dietary practices.

FBDGs can serve as an instrument of nutrition policies and programmes. Since they are based directly on diet and health relationships of particular relevance to the individual country or region, they can help address those issues of public health concern, whether they relate to dietary insufficiency or dietary excess. Food and diet are not the only components of a healthy lifestyle and it is important that other relevant messages related to health promotion are integrated into dietary guidelines.

Global strategies to reduce the burden of nutritional disorders

The prevalence of chronic diseases is increasing dramatically, with the majority occurring in developing countries. WHO proposed an integrated global strategy for the prevention and control of non-communicable diseases entitled, 'Diet, physical activity and health' in 2003. More recently WHO has highlighted the fact that chronic diseases are the leading cause of disease and disability, but are neglected elements of the global health agenda (Beaglehole et al. 2007). WHO has proposed a global goal for the prevention and control of chronic diseases to complement the MDG. The goal is to reduce by 2 per cent per year the age-specific rates of death attributable to chronic diseases, achievement of which would avert 36 million deaths by 2015. Because most of the deaths averted would be in low- and middle-income countries and would mainly affect people less than 70 years, it would bring major economic benefits and reduce the health burden of these nations. Strategies that are developed to tackle nutritional problems need to be joined up to deal simultaneously with both ends of the spectrum of nutritional disorders and need to encompass a wide range of stake holders in a joined up and integrated manner to be effective.

References

Arroyave, G., Mejia, L.A., and Aguilar, J.R. (1981). The effect of vitamin A fortification of sugar on serum vitamin A levels of pre-school Guatemalan children: A longitudinal evaluation. *American Journal of Clinical Nutrition*, **34**, 41–9.

Barker, D.J.P. (2004). The developmental origins of adult disease. In *Fetal and neonatal physiology* (eds. R.A. Polin, W.W. Fox and S.H. Abman), Third edition. W.B. Saunders, Philadelphia.

Beaglehole, R., Ebrahim, S., Reddy, S. (2007) *et al.* Prevention of chronic diseases: A call to action. *Lancet*, **370**, 2152–7

Boyle, P., Earidze, D.G., and Simans, M. (1985). Descriptive epidemiology of colo-rectal cancer. *International Journal of Cancer*, **36**, 9–18.

Cappucio, F.P. and MacGregor, G.A. (1991). Does potassium supplementation lower blood pressure? A meta-analysis of published trials. *Journal of Hypertension*, **9**, 465–73.

Colditz, G. (1999). Economic costs of obesity and inactivity. *Medicine and Science in Sport and Exercise*, **31**, S663–7.

de Onis, M., Blossner, M., Borghi, E. *et al.* (2004). Estimates of global prevalence of childhood underweight in 1990 and 2015. *Journal of the American Medical Association*, **291**, 2600–6.

Dixon, B. (1999). The paradoxes of genetically modified foods. *British Medical Journal* **318**, 547–8.

Doll, R. and Peto, R. (1981). *The Causes of Cancer.* Oxford University Press, Oxford.

Dugdale, M. (2001). Anemia. *Obstetrics & Gynaecology Clinics of North America*, **28**, 363–81.

FAO (2004). *Agricultural biotechnology: Meeting the needs of the poor?* Food and Agricultural Organization, Rome.

FAO (2006). *State of food insecurity in the world.* Food and Agricultural Organization, Rome.

FAO/WHO (1996). *Preparation and use of food-based dietary guidelines.* World Health Organization, Geneva.

Foresight (2007). *Tackling obesity: Future choices-project report.* The Stationery Office, London.

Glieberman, L. (1973). Blood pressure and dietary salt in human populations. *Ecology of Food and Nutrition*, **2**, 143–56.

Grantham-McGregor, S. (1995). A review of the studies of the effect of severe malnutrition on mental development. *Journal of Nutrition*, **125**, 2232S–8S.

Hetzel, B.S. (1987). An overview of the prevention and control of iodine deficiency disorders. In *The prevention and control of iodine deficiency disorders* (eds. B.S. Hetzel, J.T. Dunn and J.B. Stanbury). Elsevier, Amsterdam.

Horton, S. and Ross, J. (2003). The economics of iron deficiency. *Food Policy*, **28**, 51–75.

Intersalt Cooperative Research Group (1988). Intersalt: An international study of electrolyte excretion and blood pressure. *British Medical Journal*, **298**, 920–4.

Keys, A. (1980). *Seven countries: A multivariate analysis of death and coronary heart disease.* Howard University Press, Cambridge, Massachusetts.

Kris-Etherton, P.M. (1999). Monounsaturated fatty acids and risk of cardiovascular disease. *Circulation*, **100**, 1253–8.

Law, M.R. Frost, C.D., and Wald, N.J. (1991). By how much does dietary salt reduction lower blood pressure? *British Medical Journal*, **302**, 811–24.

Lissner, L. and Heitmann, B.L. (1995). Dietary fat and obesity: Evidence from epidemiology. *European Journal of Clinical Nutrition*. **49**, 969–81.

MacMohan, S., Peto, R., Cutler, J. *et al.* (1990). Blood pressure, stroke and coronary heart disease. *Lancet*, **335**, 765–74.

McKeown, T. (1976). *The modern rise of population.* Edward Arnold, London.

Muhilal, P.D., Idjrodinata, Y.R., and Karyadi, D. (1988). Vitamin A fortified monosodium glutamate and health, growth and survival of children: A controlled field trial. *American Journal of Clinical Nutrition*, **48**, 1271–6.

Martin M.J, Hulley, S.B., Browner, W.S. *et al.* (1986). Serum cholesterol, blood pressure and mortality: Implications from a cohort of 361 662 men. Lancet, **ii**, 933–6.

Mori, T.A. and Beilin, L.J. (2001). Long-chain omega 3 fatty acids, blood lipids and cardiovascular risk reduction. *Current Opinion in Lipidology*, **12**, 11–17.

Naiken, L. (2003). Keynote Paper: FAO methodology for estimating the prevalence of undernourishment. *Proceedings of the International Scientific Symposium on Measurement and Assessment of Food Deprivation and Undernutrition.* Food and Agricultural Organization, Rome.

Pharoah, P.O.D. and Connolly, D.C. (1987). A controlled trial of iodinated oil for the prevention of endemic cretinism: A long-term follow-up. *International Journal of Epidemiology*, **16**, 68–73.

Phillips, D.I.W., Lusty, T.D., Osmond, C. *et al.* (1988). Iodine supplementation: Comparison of oral or intramuscular iodized oil with potassiumiodide. A controlled trial in Zaire. *International Journal of Epidemiology*, **17**, 142–7.

Pollitt, E. (1991a). Effects of diet deficient in iron on the growth and development of preschool children. *Food and Nutrition Bulletin*, **13**, 521–37.

Pollitt, E. (199b). Iron deficiency and cognitive function. *Annual Review of Nutrition*, **13**, 521–37.

Popkin, B. (1994). The nutrition transition in low-income countries: An emerging crisis. *Nutrition Reviews*, **52**, 285–98.

Puska, P., Tuomilehto, J., Nissinen, A. *et al.* (1995). *The North Karelia Project. 20 year results and experiences.* University Press, Helsinki.

Rugg-Gunn, A.J. (1993). *Nutrition and dental health.* Oxford University Press, Oxford.

Scholl, T.O. and Johnson, W.G. (2000). Folic acid: Influence on the outcome of pregnancy. *American Journal of Clinical Nutrition*, **71**, 1295S–303S.

SCN (2004). *Fifth report on the world nutrition situation: Nutrition for improved development.* Standing Committee on Nutrition, WHO, Geneva.

Scottish Office Home and Health Department (1993). *The Scottish diet: Report of a working party to the Chief Medical Officer in Scotland.* The Scottish Office, Edinburgh.

Sen, A. (1981). *Poverty and famines: An essay on entitlement and deprivation.* Clarendon Press, Oxford.

Shetty, P. (2006). The Boyd Orr Lecture: Achieving the goal of halving global hunger by 2015. *Proceedings of the Nutrition Society*, **65**, 7–18.

Shetty, P.S. and James, W.P.T. (1994). *Body mass index: An objective measure for the estimation of chronic energy deficiency in adults.* FAO Food and Nutrition Paper, Food and Agricultural Organization, Rome.

Smith, L.C. and Haddad, L. (2000). *Explaining child malnutrition in developing countries: A cross-country analysis.* International Food Policy Research Institute, Washington.

Spurr, G.B. (1987). The effects of chronic energy deficiency on stature, work capacity and productivity. *Chronic energy deficiency: Causes and consequences.* IDECG, Lausanne.

Stoltzfus, R.J., Chwaya, H.M., Tielsch, J.M. *et al.* (1997). Epidemiology of iron deficiency anaemia in Zanzibari schoolchildren: The importance of hookworms. *American Journal of Clinical Nutrition*, **65**, 153–9.

Stolzfus, R.J., Mullany, L., and Black, R.E. (2004). Iron deficiency anemia. In *Comparative quantification of health risks: The global and regional burden of disease attributable to selected major risk factors*(eds. M. Ezzati, A. Rodgers and C.J.L. Murray). World Health Organization, Geneva.

UNICEF (1997). *The state of the world's children 1997.* Oxford University Press, Oxford.

UNICEF (2006). *The state of the world's children 2007: Women and children.* UNICEF, New York.

UNICEF/Micronutrient Initiative (2004). *Vitamin and mineral deficiency: A World progress report.* Micronutrient Initiative, Canada.

Viteri, F.E. (1997). Prevention of iron deficiency. *Prevention of micronutrient deficiencies. Tools for policy-makers and public health workers.* Institute of Medicine. National Academy Press, Washington.

WHO (1982). *Prevention of coronary heart disease.* Technical Report Series. World Health Organization, Geneva.

WHO (1990). *Diet, nutrition and the prevention of chronic disease.* WHO Technical Report Series 797. World Health Organisation, Geneva.

WHO (1995). *Physical status: The use and interpretation of anthropometry.* World Health Organization, Geneva.

WHO (2000). *Obesity: Preventing and managing the global epidemic.* World Health Organization, Geneva.

WHO (2002). *The World Health Report: Reducing risks, promoting healthy life.* World Health Organization, Geneva.

WHO (2004). *Iodine status worldwide.* World Health Organization, Geneva.

WHO (2006). *WHO child growth standards.* World Health Organization, Geneva.

WHO/FAO (2003). *Diet, nutrition and the prevention of chronic diseases.* Technical Report series 916. World Health Organization, Geneva.

WHO/UNICEF/UNU (2001). *Iron deficiency anemia: Assessment, prevention and control.* World Health Organization, Geneva.

World Cancer Research Fund/American Institute for Cancer Research (2007). *Food, nutrition, physical activity and the prevention of cancer: A global perspective.* American Institute for Cancer Research, Washington.

2.7

Infectious diseases

Davidson H. Hamer, Zulfiqar Ahmed Bhutta, and Sherwood L. Gorbach

Introduction

Infectious diseases are a major cause of morbidity, disability, and mortality worldwide. During the last century, substantial gains have been made in public health interventions for the treatment, prevention, and control of infectious diseases. Nevertheless, recent decades have seen a worldwide pandemic of the human immuno-deficiency virus (HIV), increasing antimicrobial resistance, and the emergence of many new viral, bacterial, fungal, and parasitic pathogens.

As a result of changes in a variety of different environmental, social, economic, and public health factors, morbidity and mortality due to infectious diseases have declined in industrialized countries during the last 150 years with the result being a gradual transition to chronic diseases including cardiovascular disease, diabetes mellitus, and cancer as major causes of mortality in these countries today. However, in contrast, in less developed countries, infectious diseases continue to contribute substantially to the overall burden of disease.

Detailed information on the definitions of infectious diseases, modes of transmission, and their control are provided in Chapter 12.6, by Robert J. Kim-Farley. An overview of issues related to emerging and re-emerging infections is provided in Chapter 9.17. Similarly, detailed information on diseases caused by prions, sexually transmitted infections, human immunodeficiency virus/acquired immunodeficiency syndrome (HIV/AIDS), tuberculosis, and malaria can be found in Chapters 9.11–9.15. This chapter will review the global burden of common infectious diseases in children and adults, determinants of the high infectious disease burden in resource-poor countries, and important aspects of the clinical manifestations, diagnosis, and treatment of the handful of infectious diseases that account for the major share of morbidity and mortality in children and adults worldwide.

Burden of infectious diseases

At the beginning of the twentieth century, infectious diseases were the leading cause of death throughout the world. At that time, three diseases—pneumonia, diarrhoea, and tuberculosis—were responsible for about 30 per cent of deaths in the United States. During the last century, there has been a decline in infectious diseases mortality in the United States from 797 deaths per 100 000 in 1900 to 36 per 100 000 in 1980. Despite substantial reductions in all-cause

mortality due to diarrhoeal disease and tuberculosis, pneumonia and influenza have continued to be major causes of mortality (Armstrong *et al.* 1999). Concurrent with the growth of the AIDS pandemic worldwide, there was a rise in mortality rates among persons aged 25 years and older in developed and less developed areas of the world.

In the late twentieth century, substantial reduction in child mortality occurred in low- and middle-income countries. The fall in the number of child deaths during the period of time from 1960–90 averaged 2.5 per cent per year and the risk of dying in the first 5 years of life halved—a major achievement in child survival. In the period 1990–2001, mortality rates dropped an average of 1.1 per cent annually, mostly after the neonatal period. Most neonatal deaths are unrecorded in formal registration systems and communities with the greatest number of neonatal deaths have the least information related to mortality rates and interventions. Not surprisingly therefore current global burden figures of newborn and young infant deaths are largely estimates. These figures suggest that 10.6 million children under the age of 5 years die annually and, of the 130 million births, 3.8 million die in the first 4 weeks of life—the neonatal period, with some three quarters of neonatal deaths occurring in the first week after birth. In the period 2000–2003, four communicable diseases categories accounted for 54 per cent of childhood deaths; these included pneumonia (19 per cent), diarrhoea (18 per cent), malaria (8 per cent), and neonatal sepsis or pneumonia (10 per cent) (Bryce *et al.* 2005) (Fig. 2.7.1). The distribution of these causes of mortality was similar in World Health Organization (WHO) regions with the exception of malaria, which was concentrated in sub-Saharan Africa.

The Southeast Asian region accounts for the highest number of child deaths, over 3 million, whereas the highest mortality rates are generally seen in sub-Saharan Africa. Annually, sub-Saharan Africa and South Asia share 41 and 34 per cent of child deaths respectively (Table 2.7.1) (Black *et al.* 2003). Only six countries account for half of worldwide deaths and 42 for 90 per cent of child deaths with the predominant causes being pneumonia, diarrhoea, and neonatal disorders, with surprisingly little contribution from malaria and AIDS. In all, 99 per cent of neonatal deaths occur in poor countries (estimated average neonatal mortality rate (NMR) of 33/1000 live births) and the remaining are divided among 39 high-income countries (estimated average NMR of 4/1000 live births) (Table 2.7.2).

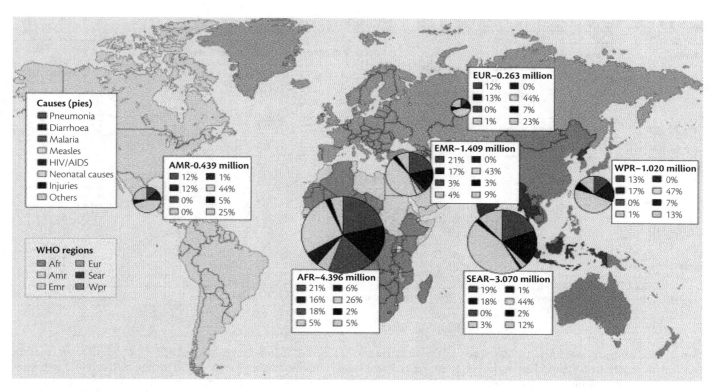

Fig. 2.7.1 Distribution of causes of child mortality worldwide; from: Bryce *et al.* (2005). WHO estimates of the causes of death in children. *The Lancet*, **365**, 1147–52.

As of the end of 2006, the Joint United Nations Programme on HIV/AIDS (UNAIDS) estimated that there were 39.5 million people living with HIV infection and that 4 million new infections occurred during 2006 along with 3 million deaths. The greatest increases in prevalence were in Central Asia and Eastern Europe while sub-Saharan Africa continued to account for nearly two-thirds of cases. In contrast to the continuing growth of the HIV/AIDS pandemic, global growth of tuberculosis slowed in the last few years. By 2004, the WHO estimated that there were 8.9 million new cases worldwide and that the incidence of tuberculosis was stable or declining in five of six WHO regions, the only exception being Africa (Nunn *et al.* 2007). Sadly, tuberculosis is responsible for approximately 10 per cent of HIV-associated deaths of children and adults in sub-Saharan Africa, despite substantial increases in the numbers of HIV-infected people receiving antiretroviral therapy in resource-poor countries.

Lower respiratory tract infections are the leading cause of DALYs worldwide, accounting for 6.4 per cent of the total. HIV/AIDS is third on the list accounting for 6.1 per cent, while diarrhoeal diseases and malaria rank fifth and ninth, accounting for 4.2 and 2.7 per cent of DALYs, respectively. In high-income countries, lower respiratory infections are the fourth leading cause of death. No communicable disease is among the top ten leading causes of DALYs in high-income countries. In contrast, pneumonia, HIV/AIDS, diarrhoea, tuberculosis, and malaria rank among the top ten causes of death and DALYs in low- and middle-income countries.

A number of factors are responsible for the decline in infectious diseases in industrialized nations during the last century. These include improved nutrition, safer food and water supplies, improved hygiene and sanitation, the introduction of antimicrobial agents, and immunizations, all of which resulted in decreased host susceptibility and reductions in disease transmission (Cohen 2000). While there have been substantial reductions in morbidity and mortality due to communicable diseases in the last century, there remain significant gaps in child and adult mortality between rich and poor countries.

Apart from the immediate causes of infections in childhood, a number of determinants contribute to the high burden of infectious diseases in developing countries. These include several distal determinants such as income, social status, and education, which work through an intermediate level of environmental and behavioural risk factors (Fig. 2.7.2). These risk factors, in turn, lead to the proximal causes of death (nearer in time to the terminal event), such as undernutrition, infectious diseases, and injury (Rice *et al.* 2000). The major social determinants affecting the mortality and morbidity of young children include poverty, crowding, poor housing conditions, malnutrition, inequity, lack of education, failure to implement breastfeeding and complementary feeding programmes, the presence of debilitating disease in addition to infections, complications of labour and LBW, inadequate health-related social behaviours and practices, and other social and cultural determinants of health.

Specific disease categories

As described above, a limited number of infectious diseases are responsible for a large proportion of the total global burden of morbidity and mortality, especially in resource-limited areas of the world. The following section will provide an overview of the major types of infectious diseases responsible for the bulk of acute and

Table 2.7.1 Regional classification of mortality rates and causes of death in children under 5 years

Region	<5 mortality rate per 1000 live births (2004)	Infant mortality rate per 1000 live births (2004)	Neonatal mortality rate per 1000 live births (2000)	Cause of death among children under 5 years					
				Neonatal Causes (2000)	HIV/ AIDS (2000)	Diarrhoea (2000)	Malaria (2000)	Pneumonia (2000)	Others (2000)
African region	167	100	43	26.2	6.8	16.6	17.5	21.1	5.6
American region	25	21	12	43.7	1.4	10.1	0.4	11.6	27.9
Southeast Asia region	77	56	38	44.4	0.6	20.1	1.1	18.1	9.9
European region	22	18	11	44.3	0.2	10.2	0.5	13.1	25.4
Eastern Mediterranean region	94	69	40	43.4	0.4	14.6	2.9	19.0	13.5
Western Pacific region	31	25	19	47.0	0.3	12.0	0.4	13.8	18.4

The World Health Report 2006: Working together for health. Geneva, World Health Organization, 2006 (http://www.who.int/whr/2006/annex/en).

chronic morbidity and mortality of children and adults worldwide. Detailed information on approaches for the prevention and control of these diseases is available in Chapter 12.6.

Acute respiratory infections (ARIs)

ARIs are classified as upper or lower respiratory tract infections. Upper respiratory tract infections include the common cold, otitis media, sinusitis, and pharyngitis while lower respiratory tract infections include laryngitis, tracheitis, bronchitis, bronchiolitis, pneumonia, and any combination thereof. ARIs are not only confined to the respiratory tract, but may also have systemic effects due to extension of infection into the bloodstream, the production of microbial toxins, inflammation, and reduced lung function.

ARIs, especially bronchiolitis and pneumonia, are the most common causes of both illness and mortality in children under 5 years with. In adults, pneumonia and influenza are major causes

Table 2.7.2 Global burden of diseases: Deaths and disability adjusted life years (DALYs), 2001

	Low and middle-income		High-income		World	
	Deaths	DALYs (3, 0)[a]	Deaths	DALYs (3, 0)[a]	Deaths	DALYs (3, 0)[a]
Total for all causes (thousands)	48 351	1 386 709	7891	149 161	56 242	1 535 871
Rate per 1000 population	9.3	265.7	8.5	160.6	9.1	249.8
Age-standardized rate per 1000[b]	11.4	281.7	5.0	128.2	10.0	256.5
Selected cause groups	Number in thousands (per cent)					
Communicable diseases[c]	17 613 (36.4)	552 376 (39.8)	552 (7.0)	8561 (5.7)	18 166 (32.3)	560 937 (36.5)
HIV/AIDS	2552 (5.3)	70 796 (5.1)	22 (0.3)	665 (0.4)	2574 (4.6)	71 461 (4.7)
Diarrhoea	1777 (3.7)	58 697 (4.2)	6 (<.1)	444 (0.3)	1783 (3.2)	59 141 (3.9)
Malaria	1207 (2.5)	39 961 (2.9)	0 (0.0)	9 (<0.1)	1208 (2.1)	39 970 (2.6)
Lower respiratory infections	3408 (7.0)	83 606 (6.0)	345 (4.4)	2314 (1.6)	3753 (6.7)	85 920 (5.6)
Perinatal conditions	2489 (5.1)	89 068 (6.4)	32 (0.4)	1408 (0.9)	2522 (4.5)	90 477 (5.9)
Protein-energy malnutrition	241 (0.5)	15 449 (1.1)	9 (0.1)	130 (<0.1)	250 (0.4)	15 578 (1.0)

Notes: Numbers in parentheses indicate percentage of column total. Broad group totals in bold are additive but should not be summed with all other conditions listed in table. *Source*: World Health Organization. Global burden of disease estimates 2001 (www.who.int/healthinfo/bodgbd2001/en/index.html).

[a] DALYs (3, 0) refer to the version of the DALY based on a 3 per cent annual discount rate and uniform age weights.

[b] Age-standardized using the WHO World Standard Population.

[c] Includes only causes responsible for more than 1 per cent of global deaths or DALYs in 2001.

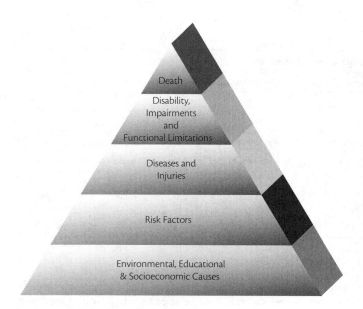

Fig. 2.7.2 Overview of the burden of disease framework. This diagram is intended for a broader scale since environmental factors can be proximate causes of death but injuries can directly cause disability or death.

of morbidity and mortality in developed as well as less-developed nations.

Global and regional epidemiology

The annual incidence in children in Europe and North America is 34–40 cases per 1000, higher than at any other time of life, except perhaps in adults older than 75 or 80 years of age. Pneumonia is the most severe and largest killer of children, causing almost 20 per cent of all child deaths globally. Recent estimates indicate that there are approximately 1.9 million pneumonia deaths annually (95 per cent confidence interval, 1.6–2.2 million), with 75 per cent of all childhood pneumonia cases occurring in just 15 countries.

Most of the deaths from ARIs are due to pneumonia. The annual incidence of pneumonia is estimated at 151 million new cases per year, of which 11–20 million (7–13 per cent) cases are severe enough to require hospitalization. Serious neonatal infections account for 30–50 per cent of neonatal mortality in different regions, and it is difficult to disentangle sepsis and deaths from pneumonia. With the inclusion of neonatal pneumonia, recent estimates indicate that pneumonia is the single largest contributor to child mortality, accounting for almost 28–34 per cent of all under-5 deaths globally. It is also important to note that in contrast to diarrhoeal deaths where mortality rates have reduced dramatically, despite the introduction of a global programme for the control of ARIs almost 15 years ago, there has been little change in overall burden of deaths from pneumonia.

There are about 4 million adults who develop pneumonia in the United States each year, of whom greater than 1 million are hospitalized. In terms of the overall burden of disease, upper and lower ARIs account for a major proportion of outpatient visits, antibiotic prescriptions, and healthcare costs in the United States and Western Europe. Despite gains in the availability and quality of healthcare in industrialized countries, ARIs, especially lower respiratory tract infections, remain a major cause of morbidity and mortality for adults and children. In fact, even today pneumonia and influenza together are the sixth most common cause for death among adults in the United States. Recovery from pneumonia in the elderly takes longer and complications and mortality are also more frequent than in younger populations. Pneumonia is one of the most common causes of hospitalization and decreased activities of daily living among the elderly. Risk factors for death from pneumonia in adults include advanced age, alcohol consumption, leucopenia, bacteraemia, hypoxemia, co-morbid conditions such as diabetes mellitus, congestive heart failure, active malignancies, and immunosuppression, and certain signs and symptoms including hypothermia, hyperthermia, tachypnoea, hypotension, and altered mental status. In addition, post-obstructive pneumonia, aspiration pneumonia, and infections due to *Staphylococcus aureus* and gram-negative bacilli are independently associated with increased mortality risk.

Many factors such as the presence of certain co-morbid medical conditions, use of certain drugs, changes in physiochemical characteristics of the non-specific host defence system such as cilia and mucus of the respiratory tract, malnutrition, and mechanical devices contribute to an increased incidence of pneumonia among the elderly. However, an important predisposing factor to the increased incidence of infections is the age-associated decline in immune responsiveness. Changes in immune response not only decrease resistance to pathogens but also contribute to increased morbidity and mortality due to respiratory infections.

Aetiology

A wide range of different bacterial and viral pathogens are responsible for community-acquired pneumonia in children and adults. Foremost among them is *Streptococcus pneumoniae*, which accounts for up to half of all cases. Other commonly encountered bacterial pathogens include *Haemophilus influenzae*, *Chlamydia pneumoniae*, *Moraxella catarrhalis*, *Legionella pneumophila*, *Mycoplasma pneumoniae*, *S. aureus*, and Gram-negative rods such as *Klebsiella pneumoniae* and *Escherichia coli* (Table 2.7.3). During recent years, the role of viral pathogens in the aetiology of acute lower respiratory tract infections has been increasingly described. While influenza is well recognized as a cause of viral pneumonia, several studies have demonstrated the importance of parainfluenza virus, respiratory syncytial virus (RSV), adenovirus, and human metapneumovirus.

Issues in presentation and diagnosis

Currently, the standard WHO algorithm for ARIs defines non-severe pneumonia as cough or difficult and fast breathing (respiratory rate of 50 breaths per minute or more for children aged 2–11 months; or respiratory rate of 40 breaths per minute or more for children aged 12–59 months) and either documented fever of above 101°F or chest in-drawing. Severe pneumonia has been defined as having cough or difficult breathing, with tachypnoea and in-drawing of the lower chest wall (with or without fast breathing); and very severe pneumonia/disease—cough or difficult breathing with one or more danger signs (central cyanosis, inability to drink, or unusually sleepy). The WHO has defined pneumonia solely on the basis of clinical findings obtained by visual inspection and setting respiratory rate cut-offs. It is recognized that mortality in children due to ARIs could be reduced by one-half if early detection and appropriate treatment could be provided.

In contrast to the simple, clinical definition of pneumonia recommended by the WHO for use in developing countries, pneumonia

Table 2.7.3 Pathogen-specific causes of childhood and adult pneumonia

Age range	Most common causative organism
Neonates (from birth to 30 days after birth)	*Streptococcus pyogenes*, *Staphylococcus aureus*, and *Escherichia coli*
Infants (from 3 weeks to 4 months)	*S. pneumoniae*
Infants older than 4 months and preschool-aged children	Respiratory viruses and *S. pneumoniae*
Children in developing countries	*S. aureus* and *Haemophilus influenzae* including non-typable strains
Adults—outpatient	*S. pneumoniae, Mycoplasma pneumoniae, H. influenzae, Chlamydiophila pneumoniae*, and respiratory viruses
Adults—inpatient	*S. pneumoniae, M. pneumoniae, C. pneumoniae, H. influenzae, Legionella pneumophila*, respiratory viruses, and aspiration
Adults—intensive care unit	*S. pneumoniae, S. aureus, L. pneumophila*, Gram-negative bacilli, and *H. influenzae*

in resource-rich countries is usually based on the presence of characteristic signs and symptoms (e.g. dry or productive cough, tachypnoea, fever, focal findings on respiratory examination), hypoxaemia, and the presence of infiltrates on chest radiograph. In general, the elderly tend to present with fewer or atypical symptoms of pneumonia than younger patients and therefore non-specific features such as fever or mental status change may be indicators of an underlying lower respiratory tract infection.

Microbiological studies can be pursued to support the diagnosis of pneumonia due to specific infectious agents and to facilitate decision making for antibiotic management. While broad spectrum empirical antimicrobial coverage is recommended in various guidelines, there is a potential risk for clinical failure and increased mortality if inappropriate antibiotic therapy is initiated. If available and adequate quality specimens can be obtained, blood cultures and sputum gram stain and culture should be performed. Rapid diagnostic tests may be useful when specific diagnoses are being considered such as RSV, influenza, or *L. pneumophila*.

Clinical approaches for the management of childhood pneumonia are significantly hampered by the lack of a gold standard, as classic microbiological methods have poor sensitivity and current algorithms lack sufficient specificity. It is therefore likely that community strategies for the recognition and management of pneumonia by ancillary health workers that rely on simple clinical criteria, other than auscultation, will overdiagnose bacterial pneumonia. There are legitimate concerns that widespread use of first-line antibiotics for all acute respiratory infections will lead to loss of effectiveness.

Evidence-based interventions

Only in the early 1980s, long after immunization and diarrhoea control programmes were launched, did the international community become aware of the epidemiological magnitude of pneumonia in children. This need for action led the WHO and UNICEF to decide that reduction of mortality from pneumonia should be the main objective of the initial ARI programme. Only about half of children with pneumonia receive appropriate medical care, and, according to limited data from the early 1990s, less than 20 per cent of children with pneumonia received antibiotics. Since early microbiological studies of lung aspirates taken from hospitalized, untreated children with pneumonia in developing countries showed that bacteria were present in more than 50 per cent of cases

and it was recognized that bacterial pathogens were responsible for the most severe cases, it became apparent that prompt treatment with a full course of effective antibiotics could be life-saving.

Antibiotic treatment of pneumonia

Although recommendations for antibiotic therapy for pneumonia are based on aetiological diagnosis, identification of the causative organism in routine clinical care is very difficult and empirical antibiotic therapy is often instituted. Guidelines for the treatment of pneumonia in immunocompetent adults in industrialized nations generally recommend a macrolide or doxycycline for outpatients; an advanced macrolide such as azithromycin or clarithromycin plus a beta-lactam or a respiratory fluoroquinolone alone for less acutely ill inpatients; and a beta-lactam plus either an advanced macrolide or respiratory fluoroquinolone for adults requiring intensive care (Mandell *et al.* 2007). The preferred treatment options must be modified for certain high-risk groups and in patients who have had recent antimicrobial therapy.

Since *S. pneumoniae* and *H. influenzae* are the most common causes of childhood pneumonia in developing countries, the WHO recommends using oral cotrimoxazole or amoxicillin as first-line drugs for the treatment of non-severe pneumonia at first level health facilities. Cloxacillin or other anti-staphylococcal antibiotics should be available to treat cases in which the initial combination fails within 48 h. Young infants with signs of pneumonia, sepsis, or meningitis should be referred to hospital for parenteral treatment. Similarly children with pneumonia and malnutrition should be referred to hospital for differential diagnosis of tuberculosis and for parenteral antimicrobial treatment for bacterial pneumonia.

The various modalities for antibiotic treatment in children according to disease severity are shown in Table 2.7.4. However, the emergence of resistance to first-line antimicrobial drugs recommended for home treatment of non-severe pneumonia has been associated with treatment failure rates as high as 22 per cent. Recent data on the failure of standard antimicrobial treatment with parenteral penicillin or amoxicillin in 24 per cent of cases for severe pneumonia among HIV-infected children in Africa are even more alarming.

The current WHO treatment guidelines for ARIs were designed before the rise of HIV infection in sub-Saharan Africa, and they do not include empiric treatment for *Pneumocystis carinii* pneumonia. Daily administration of cotrimoxazole is advocated since it reduces

Table 2.7.4 Treatment of paediatric pneumonia according to disease severity

Signs/symptoms	Classification	Treatment
Fast breathing: ≥60 breaths/min in child aged <2 months ≥50 breaths/min in child aged 2–11 months ≥40 breaths/min in child aged 1–5 years	Pneumonia	Home care
		Give appropriate antibiotics for 5 days
Definite crackles on auscultations		Soothe the throat and relieve the cough with a safe remedy
		Advise the mother when to return immediately
		Follow up in 2 days
Signs of pneumonia plus chest wall in-drawing	Severe pneumonia	Admit to hospital
		Give recommended antibiotics
		Manage airway
		Treat high fever if present
Signs of severe pneumonia plus central cyanosis, severe respiratory distress, and inability to drink	Very severe pneumonia	Admit to hospital
		Give the recommended antibiotics
		Give oxygen
		Manage airway
		Antipyretics

deaths from opportunistic infections in symptomatic HIV-infected children, including pneumonia caused by *P. carinii*. A multi-centre randomized control trial, by the APPIS Group, showed that standard empiric therapy for severe pneumonia with injectable penicillin or oral amoxicillin in severe pneumonia in infants is inadequate where HIV prevalence is high (Addo-yabo *et al.* 2004). The benefits of these guidelines would be enhanced if they could also be applied (with modification) throughout areas with high rates of HIV infection and where the pneumonia burden is high, even in HIV-negative children.

Integrated management of childhood infections (IMCI)

In the mid-1980s, WHO initiated a control programme for ARIs that focused on cases managed by health workers. The current case management of ARIs has been incorporated into the global IMCI which train health workers to recognize fast breathing, lower chest wall in-drawing, or danger signs in children with respiratory symptoms (such as cyanosis or inability to drink).

Preventive measures

Poverty, overcrowding, air pollution, malnutrition, harmful traditional practices, and delayed and inappropriate case management are important underlying determinants for high ARI case fatality rates. Preventive strategies for pneumonia include immunizing children with the pneumococcal, measles, and *H. influenzae* type b (Hib) vaccines, hand washing, reduction of the incidence of LBW, ensuring warmth after birth and appropriate feeding, promoting adequate nutrition (including exclusive breastfeeding and zinc intake), and reducing indoor air pollution (Bhutta 2007; WHO Collaborative Group on Breastfeeding 2000).

Three vaccines have the potential to substantially reduce deaths in children <5 years of age—(the Hib, measles, and pneumococcal

vaccines). Two kinds of vaccines are currently available against pneumococci: A 23-valent polysaccharide vaccine (23-PSV), which is more appropriate for adults than children, and a 7-valent protein-conjugated polysaccharide vaccine (7-PCV). The rate of invasive pneumococcal disease (IPD) has decreased among both immunized children and non-immunized adults since the introduction of heptavalent pneumococcal conjugate vaccine (PCV7) for use in infants in the United States in 2000. Moreover, newer versions of the pneumococcal conjugate vaccine might become available as early as 2008, and have the potential to significantly reduce pneumonia deaths in developing countries.

Controlled trials of hand washing promotion in child-care centres in developed countries have reported significant reduction (12–32 per cent) in rates of upper respiratory-tract infections. A community-based cluster randomized trial of hand washing promotion from Pakistan also reported that frequent hand washing (with or without soap) led to a 50 per cent reduction in pneumonia incidence and a 36 per cent lower incidence of impetigo.

About 3 billion people still rely on solid fuels, 2.4 billion on biomass, and the rest on coal, mostly in China. Globally, there is marked regional variation in solid fuel use in relation to poverty with use rates of <20 per cent in Europe and Central Asia and >80 per cent in sub-Saharan Africa and South Asia, intricately linking to poverty. More than half of all the deaths and 83 per cent of DALYs lost attributable to solid fuel use occur as a result of lower respiratory tract infection (pneumonia) in children under 5 years of age and a systematic review of the evidence for the impact of indoor air pollution on a wide range of health outcomes including pneumonia indicates substantial benefits on pneumonia prevention.

Previously, a meta-analysis of trials of daily preventive zinc supplementation showed a significant impact on pneumonia incidence (Zinc Investigators' Collaborative Group 1999). A recent update of this meta-analysis reaffirms the impact on reduction in the risk of respiratory tract infections (by 8 per cent, respectively) but not on duration of disease (Aggarwal 2007).

Public health implications

Despite the introduction of a global programme for the control of ARIs almost 15 years ago, there has been little change in overall burden of deaths from pneumonia. The bulk of deaths from childhood pneumonia disproportionately affect the poor who have higher exposure rates to risk factors for developing ARIs, such as overcrowding, poor environmental conditions, malnutrition, and also limited access to curative health services. The importance of reaching the poor with pneumonia in community settings must be underscored. Such strategies involve recognizing and ambulatory management of pneumonia in community settings through community health workers, assuring transportation and access to facilities for severe pneumonia and availability of antibiotics.

Neonatal sepsis

Sepsis and meningitis are significant causes of morbidity and mortality in newborns, particularly in preterm, LBW infants. Serious infections among newborns are estimated to cause 30–40 per cent of neonatal deaths, especially in rural populations and are associated with several risk factors.

Neonatal sepsis may be defined using clinical criteria (Table 2.7.5) and/or microbiological testing, by positive blood and/or cerebrospinal fluid (CSF) cultures. It may also be classified according to the time of onset of the disease: Early onset (EOS) and late onset (LOS). Meningitis can occur as a part of sepsis in both the early and late onset time periods or as focal infection with late-onset disease. The distinction has clinical relevance, as EOS disease is mainly due to bacteria acquired before and during delivery, and LOS disease to bacteria acquired after delivery (nosocomial or community sources). In the literature, however, there is little consensus as to what age limits apply, with EOS ranging from 48 h to 6 days after delivery.

Global and regional epidemiology

Severe bacterial infections are responsible for 460 000 deaths annually, apart from 300 000 fatalities from tetanus, many of which are due to neonatal tetanus. The reported incidence of neonatal sepsis varies from 7.1 to 38 per 1000 live births in Asia, from 6.5 to 23 per 1000 live births in Africa, and from 3.5 to 8.9 per 1000 live births in South America and the Caribbean, 6–9 per 1000 in the United States and Australia. The incidence of neonatal meningitis is 0.1–0.4/1000 live births and is higher in developing countries. Despite major advancement in neonatal care, overall case-fatality rates from sepsis range from 2 to as high as 50 per cent.

Unfortunately, hospitals in developing countries are also hot beds of infection transmission, especially multi-drug-resistant nosocomial infections. Reported rates of neonatal sepsis vary from 6.5 to 38 per 1000 live hospital-born babies and the rates of bloodstream infection range from 1.7 to 33 per 1000 live births, with rates in Africa clustering around 20 and in South Asia around 15 per 1000 live births. Factors responsible for hospital-acquired neonatal sepsis include lack of aseptic technique for procedures, inadequate hand hygiene and glove use, deficient sterilization and disinfection practices, overuse of invasive devices, re-use of disposable supplies without

Table 2.7.5 World Health Organization clinical criteria for diagnosis of neonatal sepsis and meningitis*

Sepsis	Meningitis
Symptoms	*General signs*
Convulsions	Drowsiness
Inability to feed	Reduced feeding
Unconsciousness	Unconsciousness
Lethargy	Lethargy
Fever (>37.7°C or feels hot)	High-pitched cry
Hypothermia (<35.5°C or feels cold)	Apnea
Signs	*Specific signs*
Severe chest in-drawing	Convulsions
Reduced movement	Bulging fontanelle
Crepitations	
Cyanosis	

*The more symptoms a neonate has, the higher the probability of the disease.

adequate sterilization, re-use of single-use vials, overcrowded and understaffed labour and delivery rooms, unhygienic bathing and skin care, contaminated bottle feedings, inappropriate and prolonged use of antibiotics, and lack of effective infection control practices.

Aetiology

In general, Gram-negative pathogens are responsible for a substantial proportion of EOS. In contrast to industrialized countries where group B streptococci are common causes of neonatal sepsis, *Klebsiella pneumoniae* is an important aetiology in developing countries. LOS is most commonly due to *E. coli*, *S. aureus*, *S. pyogenes*, *S. pneumoniae*, and *Salmonella* spp. The organisms causing neonatal sepsis and meningitis in developing and developed countries are listed in Table 2.7.6.

Evidence-based interventions to address neonatal infections

Child survival and safe motherhood strategies have yet to adequately address mortality in the neonatal period. The fourth Millenium Development Goal (MDG-4) commits the international community to reducing mortality in children aged <5 years by two-thirds from 1990 base figures by 2015. Real progress in saving newborns will depend upon provision of a good mix of preventive and therapeutic services.

Medical treatment

Reaching and treating sick newborn infants promptly is critical to survival. Normally, a combination of ampicillin and gentamicin is used by health staff for suspected cases of neonatal sepsis (Table 2.7.7). However, increasing antibiotic resistance among common organisms causing neonatal sepsis in both community and hospital settings presents a challenge to the selection of appropriate antibiotics. Case management of neonatal infections is mainly provided through child-health services, both in facilities and through family-community care. Scaling up of emergency

Table 2.7.6 Major bacterial causes of neonatal sepsis and meningitis

Neonatal sepsis		Neonatal meningitis	
Developing countries	**Developed countries**	**Developing countries**	**Developed countries**
Gram-negative bacilli (more common)	Gram-negative bacilli	Gram-negative bacilli (more common in neonates <1 week old)	Gram-negative bacilli
Klebsiella spp.	*Escherichia coli* (more common)	*Klebsiella* spp.	*E. coli*
E. coli		*E. coli*	
Pseudomonas aeruginosa		*Serratia marscesens*	
Salmonella spp.		*P. aeruginosa*	
		Salmonella spp.	
Gram-positive cocci (less common)	Gram-positive cocci	Gram-positive organisms	Gram-positive organisms
Staphylococcus aureus	*Streptococcus agalactiae* (Group B streptococci) (GBS) (more common)	*Listeria monocytogenes*	GBS
Coagulase-negative staphylococci (CONS)	CONS	*Streptococcus pneumoniae* (more common in neonates <1 week old)	*S. pneumoniae*
S. pneumoniae	*S. aureus*	CONS	*L. monocytogenes*
S. pyogenes		*S. aureus*	

obstetric care and sick neonatal care can be combined. Guidelines for integrated management of pregnancy and childbirth identify opportunities for assimilating maternal and neonatal care. Similarly Integrated Management of Childhood Illness (IMCI) has been widely implemented as the main approach for addressing child health in health systems. However, IMCI management guidelines do not as yet include the first week of life—the period of highest risk for child mortality, and also rely on the sick child being brought to a health facility. The recent modification of IMCI to include the neonatal period (IMNCI) and expand to community settings has now been included as a public health strategy in many countries including India. The ideal strategy would be to provide a linked

Table 2.7.7 Antimicrobial therapy of neonatal meningitis and sepsis

Patient group	Likely aetiology	Antimicrobial choice	
		Developed countries	**Developing countries**
Sepsis			
Immunocompetent children	Developed countries Group B streptococci *E. coli* Developing countries *Klebsiella* spp. *Pseudomonas* spp. *Salmonella* spp.	Ampicillin or penicillin plus an aminoglycoside	Ampicillin or penicillin plus gentamicin Or co-trimoxazole plus gentamicin
Meningitis			
Immunocompetent children (age <3 months)	Developed countries Group B streptococci *E. coli* *L. monocytogenes** Developing countries *S. pneumoniae* *E. coli*	Ampicillin plus ceftriaxone or cefotaxime	Ampicillin plus gentamicin
Immunodeficient	Gram-negative bacilli *L. monocytogenes*	Ampicillin plus ceftazidime	

strategy of care in community settings with referral to facilities in case of need.

Following the demonstration of significant reduction in neonatal mortality with the use of oral co-trimoxazole and injectable gentamicin by community health workers, this strategy could be employed in circumstances where referral is difficult. Currently in some health systems, outreach health workers, community nutrition, and child development workers are being trained to visit all mothers and neonates at home two to three times within the first 10 days, starting soon after birth, to provide home-based preventive care/health promotion and to detect neonates with sickness requiring referral. Extra contacts are proposed for LBW babies. With slight modifications, these visits can also be used to provide postpartum care to the mother as well.

Preventive measures

Preventive interventions need to bridge the continuum of care from pregnancy, through childbirth and the neonatal period, and beyond. Lack of positive health-related behaviour, education, and poverty are underlying causes of many neonatal deaths, either through increasing the prevalence of risk factors such as maternal infection or by reducing access to effective care.

Attempts to reduce the proportion of LBW births at the population level, have had limited success. Many deaths in preterm babies and in those born at term with LBW can be prevented with extra attention to warmth, feeding, and prevention or early treatment of infections. In developing countries, 90 per cent of mothers deliver babies at home without skilled health professional present. Simple low-cost interventions, notably tetanus toxoid vaccination, exclusive breastfeeding, counselling for birth preparedness, breastfeeding promotion through peer counsellors and women's groups, have been shown to reduce newborn morbidity and mortality (Darmstadt et al. 2005). Postnatally, kangaroo mother care for LBW infants, hand washing and decreased congestion in facilities, attention to environmental hygiene and sterilization, antibiotics for neonatal infections, are additional health system measures. Alcohol-based antiseptics for hand hygiene are an appealing innovation because of their efficacy in reducing hand contamination and their ease of use, especially when sinks and supplies for hand-washing are limited. Creation of a 'step-down' neonatal care unit for very LBW babies with mothers providing primary care also led to early discharge and reduction in hospital-acquired infection rates in another nursery in Pakistan. These interventions can be delivered through facility-based services, population outreach, and family-community strategies.

Early initiation of breastfeeding affects neonatal health outcomes through several mechanisms. Mothers who suckle their offspring shortly after birth have a greater chance of successfully establishing and sustaining breastfeeding throughout infancy, and also provide a variety of immune and non-immune components that accelerate intestinal maturation, resistance to infection, and epithelial recovery from infection. Prelacteal feeding with non-human milk antigens may disrupt normal physiologic gut priming. Although WHO currently recommends dry cord care for newborns, application of antiseptics such as chlorhexidine has been shown to be effective against both gram positive and gram negative bacteria and, in community studies, to reduce rates of cord infection and sepsis in newborns. A closely related issue is the need for general skin care. A randomized controlled trial of topical application of sunflower seed oil to preterm infants in an Egyptian NICU showed that treated infants had substantially improved skin condition and half the risk of late-onset infection.

At least two doses of tetanus toxoid should be given during pregnancy so that protective antibodies can be transferred to the foetus, to protect it from neonatal tetanus. Women with a history of prolonged rupture of membranes, especially if preterm, should be given prophylactic antibiotics. This approach improves neonatal outcome by increasing the latency of pregnancy. Maternal antibiotic therapy in this situation is effective in prolonging pregnancy and reducing maternal and neonatal infection-related morbidities. A multi-country study (ORACLE I) from urban centres suggested that administration of erythromycin to women with preterm premature rupture of membranes (PPROM) was associated with significant health benefits for the newborn. A domiciliary cadre of trained birth attendants potentially can be trained to recognize PPROM and provide referral and, possibly, initial antimicrobial therapy.

An important aspect of prevention of neonatal infection in developed countries relates to group B streptococcal (GBS) disease. The joint guidelines developed and implemented in the United States have led to a significant reduction in the burden of disease. The majority of newborns born to mothers with risk of GBS colonization undergo a full diagnostic evaluation and empiric therapy.

In recent years, the importance of hospital-acquired infections in newborn infants, frequently with multi-resistant organisms has been recognized. It is imperative that preventive strategies such as hand washing, reducing overcrowding and congestion, and environmental control are strictly enforced.

Meningitis in neonates, children, and adults

Acute meningitis is a potentially fatal infection caused by several microorganisms including bacteria, viruses, parasites, and fungi (Sáez-Llorens & McCracken 2003). In addition, meningitis is associated with a risk of chronic morbidity and developmental disability. Although the exact incidence of meningitis in developing countries is uncertain, case fatality rates range from 10 to 30 per cent. Even if effective treatment is provided, between 20 and 50 per cent of survivors still develop neurological sequelae. Successful outcome of neonatal meningitis relates to several factors including age, time, and clinical stability before effective antibiotic treatment, species of microorganism, number of bacteria or quantity of active bacterial products in the CSF at the time of diagnosis, intensity of the host's inflammatory response, and time elapsed to sterilize CSF cultures. The highest rates of mortality and morbidity occur following meningitis in the neonatal period.

Aetiology

The three most common bacterial pathogens, *S. pneumoniae*, *H. influenzae*, and *N. meningitidis*, account for more than 80 per cent of cases of bacterial meningitis in the United States overall, although *Listeria monocytogenes* is a greater problem for the elderly, immunocompromised, and pregnant women (Table 2.7.8). There is a relative paucity of microbiological information from developing countries, but beyond the neonatal period, the main agents of meningitis include Hib, *S. pneumoniae*, and *Neisseria meningitidis* with reported CFRs of 7.7, 10, and 3.5 per cent, respectively. Table 2.7.9 shows the common bacteria causing meningitis in developing and developed countries.

Table 2.7.8 Aetiology and treatment of bacterial meningitis

Patient group	Common organisms	Antimicrobial therapy
Immunocompetent children (age ≥3 months–18 years)	H. influenzae S. pneumoniae N. meningitidis	Developing countries: Ampicillin plus chloramphenicol
		Developed countries: Cefotaxime or ceftriaxone*
Immunodeficient, pregnant, and elderly (>50 years)	L. monocytogenes S. pneumoniae N. meningitides Aerobic Gram-negative bacilli	Ampicillin plus ceftazidime
Neurosurgical problems and head trauma	S. aureus S. pneumoniae	Vancomycin + third-generation cephalosporin

*For resistant S. pneumoniae, the American Academy of Pediatrics recommends vancomycin plus cefotaxime or ceftriaxone as empiric therapy.

Issues in presentation and diagnosis

The clinical features that may help in diagnosing meningitis are summarized in Table 2.7.10. In general, clinicians should have a low threshold for investigating and excluding meningitis in children as features may be non-specific. The clinical diagnosis can be confirmed by lumbar puncture and the examination of CSF. The CSF will have a cloudy appearance, elevated protein, increased leucocyte counts with a predominance of neutrophils, and the presence of pathogens on gram stain and/or culture provide a definitive diagnosis of bacterial meningitis. The use of latex agglutination or the S. pneumoniae C-polysaccharide antigen test (Binax NOW) may serve to confirm the diagnosis, especially if the child has been pre-treated with antibiotics (Saha et al.). A bacterial meningitis score has been shown to have an excellent negative predictive value for the presence of bacterial meningitis. If patients do not have one of the following factors—positive CSF Gram stain, CSF absolute neutrophil count ≥1000 cells/μl, CSF protein ≥80 mg/dl, peripheral blood absolute neutrophil count ≥10 000 cells/μl, or history of seizure before or at the time of presentation, they are very unlikely to have bacterial meningitis (negative predictive value = 99.9 per cent) (Nigrovic et al. 2007).

Medical treatment

The mainstay of treatment is prompt antibiotic therapy for suspected bacterial meningitis. Antibiotics need to be started before the results of CSF culture and sensitivity are available. This requires selection of an appropriate antibiotic, known to be effective against the common bacterial pathogens prevalent locally. An increasing number of β-lactamase-producing strains of Hib are resistant to ampicillin, and a smaller number of chloramphenicol acetyltransferase-producing strains are resistant to chloramphenicol. Additionally, the proportion of CSF isolates of S. pneumoniae that is non-susceptible to penicillin, ceftriaxone, and cefotaxime has also increased. Currently, the drugs for suspected or confirmed bacterial meningitis include cefotaxime (or ceftriaxone) alone or with ampicillin (preferred). If this is not available, then ampicillin + either gentamicin or chloramphenicol may be used. If sepsis is suspected, then cases should be treated with ampicillin or penicillin plus an aminoglycoside, until meningitis is confirmed. Antimicrobial therapy is described further in Table 2.7.8.

Table 2.7.9 Comparison of bacterial meningitis aetiology in children in the developing and developed world (prior to the widespread introduction of the Hib vaccine)

	Developing countries	Developed countries
H. influenzae	30%	65%
S. pneumoniae	23%	13%
N. meningitidis	28%	18%
Other organisms	19%	4%

Very early parenteral administration of corticosteroids (before or with initiation of antibiotics) significantly reduces severe adverse outcomes and case fatality rates. Similarly, there is evidence to suggest that restriction of fluids in the first 48 h may improve outcomes. While a meta-analysis of randomized, controlled trials

Table 2.7.10 Signs and symptoms of pediatric meningitis

Symptoms or presenting history	Signs
Vomiting	Stiff neck
Inability to feed and drink	Repeated convulsions
A headache or pain in back of neck	Fontanelle bulging
Convulsions	Petechiae or purpura
Irritability	Irritability
History of recent head trauma	Lethargy Evidence of head trauma
Signs of raised intracranial pressure	
Unequal pupils	
Rigid posture or posturing	
Focal paralysis in any limbs or trunk	
Irregular breathing	

has shown the benefit of steroids in all-cause bacterial meningitis, predominantly Hib meningitis, a recent study restricted to their use in pneumococcal meningitis found no significant benefits. However, there was a significantly lower rate of hearing loss in the treatment group at 3 months post-discharge. A recent Cochrane systematic review found that corticosteroids protect against severe hearing loss and neurological sequelae, and reduce mortality among adults with community-acquired bacterial meningitis in high-income countries (van de Beek *et al.* 2007). While this review found evidence of a benefit for children from resource-rich countries, there was no beneficial effect of corticosteroids for children in low-income countries.

Preventive measures

Although poverty, malnutrition, overcrowding are important risk factors for disease, delayed and inappropriate case management is a common determinant of adverse outcomes, the development of effective vaccines has been a major factor in the reduction of the burden of meningitis in the developed world. These include the Hib, pneumococcal conjugate, and meningococcal vaccines.

Haemophilus influenzae type b (Hib) vaccine

Currently three Hib conjugate vaccines are available for use in infants and young children with comparable efficacy (protective efficacy of Hib against development of laboratory confirmed invasive disease >90 per cent). All industrialized countries now include Hib vaccine in their national immunization programmes, resulting in the virtual elimination of invasive Hib disease. There is comparable impressive evidence of benefit from several developing countries following introduction of Hib vaccine and many countries are beginning to include Hib vaccine in their repertoire with GAVI support.

Pneumococcal vaccine

The older 23-valent pneumococcal polysaccharide vaccine is unsuitable for use in young children. The recent development of the 7-valent protein-conjugate polysaccharide vaccine, 9-valent and 11-valent vaccines is a major advance in the control of invasive pneumococcal disease. In the United States, the 7-PCV was included in routine vaccinations of infants and children under 2 years in 2000 and by 2001 the incidence of all invasive pneumococcal disease in this age group had declined by 69 per cent. Currently several Latin American countries are beginning to introduce pneumococcal conjugate vaccine as part of their EPI programmes.

Meningococcal vaccine

Meningococcal polysaccharide vaccine is available for A, C, W-135, and Y strains. This quadrivalent vaccine is being introduced in several developed countries as part of routine vaccine schedules, especially for adolescents who will be rooming in crowded dormitories while attending university. In many developed countries this vaccine has been replaced by the quadrivalent meningococcal conjugate vaccine, which is more immunogenic and, because it induces memory cells, is likely to lead to a longer lasting protective immune response.

Gastrointestinal tract infections

Diarrhoea, the most common manifestation of intestinal tract infections, is a leading cause of preventable death in most developing countries where its greatest impact is seen in infants and children. Infectious diarrhoea may be accompanied by numerous complications (Table 2.7.11). The financial burden associated with medical care and lost productivity due to infectious diarrhoea amounts to more than US$20 billion a year in the United States alone.

Invasive diarrhoea refers to diarrhoea caused by bacterial pathogens that invade the bowel mucosa, causing inflammation and tissue damage and may cause blood in stools (bloody diarrhoea). Invasive diarrhoea accounts for approximately 10 per cent of diarrhoeal episodes in children under 5 years of age and approximately 15 per cent of diarrhoea-associated deaths in this age group worldwide. Although less frequent, bloody diarrhoea generally lasts longer, is associated with higher risk of complications and case fatality rates, and is more likely to adversely affect a child's growth.

Global and regional epidemiology

The aetiology and severity of gastrointestinal infections are determined by several epidemiological factors. Young children and the elderly are at greatest risk for more severe disease and complications. The presence of underlying medical conditions, especially those that compromise immunity, greatly enhances the risk of acquiring an infection and its ultimate severity. Poor sanitation,

Table 2.7.11 Complications of gastrointestinal infections

Complication	Causative pathogens
Dehydration	*Vibrio cholerae*, *Cryptosporidium parvum* (especially in immunocompromised hosts), enterotoxigenic *Escherichia coli* (ETEC), rotavirus
Severe vomiting	Staphylococcal food poisoning, norovirus, rotavirus
Haemorrhagic colitis	*Campylobacter jejuni*, enterohemorrhagic *E. coli* (EHEC), *Salmonella*, *Shigella*, *V. parahaemolyticus*
Toxic megacolon, intestinal perforation	EHEC, *Shigella*, *C. jejuni* (rare), *Clostridium difficile* (rare), *Salmonella* (rare), *Yersinia* (rare)
Haemolytic uremic syndrome (HUS), thrombotic thrombocytopenic purpura (TTP)	EHEC, *Shigella*, *C. jejuni* (rare)
Reactive arthritis	*C. jejuni*, *Shigella*, *Salmonella*, *Yersinia*
Malabsorption/malnutrition	*Cyclospora cayetanensis*, *Giardia lamblia*, *C. parvum* (especially immunocompromised hosts)
Distant metastatic infection	*Salmonella*, *C. jejuni* (rare), *Yersinia* (rare)
Guillain–Barré syndrome	*C. jejuni* (rare)

inadequate water supplies, and increasing globalization of food transport systems all predispose to the development of large epidemics of food- and water-borne outbreaks of gastrointestinal disease. Seasonal or cyclic weather variations also influence the epidemiology of diarrhoeal disease and food poisoning.

Several recent reviews have evaluated diarrhoea burden and mortality rates. A review carried out two decades ago estimated that 4.6 million children died annually from diarrhoea. Kosek *et al.* have recently updated these estimates by reviewing 60 studies of diarrhoea morbidity and mortality published between 1990 and 2000 (Kosek *et al.* 2003). They concluded that diarrhoea accounts for 21 per cent of all deaths at <5 years of age and causes 2.5 million deaths per year, although morbidity rates remain relatively unchanged. Despite the different methods and sources of information, each successive review of the diarrhoea burden over the past three decades has demonstrated declining mortality but relatively stable morbidity rates. Persistent high rates of diarrhoea morbidity may have significant long-term effects on linear growth and physical and cognitive function in children. Figure 2.7.3 shows specific trends for diarrhoea in the world from 1954–2000.

Aetiology

Common aetiologies of non-inflammatory diarrhoea include enterotoxigenic *E. coli* (ETEC) and other strains such as enteroaggregative (EAEC), diffusely adhering, and enteropathogenic *E. coli, Vibrio cholerae*; non-01 choleras such as *V. vulnificus*; parasites including *Giardia lamblia, Cryptosporidium parvum*, and microsporidia; and several different virus species including rotavirus, noroviruses, and astroviruses (Hamer and Gorbach, in press). Acute inflammatory diarrhoea is the result of infection with bacterial enteropathogens such as *Shigella, Campylobacter, Salmonella* spp., enterohaemorrhagic *E. coli* (EHEC), *V. parahaemolyticus*, and *Clostridium difficile*. Among the parasites, *Entamoeba histolytica* is the most common cause of dysenteric illness although *Balantidium coli, Schistosoma*

mansoni, S. japonicum, Trichuris trichiura, hookworms, and *Trichinella spiralis* can all cause bloody, mucoid diarrhoea.

Infectious microorganisms in contaminated food and drink are the main source of travellers' diarrhoea. High-risk foods include uncooked vegetables, salsa, meat, and seafood. Tap water, ice, unpasteurized milk and dairy products, salads, and unpeeled fruits are also associated with an increased risk. Although many different pathogens may be responsible, the leading culprits are various forms of *E. coli*, particularly ETEC and EAEC. *C. jejuni* is encountered in a significant proportion of cases, particularly during cooler seasons. Viruses, *Shigella, Salmonella, Giardia, Cryptosporidium*, and *Cyclospora* spp. are responsible for a minority of travellers' diarrhoea cases.

Food poisoning is most commonly caused by the consumption of food contaminated with bacteria or bacterial toxins. Food poisoning can also be due to parasites (for example, trichinosis), viruses (e.g. hepatitis A), and other toxins (e.g. *Amanita* mushrooms). The most well-recognized causes of bacterial food poisoning are the following: *Clostridium perfringens, S. aureus, Vibrio* spp. (including *V. cholerae* and *V. parahaemolyticus*), *Bacillus cereus, Salmonella* spp., *C. botulinum, Shigella* spp., toxigenic *E. coli* (ETEC and EHEC), and certain species of *Campylobacter, Yersinia, Listeria*, and *Aeromonas*.

Issues in presentation and diagnosis

Gastrointestinal infections usually result in three principal syndromes: Non-inflammatory diarrhoea, inflammatory diarrhoea, and systemic disease. Non-inflammatory diarrhoea primarily involves the small intestine, whereas inflammatory diarrhoea predominantly affects the colon. The location of infection influences the clinical characteristics and certain diagnostic features of the diarrhoeal disease (Table 2.7.12). Thus, organisms that target the small intestine tend to produce watery, potentially dehydrating diarrhoea, while those infecting the large intestine cause bloody mucoid diarrhoea associated with tenesmus.

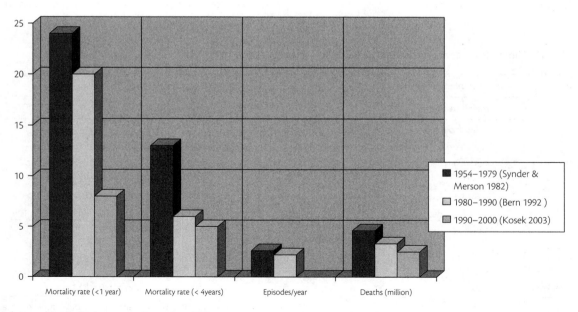

Fig. 2.7.3 Trends in worldwide diarrhoea mortality and morbidity rates.

Acute watery diarrhoea can be rapidly dehydrating, with stool losses of 250 ml/kg/day or more, a quantity that quickly exceeds total plasma and interstitial fluid volumes, and is incompatible with life unless aggressive fluid therapy can be provided. Such dramatic dehydration is usually due to rotavirus, ETEC, or *V. cholerae*, and it is most dangerous in the very young.

Persistent diarrhoea is defined as diarrhoea lasting 14 days or longer, is manifested by malabsorption, nutrient losses, and wasting, and is typically associated with malnutrition. Although persistent diarrhoea accounts for 8–20 per cent of diarrhoea episodes, it is associated with a disproportionately increased risk of death. Persistent diarrhoea more commonly follows an episode of bloody diarrhoea and is associated with a 10-fold higher risk of mortality. HIV infection is another risk factor for persistent diarrhoea in both adults and children.

Inflammatory diarrhoea is a manifestation of invasive intestinal infection that is associated with intestinal damage and nutritional deterioration, often with systemic manifestations including fever. Although clinicians often use the term bloody diarrhoea interchangeably with dysentery, the latter is a syndrome consisting of the frequent passage of characteristic, small-volume, bloody mucoid stools, abdominal cramps, and tenesmus. Agents that cause bloody diarrhoea or dysentery can also provoke a form of diarrhoea that does not present clinically with visible blood in the stool, although mucosal damage and inflammation are present and faecal blood and white blood cells are usually detectable by microscopy.

Because of the significant morbidity and costs associated with infectious diarrhoea, making a specific laboratory diagnosis can be useful epidemiologically, diagnostically, and therapeutically. A definitive diagnosis is achieved mainly through study of faecal specimens, using bacteriological culture, viral culture, or direct electron microscopy for viral particles, and identification of microbial antigens (viruses, bacteria, parasites, or toxins). DNA probes, PCR, and immunodiagnostic tests can now be used to identify several pathogens in stool specimens. Although some diseases can be diagnosed by elevations of serum antibody titres, this method is usually retrospective and often inaccurate.

Evidence-based interventions

Increased use of oral rehydration therapy, improved nutrition, increased breastfeeding, better supplemental feeding, female education, measles immunization, and improvement in hygiene and sanitation are believed to have contributed to the decline in morbidity and mortality of diarrhoea. Syndromic diagnosis provides important clues to optimal management and is both programmatically and epidemiologically relevant. The correct treatment of diarrhoea requires mothers to recognize the problem and seek medical care promptly, and that health workers give oral rehydration solution (ORS) or other fluids to prevent or treat dehydration, dispense an appropriate antibiotic when needed, provide advice on appropriate feeding, and provide follow-up, especially for children at increased risk of serious morbidity or death. In recent years, low osmolarity ORS and zinc supplementation (10–20 mg/day) have led to significantly improved diarrhea outcomes (Aggarwal 2007).

Medical treatment

Since the most devastating consequences of acute infectious diarrhoea result from fluid losses, the major goal of treatment is the replacement of fluid and electrolytes. While the intravenous route of administration has been traditionally used, ORS have been shown to be equally effective physiologically and logistically more practical and less costly to administer, especially in developing countries. ORS is the treatment of choice for mild-to-moderate diarrhoea in both children and adults, as long as vomiting is not a major feature of the gastrointestinal infection. ORS can also be used in severely dehydrated patients after initial parenteral rehydration.

Although there is no doubt about the value of ORS in treating dehydrating diarrhoea, the optimal sodium concentration of the solution remains in dispute, particularly in regard to the treatment of mild-to-moderate diarrhoea in well-nourished children in industrialized countries. The high concentration of sodium (90 mmol) in the standard WHO ORS formulation may cause hypernatraemia and even seizures in children with non-cholera watery diarrhoea. Consequently, lower concentrations of sodium and a reduced osmolarity solution have been found to be effective

Table 2.7.12 Clinical features and aetiologies of diarrhoeal diseases

Feature	Site of infection	
	Small intestine	**Large intestine**
Pathogens	*Escherichia coli* (enteropathogenic *E. coli*, enterotoxigenic *E. coli*)	*E. coli* (EIEC, EHEC)
	Cryptosporidium parvum	*Entamoeba histolytica*
	Giardia lamblia	*Shigella* spp.
	Norovirus	
	Rotavirus	
	Vibrio cholerae	
Location of pain	Mid abdomen	Lower abdomen, rectum
Volume of stool	Large	Small
Blood in stool	Rare	Common
Faecal leukocytes	Rare	Common (except in amebiasis)
Sigmoidoscopy	Normal	Mucosal ulcers, haemorrhagic foci, friable mucosa

for rehydration and not to be associated with any serious adverse clinical events (Hanh *et al.* 2001). The substitution of starch derived from rice or cereals for glucose in ORS has been another approach. Rice-based salt solutions produce lower stool losses, a shorter duration of diarrhoea, and greater fluid and electrolyte absorption than do glucose-based solutions in treating childhood and adult diarrhoea.

The provision of zinc supplements in conjunction with oral rehydration therapy serves to shorten the duration of diarrhoea and reduce the risk of subsequent episodes among children in resource-poor settings. This approach is now advocated by the WHO for the routine treatment of childhood diarrhoea in developing countries.

Dietary abstinence, the traditional approach to an acute diarrhoeal illness, restricts the intake of necessary calories, fluids, and electrolytes. During an acute attack, the patient often finds it more comfortable to avoid spicy, high-fat, and high-fibre foods, all of which can increase stool volume and intestinal motility. Although giving the bowel a rest provides symptomatic relief, continued oral intake of fluids and foods is critical for both rehydration and the prevention of malnutrition. In children, it is particularly important to restart feeding as soon as the child is willing to accept oral intake.

Because certain foods and fluids can increase intestinal motility, it is wise to avoid fluids such as coffee, tea, cocoa, and alcoholic beverages. Ingestion of milk and dairy products can potentiate fluid secretion and increase stool volume. Besides the oral rehydration therapy outlined above, acceptable beverages for mildly dehydrated adults include fruit juices and various bottled soft drinks. Carbonated drinks should be allowed to 'de-fizz' by letting them stand in a glass before ingestion. Soft, easily digestible foods are generally acceptable to the patient with acute diarrhoea.

Since most patients with infectious diarrhoea, even those with a recognized pathogen, have a mild, self-limited course, neither a stool culture nor specific treatment is required for such cases. For more severe cases, however, empirical antimicrobial therapy should be instituted, pending the results of stool and blood cultures. Gastrointestinal infections likely to respond to antibiotic treatment include cholera, giardiasis, cyclosporiasis, shigellosis, *E. coli* diarrhoea in infants, symptomatic travellers' diarrhoea, and *C. difficile* diarrhea (Table 2.7.13). The choice of antimicrobial drug should be based on *in vitro* sensitivity patterns, which vary from region to region. A fluoroquinolone antibiotic is a good choice for empirical therapy, since these agents have broad-spectrum activity against virtually all bacterial pathogens responsible for acute infectious diarrhoea (except *C. difficile*). Resistance to fluoroquinolones in South and Southeast Asia is an increasing problem.

In patients with severe community-acquired diarrhoea—characterized by more than four stools per day lasting for at least 3 days or more with at least one associated symptom such as fever, abdominal pain, or vomiting—there is a high likelihood of isolating a bacterial pathogen. In this setting, a short course of a fluoroquinolone, namely 1–3 days duration, will generally provide prompt relief with a low risk of adverse effects. Fluoroquinolones will not be effective for parasitic infections—specific antiparasitic drugs should be prescribed after identification of the offending pathogen in stool smears.

Self-treatment with an effective antimicrobial agent is advised for traveller's diarrhoea. While a fluoroquinolone is the treatment of choice, travellers to countries in Asia where resistance has become widespread should be provided with azithromycin for standby therapy.

Rifaximin may also be used but this non-absorbable antibiotic is not recommended for treatment of invasive diarrhoea, which is common among travellers to Asia, especially Thailand.

There are conflicting reports regarding the efficacy of antimicrobial drugs in several important infections, such as those caused by *Campylobacter* spp., and insufficient data for infections caused by *Yersinia and Aeromonas* spp., vibrios, and several forms of *E. coli*. In cases of EHEC, there is evidence that antibiotics are not helpful and may even be harmful.

The duration of antimicrobial therapy has not been clearly defined. While courses of anywhere from 3 to 10 days of treatment have been recommended, there are several studies that included severe forms of diarrhoea which suggested that a single dose is as effective as more prolonged therapy. For example, single-dose fluoroquinolone therapy is highly effective for infections due to *V. cholerae*, *V. parahaemolyticus*, and most *Shigella* species. On the other hand, short-course treatment of salmonella gastroenteritis with fleroxacin has not been found to be clinically beneficial. When treatment is indicated, a number of studies have shown that the combination of an antimicrobial drug and an antimotility drug provides the most rapid relief of diarrhoea.

Antimotility drugs are particularly useful in controlling moderate-to-severe diarrhoea. These agents disrupt propulsive motility by decreasing jejunal motor activity. Opiates may decrease fluid secretion, enhance mucosal absorption, and increase rectal sphincter tone. The overall effect is to normalize fluid transport, slow transit time, reduce fluid losses, and ameliorate abdominal cramping. In contrast to the potential utility of antimotility drugs, adsorbents such as kaolin, pectin, and activated charcoal are not useful for treatment of acute diarrhoea.

Loperamide is the best agent because it does not carry a risk of habituation or depression of the respiratory centre. Treatment with loperamide produces rapid improvement, often within the first day of therapy. Although there has been a long-standing concern that antimotility agents might exacerbate cases of dysentery, this has largely been dispelled by clinical experience. Patients with shigellosis, even *S. dysenteriae* type 1, have been treated with loperamide alone and have had a normal resolution of symptoms without evidence of prolonging the illness or delaying excretion of the pathogen. However, as a general rule, antimotility drugs should not be used in young children or in patients with acute severe colitis, whether infectious or non-infectious in origin.

Preventive measures

Diarrhoeal disease affects rich and poor, old and young, and those in developed and developing countries alike, yet a strong relationship exists between poverty, an unhygienic environment, and the number and severity of diarrhoeal episodes—especially for children under 5 years. Poverty also restricts the ability to provide age-appropriate, nutritionally balanced diets, or to modify diets when diarrhoea develops so as to mitigate and repair nutrient losses. The impact is exacerbated by the lack of adequate, available, and affordable medical care. Thus preventive and management strategies for diarrhoea must have an equity focus.

Malnutrition is an independent predictor of the frequency and severity of diarrhoeal illness and can lead to a vicious cycle in which sequential diarrhoeal disease leads to increasing nutritional deterioration, impaired immune function, and greater susceptibility to infection.

Table 2.7.13 Therapy of bacterial infectious diarrhoea*

	Antibiotic of choice	Dose, route, and duration	Alternative drugs
Recommended in symptomatic cases			
Shigella	Ampicillin Ampicillin-resistant strains: Trimethoprim-sulphamethoxazole (TMP–SMX)	500 mg PO q.i.d. or 1 g IV q.6h. × 3 days 50–100 mg/kg/day for children One double-strength tablet PO b.i.d. or, for children, 10 mg/kg/day TMP and 50 mg/kg/day SMX × 3 days (maximum of 320 mg/1600 mg per day)	Fluoroquinolones, nalidixic acid, azithromycin
Traveller's diarrhoea	Ciprofloxacin	500 mg PO bid × 3 days	TMP–SMX, other fluoroquinolones, azithromycin
Enteropathogenic *E. coli*, Enteroaggregative *E. coli*, and diffusely adherent *E. coli* in infants; enteroinvasive *E. coli*	TMP–SMX	As for shigellosis	Fluoroquinolones, azithromycin
Typhoid fever	Ciprofloxacin	500 mg PO b.i.d. × 7 days	Amoxicillin 1 g PO q.i.d. × 14 days; TMP–SMX; chloramphenicol 500 mg PO or IV q.i.d. × 14 days azithromycin; third-generation cephalosporins
Cholera	Tetracycline[1] Doxycycline[1]	500 mg PO q.i.d. or, for children, 40 mg/kg/day in 4 doses (max. 4g/day) × 3 days 100 mg PO b.i.d. × 3 days	Ciprofloxacin, TMP–SMX, furazolidinone, azithromycin
Salmonella (unusual cases)	Ampicillin Ampicillin-resistant strains: TMP–SMX	50–100 mg/kg/day in 4 doses × 10–14 days One double-strength tablet PO b.i.d. or, for children, 8 mg/kg/day TMP and 40 mg/kg/day SMX (max. of 320 mg/1600 mg per day) × 14 days	Ciprofloxacin 500 mg PO b.i.d. × 14 days
Not generally recommended due to lack of conclusive findings or no studies			
Campylobacter jejuni	Erythromycin	500 mg PO b.i.d. × 5 days	Ciprofloxacin 500 mg PO b.i.d. × 5 days Azithromycin 500 mg PO on day 1, 250 mg PO qd days 2–5
Yersinia enterocolitica	Fluoroquinolones, TMP–SMX, chloramphenicol		Aminoglycosides, tetracycline
Aeromonas species	TMP–SMX, third-generation cephalosporins, fluoroquinolones		Tetracycline, chloramphenicol
Vibrio, noncholera species	Tetracycline		
EPEC, EAggEC, or DAEC in adults, EHEC	TMP–SMX		
Not recommended (except in unusual cases)			
Nontyphoidal *Salmonella*			
ETEC			

*Since resistance to commonly used drugs (penicillins, TMP/SMX, and fluoroquinolones) is so widespread, it is difficult to make recommendations without knowing local susceptibility patterns of enteropathogens.
[1]Should not be administered to children less than 8 years of age.

Family knowledge about diarrhoea must be reinforced in areas such as prevention, nutrition, hand washing and hygiene, measles vaccination, preventive zinc supplements, and when and where to seek care. It is estimated that, in the 1990s, more than 1 million deaths related to diarrhoea may have been prevented each year, largely attributable to the promotion and use of these therapies.

A meta-analysis of three observational studies in developing countries shows that breastfed children under age 6 months are 6.1 times less likely to die of diarrhoea than infants who are not breastfed. Continued breast feeding during the diarrhoea episode provides nutrients the child, prevents weight loss, and improves recovery from diarrhoea. Contaminated and poor-quality complementary foods are associated with increased diarrhoea burden and stunting (Huttly 1997). Ideally, complementary foods should be introduced at age 6 months, and breastfeeding should continue for up to 2 years or even longer. Appropriate, safe, and aptly initiated complementary feeding has been shown to significantly reduce mortality in young children. Diarrhoea frequently causes fever, altering host metabolism and leading to the depletion of body stores of nutrients. These losses must be replenished during convalescence, which takes much longer than the illness does to develop. For these reasons, appropriate feeding strategies during diarrhoea episodes are a corner stone of treatment.

Probiotics, especially *Lactobacillus rhamnosus* GG, effectively reduce the frequency and duration of diarrhoea in children and adults. Probiotics are also useful for the prevention of antibiotic-associated diarrhoea.

Various studies suggest that zinc-deficient populations are at increased risk of developing diarrhoeal diseases, respiratory tract infections, and growth retardation. A meta-analysis published in 1999 showed that continuous zinc supplementation was associated with decreased rates of childhood diarrhoea (Zinc Investigator's Collaborative Group 1999), and a recent meta-analysis confirms the previous findings and indicates that zinc supplementation for young children leads to reduction in the risk of diarrhoea (by 14 per cent), serious forms of diarrhoea, and the number of days of diarrhoea per child (Aggarwal 2007).

Human faeces and contamination are the primary source of diarrhoeal pathogens. Poor sanitation, lack of access to clean water, and inadequate personal hygiene are responsible for an estimated 90 per cent of childhood diarrhoea. Promotion of hand washing reduces diarrhoea incidence by an average of 33 per cent and rigorous observational studies demonstrated a median reduction of 55 per cent in all-cause child mortality associated with improved access to sanitation facilities. Hand washing promotion strategies have also been shown to reduce diarrhoea burden with ancillary benefits in community settings.

Strict adherence to food and water precautions as outlined above will help those who travel to less developed areas of the world to decrease their risk of acquiring gastrointestinal infections. Parasitic infections, such as strongyloidiasis and hookworms, can be avoided by the use of footwear. Avoiding contact with freshwater such as rivers and lakes in endemic areas serves to prevent schistosomiasis.

Immunization represents an ideal way to prevent certain bacterial and viral diseases, but has not yet proved successful for combating many gastrointestinal pathogens. The cholera vaccine that has been available for decades suffers from low efficacy, a moderate risk of side-effects, and a short duration of action. Newer oral cholera vaccines, such as the inactivated B subunit vaccine, are highly effective for prevention of severe cholera. New rotavirus vaccines, now available for the prevention of rotaviral diarrhoea in children, have not been associated with intussusception. Measles is known to predispose to diarrhoeal disease secondary to measles-induced immunodeficiency, and it is estimated that measles vaccine at varying levels of coverage (45–90 per cent) could prevent 44–64 per cent of measles cases, 0.6–3.8 per cent of diarrhoeal episodes, and 6–26 per cent of diarrhoeal deaths among children under 5 years. Global measles immunization coverage is now approaching 80 per cent, and the disease has been eliminated from the Americas, raising hopes for global elimination in the near future, with a predictable reduction in diarrhoea as well.

Typhoid fever

Typhoid fever, a systemic disease caused by *Salmonella enterica* serovar Typhi, is an acute illness characterized by protean and non-specific symptoms, including fever and gastrointestinal infection. The systemic disease caused by *S. paratyphi* (A, B, or C) is also clinically similar; both typhoid and paratyphoid are collectively labelled as enteric fevers. The emergence of drug-resistant strains, especially multi-drug-resistant (MDR) *S. typhi*, resistant to ampicillin, chloramphenicol, trimethoprim-sulphamethoxazole, and, more recently, fluoroquinolones, is a growing problem.

Global and regional epidemiology

The global incidence of typhoid fever in 2000 was estimated to be 21.6 million cases, with more than 200 000 deaths (Crump *et al.* 2004). Approximately 12.5 million cases of typhoid fever occur annually in the developing world (excluding China), with 7.7 million cases in Asia alone. In South Asia, recent community-based studies indicate that a large proportion of cases occur in children under 5, with significant morbidity and mortality. The global case fatality rate of 1 per cent is based on conservative estimates from hospital-based fever studies; actual mortality figures may be higher in areas where referral is difficult and health services dysfunctional. Table 2.7.14 shows the regional distribution of crude typhoid incidence rates.

There have been dramatic point-source outbreaks of typhoid related to contamination of food sources or water supply. The use of contaminated ground water, consumption of street foods, and poor personal hygiene are common risk factors for infection.

Issues in presentation and diagnosis

After ingestion in contaminated food or water, *S. typhi* penetrates the small bowel mucosa and makes its way rapidly to the lymphatics, the mesenteric nodes, and finally the bloodstream. Following an initial bacteraemia, the organism is sequestered in cells of the reticuloendothelial system where it multiplies and re-emerges several days later in recurrent waves of bacteraemia, an event that initiates the symptomatic phase of infection. The incubation period ranges from 5 to 14 days.

Typhoid fever is a febrile illness of prolonged duration, characterized by hectic fever, delirium, persistent bacteraemia, splenomegaly, and a variety of systemic manifestations. Most children present with fever, headache, and abdominal discomfort, diarrhoea, sore throat, anorexia, dry cough, or myalgia and constipation. In the later phase of illness, more specific physical signs including hepatomegaly and splenomegaly may be observed. Rose spots may be seen in an early stage of the illness in fair-skinned children and large proportions have a centrally coated tongue (Bhan *et al.* 2005).

Table 2.7.14 Crude typhoid incidence rates by region, 2000

Area/region	Crude incidence*	Typhoid cases	Incidence classification
Global	178	10 825 487	High
Africa	50	408 837	Medium
Asia	274	10 118 879	High
Europe	3	19 144	Low
Latin America/ Caribbean	53	273 518	Medium
Northern America	< 1	453	Low
Oceania	15	4656	Medium

Source: Data summarized from Crump *et al.* (2004).
*Per 100 000 persons per year.

Pulse–temperature dissociation is present in some patients. In approximately 50 per cent of patients, there is no change in bowel habits; in fact, constipation is more common than diarrhoea in children with typhoid fever. As a result of recurrent waves of bacteraemia, patients with typhoid fever can develop pneumonia, pyelonephritis, osteomyelitis, septic arthritis, and meningitis. Intestinal haemorrhage and perforation, the most common complications, often occur in the third week of infection or during convalescence. The most serious complication, intestinal perforation, occurs in 0.5–3 per cent of the patients with typhoid, and because they occur most commonly in areas where optimal medical care is not readily available, it may be associated with case fatality rates ranging from 4.8 to 30.5 per cent.

Diagnosis of typhoid and paratyphoid fever requires culture of blood, bone marrow, stools, or urine to confirm growth of *S. typhi*. Laboratory findings commonly include leucopenia, thrombocytopenia, proteinurea, and elevated transaminases, but these are relatively non-specific and uncommon. In developing countries, culture facilities are expensive and mostly confined to hospitals, while most typhoid patients are diagnosed clinically and treated in outpatient settings. In other instances, serological diagnosis may be made with the Widal test. The latter, though useful, is insufficiently sensitive in endemic areas. Newer diagnostic tests have been developed, such as the Typhidot and Tubex, which detect IgM antibodies against specific *S. typhi* antigens (Bhutta 2006). Since these newer assays have not proven to have adequate sensitivity and specificity for routine use in community settings, there is a need for further refinement in serological or molecular diagnosis of the disease.

Medical treatment
In the pre-antibiotic era, typhoid fever case fatality rates approached 20 per cent. Treatment with effective antimicrobial agents—ampicillin, chloramphenicol, cotrimoxazole, and later ciprofloxacin—has progressively reduced case fatality rates to <1 per cent, except for MDR isolates. Fluoroquinolones and third-generation cephalosporins are effective in MDR typhoid but over the last few years there have been increasing reports in Asia of *S. typhi* strains with reduced fluoroquinolone susceptibility. The presence of nalidixic acid resistance *in vitro* is associated with clinical treatment failures with fluoroquinolones. Alternative therapies including azithromycin or third-generation cephalosporins are recommended in these circumstances. Given the considerable morbidity and higher mortality rates reported with MDR typhoid in children, it is imperative that appropriate antibiotic therapy be instituted promptly and, when the appropriate facilities are available, treatment choices should be guided by susceptibility testing.

Preventive measures
Detection of sources of infection related to recent typhoid fever in household contacts, commercial food handlers, or contaminated drinking water sources is essential to design effective preventive measures for disease containment.

Although the old whole-cell-inactivated typhoid vaccine has been withdrawn because of side effects, there are two licensed vaccines for prevention of disease: Ty21a (an attenuated strain of *S. typhi* administered orally) and Vi (the purified bacterial polysaccharide vaccine, given parenterally). These two vaccines have comparable protective efficacy and while they have been largely used for travellers, recently the Vi vaccine has been used for school vaccination programmes in large public health settings in Asia. For younger children and infants the Vi conjugate vaccine has been shown to provide a high degree of protection in a series of studies in Vietnam. However, the conjugate vaccine has as yet not been produced for public health use.

Dengue fever
In recent years, dengue fever, a mosquito-borne arboviral disease, has become one of the most common and rapidly spreading vector-borne diseases (after malaria) and thus now represents a major international public health concern. The dengue virus belongs to the genus *Flavivirus* (single-stranded, non-segmented RNA viruses), which includes four serologically distinct serotypes (DEN-1, DEN-2, DEN-3, and DEN-4). Variations in virus strains within and between the four serotypes influence disease severity. There is limited protection across serotypes. Secondary infections (particularly with serotype 2) are more likely to result in severe disease and dengue haemorrhagic fever.

Global and regional epidemiology
Humans and mosquitoes are the principal hosts of dengue virus, although some non-human primates can also be infected. Dengue epidemics occur during the warm, humid, rainy seasons, which favour breeding conditions for the mosquito vector, *Aedes aegypti*. More than two-fifths of the world's population (~2.5 billion) lives in areas potentially at risk for dengue, which is endemic in more than 100 countries across the globe, with tropical areas of Asia, the Western Pacific, Latin America, and the Caribbean being the most seriously affected regions.

In some case series, dengue fever has been reported as the second most frequent cause of hospitalization (after malaria) among travellers returning from the tropics. It causes an estimated 100 million illnesses annually, including 250 000–500 000 cases of dengue haemorrhagic fever—a severe manifestation of dengue—and 24 000 deaths (Deen *et al.* 2006). Around 95 per cent of cases occur in children less than 15 years of age, with infants representing 5 per cent of the cases.

Issues in presentation and diagnosis
The incubation period can vary from 3 to 14 days (typically between 5 and 7 days) and viraemia can persist up to 12 days (typically 4–5 days). Fever usually lasts for 5–7 days; fevers persisting

beyond 10–14 days suggest another diagnosis. The clinical features of dengue vary with patient age. Most dengue infections, especially in children, are minimally symptomatic or asymptomatic (Fig. 2.7.4). Children may also present with atypical syndromes such as encephalopathy and fulminant liver failure.

Classic dengue fever is characterized by a high fever of abrupt onset, sometimes with two peaks (saddle back fevers), severe myalgias, arthralgia, retro-orbital pain, headaches, and any of the three types of rashes, including a petechial rash, diffuse erythematous rash with isolated patches of normal skin, and a morbilliform rash, haemorrhagic manifestations, and leucopenia. Other manifestations include flushed facies, sore throat, cough, cutaneous hyperesthesia, and taste aberrations. Convalescence may be prolonged and complicated by profound fatigue and depression.

When the only haemorrhagic manifestation is provoked (by a tourniquet test), the case is categorized as Grade I dengue haemorrhagic fever, but a spontaneous haemorrhage, even if mild, indicates Grade II illness. Grades III and IV dengue haemorrhagic fever (incipient and frank circulatory failure, respectively) represent dengue shock syndrome which is characterized by sustained abdominal pain, persistent vomiting, sudden change from fever to hypothermia, alteration of consciousness, and a sudden drop in platelet count. Around 40 per cent of patients also have enlargement and tenderness of the liver. Rare presentations of infection include severe haemorrhage, severe hepatitis, rhabdomyolysis, jaundice, parotitis, cardiomyopathy, and variable neurological syndromes.

Infection with one serotype is thought to produce lifelong immunity to that serotype but only partial immunity to the others. Previous infection with a specific serotype followed by infection with a new serotype greatly increases the risk of dengue haemorrhagic fever.

Dengue virus serotypes are distinguishable by complement-fixation and neutralization test. Other diagnostic tests for patients with dengue include packed cell volume, platelet count, liver function tests, prothrombin time, partial thromboplastin time, electrolytes, and blood gas analysis. Laboratory findings commonly associated with dengue include leucopenia, lymphocytosis, increased concentration of liver enzymes, and thrombocytopenia. Diagnosis can be confirmed with several laboratory tests, especially the haemagglutination inhibition test and IgG or IgM enzyme immunoassays. Platelet counts and haematocrit determinations should be repeated at least every 24 h to allow prompt recognition of the development of dengue haemorrhagic fever and institution of fluid replacement. Diagnostic criteria for dengue fever are provided in Table 2.7.15.

Evidence-based interventions

Rapid urbanization has led to an increase in the environmental factors that contribute to the proliferation of *Aedes* mosquitoes. These include uncontrolled urban development, inadequate management of water and waste, presence of a range of large water stores, and disposable, non-biodegradable containers that become habitats for the larvae. These factors can change a region from non-endemic (no virus present) to hypoendemic (one serotype present) to hyperendemic (multiple serotypes present).

Medical treatment

No specific therapeutic agents exist for dengue fever apart from analgesics and medications to reduce fever. Treatment is supportive; steroids, antivirals, or carbazochrome (which decreases capillary permeability) have no proven role. In contrast, ribavirin, interferon alpha, and 6-azauridine have shown some antiviral activity *in vitro*. Mild or classic dengue is treated with antipyretic agents such as acetaminophen, bed rest, and fluid replacement (usually administered orally and only rarely parenterally); most cases can be managed on an outpatient basis.

The management of dengue haemorrhagic fever and the dengue shock syndrome is purely supportive. Aspirin and other non-steroidal anti-inflammatory drugs should be avoided owing to the increased risk for Reye's syndrome and haemorrhage.

Preventive measures

In the absence of a vaccine, control of the vector mosquito, *Aedes aegypti*, is the only effective preventive measure. At a personal level, the risk of mosquito bites may be reduced by the use of protective clothing and repellents. The single most effective preventive measure for travellers in areas where dengue is endemic is to avoid mosquito bites by using insect repellents containing *N*,

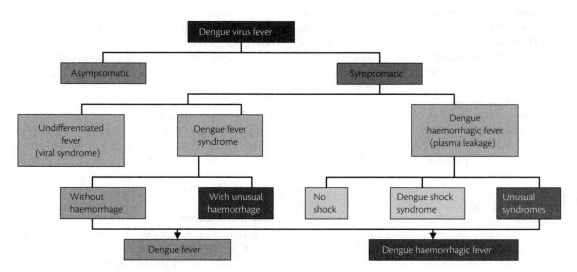

Fig. 2.7.4 WHO classification of symptomatic dengue infection.

Table 2.7.15 Diagnostic criteria for dengue fever

Dengue fever

Acute illness with two or more of:

Headache, retro orbital pain, myalgia, arthralgia, rash, haemorrhagic manifestations, and leucopenia

WHO definition for dengue haemorrhagic fever (WHO 2006)

◆ Fever

◆ Platelet count ≤100 000/mm³

◆ Haemorrhagic manifestations

◆ Evidence of plasma: Leakage caused by increased vascular permeability manifested by at least one of the following:

◆ Elevated haematocrit (≥20 per cent over baseline or a similar drop after intravenous fluid replacement),

◆ Pleural or other effusion (e.g. ascites)

◆ Low protein

Dengue shock syndrome

Criteria for dengue haemorrhagic fever:

◆ Pulse pressure <20 mm Hg or

◆ Hypotension (defined as systolic pressure <80 mm Hg for those aged <5 years or <90 mm Hg for those >5)

Probable diagnosis

At least one of following:

◆ Supportive serology

◆ Occurrence at same location and time as confirmed cases of dengue fever

Confirmed diagnosis

At least one of following:

◆ Isolation of dengue virus

◆ Four-fold or greater increase in serum IgG or increase in IgM antibody

◆ Detection of dengue virus or its genomic sequences by reverse transcription.

N-diethyl-3-methyl-benzamide (DEET) or picaridin. The insect repellents should be used in the early morning and late afternoon, when *Aedes* mosquitoes are most active.

At a public health level, the risk of dengue fever outbreaks can be reduced by removing neighbourhood sources of stagnant water or by using larvicides (especially for containers that cannot be eliminated), and predatory crustaceans.

Live attenuated tetravalent vaccines are being evaluated in phase 2 trials. Preliminary results have demonstrated 80–90 per cent seroconversion rates in humans. New approaches to vaccine development being studied include infectious clone DNA and naked DNA vaccines. These vaccines offer promise in terms of protection against all serotypes as well.

Parasitic infections

A broad range of parasites plague humans worldwide. While certain parasites, such as the *Plasmodium* species that cause malaria, are well recognized and have received intensive international support for research and programmatic control interventions, others are considered among the world's most neglected diseases.

Some of the main neglected tropical parasitic diseases include the protozoan infections: Human African trypanosomiasis, visceral leishmaniasis, and American trypanosomiasis (Chagas disease) and helminthic infections such as the soil-transmitted nematodes (ascariasis, hookworms, trichuriasis), schistosomiasis, lymphatic filariasis, onchocerciasis, and dracunculiasis.

Of the 20 major helminth infections of humans, the commonest are the geo-helminths. Roundworms, members of the phylum Nematoda, are responsible for an estimated 1 billion or more human infections. In many low-income countries, it is more common to be infected than not. Indeed, a child growing up in an endemic community can be infected soon after weaning, and continue to be infected and constantly re-infected for life.

Global and regional epidemiology

Recent global estimates indicate that more than a quarter of the world's population is infected with one or more helminths. The geographic distribution of roundworms in many tropical and subtropical regions closely parallels socioeconomic and sanitary conditions. In locales where several species of intestinal parasites are found, coinfection with *Ascaris lumbricoides, Trichuris trichiura,* and hookworms is common. In low- and middle-income countries, about 1.2 billion people are infected with the roundworm, *Ascaris lumbricoides,* while more than 700 million are infected with hookworm (*Necator americanus* or *Ancylostoma duodenale*) or whipworm (*Trichuris trichiura*) (Hotez *et al.* 2004). In 2002, the WHO estimated that 27 000 people die annually from geo-helminthic infections. Many investigators, however, believe that this figure is an underestimate. It has been estimated that 155 000 deaths annually occur from these infections (CFR 0.08 per cent).

Issues in presentation

Children of school age are at greatest risk from the clinical manifestations of disease. Studies have shown associations between helminth infection and undernutrition, iron deficiency anaemia, stunted growth, poor school attendance, and poor performance in cognition tests. Some 44 million pregnancies are currently complicated by maternal hookworm infection, placing both mothers and children at higher risk of anaemia and death during pregnancy and delivery. Intense whipworm infection in children may result in trichuris dysentery syndrome, the classic signs of which include bloody diarrhoea, anaemia, growth retardation, and occasionally rectal prolapse. Heavy burdens of both roundworm and whipworm are associated with protein energy malnutrition and deficiencies of certain micronutrients such as vitamin A.

Medical treatment

The WHO recommends the use of albendazole, mebendazole, pyrantel pamoate, and levamisole (Table 2.7.16). Both benzimidazoles, albendazole, and mebendazole have high efficacy against roundworm and moderate efficacy against whipworm. Single-dose mebendazole is much less effective against hookworm, with cure rates typically below 60 per cent.

Preventive measures

Better sanitation reduces soil and water transmission as transmission of geohelminths depends on transmission in environments contaminated with egg-carrying faeces. The provision of adequate sanitation is the only definitive intervention to eliminate helminthic

Table 2.7.16 Diagnosis and treatment of major intestinal nematode infections

Organism	Type of specimen	Specimen preparation	Size of eggs or larvae (μm)	Drug of choice	Alternative therapies
Trichuris trichiura	Stool	Direct smear or concentration	50–54 × 23	Mebendazole, 100 mg orally (PO) twice daily (bid) × 3 days	Albendazole, 400 mg PO once
Ascaris lumbricoides	Stool	Direct smear or concentration	45–70 × 35–50	Mebendazole, 100 mg PO bid × 3 days or Albendazole, 400 mg PO once or Pyrantel pamoate, 11 mg/kg PO once (max 1 g)	Piperazine citrate, 75 mg/kg bid (max 1 g) by nasogastric tube × 2–3 days until resolution of obstruction
Ancylostoma duodenale Necator americanus	Stool	Direct smear or concentration	55–70 × 35–45	Mebendazole, 100 mg PO bid × 3 days	Albendazole, 400 mg PO once or Pyrantel pamoate, 11 mg/kg PO × 3 days (max 1 g)
Enterobius vermicularis	Adhesive tape preparation	Direct microscopy	50–60 × 20–30	Mebendazole, 100 mg PO once or Pyrantel pamoate, 11 mg/kg PO once Repeat in 2 weeks	Albendazole, 400 mg PO once Repeat in 2 weeks
Strongyloides stercoralis	Stool, duodenal aspirate	Concentration or Baermann method	400–500 × 15	Ivermectin, 150–200 μg/kg PO × 1–2 days*	Thiabendazole, 25 mg/kg PO bid × 2 days (max 3 g/day)

*Intrarectal ivermectin is an option for treatment of high-grade strongyloidiasis.

infections, but to be effective it should cover a high percentage of the population. With high costs involved, implementing this strategy is difficult where resources are limited. Both the World Bank and WHO promote helminth control programmes and considers it as one of the most cost effective strategies to improve health in developing countries. These programmes emphasize mass drug administration as a major component of control.

Recommended drugs for use in public health settings include albendazole (single dose: 400 mg, reduced to 200 mg for children between 12 and 24 months), or mebendazole (single dose: 500 mg), as well as levamisole or pyrantel palmoate. Programmes aim for mass treatment of all children in high-risk groups (communities where worms are endemic) with antihelmintic drugs every 3–6 months. A recent systematic review of randomized controlled trials found that deworming increases haemoglobin by 1.71 g/l (95 per cent confidence interval 0.70–2.73), which could translate into a small (5–10 per cent) reduction in the prevalence of anaemia (Gulani et al. 2007).

Home delivery of antihelminthics is problematic for several reasons and thus school-based deworming programmes are preferred. These have been showed to boost school participation and are practical as schools offer a readily available, extensive, and sustained infrastructure with a skilled workforce that can be readily trained. In Kenya, such a programme reduced school absenteeism by a quarter, with the largest gains among the youngest children. Perhaps even more importantly, this study showed that those children who had not been treated benefited from the generally lowered transmission rate in the schools. These school-based programmes have resulted in improvements in overall nutritional status, growth, physical fitness, appetite, anaemia, and cognitive development. The above measures must be coupled with community behaviour change strategies with the aim of reducing contamination of soil and water by promoting the use of latrines and hygienic behaviour. Without a change in defecation habits, periodic deworming cannot attain a stable reduction in transmission.

Conclusion

The global burden of infectious diseases contributing to childhood and adult mortality is considerable. The situation is further compounded by increasing antimicrobial resistance and the emergence of newer infections with viruses such as avian influenza (H5N1) and the coronavirus responsible for the severe acute respiratory syndrome (SARS). Although the contribution of neonatal infections to overall child mortality has only recently been recognized, the persistent global burden of deaths due to diarrhoea and pneumonia underscore the need for improved public health strategies for change. There are interventions that can make a difference to childhood and adult infectious diseases (Table 2.7.17). What is needed is their implementation at scale to populations at greatest risk. This will require not only biomedical approaches but measures to address the social determinants of disease.

Table 2.7.17 Public health interventions and their effect on diseases

Major intervention	Disease prevented or treated
Effective antenatal care	Neonatal sepsis and meningitis, pneumonia
Skilled maternal and neonatal care	Neonatal sepsis and meningitis, neonatal tetanus
Maintenance of good personal hygiene	Neonatal sepsis and meningitis, diarrhoea, typhoid fever
Antimicrobial therapy	Neonatal sepsis, meningitis, bacteraemia, diarrhoea, pneumonia, typhoid fever, malaria, helminths
Vaccines	Pneumonia, typhoid fever, meningitis, bacteraemia
Oral rehydration therapy	Diarrhoea
Vitamin A	Diarrhoea, measles, malaria
Zinc	Diarrhoea, pneumonia, malaria
Provision of safe water, sanitation, and hygiene	Neonatal sepsis and meningitis, diarrhoea, pneumonia, typhoid fever, helminths
Breast feeding	Neonatal sepsis and meningitis, diarrhoea, pneumonia
Complementary feeding	Neonatal sepsis, diarrhoea, pneumonia
Intermittent preventive therapy in pregnancy	Malaria
Insecticide-treated nets	Malaria
Integrated vector control	Malaria, dengue, other vector-borne diseases

References

Addo-Yobo, E., Chisaka, N., Hassan, M. et al. (2004). Oral amoxicillin versus injectable penicillin for severe pneumonia in children aged 3 to 59 months: A randomised multicentre equivalency study. The Lancet, 364, 1141–1148.

Aggarwal, R., Sentz, J., and Miller, M.A. (2007). Role of zinc administration in prevention of childhood diarrhea and respiratory illnesses: A meta-analysis. Pediatrics 119, 1120–30.

Armstrong, G.L., Conn, L.A., and Pinner, R.W. (1999). Trends in infectious disease mortality in the United States during the 20th century. Journal of the American Medical Association, 281, 61–6.

Bhan, M.K., Bahl, R., and Bhatnagar, S. (2005). Typhoid and paratyphoid fever. The Lancet, 366, 749–62.

Bhutta, Z.A. (2006). Current concepts in the diagnosis and treatment of typhoid fever. British Medical Journal, 333, 78–82.

Bhutta, Z.A. (2007). Dealing with childhood pneumonia in developing countries: How can we make a difference? Archives of Diseases of Childhood, 92, 286–8.

Black, R.E., Morris, S.S., and Bryce, J. (2003). Where and why are 10 million children dying every year? The Lancet, 361, 2226–34.

Bryce, J., Boschi-Pinto, C., Shibuya K. et al. (2005). WHO estimates of the causes of death in children. The Lancet, 365, 1147–52.

Cohen, M.L. (2000). Changing patterns of infectious disease. Nature, 406, 762–7.

Crump, J.A., Luby, S.P., and Mintz, E.D. (2004). The global burden of typhoid fever. Bulletin of the World Health Organization, 82, 346–53.

Darmstadt, G.L., Bhutta, Z.A., Cousens, S. et al. (2005). Lancet Neonatal Survival Steering Team. Evidence based cost-effective interventions: how many newborn babies can we save? The Lancet, 365, 977–88.

Deen, J.L., Harris, E., Wills, B. et al. (2006) The WHO dengue classification and case definitions: time for a reassessment. The Lancet, 368, 170–173.

Gulani, A., Nagpal, J., Osmond, C. *et al.* (2007). Effect of administration of intestinal anthelminthic drugs on haemoglobin: Systematic review of randomised controlled trials. *British Medical Journal,* **doi: 10.1136,** 1–6.

Hamer, D.H. and Gorbach, S.L. Gastrointestinal infections. In (eds. D.A. Warrell, T.M. Cox, and J.D. Firth). *The Oxford textbook of medicine,* 5th edition. Oxford University Press, Oxford, England; in press.

Hanh, S.K., Kim, Y.J., and Garner, P. (2001). Reduced osmolarity oral rehydration solution for treating dehydration due to diarrhoea in children: A systematic review. *British Medical Journal,* **323,** 81–5.

Hotez. P.J., Brooker, S., Bethony, J.M. *et al.* (2004). Hookworm infection. *New England Journal of Medicine,* **351,** 799–807.

Huttly, S.R., Morris, S.S., and Pisani, V. (1997). Prevention of diarrhoea in young children in developing countries. *Bulletin of the World Health Organization,* **75,** 163–74.

Kosek, M., Bern, C., and Guerrant, R.L. (2003). The magnitude of the global burden of diarrheal disease from studies published 1992–2000. *Bulletin of the World Health Organization,* **81,** 197–204.

Mandell, L.A., Wunderink, R.G., Anzueto, A. *et al.* (2007). Infectious Diseases Society of America/American Thoracic Society consensus guidelines on the management of community-acquired pneumonia in adults. *Clinical Infectious Diseases,* **44,** S27–S72.

Nigrovic, L.E., Kupperman, N., Macias, C.G. *et al.* (2007). Clinical prediction rule for identifying children with cerebrospinal fluid pleocytosis at very low risk of bacterial meningitis. *Journal of the American Medical Association,* **297,** 52–60.

Nunn, P., Reid, A., and De Cock, K.M. (1997). Tuberculosis and HIV infection: The global setting. *Journal of Infectious Diseases,* **196** (Suppl 1), S5–S14.

Rice, A.L., Sacco, L., Hyder, A. *et al.* (2000). Malnutrition as an underlying cause of childhood deaths associated with infectious diseases in developing countries. *Bulletin of the World Health Organization,* **278,** 1207–21.

Sáez-Llorens, X. and McCracken, G.H. (2003). Bacterial meningitis in children. *The Lancet,* **361,** 2139–48.

Saha, S.K., Darmstadt, G.L., Yamanaka, N. *et al.* (2005). Rapid diagnosis of pneumococcal meningitis: Implications for treatment and measuring disease burden. *Pediatric Infectious Disease Journal,* **24,** 1093–8.

Van de Beek, D., de Gans, J., McIntyre, P. *et al.* (2007). Corticosteroids for acute bacterial meningitis. *Cochrane Database of Systematic Reviews,* CD004405.

WHO Collaborative Study Team on the Role of Breastfeeding on the Prevention of Infant Mortality (2000). Effect of breastfeeding on infant and child mortality due to infectious diseases in less developed countries: A pooled analysis. *The Lancet,* **355,** 451–5.

Zinc Investigators' Collaborative Group (1999). Prevention of diarrhea and pneumonia by zinc supplementation in children in developing countries: Pooled analysis of randomized controlled trials. *Journal of Pediatrics,* **135,** 689–97.

2.8

The global environment

Anthony J. McMichael and Hilary J. Bambrick

Introduction

We, the human species, have reached an unfamiliar crossroads with respect to the health risks posed by the external environment. We not only continue to face the health risks posed by long-familiar forms of environmental contamination, but now also face an emerging range of larger-scale and more systemic environmental hazards. As the sheer size and economic intensity of human endeavour, globally, has escalated in recent decades, its impact on the natural systems and processes of the global environment has increased—and, in consequence, environmental changes at that larger scale are becoming evident (Kennedy 2006).

These changes, such as global climate change, freshwater depletion, soil erosion, and the loss of species, are occurring on an unprecedented scale. They represent a weakening of Earth's life-support systems, a weakening of the foundations of biological health and life upon which human health ultimately depends. They therefore pose current and future risks to human health. Meanwhile, the ongoing increases in interconnectedness and 'globalization' of economic systems, trade, food systems, cultural diffusion, human mobility, electronic communication, and the spread of infectious agents are adding further to the contemporary emergence and strengthening of macroscopic influences on population health and disease.

These human-induced 'global environmental changes' are thus expanding the topic scope of 'environment and health'. Contamination by additives (chemicals, radiation, microbes) has long been the main source of environmental risks, and it remains so in many of the world's poorer and more vulnerable communities and populations. Meanwhile, populations everywhere are beginning to encounter this further dimension of health risk from larger-scale disruptions of environmental and ecosystem processes. Food yields, for example, are becoming less secure, and infectious disease occurrence is becoming more varied and volatile.

In essence, whereas traditional environmental hazards to human health mostly arise from the unintended *addition* of contaminants to air, water, soil, or food—or from excessive exposure to naturally occurring environmental factors (e.g. solar radiation)—these emerging larger-scale hazards arise from the *loss* of environmental attributes such as stability, productivity, regenerative and absorptive capacity. This added depth, indeed qualitative extension, to the category 'environmental health' necessitates some new and modified research strategies. It also requires a shift in how we think about and apply preventive strategies.

Implications for research concepts and methods

During the past half-century, the environment has mostly been treated by public health researchers and practitioners in a reductionist, itemized fashion. The health risks associated with specific physical, chemical, or microbiological agents have been characterized and quantified, one by one, and targeted interventions to reduce those risks have then been formulated and evaluated. This has been an important and fruitful strategy for the detection, characterization, and quantification of the health risk of each new contaminant and other agents entering the environment—and for the subsequent risk management strategy, often by setting exposure standards. This 'classical' type of environmental epidemiological study has often assumed the risk to be mediated by a straightforward causal relation between the specified exposure and health outcome, exhibiting either linear or curvilinear risk function. From such modelled relationships, the health risks at different doses can be estimated.

That focus and strategy of research (risk identification and assessment) and risk management remains important. As industrialization, agricultural production, and overall economic development have spread and intensified around the world, many new and often localized exposures to specific chemical and physical agents have resulted. New technologies—such as the use of mobile phones—can entail specific new exposure hazards. Vigilance is necessary on the research and policy fronts in relation to all such specific physical, chemical, and microbiological hazards to human health.

For all environmental exposures, old and new, there is the opportunity to study the relations with health outcomes at one or several levels of aggregation. Where widely-acting environmental exposures (e.g. urban air pollution and the post-Chernobyl ionizing radiation exposure) impinge on whole communities fairly evenly, it is appropriate for whole communities or populations to be the unit of analysis. Similarly, many epidemiological studies have estimated the percentage change in the study population's death rate associated with each unit increase in level of ambient air pollution. Other environmental exposures may impinge unevenly between individuals, with considerable difference in the 'dose' received. In such situations it is desirable to compare sets of individuals for whom estimates of individual-level exposure are possible. Conveniently, some such exposures are measurable at the individual level (via concentrations in blood, urine, saliva, or hair; or with molecular biomarkers), and this allows their associated health risks to be estimated at varied levels of received dose.

It is likely that much of the research on the health risks posed by global environmental changes will be conducted at the level of population or community. If climate change affects the altitude of transmission of malaria within a highland region, the primary research question is whether there has been an observable change in the physical range of malaria occurrence. Subsequent questions about which age-groups, families, or communities have been most affected are of interest, but are not specific to the climate change issue. Similarly, if heat-waves become more frequent and more severe under climate change conditions, there is need for research to assess how the exposure of populations to unusually high temperatures or unusually long heat-waves affects the immediate rates of death—overall, by specified cause, and for relevant identifiable sub-populations (age, sex, socioeconomic position, urban versus rural, etc.).

This type of research question refers to indices of the exposure and vulnerability of whole communities in relation to an environmental change entailing the disturbance of a natural system (e.g. the world's climate) that reflects the pressures exerted by human societies as a consequence of their way of living. The research and risk assessment question has a clear 'ecological' character. This has fundamental implications for how we could, indeed should, think about reducing or averting the risk to health.

Thinking 'ecologically'

The advent of a range of larger-scale environmental influences on human health is requiring researchers as public health practitioners to think in ecological terms. (The word 'ecological', here, refers to understanding relations within and between communities of living organisms, and between them and their physical environment. It does *not* refer to the regrettably mislabelled 'ecological studies', as classified by epidemiology textbook orthodoxy.) This need to think more ecologically will require an enhanced understanding of how these complex environmental systems are changed by human actions, and by what pathways, both direct and indirect, these changes then affect health.

To estimate the current and, importantly, the future health consequences of these systemic changes will require advances in many of our research methods. This would include developments in the following: Spatial analysis; time-series analysis; and techniques of modelling (both statistical and process-based) to estimate future health risks, handle uncertainties inherent in future scenarios, define the parameters of future 'health risk', and explore how the combined impact of concurrent environmental and social changes affects health risks.

An appropriate response to this challenge will also enrich research and policy thinking in other domains. For example, if in considering the health impacts of the urban environment we view cities as no more than an aggregation of specific 'toxic' exposures (lead from petrol, air pollutants, noise levels, road trauma, etc.), then we only address part of the health impact agenda. By viewing the city as a system that reflects and affects human ecology, the urban environmental health calculus then also includes consideration of how city design and transport systems affect physical activity (and obesity); access to, and type of, food retail outlets; mental health stresses in suburbia; infectious disease contact networks; and the release of greenhouse gases with their subsequent climate-changing and, hence, health consequences.

In summary, human-induced changes in the environment at large—the human-built environment, the globalizing geopolitical and economic environment, and the natural systems of the biosphere—pose major new challenges for epidemiologists and public health practitioners. The environmental health agenda of the twenty-first century will encompass much more than it did during the preceding two centuries. During those centuries, industrialization and urban living gathered momentum and affected local environments. Contemporary China provides a compelling reminder of how extensively such activities can contaminate environments and endanger health. Today, the scale of those human activities and their resultant pressures on the environment are affecting the environment and its natural systems at global and regional levels.

The 'environment'—local and global

History of evolution of ideas about environment and health

Concern over environmental conditions substantially shaped the historical evolution of public health and its core research discipline, epidemiology. In nineteenth-century Britain, there was a need to understand and remedy, for example: Toxic hazards in locally-brewed alcoholic drinks, the cholera outbreaks in London, mortality differentials between contrasting geographic and socioeconomic groups, and various specific occupational exposure hazards.

During earlier centuries, there persisted the age-old belief that disease reflected God's retributory judgement on the human condition. Then, in the seventeenth century, new philosophical perspectives emerged as the foundations of modern empirical science were laid in Western Europe. Francis Bacon argued for scientific enquiry based on empirical observation and comparison. René Descartes propounded a reductionist framework for studying the external 'machine-like' world.

This Enlightenment thinking about the role of scientific enquiry, the rise of inductive logic (drawing generalized inferences about relationships and physical laws from specific sets of observations), and a utilitarian approach to the fruits of scientific enquiry nurtured a more activist approach to managing the environment. Consequently, the 'social hygiene' movement arose in late seventeenth-century Europe, seeking to improve and cleanse the environment. Major social expenditures were required, ranging from draining marshes, removing urban refuse, and improving roadways.

In the wake of the French Revolution, social ideologies gave greater emphasis to egalitarianism. There was recognition that the widespread damaging environmental impacts of intensified mechanized production methods, crowding, and the disposal of wastes and excreta impinged heavily on the health of urban-industrial populations. In Britain, for more pragmatic and utilitarian reasons, the Sanitary Idea emerged in the 1840s in response to the perceived chronic poverty, illness, and debilitation of the urban workforce. The sanitary engineering idea also became linked with early notions of urban sustainability—including the recycling of sewage, attaining local self-sufficiency in food production, and achieving full employment. Later that century, in England, Ebenezer Howard's ideal of smaller decentralized 'garden cities', with green-belts and with residential areas separated from work zones, became popular as a means of countering the health-endangering miasmas emanating from dank, dirty, and crowded urban-industrial environments.

Meanwhile, improvements in nutrition, the urban environment and general social progress were ushering in the first public health revolution (McKeown *et al.* 1972). Other health gains arose via changes in human social organization and economic practices. For example, the mechanization of European agriculture from the mid-eighteenth century, with increased fodder production, stimulated a growth in cattle herds. This caused a reduction in human malaria, since the malaria-transmitting anopheline mosquitoes much prefer their blood-meals from cattle than from humans.

The spectacular rise of bacteriology in the 1880s caused a frameshift in perspective. Microbes were now deemed to be the primary cause of disease. This influential 'Germ Theory', along with new theories of cell biology and heredity, of micronutrient deficiencies, and the medicalization of child-bearing and child-rearing, all refocused the health sciences on the individual. Ideas of shared environmental exposures and the resultant shared health risks receded.

The model of specific causation—and hence prevention and treatment—of disease inherent in the Germ Theory prevailed early in the twentieth century. However, some counterbalancing of ideas arose from new knowledge about the vector-based transmission (by mosquitoes, ticks, biting flies, etc.) of major diseases such as malaria, schistosomiasis, dengue fever, yellow fever, and leishmaniasis. This underscored the important influences of wider environmental and ecological conditions. It led to new environmental management strategies in tropical and subtropical regions, including the spraying of mosquito breeding sites with DDT, control of surface water, and the control of alternative mammalian host species.

By the mid-twentieth century, the spread of industry and motorized transport had greatly increased local environmental exposures. Major urban air pollution episodes occurred, and these helped stimulate new environmental legislation in Western countries during the 1960s and beyond. Meanwhile, in her iconic book *Silent Spring*, Rachel Carson (1962) focused attention on a new concern—the apparently pervasive ecological damage caused by the bioaccumulation of pesticides, such as DDT and other chlorinated hydrocarbons. Concentrations of these human-made chemicals increased up the food chain. Humans, she argued, were on notice that such human-made chemicals, rippling through the natural world, would eventually damage human biology.

In the 1970s, the recognition of 'acid rain' heightened awareness that some types of environmental health hazards were transcending landscapes and national boundaries. As the increasing fire power of modern epidemiology began to yield information about health risks from long-term follow-up studies of occupational cohorts, new concerns also arose about the health hazards posed by cumulative exposure to various industrial and agricultural environmental contaminants. These included, especially, the environmentally persistent chlorinated hydrocarbons and several heavy metals (especially lead and cadmium). Exposures to these agents can, variously, impair the immune system, reproductive system, and neurological system—along with liver and kidney functioning and bone architecture.

During the 1970s and 1980s, concerns about chemical pollution of the environment and other forms of environmental damage assumed more of a 'life of their own' in public discourse. This is evident in much of the language of the UN's famous 1972 Stockholm Conference on the Environment, and in the orientation of the report *Our Common Future*, in 1987, from the UN's World Commission on Environment and Development (the 'Brundtland Commission')

(World Commission on Environment and Development 1987). Both were particularly concerned to explore how environmental conservation and quality could be achieved in concert with the anticipated, and desired, increases in economic development.

In high-income countries, epidemiologists and the health sector at large became preoccupied with new insights and new ways of studying the health risks arising from specific individual-level behaviours and exposures, including cigarette smoking, alcohol consumption, aspects of the 'Western' diet, oral contraceptive use, sexual behaviours, personal solar exposure, and domestic chemical exposures. There was a partial eclipse of research interest in understanding how aspects of the ambient environment affect rates of disease.

Acting as a modern Isle of Iona, air pollution epidemiology largely kept alive an interest in understanding how changes in types and levels of ambient environmental exposure affected health outcomes in whole communities. Then, in the late 1980s and the 1990s, it began to emerge that there was yet another—different and larger—category of environmental hazard looming over human health. That is the major focus of this chapter.

Current burden of disease due to environmental exposures

The World Health Organization estimates that one-quarter of the global burden of disease is due to modifiable environmental factors in air, water, soil, and food (Prüss-Üstün & Corvalán 2006). The figure in children is higher, over one-third—and predominantly from diarrhoeal disease, lower respiratory infections, unintentional injuries, and malaria. This environment-related burden is much greater in low-income than high-income countries: An estimated 25 per cent of deaths in developing regions versus 17 per cent in developed. Comparing low-income to high-income countries, healthy life-years lost to environmentally caused disease are 25 times higher for road crashes, 140 times higher for diarrhoeal diseases, and 800 times higher for respiratory infections. Children in developing countries lose an estimated eight times more healthy life-years from environmental diseases than do their developed country counterparts.

These environmental hazards remain enormously important in lower income countries, especially in socioeconomically and politically disadvantaged communities. Technically, many of them can be managed or eliminated on a local basis. But this requires political will and resources, and a moral or ideological responsiveness to the existence of health inequalities.

Meanwhile, these ongoing environmental health hazards are being supplemented, increasingly, by the emergence of health risks due to changes in the 'global environment'. Those changes are occurring at a much larger scale, and involve various systemic disturbances and shifts that have direct and indirect consequences for human health. The best-known, and the most important with respect to the future sustainability of health-supporting conditions for human populations, are the 'global environmental changes' (GEC) such as climate change, biodiversity loss, and degradation of food-producing ecosystems on land and in the oceans.

These GECs can be thought of as a major component of a wider set of 'global changes' that typify the growing scale, speed, and intensity of changes in environmental, social, economic processes and conditions in the world at large. That larger set is shown schematically in Fig. 2.8.1.

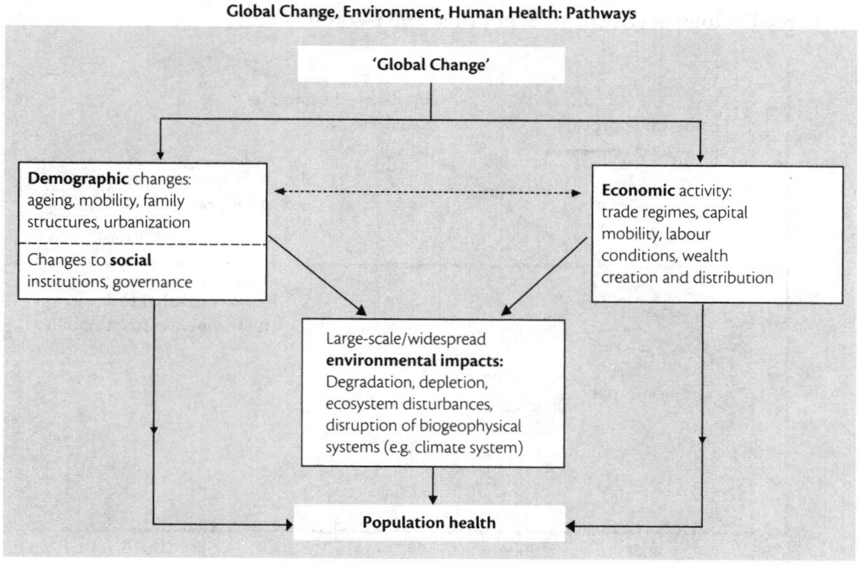

Global Change, Environment, Human Health: Pathways

Fig. 2.8.1 Schematic diagram of major domains of 'global change'. Demographic, social, and economic variables generate and influence the pressures on the natural environment. Those variables and associated large-scale environmental changes affect human health.

Global environmental changes: Larger and systemic influences on population health

There is an urgent need for a fuller understanding of how human-induced global environmental changes pose risks to human health. These large-scale hazards to health have arisen from the disruption or depletion of complex biophysical and ecological systems that is now occurring on an increasing scale as a result of expanded and intensified human economic activity.

These emerging global environmental changes entail the *loss* of natural environmental capital and *disruption* of ecosystems. That type of human impact on the environment is qualitatively distinct from the more familiar process of (mostly time-limited and reversible) local environmental *contamination*. The elucidation of these hazards to health requires more than the mono-disciplinary and single-factor approaches that have generally served epidemiologists, toxicologists, and environmental scientists well in the past.

It is important, here, to clarify the nature and the dimensions of this recent development in the ways in which human activities are now altering many aspects of the structure and functioning of the natural world.

The 'ecological footprint'

A widely used measure of human impact on the environment is the 'ecological footprint'. This relates directly to the more familiar concept of environmental 'carrying capacity'—i.e. how many individuals can be sustained over time by a specified unit of land area. The 'footprint' reverses the arithmetic: It asks how many units of environment are required to meet the needs (or wants) of a specified unit of human population—an individual, community, city, or population.

Several recent assessments have been made of the global human population's aggregated 'footprint' on Earth's environment. The consistent conclusion is that humanity is collectively consuming more materials and generating more waste than the natural environment can supply and absorb, respectively, on a recurrent basis. That is, we are operating in 'ecological deficit', depleting Earth's stocks of natural environmental 'capital'—in order to meet our now excessive demands on the environment.

The World Wide Fund for Nature (WWF) has estimated the world population's ecological footprint by analysing trends in stocks and flows at national level over recent decades, focusing particularly on major categories of ecological systems, including freshwater, marine, and forest ecosystems. Figure 2.8.2 shows the WWF's estimation for the period 1961–2003. The size of the human footprint is expressed as the number of Planet Earths needed to meet the total environmental demands. Beyond the year 2003, the figure comprises three scenario-based estimates of future aggregate environmental demands, assuming that the specified economic development, policy, and technology trajectories will apply.

A separate recent analysis, comparing national indices (Dietz *et al.* 2007), concludes that population size and rising affluence (with its associated patterns of production and consumption) are the principal drivers of humanity's pressures on the natural environment. Other commonly postulated determinants such as the extent of urbanization, type of economic structure, and population age distribution were found to have relatively little effect. The analysis also found that higher levels of education and life expectancy were not associated with elevated environmental pressures. This finding suggests that some important aspects of human well-being can be improved without significant risk to the environment.

Of course, a prime purpose for seeking to understand the health consequences of human-induced changes to the global environment is to enrich the evidence base for policy-making. Big decisions need to be made about the choice of technologies and the form of physical and social development. How should we generate energy? How can our cities be made sustainable and socially congenial? What forms of transport should we use? What aspects of trade should be encouraged, and what aspects discouraged?

That last question leads to consideration of one of the major other 'global' developments in today's world that is exerting increasing influence on human health—international trade. This, in concert, with an increasing international cultural diffusion that is influencing patterns of consumer preference and behaviours, is a good illustration of the category of emerging large-scale influences on human health that are not primarily mediated by changes in the natural environment.

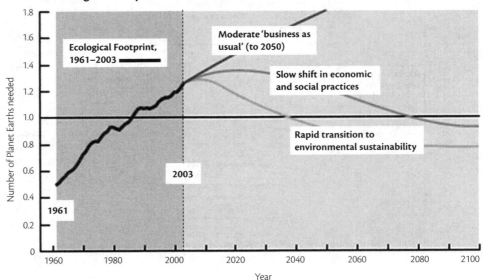

Fig. 2.8.2 Estimated time-trends in the total human ecological footprint, expressed as the changing number of Planet Earths needed for 1961–2003 (data-based) and 2003–2100 (scenario-based) (WWF International 2006).

International trade, globalization, and health

Historically, various environmental health hazards have arisen from rapid urban immigration (where crowding and poor sanitation can amplify infectious disease transmission, for example) and from localized pollution due to the rapid expansion of poorly regulated industry. Many of these hazards have been of a relatively simple, direct-acting, kind. Today, increasingly, intensive international trade, especially in food and therapeutic goods, presents new and complex challenges to global environmental health.

Food producers are under increasing pressure to be economically competitive—usually to produce the most food for the least cost. Increasingly mechanized production may be economically cheap in conventional market terms, but it often requires more energy to produce the food than is available from the food produced. The environmental consequences, many of which pose health risks, include a growing contribution to global greenhouse gas emissions (FAO 2006). Other intensive farming practices, such as the use of hormones and antibiotics to promote animal growth, can both damage the environment and produce food that is potentially unsafe.

Today's 'factory farmed' meat has a very different lipid profile from the wild-animal meat that was consumed during much of our species' evolutionary history. The latter type of meat has much lower saturated fat content and is higher in omega-3 fatty acids (the so-called 'fish oils') (McMichael 2005). Further, people in many countries are now consuming considerably more meat (currently 125 kg annually per capita in the United States) (Brown 2005) than would have been available in earlier times, and they expend less energy to get it. This systemic energy imbalance in our modern way of life further underpins the global obesity epidemic.

Industrial agriculture, now spreading worldwide with ever increasing pressure to become more and more economically 'efficient' poses additional health risks via the extensive use of fertilizers and pesticides, feed formulations that include animal tissues, arsenic and antibiotics, and the consequent environmental pollution (Bambrick 2004). Complex and 'unnatural' food chains—whereby herbivores such as cattle are fed the remains of other animals—continues in some countries (and indeed is deemed to be acceptable

practice under international standards applied by the World Trade Organization). Such practices continue despite the UK 'mad cow' (bovine spongiform encephalopathy) epidemic disaster of the 1990s. That economic and public health disaster was caused by feeding mammalian (cattle and sheep) offal to cattle—and it resulted in the transmission of the novel infectious agent, or prion, to human consumers, causing the neurodegenerative disorder 'variant Creutzfeldt–Jakob disease' (Nathanson *et al.* 1997).

Chickens are commonly fed fish-meal from unintended by-catch, much of which is shark that is so high in mercury content that it is unfit for human consumption (Bambrick & Kjellström 2004). Insufficient research attention has been paid to studying the human health risks that might result from eating such chickens, or their eggs. Similarly intensive practices are being applied, increasingly, to various forms of aquaculture, with the same potential for contamination of the human food supply. Where aquaculture employs netted enclosures in the open ocean, antibiotics, pesticides, and disease can spread freely to non-farmed areas.

Food, as an increasingly global commodity, often has such complex and multidirectional pathways that it obscures the origins of individual ingredients in manufactured items. This poses difficulties of four main kinds: (i) Identifying an outbreak (which may occur in disseminated fashion) of a food-borne disease; (ii) responding to it by recalling all affected items; (iii) determining where in the supply chain the contamination occurred; and (iv) implementing prevention, since legislation at the place of origin may be inadequate or not enforceable.

Even as these various economic pressures and practices in an increasingly competitive global marketplace are jeopardizing various aspects of foods safety, the international trade rules applied by the World Trade Organization seriously limit the capacity of individual countries to employ domestic legislation to protect public health (such as by restricting imports) (Bambrick 2004). Such trade agreements seek primarily to limit non-tariff barriers to trade. However, they may also erode food safety, because nations importing food are discouraged from setting regulatory standards higher than the often low standards of the exporting nation.

Similar problems—complexity in origin, multidirectional trade, and pressures to reduce regulatory standards—exist in the international trading of therapeutic goods, including human blood and plasma products. For example, some rich countries rely on blood and plasma purchased from the poor in developing countries, both to shore up their national supply and to manufacture blood-derived therapeutic products for subsequent export (Bambrick *et al.* 2006).

Global environmental change: Definition, context, significance

Human pressures on the Earth System

The various above-mentioned human-induced changes to natural environmental (biophysical and ecological) systems are a consequence of the aggregated regional and global pressures exerted by the continuing growth in human population size and economic activity. They accompany, and to some extent are caused by, aspects of 'globalization', as social, economic, cultural, technological, and political connectedness increases among human societies around the world. The total environmental impact of humankind is now so great that it is inducing changes in components of the Earth System (Millennium Ecosystem Assessment 2005). For key environmental parameters, the Earth System has recently moved well outside the range of natural variability that applied over the last half million years or so. This is unprecedented in human experience.

The Earth System is now becoming a major focus of interdisciplinary study. It is a self-regulating system that comprises physical, chemical, biological, and human components. The interactions and feedbacks between component parts of the geosphere and biosphere are complex and exhibit multi-scale temporal and spatial variability. Recently, and for the first time, human activities have begun significantly to alter Earth's atmosphere, land surface, oceans, coasts, biological diversity, hydrological and biogeochemical cycles. These anthropogenic changes are now equalling some of Nature's great forces in extent and impact. Human activities have, for example, approximately doubled the amount of activated nitrogen (ammonia and other nitrogen compounds) that is produced each year. Many of these global environmental changes (GEC), including global climate change (Rahmstorf *et al.* 2007)—appear to be accelerating.

The manifestations of these changes are many. Forest cover is declining in many tropical regions. There is a widespread and continuing loss of productive agricultural and pastoral soil on all continents. With industrialized fishing fleets, we have over-fished most of the large ocean fisheries. Farming and industrial activities have severely depleted many of the great aquifers upon which the future of irrigated agriculture and urban sustainability depends. The widespread use of nitrogenous fertilizer, along with fossil fuel combustion, has doubled the rate at which activated nitrogenous compounds enter the global environment. Most irreversible of all, human pressures are extinguishing whole species and many local populations at an historically unprecedented overall rate. Indeed, we are, in reality, perpetrating the Sixth Great Extinction to have occurred since vertebrate life emerged on Earth around a half billion years ago (Leakey & Lewin 1995).

These GECs represent a reduction in the capacity of the natural environment to supply and replenish resources, absorb, and recycle the wastes products of the activities of humans and other animals (e.g. cattle, pigs), and to provide climatic–environmental stability

---

Box 2.8.1 the main types of global environmental changes

- Changes to atmospheric composition and, therefore, function:
  - Greenhouse gas accumulation, leading to climate change
  - Stratospheric ozone depletion
- Changes to food-producing ecosystems:
  - Land cover, soil fertility
  - Coastal and marine ecosystem stocks
- Biodiversity changes:
  - Loss/extinction
  - Redistribution (invasion)
- Internal rearrangements (balance)
- Changes to cycles of elements (especially N, P, S)—in addition to the carbon cycle (climate change)
- Changes to the hydrological cycle, and depletion of freshwater supplies
- World-wide dissemination of persistent organic pollutants (POPs)
- Urbanization
- Desertification

---

and physical buffering processes. This diminution of capacity results from changes to the structure, composition, and function of Earth's biophysical and ecological systems (i.e. 'life-support systems').

Global environmental changes: Types, inter-relations

The various GECs that are symptoms of this human overloading of the Earth System are listed in Box 2.8.1. They are 'global' in one or other of two senses. Some, such as climate change and stratospheric ozone destruction, are spatially integrated at world scale. Others such as species extinctions and land degradation occur via the worldwide aggregation of local changes.

Figure 2.8.3 illustrates the main pathways by which GECs can affect human health (Earth System Science Partnership 2006). Neither the set of pathways nor the categories of health impacts shown are exhaustive. For example, many of the impacts shown would also be associated with mental health problems (e.g. post-traumatic stress disorders, suicides), while other environmental changes would result in conflicts or refugee flows in response to depleted resources. In the complex real world of human politics and culture there are also, of course, many important modulating 'non-environmental' influences on these GEC-related health risks.

The area with particular need for research is shown within the grey-shaded rectangle. Much research remains to be done on the health consequences of stratospheric ozone depletion and global climate change. However, that research domain needs less 'affirmative action' than do the relationships shown in the grey area—many of which are intrinsically complex, entailing perturbations of ecosystems and feedbacks between concurrent environmental change processes. Some of the complexity inherent in tackling the health impacts of global environmental change is discussed in Box 2.8.2.

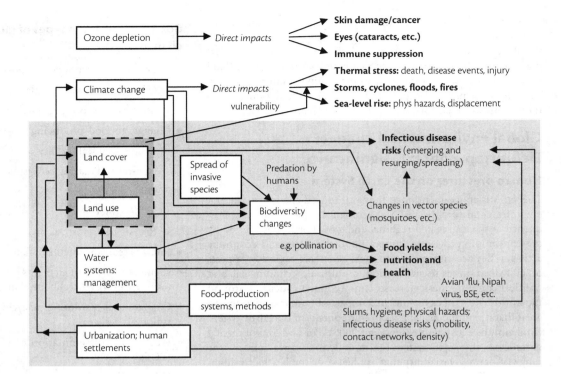

Fig. 2.8.3 Schematic diagram of the main types of biogeophysical pathways by which Global Environmental Changes (shown in red) can affect human health. From Earth System Science Partnership: Global Environmental Change and Human Health project (2006).

Box 2.8.2 Millennium Development Goals: The nexus between GECs, sustainability, human well-being, and health

At the turn of the century, the United Nations embraced a set of eight Millennium Development Goals (United Nations 2000). The first six of these seek reductions in poverty, illiteracy, gender inequality, malnutrition, child deaths, maternal mortality, and major infectious diseases. The seventh goal seeks 'environmental sustainability'. While highlighting several areas of major challenge to human health, this itemization of goals creates a disconnect that all-too-easily separates environmental considerations from health considerations.

Poverty, for example, cannot be eliminated against a counter-current of degraded and non-productive environments, especially when the environmental deficits impinge primarily on the poor and exacerbate the risks of disease. Likewise, adequate food and freshwater supplies require soil fertility, climatic stability, river flows, and various ecological functions (e.g. pollination). Infectious diseases cannot be contained in conditions of climatic instability, land disturbance, environmental refugee flows, and environment-related poverty.

Further, the goal of 'environmental sustainability' must extend well beyond addressing traditional, long-standing, physical, chemical, and microbiological hazards in local environments—even though those exposures remain important, particularly as accompaniments to industrialization and urbanization in lower income countries, and have the greatest impact on poor and vulnerable communities (Butler & McMichael 2005). Lower income groups have been most affected by air pollution in Sao Paulo, leaded house paint in inner-urban USA, and isocyanate poisoning in Bhopal, for example (McMichael 2002). These localized hazards, while serious, are remediable; they do not entail an enduring, perhaps permanent, loss of natural environmental capital.

The health risks from *global* environmental changes also impinge unequally, both within and between populations. Further, the health risk disparities due to climate change, agroecosystem degradation, freshwater shortages, and other GECs may well increase in coming decades, reflecting differences in location, economic conditions, social and human resources, political power, and the extent of direct dependency on local environments (Prüss-Üstün & Corvalán 2006). Most arable land has now been privatized, and access to stocks of wild species (fish, land-animals, wild plants) is declining as population pressures and commercial activities intensify. Freshwater is increasingly being privatized as natural sources become depleted or degraded.

Health risks from global environmental changes

Climate change

Global climate change is the most widely recognized of the GECs. It is becoming generally understood that our prevailing pattern of energy generation and use, and of agricultural (including livestock) production, is increasing the concentration of energy-trapping (greenhouse) gases in the lower atmosphere. That additional trapped energy manifests as heat, which then warms the Earth's surface. This human-driven increment in the atmosphere's natural 'greenhouse' capacity (which achieves a warming of around 33°C) keeps the planet comfortably above freezing point. The human-generated greenhouse gases comprise, principally, carbon dioxide, methane, nitrous oxide, and industrial halocarbons.

The reality of human-induced climate change is now largely agreed by climate scientists around the world. Nevertheless, many details remain in relation to process, timing, and the uncertainty of critical thresholds that may be reached. The Fourth Assessment Report of the Intergovernmental Panel on Climate Change (IPCC 2007) concludes that there is at least 90 per cent certainty that the unusual warming in recent decades has been mostly due to human actions.

During the last century, the world's average surface temperature increased by approximately 0.6°C; two-thirds of that warming occurred after 1975. Other evidence shows that climate variability has increased in various regions. Further warming of 1.8–4.0°C (including another 0.6°C rise already in the pipeline) is forecast for this century (Fig. 2.8.4). The actual outcome will depend largely on how human societies adjust their energy metabolism and agricultural practices over coming decades. Rainfall patterns will also change. Importantly, there will also be a generalized increase in variability of weather patterns, although this will itself vary by geographic region. Indeed, all these anticipated changes in climatic conditions will vary by region.

The IPCC's Fourth Assessment Report is, a year or two further on, widely viewed as being rather conservative in its projections. In large part this reflects the fact that it had necessarily had a 'cut-off' date for admissible published evidence in early 2006. Subsequent evidence during 2006–2007 has pointed to an apparent acceleration in emissions, warming, glacier melting, and sea level rise (Rahmstorf *et al.* 2007).

This ongoing warming is affecting physical and biotic systems. More than 90 per cent of the significant changes to physical and biological systems observed since 1970 are consistent with warming (IPCC 2007b). Ice-sheets are melting faster than foreshadowed in the previous assessment; long-term drying is already emerging in southern and western Africa, southern Europe, India, and Australia (IPCC 2007a). The seasonal cycles of birds, bugs, butterflies, bears, and buds are changing, and are getting out of kilter with one another: Many finely tuned ecological systems are becoming uncoupled (IPCC 2007b).

Much early public discussion about climate change focused on risks to economic growth, physical infrastructure, and recreational amenities. The real risk is more profound. Climate change is a serious threat to the physical and ecological systems upon which biological function and health depend. That is, it endangers health and life on Earth. From an anthropocentric view, the public health task is to address prevention at two distinct levels. The essential primary prevention task, by definition, is to reduce global greenhouse gas emissions. However, since climate change is already occurring and more change is inevitable ('committed'), we must also develop strategies to lessen the adverse impacts on health.

Health effects of climate change

The health effects of global climate change are, in small part, with us already—but are difficult to identify and attribute at this early stage. Now and, increasingly, in the future, they will occur via various direct and indirect pathways (see Fig. 2.8.5, and also Fig. 2.8.3) (McMichael 2006). Some effects would be immediate, some would be delayed. The impacts will vary between regions and populations,

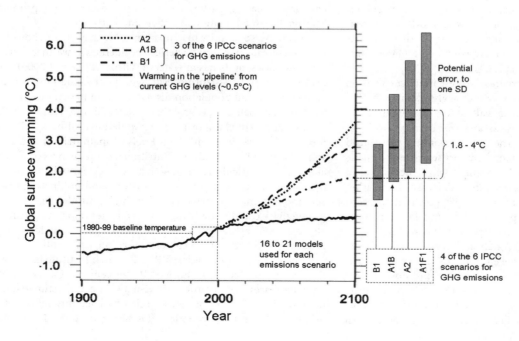

Fig. 2.8.4 Recent and projected (modelled) future change in average Earth-surface temperature. *Source*: modified from IPCC Fourth Assessment Report (Meehl *et al.* 2007). The four scenarios included here span the full range (1.8–4.0°C) between the best (central) estimates of the six scenarios used in the original modelling.

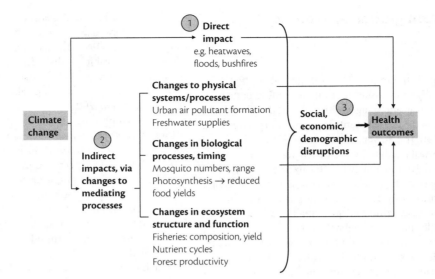

Fig. 2.8.5 Schema of main pathways by which climate change can affect human health.

in particular as a function of the geographic pattern of climatic trends and events and the vulnerability of the local population, which would be affected by, for example, the underlying burden of chronic disease, poverty levels, and the capacity of local infrastructure to respond to environmental change.

Some health outcomes in some populations would be beneficial. For example, some low-latitude regions may become too hot for mosquitoes, and winter cold periods would become milder in various temperate-zone countries where death rates currently tend to peak in wintertime. However, there is a broad consensus that most of the anticipated health effects of climate change would be adverse (McMichael 2006; IPCC 2007b). The direct health effects would include changes in mortality and morbidity from altered exposures to thermal extremes; the respiratory health (including asthma) consequences of increased exposures to photochemical pollutants and aeroallergens; and the physical hazards of the increased occurrence of storms, floods, or droughts, in at least some regions. Intensified rainfall, with flooding, can overwhelm urban wastewater and sewer systems, leading to contamination of drinking water supplies. This is most likely in large crowded cities where infrastructure is old or inadequate (Box 2.8.3).

Over time, as climate change progresses, these indirect effects on health are likely to have a relatively greater aggregate impact than the direct effects. These would include alterations in the range and activity of vector-borne infectious diseases (for example, malaria, dengue fever, and leishmaniasis). The vector organisms that spread these diseases (for example, mosquitoes) are very sensitive to climatic conditions, as is the parasite's development while incubating in the vector: Increased ambient temperature decreases incubation period. Scenario-based modelling studies suggest that the geographic zone and seasonality of potential transmission of malaria and dengue fever will increase in many parts of the world.

In temperate Europe and North America, climate-sensitive vector-borne infections include tick-borne encephalitis and Lyme disease. There is uncertainty, and debate, over whether and how climate change will affect patterns of transmission of these tick-borne infections. In Australia, studies have shown that rainfall patterns (especially in association with the El Niño cycle), temperature, tidal movements, and the ecology of vertebrate host species influence outbreaks of mosquito-borne Ross River virus disease, the major Australian arboviral infection.

Changes in climatic conditions will also affect the rates of transmission of many person-to-person infections, especially food- and water-borne pathogens. *Salmonella*, and various other bacteria that cause food poisoning, proliferate more rapidly at higher temperatures. A weaker seasonal relationship exists for infection by *Campylobacter*. Diverse studies have shown that short-term temperature increases are followed by increased notifications of non-specific food-poisoning in the United Kingdom (Bentham & Langford 2001) and of diarrhoeal diseases in Peru and Fiji (Checkley *et al.* 2000; Singh *et al.* 2001). Simple monotonic associations exist between temperature and salmonellosis notifications in European countries (Kovats *et al.* 2004) and Australia (D'Souza *et al.* 2004). Outdoor temperatures might also affect exposures via seasonal changes in eating patterns (e.g. eating foods more prone to Salmonella contamination at buffets and barbecues).

Cholera is also sensitive to temperature. Much evidence shows that the cholera-causing *Vibrio* bacterium proliferates in warmer water in lakes, estuaries, and coastal waters (Wilcox & Colwell 2005). The combination of persistent poverty (with poor sanitation), warmer temperatures, and population displacement in poorer regions will tend to exacerbate the occurrence of cholera in the future.

Of great potential importance to population health, especially in food-insecure regions with high levels of malnutrition and child stunting, would be the adverse nutritional consequences of regional declines in agricultural productivity. Crop yields will be affected by changes in temperature, soil moisture, and pollinating insect activity. In temperate regions and at high latitudes, agricultural productivity could initially increase, while declining in agriculturally marginal areas (IPCC 2007b) Such changes in local food production will affect food choices, nutrition, and health.

Research by the International Rice Research Institute has shown that rice yields decline by around 10 per cent per 1°C rise in the growing-season temperature. Above a 3°C rise, it is estimated that net global production of cereal grains by later this century will decline by around one-twentieth (Fischer *et al.* 2005). The level of

Box 2.8.3 Climate change will exacerbate existing health inequalities

The impact of climate change will differ between rich and poor countries. It will disproportionately affect diseases which already place major health burdens on poorer countries. Many of the 30 most significant causes of premature death around the world are closely linked with the environment and will be substantially and directly affected by climate change (Fig. 2.8.6). Poor countries already suffer many times the burden than richer countries.

Malaria, for example, leads to more than 10 000 times as many years of life lost in the poorest 20 per cent of countries than in the richest 20 per cent. Deaths among young children from diarrhoeal disease and from malnutrition—both closely related to climate—are likely to increase with further stress on water supplies and reduced crop yields. Many other important causes could be affected indirectly; increased depression and suicide among rural populations and farmers with prolonged drought, or more deaths resulting from wars over scarcer resources. Other mosquito-borne diseases and diarrhoeal diseases are responsible for between one and three thousand times more years of life lost in the poorest compared to the richest countries and, being directly dependent on climate, are predicted to increase with climate change.

The poorest countries will not only be exposed to heightened disease risks from climate change, but will have least capacity to adapt technologically, and their health systems will be least able to respond.

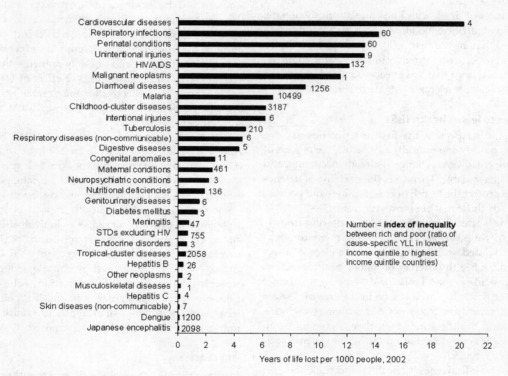

Fig. 2.8.6 The 30 most significant causes of premature death worldwide (years of life lost: YLL), and also showing an index of inequality between rich and poor countries. YLL data from WHO (2007).

decline in many already food-insecure populations in low-latitude regions is estimated at around 10–20 per cent (Lobell & Field 2007). Droughts and floods could further impair local production. Declines are also projected for wild fisheries and, perhaps, aquaculture production (IPCC 2007b).

There is a potentially very large, but more diffuse and harder-to-quantify, category of risk to health. Climate change will inevitably adversely affect physical and psychological health in the wake of loss of livelihoods, displacement of population, and economic disruption. This will occur particularly because of rising sea levels

(for example, small island states, coastal Bangladesh, and the Nile Delta), agroecosystem decline, and freshwater shortages.

Detecting health impacts

Initially, most climate-induced health impacts will be difficult to detect. If an ice-sheet melts it must be because its environment is warmer. If plants flower early, that almost certainly reflects changed climatic conditions. However, evidence that malaria is moving higher in East African highlands (Patz *et al.* 2002) could reflect the associated warming—or it could reflect changes in land use, population movements, mosquito spray programmes, antimalarial drug resistance, or all of the above.

Further, human health is often well buffered by culture, behaviour, and healthcare. The signal is thus hidden. For example, if climate change affects local grain yields, then (unlike polar bears no longer able to catch prey because of the receding ice floes) humans can trade or switch to other crops. Either the evidence or the actual occurrence of health impact can thus be masked or deferred, making detection more difficult.

Various infectious diseases are quite probably now responding to climatic changes. Viewed together, the recent shifts in physical range of malaria (sub-Saharan Africa), tick-borne encephalitis (Sweden), and the schistosomiasis water-snail (eastern China)—all associated with warming—and the changing seasonal and inter-annual pattern of some enteric bacterial infections (cholera, other vibrios, salmonellosis) suggest that climate change is now affecting at least some infectious diseases (McMichael *et al.* 2006; McMichael & Woodruff 2007).

Meanwhile, using a rather conservative statistical formula confined to four causes of death with known relations to climatic variables (malaria, malnutrition, flooding, and diarrhoeal disease), WHO has estimated that, by the year 2000, around 150 000 deaths from those causes were occurring annually in low-income countries because of the climate change that had already occurred (relative to the 1961–1990 global climate average) (McMichael *et al.* 2002).

Adaptive strategies to lessen health risks

From a public health perspective, the first order of business for society is to curb, as quickly and radically as possible, the process of global climate change. However, change is already occurring, and some more is now unavoidable. Therefore, the next line of defence is to take actions to protect the health of communities and populations, and particularly those that are most vulnerable.

Climate change will affect health primarily by altering (mostly increasing or intensifying) various existing climatic–environmental exposures and related social conditions that already affect human health. Existing health systems and public health practices should therefore provide a good basis for developing a stronger coping capacity. One particular need will be in the area of disaster preparedness. If the severity or frequency of heat-waves, cyclones, floods, landslides, and bushfires increases, then there will be an increase in the episodic acute demands on the health system's accident-and-emergency services.

To achieve long-term effectiveness of health protection, however, adaptive strategies will be needed that extend across sectors. These would include:

◆ Public education about the health risks of climate change;

◆ Early-alert systems for impending weather extremes;

◆ Community-based neighbourhood support/watch schemes;

◆ Better (i.e. climate-proofed) housing design and urban planning;

◆ Disaster preparedness, and an enhanced health-system 'surge' capacity;

◆ Expanded infectious disease control programmes (vaccines, vector control, rapid case treatment);

◆ Improved surveillance of risk-indicators and health outcomes; and

◆ Appropriate workforce training and career development.

Stratospheric ozone depletion

Stratospheric ozone depletion is a separate phenomenon from greenhouse gas accumulation in the lower atmosphere (troposphere). It results in an increase in ultraviolet irradiation (UVR) at the Earth's surface. The major ozone-destroying chemicals, chlorofluorocarbons (CFCs), have been used as refrigerants and propellants since the 1920s. They were first suspected of damaging atmospheric ozone in the 1970s. Rapid international response ensued, with the signing of the Vienna Convention for Protection of the Ozone Layer in 1985, followed by the Montreal Protocol in 1987 mandating a global phasing out of CFCs. Compliance has been good, though not complete.

Because of their long atmospheric lifetimes, the increase in UVR exposure is yet to peak, sometime within the next decade, and then decline slowly back to normal levels by around mid-century. Meanwhile, the increased exposure to the ultraviolet B radiation (UBV) is expected to cause slight increases in the severity of sunburn and the incidence of skin cancers in fair-skinned populations, and various eye disorders (such as cataracts) are expected to increase (Lucas *et al.* 2006). Some UVR-induced suppression of immune functioning may also result, thus increasing susceptibility to infectious diseases and possibly reducing the efficacy of some vaccines. That immunosuppressive effect of UVR, both local and systemic, may be protective for the development of autoimmune diseases, particularly multiple sclerosis (McMichael & Hall 1997; Ponsonby *et al.* 2002).

Exposure to a certain amount of UVR is beneficial to other aspects of health, particularly by enabling the synthesis of vitamin D via conversion of precursors in the skin. This vitamin assists calcium absorption and is essential for skeletal health, particularly the prevention of rickets, osteomalacia, and osteoporosis.

The regional population health impacts of stratospheric ozone depletion will depend on changes in individual-level received exposure to UVR, and this will vary according to: (i) the amount and wavelength constitution of changes in UVR flux at the Earth's surface—which is influenced by latitude, cloud cover, and stratospheric ozone; (ii) skin pigmentation, with darker skin being more protective than lighter skin; and (iii) cultural practices and behaviour, determining, for example, how much outdoor activity is undertaken and how much skin is exposed.

Skin cancers

Estimates made in the 1990s indicated that the increased exposure to UBV would cause basal cell carcinoma incidence to increase, temporarily, by around 15–20 per cent at mid–high latitudes, but to increase very much less at intermediate latitudes. The estimated percentage increases in incidence of squamous cell carcinoma would be twice as great as for basal cell carcinoma. One widely cited study, using integrated mathematical modelling, estimated that non-melanoma skin cancer rates would rise to a peak excess incidence of approximately 10 per cent in the United States and Europe around the middle of the twenty-first century (Slaper *et al.* 1996).

Eye health

Acute exposure to a high dose of UVB results in acute inflammation of the cornea and conjunctiva (photokeratitis and photoconjunctivitis or snow blindness). Chronic exposure is one risk factor for the development of pterygium (a fleshy, wing-shaped growth on the eye's medial surface).

Cataracts are extremely common among older age groups in some populations and cause visual impairment, ranging up to complete blindness. They are associated with an increased risk of mortality in both developed and developing countries. Chronic UVR exposure, especially to UVB, appears to be an important cause of cortical and posterior subcapsular cataract, whereas intense exposure in childhood and young adulthood may cause nuclear cataracts (Neale *et al.* 2003). Even a marginal impact of increased UVB exposure on the incidence of already-common cataract would significantly affect population health.

Indirect and ecological effects

A potentially important, although indirect, health detriment could arise from UVB-induced impairment of photosynthesis on land (terrestrial plants) and at sea (phytoplankton, as the base of the marine food web). Although such effects could reduce the world's food yields, few relevant data are yet available.

Biodiversity: Losses and invasions

Through humankind's spectacular reproductive and technological 'success', the natural habitats of many other species have been occupied, damaged, or eliminated. Biologists estimate that this ongoing human-induced mass extinction may cause extinction of around one-third of all species alive in the 1800s by the end of this century (Pimm *et al.* 1995). The rate of species loss in today's world is three to four orders of magnitude faster than the natural background rate of extinction.

The loss of various key species would weaken whole ecosystems. This would have consequences that would often be adverse to human interests, such as changing the ecology of vector-borne infections and of food-producing systems that depend on pollinators and the predation of pests, and impairing the cleansing of water and the circulation of nutrients that normally cycle through ecosystems. Much genetic and phenotypic material would also be lost. To maintain the hybrid vigour and environmental resilience of 'food' species, a diversity of wild species is needed as a source of genetic additives. Further, a high proportion of modern medicinal drugs in Western medicine has natural origins, and many defy synthesis in the laboratory. Scientists test thousands of novel natural chemicals each year, seeking new drugs to treat HIV, malaria, drug-resistant tuberculosis, and cancers.

The obverse of this problem of species losses is the accelerating spread of 'invasive' species. This is occurring particularly in response to environmental disturbance and change and to the increased intensity of long-distance trade, tourism, and migration. These are discussed further, below. Another example comes from the vast proliferation of water hyacinth (a decorative plant from Brazil) in Lake Victoria, eastern Africa, which has reportedly extended the breeding grounds for the water snail that transmits schistosomiasis.

Field studies have shown how depletion of certain mammalian species within complex ecological communities boosts the intensity of replication and transmission of certain microbes that can infect humans (e.g. the spirochaete *Borrelia burgdorferi* that causes Lyme Disease), or leads to a greater exposure of humans, no longer protected by other biteable targets, to disease-transmitting mosquitoes (Dobson *et al.* 2006).

Land-use and sea-use changes: Consequences for food and malnutrition

The increase in land degradation has great implications for food supplies and therefore for nutrition, child growth and (physical and neurocognitive) development, and health. During recent decades the combination of erosion, desiccation, and nutrient exhaustion, plus irrigation-induced water-logging and salinization, has seriously degraded up to around one-third of the world's 1.5 billion hectares of readily arable farmland (Millennium Ecosystem Assessment 2005).

The 'Green Revolution', which fed much of the expanding human population during the 1960s to the 1980s, depended on laboratory-bred, high-yield cereal grains, fertilizers, groundwater, and arable soils. In retrospect, those productivity gains appear to have come substantially at the expense of using up environmental and ecological 'capital'—especially topsoil and groundwater. Today, as greater food yields are pursued to feed an increasing population, an estimated 850 million people are malnourished (FAO 2005).

Meanwhile, at sea, many of the world's great fisheries are now on the brink of being overexploited. The United Nations' Food and Agriculture Organization (FAO) estimates that the sustainable fish-catch limit has been neared—around 100 million tonnes per year (FAO 2002).

Changes to global element cycles (e.g. nitrogen and phosphorus)

An under-remarked category of global environmental change is the changing and intensification of cycling of elements and associated compounds through the biosphere. There is an emerging view among expert scientists that the build-up of activated nitrogen (ammonia and other nitrogen compounds) is beginning to pose a substantial threat to the composition and functioning of aspects of the natural world around us. The agricultural (including livestock) sector is a major source of disturbance to these global and regional cycles.

Intensive agriculture affects water quality not only by increasing the sediment load, but by leaching nutrients and agricultural chemicals and toxic chemicals into streams and rivers. Since 1960, there has been a sevenfold increase, globally, in fertilizer application and a 70 per cent increase in irrigated cropland area (Millennium Ecosystem Assessment 2005; Earth System Science Partnership 2006). Agricultural fertilizer use and livestock excreta comprise the largest source of excess nitrogen and phosphorus entering waterways and coastal zones. Indeed, humans now generate as much biologically activated nitrogen as do all of Nature's pathways—volcanoes, lightning, vegetation, and others. Indeed, the human contribution, especially from nitrogenous fertilizers, is on track to increase by a further 65 per cent by 2050. We are thereby changing the chemistry of soils and waterways widely around the world.

This poses various risks to human health, both direct and indirect, including:

◆ Diminished crop yields (soil nitrification and acidity), posing risks to nutritional sufficiency

◆ Eutrophication (nitrates and phosphates) of waterways, potentiating cholera outbreaks (via planktonic blooms, the natural reservoir for the cholera vibrio)

◆ Stomach cancer (nitrate ingestion)—long hypothesized, but not clearly resolved

- Nitrogen oxides as ambient (and domestic) air pollutants
- Methaemoglobinaemia ('blue babies')

Depletion of freshwater supplies

The issue of large-scale changes in the supply and quality of freshwater is fundamental to the health of the environment, and it has intersections with various other global environmental changes (Millennium Ecosystem Assessment 2005). The basic problem, of course, is that the growth in human numbers and the intensification of industrial and food production processes (irrigation, livestock production, etc.) means that the renewable supply of freshwater in many parts of the world is now being exceeded. Hence the diminution of flows in many great rivers, and the decline in aquifers (including 'fossil water' from the previous glaciations).

As the world's climate changes, mountain glaciers are shrinking on all continents, and some river flows are, therefore, being diminished. Further, in a warmer world, run-off from rain is affected, both because evaporation is more rapid and soil surfaces have undergone change.

Freshwater is critical to many aspects of health: Domestic hygiene, food production, food processing and cooking, and sanitation systems. The storage of freshwater has consequences for mosquito populations and, hence, diseases such as malaria and dengue fever. The building of canals (e.g. in China) affects the probabilities of spread of water-snails and, hence, schistosomiasis.

The Millennium Assessment (2005) concludes that:

Current patterns of human use of water are unsustainable. From 5% to possibly 25% of global freshwater use exceeds long-term accessible supplies and is met through engineered water transfers or the overdraft of groundwater supplies. More than one billion people live in areas without appreciable supplies of renewable freshwater and meet their water needs in this way.

Persistent organic pollutants

Various chemical pollutants, particularly the chlorinated organic chemicals such as the polychlorinated biphenyls (PCBs), persist within the environment and have become globally pervasive. They are referred to as persistent organic pollutants, or 'POPs'. The semi-volatile members of this class of chemicals undergo a type of serial distillation process in the atmosphere, as they pass from 'cell' to 'cell', moving from low to high latitudes. Via this intriguing process, they ultimately emerge at higher concentrations in living creatures at the circumpolar regions than in their counterpart at lower latitudes where the chemicals are produced, used, and released.

Some of these environmentally persistent chemicals are likely to affect neurological, immune, and reproductive systems in humans, who obtain their food at the top of the increasingly contaminated food chain. Weakening of ecosystems—as perhaps foreseen by Rachel Carson in *Silent Spring* in 1962—may also occur, resulting in various flow-on environmental health effects in human populations.

GECs and infectious disease: A global transition in human–microbe relations?

There has been a recent and continuing increase in tempo in the emergence and spread of infectious diseases in human populations. This has occurred since the mid-1970s, across all continents. Approximately 40 previously unknown or unrecognized infectious

diseases in humans have been identified (Institute of Medicine 2003).

In the decade between 1994 and 2003, the following human infectious diseases have emerged:

2003	Severe acute respiratory syndrome (SARS)
1999	Nipah virus
1997	H5N1 flu virus (avian influenza) Variant Creutzfeldt–Jakob disease (human 'mad cow disease')
	Australian bat lyssavirus
1995	Human herpes virus 8 (Kaposi sarcoma virus)
1994	Sabia virus (Brazil) Hendra virus

This development suggests that, today, a critical combination of social and technological change, intensity of human action, and disruption of environments is creating a new round of ecological opportunities for many previously unknown or unrecognized infectious agents (see also Box 2.8.4). That combination includes: Increased human mobility, more long-distance trade, intensification of food production, more large dam and irrigation projects, accelerating urbanization, extended sexual contact networks, antibiotic over-use, expanding numbers of refugees, and the exacerbation of poverty in inner-urban ghettos, shanty towns, and in poor undernourished populations everywhere. All these trends have great consequences for the emergence and spread of infectious diseases (Weiss & McMichael 2004).

The intensification of livestock production provides an important example. We have seen the emergence in recent decades of various new infectious agents that have crossed from 'food' animals to humans—such as mad cow disease (bovine spongiform encephalopathy) and its human variant Creutzfeldt–Jakob disease, Nipah virus disease (from pig farming in Malaysia), severe acute respiratory syndrome (SARS) apparently from animals brought into the wet food markets of East Asia, and highly pathogenic H5N1 avian influenza apparently from poultry production processes in southern China and Southeast Asia.

These outbreaks reflect, more generally, the transformation and intensification of agriculture and livestock production, especially 'factory farming' on a large scale. Industrialized crop and animal production is increasing rapidly near the urban centres of Asia, Africa, and Latin America. In this way the traditional relations between small farmers, their animals, and the local environment are being broken, disrupting environments, livelihoods and community structures, and mobilizing 'new' human-infecting microbes—and often in socioeconomic and political environments that are slow to detect and respond to a new threat.

As humans encroach further into pristine environments, new contacts between wild fauna, insect vectors, domesticated livestock, and humans occur. This increases the risk of cross-species infection. An example of such contact followed the establishment of large commercial piggeries close to the tropical forest in Perak, northern Malaysia. There, in 1997–98, the Nipah virus first crossed over from fruit bats (flying foxes, *Pteropus* species) to pigs and thence to pig farmers (Daszak *et al.* 2006). That zoonotic infection illustrates how the conjunction of intensified animal husbandry in association with large-scale environmental change and ecosystem disruption can potentiate a new zoonotic infection. In that case, forest-clearing and, perhaps, El Niño regional drying reduced the natural forest fruit supplies for bats, the natural reservoir of the virus. The presence of pig-farming, in cleared forest settings with associated fruit orchards, acted as an alternative food source for the bats, which then infected the pigs and, thence, the pig farmers.

More generally, the clearance and fragmentation of forest has increased the exposure of rural populations in low-income countries to a number of infectious diseases, such as various newly encountered arenaviruses that cause haemorrhagic fevers in South American populations. Other research in the Peruvian Amazon has shown that the abundance of *Anopheles darlingi* mosquitoes, the major local malaria vector, increases by several orders of magnitude over locations with progressively intensive levels of forest clearance (Patz *et al.* 2000).

On the social–behavioural front, especially in the urban environment, relaxation of traditional cultural norms has yielded newer, freer, patterns of human behaviour, including in relation to sexual activities and illicit drug use. Modern medical manoeuvres, including blood transfusion and organ transplantation, also create new opportunities for viruses to pass from person to person.

Long-distance trade amplifies the dissemination of various infectious diseases. Outbreaks of the potentially lethal toxin-producing *E. coli* O157 in North America and Europe in the 1990s were caused by contaminated beef imported from infected cattle in Latin America. Large development projects, particularly dams, irrigation schemes, and road construction, often potentiate the spread of infectious diseases spread by vectors or intermediate hosts, such as malaria, dengue fever, and schistosomiasis.

Meanwhile, as discussed above, a new and longer shadow is now falling over future infectious disease risks by human-induced changes in the world's climate (Dobson *et al.* 2006).

Box 2.8.4 Major factors affecting the emergence and spread of infectious diseases in humans

- Population growth and density (often accompanied by peri-urban poverty)
- Urbanization: Changes in social and sexual relations
- Globalization of travel and trade (distance and speed)
- Intensified livestock production
- Live animal food markets: Longer, faster, supply lines
- Changes to ecosystems (deforestation, biodiversity loss, etc.)
- Global climate change
- Biomedical exchange of human tissues (transfusion, transplantation)
- Misuse of antibiotics (humans and domestic animals)
- Increased human susceptibility to infection: Due to population ageing, HIV infection, intravenous drug use, increased UVR exposure from ozone depletion

---

Research: Scope, methods, policy role

Categories of research question

From the preceding text it is clear that this is a complex and challenging domain in which to conduct research to identify causal relations, assess health risks, and develop and evaluate interventions. With complexity comes uncertainty, and this, in turn, requires some new ways of thinking about and communicating research results. It has implications, of course, for policy development. When uncertainties are considerable, and risks to health are potentially great, what is the role of precaution?

There are three broad categories of epidemiological research task—which can be thought of as inspection, detection, and projection. Much of that research needs to be conducted in collaboration with other disciplines. The research tasks are:

1. Study the 'baseline' relations between a specified health outcome and natural variations in climatic–environmental conditions. This research extends the information base, which, in turn, is needed for each of the next two categories of research.

2. Seek early evidence of changes in rates of occurrence of disease or disease risk factors (e.g. mosquito population range or altered allergy seasons) that are reasonably attributable to recent local environmental or climatic change.

3. Use the baseline information to estimate how future scenarios of climatic–environmental change (generated from scenarios of future human pressures on the environment) will affect the rate and/or range of occurrence of specified health outcomes.

The third of these research areas is complex, and relatively unfamiliar to mainstream epidemiology and population health research. It will often require high-level integrated mathematical modelling. That integration can be of two main types—vertical integration (along the central causal chain), and horizontal integration (which brings into the calculus other non-climate variables and processes that may modify steps in the central causal chain).

Integrated assessment of health impacts

The impacts of environmental change on human health and survival are a long way 'to the right' in the causal chain. Most of the research done to date in this 'global environmental' domain has been in relation to climate change. The following discussion therefore uses climate change-related research as the template for thinking more generically about the risk assessment challenges.

Most research energy in the realm of integrated assessment has been (understandably) expended further to the left of the causal chain. This has sought to enhance the capacity of climate models to provide valid and more precise estimates of the impact of plausible scenarios of future global greenhouse gas emissions on future climate projections. Once this step is deemed satisfactory, those modelled climate change 'output' scenarios can be used to model future changes in health-determinant variables: Mosquito populations, flood patterns, local food production, the likely duration and frequency of heat-waves, and so on. These 'exposures' are then applied to the existing, known, exposure–effect (dose–response) relationships, to estimate changes in probabilities of health outcomes.

A more sophisticated approach incorporates into the model, via 'horizontal integration', information about ongoing trends in other determinants of health outcomes for which reasonable extrapolation of future trends is possible. Examples would be demographic trends in age structures, likely future uptake of domestic air-conditioning by 2050; advent of relevant vaccines and likely consequent population immunity, and the introduction and extension of deliberate and specific 'adaptive' changes such as mosquito control programmes, heat-wave warning systems, and flood protection measures.

Integrated assessment, as currently practised, is (mostly) inherently conservative in that it assumes future smooth changes in both climatic mean conditions and variability. Step-changes and the consequences of passing critical thresholds are much less easy to foresee and model. This can be illustrated by considering the integrated-assessment modelling of climate change impacts on regional cereal grain yields. This modelling has been based on physiological models of how temperature and soil moisture affect plant growth, and has not been able to take account of, for example, a change in the pattern of outbreaks of plant pests and diseases or a change in patterns of extreme weather events (floods, storms, etc.)—events that would be rather stochastic. Further, it is also not possible to include projections of those types of social and technological changes that are not reasonably foreseeable.

Adaptations to reduce health risks: Further dimension for integrated modelling

Human-induced climate change is occurring this decade, and more change is unavoidable because of the time-lags in this complex process. Hence, beyond steps taken to curtail greenhouse gas emissions, there is need for societies to take health protecting 'adaptive' actions.

There are two main categories of adaptation. These are: (i) spontaneous (e.g. physiological adaptation to higher temperature; ongoing improvements in housing; unscheduled discovery of effective vaccines); and (ii) planned (e.g. heat-wave warnings; improved mosquito control programmes; public education about hazards).

Research on climate change impacts has, to date, mostly used rather simple assumptions about possible adaptive responses (behavioural, technological, health, and economic). Little attention has been paid to considering how health systems and other social institutions might respond to climate change, or how these might interact to reduce exposure and enhance adaptive capacity.

Enriching mitigation and adaptation policy decisions

Elucidating the risks to population health from GEC will enable better informed social policy responses. Policy decisions must encompass the following:

1. Mitigation policies aimed at stopping detrimental environmental change. (Concern over health risks motivates many people to address the issue of climate change and other environmental changes. Research that enriches the evidence of health risks should therefore add further rationale and stimulus to the policy discussion of mitigation strategies.)

2. Adaptive strategies, policies, and measures to reduce current and future adverse health impacts of global environmental changes.

3. 'Portfolio' solutions that combine mitigation and adaptation (such as solar power for home, clinics, schools, agriculture, and small businesses; water purification; pumping and crop irrigation; desalination, public transport).

While GECs occur at global/worldwide scale, many of the health impacts will be site-specific and path-dependent; that is, they will depend on local circumstances. For example, malaria epidemics

occur following rainy seasons in some regions, but during droughts (with local stasis of water) in others. Therefore, as ever, public health interventions must be designed at a scale and of a kind that is appropriate to the health outcome of local concern.

Interventions will be required at local, national, regional, and global scales. Research will therefore have maximum translational impact if, in aggregate, it spans all of these levels.

Implications for public health policy and practice

It is evident from this chapter that there are very many, often complex and interacting, ways in which human-induced changes to the environment-at-large affect—and will increasingly affect—risks to health. Beyond slowing, ceasing, or reversing the environmental change itself, the main task for the health sector is to take actions to minimize the translation of those risks into actual adverse health outcomes. A central consideration, and one that should help guide the priorities for action, is the differential vulnerability of sub-populations and groups.

Population vulnerability

The vulnerability of a particular population, sub-population, or local group to the potential health impacts of GEC depends is a function of: (i) the extent of the external exposure; (ii) the 'constitutional' sensitivity of the population/group and its support structures; and (iii) the level of adaptive resources and capacity. In more detail:

1. Magnitude of exposure to environmental change: This includes changes in both average environmental conditions and in the extent of their variability. Repeated weather extremes (e.g. repeated heavy rains) or sequential extremes (such as prolonged drought followed by heavy rains and flooding) can deplete a community's coping mechanisms and resources thereby increasing vulnerability to stresses.

2. Extent to which health status, or the natural or social systems on which health outcomes depend, are sensitive to ('susceptible' to) the environmental change: This refers, in essence, to the form of the exposure–response relationship for that 'target' entity. The sensitivity of ecosystems (e.g. agroecosytems) may also be important if the environmental stresses are likely to alter essential health-supporting functions such as water supplies, food production, carbon sinks, and stabilization of infectious disease transmission.

3. Adaptive capacity: This reflects resources and actions, both potential and those already in place, to reduce the extent of incurred adverse health outcome. A simple example is that the prevalence of air-conditioning within an urban area will help to reduce the impacts of heat extremes. The effectiveness of any existing adaptive interventions partially determines the above-mentioned exposure–response relationship.

In general, the vulnerability of a population depends on the level of material resources, effectiveness of governance and civil institutions, quality of public health infrastructure, access to relevant local information, and pre-existing burden of disease (Woodward et al. 2001). Indeed, a mix of individual, community, political, social, economic, cultural, and geographical factors determine vulnerability. These factors are not uniform across a region or nation; rather, there are geographic, demographic, and socioeconomic differences. Hence, the effective targeting of prevention or adaptation strategies requires understanding which demographic or geographic sub-populations may be most at risk.

One particular challenge in developing adaptation strategies is the issue of scale. The drivers of, and hence the potential for response to, GEC can operate at international, national, and local levels. Ozone depletion is a global issue, with chlorofluorocarbons (CFCs) produced locally affecting global stratospheric concentrations. Deforestation, international trade, and travel have local, national, regional, and international environmental and social impacts. These can influence the emergence of infectious diseases across these scales. Infectious diseases emerging in one part of the world can affect nations throughout the world. Clearly, the choice of effective interventions requires understanding of the scale at which the drivers of change and health outcomes occur.

Preventive strategies: Examples in relation to climate change

Many local actions can be taken to reduce the vulnerability of communities and whole populations to the health hazards of climate change. Climate change will act primarily by intensifying many of the existing climatic–environmental exposures and associated social and ecological conditions that affect human health. Hence, existing health systems and public health practices ought to provide a good base for adaptive strategies to reduce health impacts.

Major components of the health sector task—which will vary considerably between regions and countries—are as follows:

1. Preventive programmes, such as vaccines, mosquito control, food hygiene and inspection, nutritional supplementation

2. Public education (including via doctors' waiting rooms and hospital clinics)

3. Surveillance of disease occurrence and disease risk factors

4. Forecasting of likely future health risks, from:

    a. Projected climate change

    b. Mitigation and adaptation strategies

5. Health sector workforce training and in-career development

6. Minimization of greenhouse gas emissions from health system infrastructure

To achieve long-term effectiveness, adaptive strategies must extend well beyond the formal health sector, to include:

1. General public education about the health risks of climate change

2. Early-alert systems for impending weather extremes

3. Community-based neighbourhood support/watch schemes, to protect the most vulnerable

4. Better (climate-proofed) housing design, urban planning, water catchment, agricultural extension services (improved farming practices)

5. Disaster preparedness, including health-system 'surge' capacity

Beyond these adaptive strategies lies the greater preventive challenge of slowing, then averting, climate change via radical and far-sighted policy decisions at national and international levels. Health professionals everywhere have both the opportunity (via their knowledge, community engagement, and policy influence) and the responsibility to help make this happen.

Conclusion

The relations between human population health and the conditions of the social and natural environments is a profound and long-term one—and is at the core of the quest for sustainability. This fundamental ecological relationship is buffered by culture, and it therefore often lacks the immediacy that is apparent elsewhere in nature. However, viewed in ecological and population-level terms, the limits to, and the characteristics of, a population's health profile are determined in the medium-to-longer term by environmental conditions.

Over the past half-century there has been a growing awareness of the health risks that arise from environmental exposures, including from modern industrial and agricultural practices. This spectrum of health hazards encompasses toxicological, physical, and micro-biological exposures, all usually confined within a localized setting. Local air pollution, environmental tobacco smoke, and pesticide residues in local food produce are familiar examples. Such localized environmental hazards remain important public health issues, particularly in many developing countries.

Today, however, as the scale of human impact on the world's environment increases, larger scale and more complex changes in ecological and biogeophysical systems portend potentially greater, and longer lasting, risks to human health and survival. The aggregate pressures of human societies, regionally and globally, are now disrupting and depleting various of the planet's large-scale natural environmental systems—as evidenced by greenhouse gas accumulation and climate change, stratospheric ozone depletion, depletion of freshwater supplies, degradation of fertile land, depletion of ocean fisheries, marked changes to the cycling of several elements (especially nitrogen and its biologically activated forms), loss of biodiversity and associated disruptions of ecosystems, and, via biophysical processes, the global dispersion of persistent organic pollutants.

These global environmental changes are unprecedented in human experience, at least at this scale, and some of them (such as climate change, stratospheric ozone depletion, and the global amplification of activated nitrogen) are new at any scale. The increasingly urgent challenge for public health researchers and practitioners is to understand how today's remarkable human-induced changes to larger-scale environmental systems are influencing—and are likely to influence increasingly—the health of populations around the world.

The modern 'environmental health' agenda therefore must address these larger, increasingly prominent, systemic influences on human health. This requires broad, collaborative, engagement across disciplines and across cultures and economies. The need for global research capacity-building in this domain is both urgent and crucial. The need for public and policy receptivity to these dimensions, with their often longer time horizons, is equally critical.

References

Bambrick, H. (2004). *Trading in food safety: The impact of trade agreements on quarantine in Australia*. The Australia Institute, Canberra.

Bambrick, H. and Kjellström, T. (2004). Good for your heart but bad for your baby? Revised guidelines for fish consumption in pregnancy. *The Medical Journal of Australia*, **181**(2), 61–62.

Bambrick, H., Faunce, T., and Johnston, K. (2006). Potential impact of the AUSFTA on Australia's blood supply. *The Medical Journal of Australia*, **185**(6), 320–3.

Bentham, G. and Langford, I.H. (2001). Environmental temperatures and the incidence of food poisoning in England and Wales. *International Journal of Biometeorology*, **45**(1), 22–6.

Brown, L. (2005). *Learning from China: Why the Western Economic Model will not work for the world [online]*, Earth Policy Institute. www.earth-policy.org/Updates/2005/Update46.htm.

Butler, C. and McMichael, A. (2005). Environmental Health. In (eds. B. Levy and V. Sidel) *Social injustice and public health*, pp. 318–36. Oxford University Press, Oxford.

Carson, R. (1962). *Silent spring*. Houghton Mifflin, Boston.

Checkley, W., Epstein, L.D., Gilman, R.H. *et al.* (2000). Effects of El Niño and ambient temperature on hospital admissions for diarrhoeal diseases in Peruvian children. *Lancet*, **355**, 442–50.

D'Souza, R.M., Becker, N.G., Hall, G. *et al.* (2004). Does ambient temperature affect foodborne disease? *Epidemiology*, **15**(1), 86–92.

Daszak, P., Plowright, R., Epstein, J.H. *et al.* (2006). The emergence of Nipah and Hendra virus: pathogen dynamics across a wildlife-livestock-human continuum. In *Disease ecology: Community structure and pathogen dynamics* (eds. S.K. Collinge and C. Ray), pp. 186–201 Oxford University Press, New York.

Dietz, T., Rosa, E., and York, R. (2007). Driving the human ecological footprint. *Frontiers in Ecology and the Environment*, **5**, 13–18.

Dobson, A., Cattadori, I., Holt, R. *et al.* (2006). Sacred cows and sympathetic squirrels: The importance of biological diversity to human health. *PLoS Medicine*, **3**, e231–45.

Earth System Science Partnership (2006). *Global environmental change and human health (GEC&HH)*. http://www.essp.org/en/joint-projects/health.html.

FAO (2005). *The state of food and agriculture*, United Nations.

FAO (2006). *Livestock's long shadow. Environmental issues and options*, 414 pages. FAO, Rome.

Fischer, G., Shah, M., Tubiello, F.N. *et al.* (2005). Socio-economic and climate change impacts on agriculture: An integrated assessment, 1990–2080. *Philosophical transactions of the Royal Society of London. Series B, Biological sciences*, **360**(1463), 2067–83.

Institute of Medicine (2003). *Microbial threats to health: Emergence, detection, and response*, Institute of Medicine of the National Academies. http://www.iom.edu/CMS/3783/3919/5381.aspx.

IPCC (2007a). *Climate change 2006, Vols. I, II, and III. IPCC Third Assessment Report*. Cambridge University Press. New York.

IPCC (2007b). *Climate change 2007: Climate change impacts, adaptation and vulnerability. IPCC WGII Fourth Assessment Report*, Intergovernmental Panel on Climate Change. http://www.ipcc-wg2.org/index.html.

Kennedy, D. (ed.) (2006). *The state of the planet 2006–2007*. Island Press, Washington DC.

Kovats, R.S., Edwards, S.J., Hajat, S. *et al.* (2004). The effect of temperature on food poisoning: a time-series analysis of salmonellosis in ten European countries. *Epidemiology and Infection*, **132**, 443–53.

Leakey, R. and Lewin, R. (1995). *The Sixth Extinction: Pattern of life and the future of mankind*. Doubleday, New York.

Lobell, D.B. and Field, C.B. (2007). Global scale climate-crop yield relationships and the impacts of recent warming. *Environmental Research Letters*, **2**(014002).

Lucas, R., Repacholi, M., and McMichael, A. (2006). Is the current public health message on UV exposure correct? *Bulletin of the World Health Organization*, **84**(6), 485–91.

McKeown, T., Brown, R.G. and Record, R.G. (1972). An interpretation of the modern rise of population in Europe. *Population Studies*, **26**(3), 345–82.

McMichael, A. (2002). The urban environment and health in a globalising world: Issues for developing countries. In *Urban health in the third world* (ed. R. Akhtar), pp. 423–46. APH Publishing, New Delhi.

McMichael, A. (2005). Integrating nutrition and ecology: Balancing the health of humans and biosphere. *Public Health Nutrition*, **8**, 706–15.

McMichael, A. and Hall, A. (1997). Does immunosuppressive ultraviolet radiation explain the latitude gradient for multiple sclerosis? *Epidemiology*, **8**, 642–5.

McMichael, A. and Woodruff, R. (2007). Climate change and infectious disease. In *Social ecology of infectious disease* (eds. K. Mayer and H. Pizer). Academic Press, New York.

McMichael A.J., Campbell-Lendrum D., Kovats S. *et al.* Climate Change. In: Ezzati M, Lopez AD, Rodgers A, Mathers C (eds.) *Comparative Quantification of Health Risks: Global and Regional Burden of Disease due to Selected Major Risk Factors*. Geneva: World Health Organization; 2004. pp. 1543–1650.

McMichael, A.J., Woodruff, R.E., and Hales, S. (2006). Climate change and human health: Present and future risks. *Lancet*, **367**(9513), 859–69.

McMichael, T., Campbell-Lendrum, D., Kovats, S. *et al.* (2002). *Comparative risk assessment for climate change.*

Meehl, G.A., Stocker, T.F., Collins, W.D. *et al.* (2007). Global climate projections. In *Climate change 2007: The physical science basis. Contribution of working Group I to the fourth assessment report of the Intergovernmental Panel on Climate Change* (eds. S. Solomon, D. Qin, M. Mannin, Z. Chen, M. Marquis, K.B. Averyt *et al.*). Cambridge University Press, Cambridge, United Kingdom and New York, NY, USA.

Millennium Ecosystem Assessment (2005). *Ecosystems and human wellbeing: Synthesis*. Island Press, Washington, DC.

Nathanson, N., Wilesmith, J., and Griot, C. (1997). Bovine spongiform encephalopathy (BSE): Causes and consequences of a common source epidemic. *American Journal of Epidemiology*, **145**(11), 959–69.

Neale, R.E., Purdie, J.L. *et al.* (2003). Sun exposure as a risk factor for nuclear cataract. *Epidemiology*, **14**(6), 707–12.

Patz, J.A., Graczyk, T.K., Geller, N. *et al.* (2000). Effects of environmental change on emerging parasitic diseases. *International Journal for Parasitology*, **30**(12–13), 1395–405.

Patz, J.A., Hulme, M., Rosenzweig, C. *et al.* (2002). Climate change - regional warming and malaria resurgence. *Nature*, **420**(6916), 627–8.

Pimm, S., Russell, G., Gittleman, J. *et al.* (1995). The future of biodiversity. *Science*, **269**, 347–50.

Ponsonby, A.L., McMichael, A., and van der Mei, I. (2002). Ultraviolet radiation and autoimmune disease: insights from epidemiological research. *Toxicology*, **181–182**, 71–8.

Prüss-Üstün, A. and Corvalán, C. (2006). *Preventing disease through healthy environments. Towards an estimate of the environmental burden of disease*. World Health Organization, Geneva.

Rahmstorf, S., Cazenave, A., Church, J. *et al.* (2007). Recent climate observations compared to projections. *Science*, **316** (5825), 709.

Singh, R.B., Hales, S., de Wet, N. *et al.* (2001). The influence of climate variation and change on diarrheal disease in the Pacific Islands. *Environmental Health Perspectives*, **109**(2), 155–9.

Slaper, H., Velders, G.J.M., Daniel, J.S. *et al.* (1996). Estimates of ozone depletion and skin cancer incidence to examine the Vienna Convention achievements. *Nature*, **384**(6606), 256–8.

United Nations (2000). *Millennium development goals*. New York.

Weiss, R.A. and McMichael, A.J. (2004). Social and environmental risk factors in the emergence of infectious diseases. *Nature Medicine*, **10**(12 Suppl), S70–6.

WHO (2007). *Global burden of disease statistics*. Last updated, date accessed 30 April 2007. http://www.who.int/healthinfo/bod/en/index.html.

Wilcox, B.A. and Colwell, R. (2005). Emerging and re-emerging infectious diseases: biocomplexity as an interdisciplinary paradigm. *Ecosystem Health*, **2**, 244–57.

Woodward, A., Hales, S., and de Wet, N. (2001). *Climate change: Potential effects on human Health in New Zealand*. Report prepared for the Ministry for the Environment as part of the NZ Climate Change Programme. Wellington. pp. 1–22. http://www.mfe.govt.nz/ publications/climate/effect-health-sep01/effect-health-sep01.pdf.

World Commission on Environment and Development (1987). *Our common future: Report of the World Commission on environment and development*, United Nations, 317 pages, Oxford University Press, Oxford.

WWF International (2006). Living planet report 2006. World Wildlife Fund International, Gland, Switzerland. http://assets.panda.org/downloads/ living_planet_report.pdf.

2.9

Health services as determinants of population health

Martin Gulliford

Abstract

This chapter evaluates the relationship between health services and public health and asks 'what is the role of health services in improving population health?'. Traditional thinking in public health has been sceptical of the value of health services at improving health. This stems from recognition of the importance of wider determinants of health, the limited effectiveness of healthcare interventions, and the importance of iatrogenic illness. A number of efficiency-oriented strategies have been developed to increase the health gains from healthcare including needs assessment, health technology assessment and cost-effectiveness analysis, implementation research to promote the uptake of research findings, and strategies to improve the organization and delivery of healthcare. Estimates suggest that healthcare now adds about 5 years to life expectancy at birth in high-income countries. Application of similar techniques to the health problems of middle- and low-income countries suggests that about a quarter of the overall burden of disease in these countries could be prevented through implementation of packages of low-cost but highly effective interventions. Investment in these health interventions would be justified by the economic benefits associated with improved population health. Implementation of the essential package of care approach is hampered by the relative or absolute lack of health services for poor populations in middle- and low-income countries. The distribution of health services in middle- and low-income countries generally shows substantial pro-rich inequity and the financial costs of accessing healthcare may further impoverish poor households. Primary care, with its emphasis on universality and affordability, has been successfully implemented in some countries with favourable health outcomes. In high-income countries, where universal coverage and equitable access to primary care have been more widely achieved, pro-rich inequity exists in accessing preventive medical interventions and specialist care for more serious illnesses. These inequities may contribute to some adverse health outcomes in lower socioeconomic groups. Public health specialists should advocate principles of efficiency and equity and contribute to realizing these through participation in processes of needs assessment, health technology assessment, quality improvement, and facilitating access to needed healthcare for all groups.

Introduction

Healthcare represents one of the largest investments that societies make in the health needs of the population but the role of health services in improving population health is disputed. According to one argument, healthcare should not be regarded as one of the determinants of population health because it is largely ineffective at prolonging life and even causes premature mortality through iatrogenic disease (Illich 1976). A more mainstream view is that health services play an important role in delivering clinical interventions for the treatment and cure of disease, as well as population interventions for the prevention of disease and promotion of health. Health services represent one of three key areas of public health activity alongside health protection and health improvement (Faculty of Public Health 2007). Public health specialists often play an important role in planning and managing health services. This chapter evaluates the relationship between healthcare and public health; it asks 'What is the role of health services in improving population health?'

Definition of healthcare

The boundaries of health services and health systems are difficult to define (Box 2.9.1). Broader definitions encompass 'all the activities whose primary purpose is to improve or maintain health' (Murray & Frenk 2000). This includes interventions that are not implemented through healthcare services including, for example, improvements to road and vehicle safety. In this chapter, multi-sectoral interventions are considered to contribute to health improvement and not healthcare (Box 2.9.2). The objective of this chapter is to evaluate whether healthcare contributes to population health independent of intervention on wider determinants of health.

Health services at different levels of economic development

In order to set the chapter in context, Table 2.9.1 provides illustrative data for health services indicators for several countries at different levels of economic development (World Bank 2006). It is clear that the countries with the lowest-incomes and worst health

Box 2.9.1   Definitions of health systems, healthcare, and health services

◆ **Health systems:** (i) All the activities whose primary purpose is to improve or maintain health (Murray and Frenk 2000); (ii) the economic, fiscal, and political management method that nations use to run the national healthcare services (Last 2007) (iii) a local or regional group of organized health services (Last 2007)

◆ **Healthcare:** Services provided to individuals or communities by agents of the health services or professions to promote, maintain, monitor, or restore health. Healthcare is not limited to medical care, which implies therapeutic action by or under the supervision of a physician. The term is sometimes extended to include self-care (Last 2001)

◆ **Health services:** Services that are performed by healthcare professionals, or by others under their direction, for the purpose of promoting, maintaining, or restoring health. In addition to personal healthcare, health services include measures for health protection, health promotion, and disease prevention (Last 2001)

also have the smallest share of resources committed to health services. In the high-income countries, per capita expenditure on health is some 200 times greater than in the low-income countries and health conditions, measured in terms of life expectancy at birth, are substantially better. These variations among countries illustrate enormous inequality in distribution of healthcare resources at the global level.

Table 2.9.1 also illustrates considerable variation among countries in the same income category. There is variation in the overall level of resources devoted to the health sector; in the relative proportions of public and private sector spending; as well as variation among countries in health outcomes at a given level of expenditure on health. Among middle-income countries, Costa Rica has been successful at mobilizing resources for health and life expectancy is higher than expected. Among the high-income countries, the United States is unusual in having exceptionally high health expenditure but life expectancy is lower than expected. These variations reflect, to a greater or lesser extent, the prevailing philosophies

Box 2.9.2   Aspects of health

Healthcare need	Capacity to benefit from health care (Stevens *et al.* 2004)
Health improvement	Population health benefit associated with intervention on the determinants of health
Health gain	Individual or population health benefit associated with healthcare intervention
Health outcome	Change in individual or population health status associated with utilization of needed healthcare

that shape societal views of the purpose of health services as well as the policies, institutions, and community responses to questions of health and healthcare.

Concepts and values in healthcare

Purpose and value of health services

Health services serve several objectives. Health services can improve health by preventing or delaying the onset of disability or death; they contribute to relieving pain and suffering; healthcare is also valued for providing information concerning diagnosis and prognosis. Healthcare is concerned more generally with how individuals' lives will begin and end and with what opportunities they will have in between. The US Presidents' Commission (President's Commission for the Study of Ethical Problems in Medicine and Biomedical and Behavioural Research 1983) observed that healthcare is valued beyond its immediate benefits 'touching on countless important and in some ways mysterious aspects of personal life investing it with significant value as a thing in itself'. Healthcare represents a tangible expression of the value placed on life and health.

For individuals, as well as for private providers and commercial interests, healthcare is valued as a private good that can be utilized to preserve or improve health. Despite this, markets generally fail to provide a satisfactory distribution of healthcare. The risk of illness is unpredictable, the costs of healthcare can be extremely high, and consumers may have limited information on which to base choices. For these reasons, communities and national governments are usually involved in arrangements for the delivery of healthcare in order to pool risks and regulate healthcare markets. However, healthcare often yields benefits that extend beyond individual recipients. For example, the treatment of pulmonary tuberculosis has value in controlling the spread of disease to others. Such positive externalities may be valued more by communities than by individuals. Societies therefore value healthcare as a merit good, which is typically under-utilized when distributed by market forces that allow individuals to value only the personal benefits they obtain. Extending this argument, healthcare may contribute to generating public goods that benefit all. Thus, the eradication of smallpox, or the control of antimicrobial drug resistance, offer benefits that are freely accessible to the global population with a value extending beyond national boundaries (Smith *et al.* 2003).

Dimensions for evaluation

The diverse objectives, and the complex organization and delivery of healthcare, require evaluation on several different conceptual dimensions. Maxwell's (1984) framework of six dimensions is frequently used (Box 2.9.3). Each of Maxwell's dimensions represents a complex, multi-faceted concept that is not easily defined. The dimensions can be broadly grouped into those associated with efficiency, including efficiency and effectiveness; and those associated with equity, including equity and access. Relevance to need, and social acceptability, contribute to the definition of both efficiency and equity. The relative importance assigned to the concepts of efficiency and equity is important in shaping health services and is the subject of significant ideological debate concerning how the inputs and outputs of health services should be organized and valued.

Table 2.9.1 Health expenditures and health services indicators at different levels of economic development around 2003–2004

	Gross national income per capita (2004 US$)	Health expenditure (per cent GDP)	Public expenditure (per cent total)	Health expenditure per capita (US$)	Doctors per 1000 population	Hospital beds per 1000 population	Life expectancy at birth years)
Low-income							
Kenya	480	4.3	38.7	20	0.1	1.6	48
Pakistan	600	2.4	27.7	13	0.7	0.7	65
Middle-income							
Albania	2120	6.5	41.7	118	1.3	3.1	74
Costa Rica	4470	7.3	78.8	305	1.3	1.4	79
Indonesia	1140	3.1	35.9	30	0.1	0.7	67
High-income							
Japan	37050	7.9	81.0	2662	2.0	14.3	82
United Kingdom	33630	8.0	85.7	2428	2.2	4.2	79
United States	41440	15.2	44.6	5711	2.3	3.3	77

Source: World Bank (2006).

Ideological and philosophical drivers

On the input side, obtaining needed healthcare is regarded at one extreme as the responsibility of individuals and families. This is often the case in low-income countries where government or externally funded health services may not be available and families necessarily make out-of-pocket payments to private providers or do not obtain healthcare (van Doorslaer *et al.* 2006b). In high-income countries, obtaining needed care is sometimes also viewed primarily as an individual responsibility with the government, representing the organized efforts of society, having a minimal role in the regulation of the healthcare market. This libertarian view is most evident in the organization of healthcare in the United States (Blake *et al.* 2003). One proposed justification is that taxation to provide healthcare for others infringes against individuals' freedom of choice. From this perspective, fairness only concerns basic opportunities to compete for health resources and does not require that a fair distribution of healthcare be realized. As greater income and wealth are generally associated with better access to healthcare but with fewer health needs, this libertarian approach will not usually lead to an equitable distribution of healthcare. This is in contrast to the more egalitarian approach that has prevailed in most high-income countries with the ideal of universal eligibility to comprehensive services and the objective of equity of access to healthcare (Mossialos *et al.* 2003).

A separate set of tensions concerns how the outputs of healthcare should be distributed. According to utilitarian doctrine, society in general and health services in particular should aim to maximize the health gains obtained across all individuals. This idea is summed up by the slogan 'the greatest good for the greatest number'. This utilitarian approach is sometimes regarded as 'the guiding principle for many of the decisions and actions of public health professionals' (Last 2007, p. 385). The objective of maximizing the health gain to be achieved from the available resources is closely related to the economic principle of efficiency. Resources for health will be used most efficiently when health gain is maximized (Box 2.9.3).

The simple form of utilitarianism is problematic. This approach only requires that the sum of health gains in a population should be maximized, it does not require that all individuals receive a fair distribution of potential benefits from healthcare. This is in contrast to approaches based on concepts of human rights and social justice in which each individual is considered to have a right to health. According to this approach, all individuals are considered to be entitled to healthcare even when the contribution this makes to the aggregate benefit of the wider community does not require that they receive it (Dworkin 1977). The rights to health and medical care are recognized in the Universal Declaration of Human Rights (United Nations 2007). The International Covenant on Economic, Social and Cultural Rights goes further and requires that governments create 'conditions which would assure all medical services and medical attention in the event of sickness' (Office of the High Commissioner for Human Rights 2007). These international statements do not guarantee that access to needed services will be possible for all individuals but they are important in offering a degree of protection to marginalized and vulnerable groups. An approach

---

Box 2.9.3 Dimensions for evaluation of health services

Effectiveness	Extent to which a healthcare intervention achieves the intended outcome (Last 2007)
Efficiency	Outcome achieved in relation to expenditure of resources (Last 2007)
Equity	Fairness, or justice, in respect of treatment of different individuals or groups (Last 2007)
Access	Extent to which services are available, can be utilized, deliver needed services, and achieve appropriate outcomes (Gulliford *et al.* 2002)
Appropriateness	Relevance to need (Maxwell 1984)
Responsiveness	Social acceptability (Maxwell 1984)

Source: Maxwell (1984).

based on human rights favours a just or equitable distribution of healthcare over the maximization of potential health gains across the population. The pursuit of equity is also justified in terms of Rawl's theory of justice as fairness which proposed that a just society will be arranged so as to achieve fair equality of opportunity, with inequalities only permitted if they are of the greatest benefit to the least-advantaged members of society (Daniels *et al.* 2004). Based on the concepts of human rights and social justice, equity may be regarded as a moral value which health services should strive to promote (Braveman *et al.* 2001). Efficiency will often be compromised through this approach, as for example, if equitable access to specialist services is to be provided in sparsely populated rural areas, or if insulin therapy for insulin-dependent diabetes is to be ensured in low-income country settings.

The conflicting principles underlying the financing and delivery of healthcare outlined in this section are apparent in the differing approaches to provision of health services in different countries. Existing health systems result from compromises that are made through the policy process. In the healthcare systems of high-income countries, collective healthcare provision based on universal eligibility is favoured but individuals may not be prevented from purchasing healthcare privately. Equity of access is an objective, but this is only to the extent to which it is considered acceptable to compromise efficiency. In other systems, such as the United States or in middle-income countries, private financing of healthcare through insurance or out-of-pocket payments may predominate, but governments may facilitate access to basic health services for vulnerable groups such as the poor and elderly.

In the following sections, approaches to the relationship between health services and population health are divided into those that are predominantly motivated by the pursuit of efficiency and those driven by the goal of greater equity. Two specific questions are addressed: 'How do health services aim to optimize health gains?' and 'How do health services ensure an optimal distribution of health gains?'

Efficiency-driven approaches

Underlying problems

Lack of effectiveness

A basic assumption underlying the efficiency-driven approach is that utilization of healthcare is associated with health gains. This assumption was challenged by Illich who claimed that 'a vast amount of contemporary clinical care is incidental to the curing of disease, but the damage done by medicine to the health of individuals and populations is very significant' (Illich 1976, p. 23). Illich acknowledged that medicine has some effect in preventing and curing infectious diseases through the use of vaccinations and antimicrobial drugs but he argued that the historical reductions in mortality from infectious diseases in high-income countries occurred before these technologies became available. In his opinion, treatment of non-communicable diseases such as cancer and cardiovascular disease was of negligible benefit and may cause considerable harm (Illich 1976).

Illich's interpretation was supported by McKeown's (1979) analysis of historical trends in mortality in Britain. This analysis was important in identifying the limited role of medicine as a determinant of health in the historical era. For example, relative reductions in mortality between 1881 and 1950 ranged from 30-fold for tuberculosis,

20-fold for digestive diseases, and 15-fold for respiratory disease (Office for National Statistics 1998). Most of these reductions occurred before widespread use of specific antimicrobial treatment after 1945. These trends support the interpretation that environmental influences, particularly improved nutrition, clean water supplies, and better housing and sanitation, were largely responsible for historical reductions in mortality from infectious diseases in high-income countries with limited gains from health service interventions (McKeown 1979).

Consistent with McKeown's analysis, the historian Wooton suggested that before the late nineteenth century medical practice had little capacity to improve health, and was generally only harmful (Wooton 2006). It was only through the development of the germ theory of infectious disease causation, and its practical application in antiseptic surgery from 1865 onwards, that medicine first began to implement procedures that gave greater benefit than harm. Wooton (2006) argued that in the historical era, progress in medicine was largely confined to the development of a body of scientific knowledge concerning health and disease. This knowledge was not translated into practical applications and consequently medicine did not develop as a technology for improving health until more recent decades.

A similar argument was developed earlier by Cochrane in his book *Effectiveness and Efficiency* (Cochrane 1972). Cochrane commented on the rising costs of medical care and the dominance of treatment of established disease over preventive medicine. He showed that in many instances there was little evidence available concerning whether medical interventions were beneficial, ineffective, or harmful. When randomized controlled trials were conducted, they often showed that benefits of intervention were smaller than anticipated and unexpected adverse effects of treatment were not uncommon. For example, one large clinical trial showed that routine use of corticosteroid drugs in patients with head injury was associated with a relative increase in mortality of 15 per cent (95 per cent confidence interval 7–24 per cent) (Roberts *et al.* 2004). Cochrane advocated a now generally accepted view that all healthcare interventions should be tested in randomized controlled trials, and the results of all such trials should be systematically collected, analysed, and implemented in clinical practice. He advocated greater emphasis on applied research, rather than pure scientific research with little potential for benefit to patients or the public.

The dissociation between the scientific prestige associated with different medical specialities and their potential for improving health was noted by McKeown in his Introduction to *The Role of Medicine* (McKeown 1979). Tradition and professional opinion were, for a long time, the main drivers of clinical practice and the organization and delivery of medical care. However, tradition came under attack through research from epidemiologists and social scientists that questioned the effectiveness of widely used procedures, demonstrated inexplicable variations in clinical practice, widespread problems with medical errors and poor quality of care, and showed that methods for organizing and delivering care were not consistent with patients' wants and needs.

Quality of care and variations in practice

'Quality of care' is a wide ranging concept that includes departures from optimal standards of healthcare judged on any of Maxwell's dimensions (Maxwell 1984). In Donabedian's framework (Donabedian 2003), quality may be assessed in terms of the organizational structures for care, the processes of care that are delivered, or the health outcomes of care.

Problems with quality of care are often revealed through variations in the organization and delivery of care. For example, in Brazil 72 per cent of women giving birth in private clinics had Caesarean sections, compared with 31 per cent in public hospitals; yet, 70–80 per cent of women in either setting expressed a preference for vaginal delivery (Potter *et al.* 2001). In Pakistan, 68 per cent of subjects in a household survey had received one or more injections for treatment of acute symptoms in the preceding 3 months, with an average of 13.6 injections per person per year. A new needle was reportedly used in only 53 per cent of instances (Janjua *et al.* 2005). In Trinidad in 1993, 59 per cent of diabetic patients with hypertension were treated with a combination of reserpine, clopamide, and dihydroergocristine; this combination was rarely used in neighbouring islands (Mahabir & Gulliford 2005). In England in 2000, 26 per cent of patients diagnosed with 'influenza' in primary care, and 13 per cent with 'common colds', were prescribed antibiotics (Ashworth *et al.* 2004). At different family practices the proportion prescribed antibiotics ranged from 0 to 97 per cent for influenza and 0 to 84 per cent for common colds (Ashworth *et al.* 2005).

Variations such as these may originate in uncertainty concerning the optimal use of specific medical interventions. This uncertainty permits the outcome of clinical decisions to be influenced by factors such as the supply of medical services, or practitioner and patient preferences, leading to wide and often idiosyncratic variations in practice. Variations in practice may result in health resources being used inefficiently; in patients being treated in ways that are contrary to their expressed preferences; in the widespread use of potentially harmful procedures; or patients being denied the potential benefits of effective therapy.

Iatrogenic illness and patient safety

Iatrogenic illness and problems with patient safety represent a particular set of concerns with quality of care. Errors in medical care have been shown to be common, especially in hospital settings. In the US Harvard Medical Practice Study of 30 121 subjects from 51 acute hospitals in 1984 (Brennan *et al.* 1991), injuries caused by medical management occurred in 3.7 per cent of hospital admissions. A quarter of these adverse events were judged to be caused by negligence; 2.6 per cent were permanently disabling, and 13.6 per cent led to death. Based on these results, it was estimated that there may be between 44 000 and 88 000 deaths in the United States annually from errors in medical care (Kohn *et al.* 2000). In primary care, there may be significant errors in 0.1–1 per 100 consultations (Bhasale *et al.* 1998). These include delays in diagnosis, wrong diagnoses, errors in prescribing, failure to prescribe needed treatment, and difficulties with communication and referral (Bhasale *et al.* 1998).

Healthcare-associated infections are an increasing problem. In England in 2006, there were 55 681 cases of *Clostridium difficile* infection in people aged 65 years and over, generally associated with broad-spectrum antibiotic use in hospitals (Health Protection Agency 2007). Over-utilization of antimicrobial drugs is leading to the emergence of organisms that show multiple resistance, leading to healthcare-acquired infections that are difficult to treat. In England and Wales, the number of methicillin-resistant Staphyloccus aureus (MRSA) related deaths increased from 669 in 2000 to 1168 in 2004 (Office for National Statistics 2006). Multi-drug-resistant tuberculosis has emerged as an important threat with an estimated 450 000 cases worldwide in 2006 (World Health Organization 2007a).

Misallocation of resources and problems in service organization and delivery

The World Health Report for 2000 characterized health services as often 'poorly structured, badly led, inefficiently organized, and inadequately funded' (World Health Organization 2000) (p. xiv). A common problem is over-allocation of resources to hospitals. In high-income countries about 70 per cent of health services expenditure is on hospital services. This pattern of expenditure has been exported to middle- and low-income countries, often in the form of development projects that provide hospital infrastructure, not always accompanied by the required running costs. Hospital-based services generally deliver interventions of low cost-effectiveness compared with those delivered in primary care (World Bank 1993). Other problems concern the relationship between public and private sectors with doctors employed in the public sector often 'moonlighting' in private clinics, or charging for services provided in public clinics (World Health Organization 2000). The private sector may be inadequately regulated. There is often a lack of respect for the comfort, dignity, and concerns of patients (Phillips 1996).

Proposed solutions

Clinical effectiveness and health technology assessment

Cochrane's book *Effectiveness and Efficiency* was influential in leading to the development of strategies for improving clinical effectiveness, including the promotion of 'evidence-based medicine' grounded in the belief that clinical decision-making should be informed as far as possible by the results of well-conducted randomized controlled trials (RCTs) that provide evidence for the effectiveness of interventions (Sehon & Stanley 2003). This requires that the results of all available RCTs should be summarized in the results of systematic reviews and meta-analyses such as those produced by the Cochrane collaboration. This approach has been extended to cover not just therapeutic interventions but diagnostic techniques, screening strategies, and methods for delivering care under the more general heading of health technology assessment.

Health technology 'includes any method used to promote health, prevent and treat disease and improve rehabilitation or long-term care' (The NHS Health Technology Assessment Programme 2007). Health technology assessment includes evaluation of both the effectiveness and resource use associated with new medical technologies. Cost-effectiveness analysis is now commonly integrated into the implementation of randomized controlled trials so that the cost per unit benefit from an intervention may be estimated. Cost-utility analysis allows the health benefits from different interventions to be compared using a common metric such as the quality-adjusted life year (QALY). This permits more explicit comparison of the benefits obtained, and the resources used by different interventions, thus informing choices made in resource allocation decisions. Processes for assessing population health needs have also been made more explicit, based on the incidence and prevalence of disease and the effectiveness of interventions, so that health services can be designed to deliver services that are relevant to the population's health problems (Stevens *et al.* 2004).

Quality improvement, implementation research, and patient safety

The increasing availability of objective evidence concerning effective treatment for different conditions has been associated with increased evaluation of medical care against agreed standards. It is clear that there is widespread failure to achieve standards of good clinical practice or to implement fully interventions that have been shown to be effective in randomized controlled trials. For example, the technique of cumulative meta-analysis showed a delay of many years between evidence of efficacy and implementation of thrombolytic therapy in myocardial infarction (Lau *et al.* 1992). These problems have given rise to a new area of research known as 'implementation research' that aims to evaluate and identify methods to encourage health professionals to practice in accordance with evidence-based guidelines (Eccles *et al.* 2005). Studies in implementation research typically combine a range of interventions such as the provision of guidelines, invitations to educational meetings, provision of advice from respected peers, or the inclusion of prompts in the medical record. Such combinations of interventions commonly offer modest benefits in terms of promoting evidence-based practice (Oxman *et al.* 1995). In the United Kingdom, the government recently introduced a system of contractual financial incentives to encourage family doctors to deliver specified processes of care and designated intermediate outcome targets in their patients, with a main emphasis on chronic illness management (Roland 2004). Initial results appear to be impressive (Doran *et al.* 2006).

Alongside quality improvement initiatives, and requiring similar techniques for implementation, there have been specific initiatives to increase patient safety. In some countries, special organizations have been set up with the brief of improving patient safety through surveillance of critical events, identifying risks, and feeding back information to improve services. In 2004, the World Health Organization launched a World Alliance for Patient Safety with a headline campaign of 'Clean Care is Safer Care' focusing on safe blood transfusion, injection and immunization, safer clinical procedures, clean water, sanitation, and hand hygiene (World Alliance for Patient Safety 2007).

Systems redesign and service organization and delivery research

The focus of health technology assessment is primarily at the micro-level of the interaction between individual patients and health professionals. Increasingly, the organizational context in which care is delivered is viewed as important in influencing the effectiveness and efficiency of care (Sheldon 2001). Whether services are delivered in primary or secondary care, by physicians or nurses, by specialist teams or generalists may be important in influencing the costs and outcomes. The size and workload of an organization, its staffing levels, the management strategies, and organizational culture may also influence the quality and safety of services (Mannion *et al.* 2005). Consequently, there has been an expansion of social-science-based research into organization and delivery of health services. This includes investigation of the nature of patient and carer interactions with the health system, the roles of the healthcare workforce, or the impact of organizational change on the various dimensions of quality of care (Fulop *et al.* 2003). At the same time, there has been a much greater interest in experimentation with different models of organizing care including transferring care from hospital to primary and community settings, utilizing staff with different types of training, or integrating specialist skills into primary care service delivery. Such changes have sometimes been facilitated by health sector reforms that remove commissioning and service planning functions from the hands of service providers.

Redesign and modernization of service delivery have been particularly important in the management of chronic conditions.

Health services have been designed traditionally to deal with acute episodes of illness but most contacts with health services are now for chronic conditions (Bodenheimer *et al.* 2002). More than two-thirds of adults in high-income countries have one or more chronic conditions, and chronic conditions account for 80 per cent of primary care consultations and 60 per cent of hospital bed days. The management of chronic conditions requires ongoing surveillance of patients' condition, management of risk factors, early detection of complications, and education of patients so that they can actively manage their own illness and reduce risk through appropriate lifestyle and behavioural changes. Traditionally designed health services are often very ineffective at delivering services that can achieve these outcomes. The US Institute of Medicine referred to a 'quality chasm' representing the discrepancy between the potential for delivering effective care and the reality of chronic illness management (Institute of Medicine 2005). This has led to the development of new models of service delivery in chronic illness care with a focus on developing care in primary settings, linking appropriately trained staff skilled in education and promoting self-care, with easy access to specialist advice, supported by reliable and easy to use clinical information systems (Bodenheimer *et al.* 2002).

Healthcare and population health

Perceptions of the role of health services as determinants of population health have evolved. Historically, medical care was of limited importance as a determinant of health; medical care was often ineffective and had a considerable capacity for causing harm. In the twentieth century however, the pace of technological innovation accelerated and from 1948 onwards the application of randomized controlled trials to evaluate the effectiveness of health technologies was increasingly accepted. Effective interventions came to be widely used. These included vaccination and immunization against infectious disease, screening for early stages of cancer, treatment of risk factors for cardiovascular disease, or treatment services for the major causes of mortality. The impact of the widespread implementation of such interventions on population health is difficult to evaluate because of the contribution of wider and more powerful determinants of population health cannot be readily controlled as they might be in a randomized trial. Three main approaches have been used to evaluate the impact of healthcare on population health indicators.

'Avoidable' mortality

The 'avoidable' mortality argument is that if a given condition is amenable to medical intervention, then there should be few or no deaths from the condition. Mortality rates may be used as sentinel indicators of the effectiveness of healthcare services. For example, if surgical services are effective then there should be few deaths from acute appendicitis, cholecystitis or abdominal hernia. This approach was developed and implemented most extensively by Holland and co-workers (Holland 1991) who mapped the distribution of 'avoidable' deaths in Europe. The approach has been extended to monitoring of morbidity and health service utilization in routinely published indicator datasets. However, the approach suffers from the limitations that definition of 'avoidability' may often be grounded in low level evidence, and there are few health conditions for which the wider determinants of health are not important in determining the distribution of mortality.

Time-series analysis

If a health service intervention is implemented across a population over a short space of time, changes in trends in mortality or morbidity may be used to evaluate the effectiveness of the intervention. There have been well-documented reductions in the incidence of infectious diseases following the implementation of new vaccination programmes. There have also been changes in mortality from cancer following the implementation of screening programmes. This approach is complicated by underlying secular trends in disease incidence as well as by changes over time in the effectiveness of case management.

Modelling

Modelling approaches to the evaluation of health service effectiveness vary in their sophistication but all utilize evidence concerning the incidence and prevalence of disease, the effectiveness of clinical interventions, and the expected coverage and quality of services in the population at risk. This information is used to estimate the contribution of medical care to real or projected changes in mortality or other health outcomes in populations of interest.

Healthcare and population health: High-income countries

Bunker and colleagues (Bunker *et al.* 1994) modelled the contribution of medical care to life expectancy in the US population. Examples of their estimates are shown in Table 2.9.2. Their report concluded that medical care, including preventive and treatment services, contributed about 5 years additional life expectancy in the United States with potential for gain of an additional 1.5–2 years if effective interventions were implemented more completely, with improved population coverage and higher standards of care. In a more recent study, Cutler *et al.* (2006) estimated changes in life expectancy at birth in the United States between 1960 and 2000. The cumulative increase in life expectancy during this period was 6.97 years with reduced mortality from cardiovascular disease accounting for 4.88 years (70 per cent) and reduced rates of infant deaths accounting for 1.35 years (19 per cent). Based on Bunker's estimates, as well as analyses of the decline in mortality from cardiovascular disease (Unal *et al.* 2004), Cutler *et al.* (2006) attributed

half of this increased life expectancy to more effective medical intervention. Several examples illustrate the substantial benefits to be obtained from effective medical care.

Survival with human immunodeficiency virus (HIV)

The first illustration concerns the survival of people who are infected with HIV. Lohse *et al.* (Lohse *et al.* 2007) compared the survival of HIV-infected individuals in Denmark with that of controls matched for age, sex, and place of residence drawn from the general population. The estimated median survival of incident HIV cases after 25 years of age was 7.6 years in 1995–6, 22.5 years in 1997–1999, and 32.5 years in the period 2000–2005. This dramatic improvement in survival following diagnosis was attributed to the introduction of highly active antiretroviral therapy (HAART). This improvement is all the more remarkable when it is remembered that HIV was first identified in 1984. This example illustrates the capability of medical care to change the clinical course of a condition. In this case HIV became a chronic disease requiring active medical therapy over many years, with a prognosis similar to that of a diagnosis of insulin-treated type 1 diabetes mellitus. Indeed, before insulin treatment became available, the prognosis of type 1 diabetes was similar to, or worse than that of HIV infection in the pre-HAART era.

Breast cancer mortality

Another example concerns mortality from breast cancer, the most frequent cancer among women in high-income countries. In the United Kingdom, population-based mammographic screening was introduced for women aged 50–64 years after 1988. The decision to introduce screening was based on strong, but disputed, evidence from randomized controlled trials (Gotzsche & Olsen 2000; Nystrom *et al.* 2002). Around this time, there was also accumulating evidence for increasing survival following clinical diagnosis through more effective use of specific therapies, including the oestrogen receptor antagonist tamoxifen. An analysis of breast cancer mortality for women aged 55–69 years in England and Wales, showed an estimated 21.3 per cent reduction in breast cancer mortality between 1990 and 1998 compared with the predicted trend (Blanks *et al.* 2000). The authors estimated that approximately one-third of this decrease could be attributed to breast cancer screening with two-thirds of the reduction attributed to improved treatment.

Table 2.9.2 Measuring the effects of medical care. Estimated increases in life expectancy for the population from clinical preventive and curative services

Examples: Condition treated	Relevant population	Estimated gain in life years in those receiving the service	Estimated gain in life expectancy distributed across the US population	
			Current	Potential
Cervical cancer screening	Adult women	96 days	2 weeks	1 week
Immunization for diphtheria	All children	10 months	10 months	0
Cervical cancer treatment	Affected women	21 years	2 weeks	1 week
Ischaemic heart disease	Affected adults	14 years	1.2 years	6–8 months
Appendicitis	Affected individuals	50 years	4 months	0
Trauma	Affected individuals	24–38 years	1.5–2 months	3–4 months
Estimated overall gain from preventive and curative services			5 years	1.5–2 years

Source: Bunker *et al.* (1994).

Allgood *et al.* (2008) compared women who died of breast cancer with control women who did not die and found that attending for breast screening was associated with between a 35 and 65 per cent reduction in odds of mortality depending on assumptions. Cancer Research UK (2008) reported that 5-year survival of women diagnosed with breast cancer increased from 52 per cent in 1971–3 to 80 per cent in 2001–3. The example of breast cancer, illustrates the difficulty of analysing longer term outcomes of health service interventions. Analysis required estimation of the secular trend, in this case increasing, as well as separate effects of a population screening intervention and the outcomes of improved clinical treatment.

Coronary heart disease (CHD) mortality

These same difficulties are also evident in the third example, which concerns the impact of healthcare on declining mortality from coronary heart disease. In Finland, as in a number of other high-income countries, coronary heart disease mortality has been declining since the 1960s. During the 1980s and 1990s, a number of new therapies were introduced, whose effectiveness had been demonstrated in large randomized controlled trials. These included more effective drug therapy for patients with myocardial infarction, angina or heart failure as well as coronary artery bypass surgery for patients with angina. There were also declining trends in the major risk factors for CHD including elevated cholesterol and blood pressure levels and cigarette smoking. Based on observed trends in risk factors and uptake of specific therapies, Laatikainen and colleagues (Laatikainen *et al.* 2005) estimated that about 53 per cent of the reduction in CHD mortality in Finland between 1982 and 1997 could be attributed to changes in risk factor levels, while 23 per cent could be attributed to more effective medical care, including secondary prevention, in those affected by the condition. In England and Wales, coronary heart disease mortality declined by 62 per cent in men and 45 per cent in women between 1981 and 2000, and about 42 per cent of the decline was attributed to medical intervention (Unal *et al.* 2004).

These analyses of CHD trends and their determinants raise important questions concerning the priority to be given to prevention efforts through population strategies as compared to healthcare intervention, contributing 'high risk' approaches to primary prevention and to secondary and tertiary prevention in those with established disease. Comparison of the potential costs and outcomes of population strategies for primary prevention, as compared to medical care intervention, should generally favour the former. However, the dominant epidemiological approach to evaluation, the randomized controlled trial, lends itself most readily to the evaluation of medical care interventions. The application of epidemiological designs to the evaluation of population-wide prevention strategies has generally given disappointing results (Ebrahim & Smith 2001). This may have encouraged epidemiologists to give undue priority to medical care interventions with less attention given to the implementation and evaluation of population strategies. For example, Wald and Law (Wald & Law 2003) used the results of meta-analyses of clinical trials to support the concept that a 'polypill' containing a number of effective but low-cost pharmaceuticals (a statin, three blood pressure-lowering drugs, as well as aspirin and folic acid) may have the potential to prevent up to 80 per cent of stroke and coronary heart disease deaths. However, a pill is not a panacea for a lifetime of exposure to unhealthy risks and a strategy grounded in the high-risk approach may not be appropriate for population-wide implementation.

Healthcare and population health: Middle- and low-income countries

Immunization

In high-income countries, environmental changes associated with economic development mostly occurred before effective medical interventions became available. This was not true for the low-income countries and did not always apply to the poor in middle-income countries. The health gains from clinical and public health interventions that were provided through health services in these countries were more obvious than in the high-income countries, and this was especially so for the effects of immunization programmes.

Between 1967 and 1977, the World Health Organization organized a programme to eradicate smallpox, based on systematic delivery of smallpox vaccination to populations at risk. In 1967, there were up to 2 million deaths from smallpox annually, but there have been no naturally occurring cases since 1977. The additional cost of the smallpox eradication programme was modest (Fenner *et al.* 1988). The success of this programme showed that the widespread use of a highly effective but low-cost intervention had the potential to have a major impact on mortality. Following on from the smallpox eradication programme, the WHO established the Expanded Programme on Immunisation (EPI). This aimed to deliver immunization against polio, diphtheria, pertussis, measles, tetanus, and BCG against tuberculosis to children as well as tetanus immunization for pregnant women, achieving 80 per cent coverage for the main vaccines in children since 1990 (World Health Organization 2007b). The EPI programme was estimated to reduce the overall burden of disease among children under 5 by 20–25 per cent (World Bank 1993). The Global Polio Eradication Initiative has been successful in further reducing the spread of polio, with only four countries (Afghanistan, Pakistan, India, and Nigeria) still experiencing indigenous polio transmission in 2006. Between 1988 and 2005 an estimated 5 million people avoided long-term disability from Polio as a result (Global Polio Eradication Initiative 2006). Immunization programmes are now being extended to include additional vaccines including hepatitis B and *Haemophilus influenzae* type B (World Health Organization 2007b). For example, a decrease in *Haemophilus influenzae* type B disease burden was recorded in South Africa following the introduction of the new vaccine (von Gottberg *et al.* 2006).

Investing in Health

Building on the success of immunization programmes, the World Bank's World Development Report for 1993 (World Bank 1993) applied the tools of needs assessment, health technology assessment, and cost-effectiveness analysis to modelling potential solutions to a wider range of health problems in middle- and low-income countries. The motivation behind the report was summarized in its title, *Investing in Health*. A healthy population is a major resource that can contribute to stronger economic growth and improving standards of living (Bloom *et al.* 2004). On average, each 10 per cent increase in life expectancy at birth in a country is associated with an increase in economic growth of 0.3–0.4 per cent per year (Commission on Macroeconomics and Health 2001). Improved health can lead to greater productivity because there are more economically active adults, fewer dependent adults affected by illness, children who are better able to participate in education enhancing their productivity as adults, and rising expectations of longevity providing a motivation to save for later life.

The 1993 World Bank Report argued that existing resources for healthcare were utilized extremely inefficiently and that major health gains could be achieved through focused investment in limited packages of highly effective but low-cost clinical interventions and public health measures delivered through health and other services. This investment could be justified in economic terms through the benefits it could bring to productivity and economic growth.

The Global Burden of Disease study and the Disease Control Priorities project were influential in identifying, quantifying, and prioritizing needs for healthcare intervention in countries at different levels of development (Lopez *et al.* 2006). Using information about the burden of disease and the cost-effectiveness of different interventions it was possible to model the health gain, measured in terms of disability adjusted life years (DALYs), that could result from different interventions and identify priorities for investment. The World Development Report estimated that a gain of DALYs equivalent to about 25 per cent of the burden of disease in middle- and low-income countries could be achieved through implementation of programmes of low-cost public health interventions, partly delivered through health services, as well as essential cost-effective clinical services (Table 2.9.3) (World Bank 1993). A recommended package of essential measures included extended and increased uptake of immunization, improved nutrition education and micronutrient supplementation, treatment of sick children, and reproductive health interventions including prevention and treatment of sexually transmitted diseases and safe motherhood. It was estimated that significant health gains could be achieved with little additional overall cost to governments, through disinvestment from public spending on what it termed 'discretionary clinical services', including interventions of low cost-effectiveness delivered in hospital settings.

Developments from *Investing in Health*

The 1993 World Development Report contributed to an important shift in thinking in several respects. Providing health services to the poor in middle- and low-income countries was no longer to be regarded as a weak form of buffering against the consequences of poverty. Instead, delivering health interventions to the poor was viewed as attacking the causes of poverty and contributing towards establishing conditions that could lead to economic growth, providing households with a route out of a continuing cycle of poverty and illness. Following on the publication of the Report, the World Health Organization established a Commission on Macroeconomics and Health (2001) whose report endorsed the importance of preventing and treating disease as a means of promoting wealth as well as health. This facilitated the mobilization of resources for health in middle- and low-income countries. A Global Fund was established to attract funds to be directed towards programmes for the prevention and treatment of AIDS, TB, and malaria (The Global Fund 2007). The Global Alliance on Vaccines and Immunisation (GAVI) was set up to promote immunization programmes in the poorest countries through both public and private sector funding (GAVI Alliance 2007).

The 1993 Report was also important in encouraging a more explicit approach to rationing of services and priority setting for health investment, justified by the extent of health gains that could be achieved through this approach. For example, it is estimated that for a cost of US$1 million the loss of 50 000 to 500 000 DALYs could be averted through extended vaccine coverage, the loss of 50 000 to 125 000 DALYs could be averted through improved malaria treatment programmes (Jamison *et al.* 2006). Estimates such as these encouraged governments to retreat from the ideal of universal access to comprehensive services and to promote instead

Table 2.9.3 Actual and proposed allocation of public expenditure on health in developing countries and potential health gains, 1990

Package component	Proposed spending on package ($ per capita)	Estimated actual spending 1990	Reduction in disease burden	
			Per cent	Millions of DALYs
Public health Immunization (EPI plus[a]), school health interventions, HIV/AIDS prevention, tobacco and alcohol control, nutrition and family planning education, STD[b] control, malaria (selected prevention measures)	5	1	6	77
'Essential' clinical services Treatment of TB, maternal health and safe motherhood, family planning, integrated management of childhood illness, treatment of sexually transmitted diseases, malaria treatment, non-communicable diseases and injuries (selected early screening and secondary prevention)	10	4–6	19	225
'Discretionary' clinical services All other services including low-cost-effectiveness treatment of cancer, cardiovascular disease, major trauma, neurological and mental health conditions	6	13–15		
Total	21	21	25	302

[a] EPI plus, Expanded Programme on Immunisation with additions (see text for explanation)
[b] STD, sexually transmitted disease
Sources: World Bank (1993) and World Health Organization (2000).

the notion of universal access to essential services (World Health Organization 2000). Updated estimates were published for the global burden of disease and risk factors (Lopez *et al.* 2006) and revised estimates for the costs and effectiveness of different packages of intervention were published (Jamison 2007; Laxminarayan *et al.* 2006). These included a growing appreciation of the present and likely future impact of chronic non-communicable diseases affecting adults in middle- and low-income countries, together with a recognition that selected interventions for these conditions could be very cost-effective.

The thinking of *Investing in Health* was also influential in high-income countries. For these countries, a major implication is that appropriate healthcare as well as population strategies to promote health are an increasingly important investment in order to contain the costs associated with an ageing population affected by a high prevalence of chronic illness. In the United Kingdom, the Treasury commissioned a former chief executive of a leading bank to examine the case for increasing investment in health services (Wanless 2004). His report recognized the increasing costs associated with chronic conditions and argued for the need 'to invest in reducing demand by enhancing the promotion of good health and disease prevention' (p. 3) with 'health services evolving from dealing with acute problems through more effective control of chronic conditions to promoting the maintenance of good health' (p. 10) (Wanless 2004).

Criticisms of *Investing in Health*

The approach of *Investing in Health* was grounded in modelling the potential health gains that might be achieved through optimal use of specific interventions. This approach was endorsed by the later World Health Report 2000 (World Health Organization 2000) and by the report of the Commission on Macroeconomics and Health (Commission on Macroeconomics and Health 2001). Nevertheless, there is a concern that anticipated benefits from essential packages of care have not been fully realized, leading to two main types of criticism of the approach. First, there are technical criticisms of the methods used in estimating the costs and outcomes of intervention in different conditions. Several important assumptions are disputed. The estimation of DALYs in the 1993 report utilized weights that assigned greater value to life years of economically active adults than infants or older people. The same discount rate was used across different countries, but low-income countries would generally value present benefits more highly than high-income countries. Costs of intervention were estimated as average rather than marginal costs (Williams 1999). The balance of costs and benefits may vary in different settings. This is illustrated by the observation that there have been no cases of wild-type poliomyelitis in the United States since 1979, but polio control costs US$230 million annually, and there are an average of nine polio cases per year linked to oral polio vaccine (Taylor *et al.* 1997). While these methodological criticisms are important at the margin, they do little to vitiate the general conclusion that if effective low-cost interventions were employed more efficiently there would be considerable health gains.

A second type of criticism concerns the lack of a well-developed strategy for implementation of essential packages of care. Proposed disinvestment from regressive, specialist services of low-cost effectiveness is unlikely to prove politically acceptable in most countries (Gwatkin *et al.* 2004). Investment in essential packages of intervention requires appropriate policies and structures that will support the financing and delivery of services, especially for the poor. Cost-effectiveness analysis is useful in defining the set of interventions that should be delivered by health services but has a more limited role in defining the systems that should be developed to implement them. This is illustrated by the debate concerning the appropriateness of the strategy for polio eradication (Taylor *et al.* 1997). The resources allocated to short-term intensification of polio vaccination activity may have been better invested in long-term efforts to strengthen health systems that can deliver interventions for a range of priority conditions (Taylor *et al.* 1997). The counter-argument is that the Polio Eradication strategy is implemented with a subsidiary aim of strengthening heath systems, and some empirical evidence from a range of low-income countries suggests that this has been achieved, although possibly to a more limited extent than was possible (Loevinsohn *et al.* 2002). Both arguments point to the need for the development of health systems that offer access to affordable care to everyone.

Equity-driven approaches

Equity-driven approaches to health services are primarily motivated by a concern for social justice. Equity requires that all individuals or groups in the population should be treated fairly, with a just distribution of the costs of providing services, as well as a fair distribution of the benefits obtained through utilization of health services. The data shown in Table 2.9.1 illustrate substantial inequity in the distribution of health resources between rich and poor countries. This global inequity is sometimes addressed through the concept of the right to health. For example, facilitating access to essential medicines, such as antiretroviral therapy, represents a practical means of approaching the realization of the right to health (Hogerzeil 2006).

More than 150 countries recognize the right to the highest attainable level of health; yet, most societies tolerate inequalities in the determinants of health to a varying extent. The unequal distribution of determinants, especially income and education, fosters the development of inequalities in health. Inequality in the distribution of income between groups in a country may be summarized using the Gini coefficient, which provides a numerical index of inequality ranging in value from zero, indicating perfect equality in income, to one indicating maximal inequality in income distribution. Gini coefficients for countries generally fall in the range 0.2–0.6. There is evidence that more unequal societies have worse health (Wilkinson & Pickett 2006).

Health and normal functioning are necessary prerequisites of the fair equality of opportunity that is required in a just society (Daniels *et al.* 2004). Therefore, health systems should be organized so as to minimize inequalities in health and improve the health status of all groups in a population (Daniels *et al.* 2004). Universal access to healthcare is the objective, but 'What is access to healthcare?' and 'How can we judge whether a just distribution of access to care has been realized?'

Access to healthcare

In general terms, 'access to healthcare' is said to exist when individuals or families can mobilize the resources they need to preserve or improve their health (Gulliford *et al.* 2002). At the simplest level, having access to healthcare may be judged in terms of the availability of services (Box 2.9.4). This may include the geographical proximity or physical accessibility of services. Availability may also

Box 2.9.4 Dimensions of access to healthcare		
Dimension of access	**Meaning**	**Potential indicators**
Availability	Whether there is an adequate supply of health services in an area	◆ Number of physicians or nurses per 1000 population ◆ Number of hospital beds per 1000 population ◆ Distance to nearest primary care provider ◆ Distance to nearest hospital
Utilization	Whether health services are utilized	◆ Primary care consultations for 1000 population ◆ Hospital admissions per 1000 population
Relevance to need	Whether appropriate services are received by people who need them	◆ Proportion of births attended by trained healthcare professional ◆ Proportion of subjects with elevated blood pressure who receive antihypertensive therapy
Outcomes	Whether achievable health outcomes are realized	◆ Maternal mortality rate ◆ Mortality rate from appendicitis

encompass the supply of services in terms of the numbers of doctors, nurses, or hospital beds per 1000 population (Table 2.9.1). At the next level, gaining access to healthcare means that services are utilized when they are needed. There may be considerable barriers to the uptake of services even when these are available. Obstacles to utilization include financial barriers, such as the costs to individuals or households of utilizing care; physical barriers, including distance or difficulties of travel; personal barriers, as when services are not viewed as culturally appropriate, socially acceptable or consistent with personal beliefs; or organizational barriers, as when there are difficulties obtaining a consultation, or delays in receiving needed treatment, because of waiting lists or limited capacity of services (Aday & Anderson 1981; Pechansky & Thomas 1981). Utilization of services only offers benefit when care provided is relevant to need and is effective in addressing people's health problems (Box 2.9.4). Finally, access to healthcare should deliver effective care that meets people's health needs and achieves the intended health outcome.

Equity in access to healthcare

Equity in healthcare can be evaluated in several different ways (Box 2.9.5). An important distinction, which is attributed to Aristotle, is the one between horizontal as compared to vertical equity (Gillon 2005). Horizontal equity requires that equals should be treated in proportion to their equality, while vertical equity requires that unequals should be treated in proportion to their inequality. It is generally easier to evaluate horizontal equity, as this requires that all people with the same needs have access to the same services, 'equal access for equal need'. Horizontal inequity in access to healthcare, like inequality in income or health, is often measured using Gini-like metrics known as concentration indices (Wagstaff et al. 1991; Mackenbach & Kunst 1997).

In reality, different groups in a population often have different needs and require appropriately differentiated services. This is evident, for example, in the healthcare needs of indigenous peoples in Australia whose life expectancy at birth is some 17 years shorter than that of the general population. Mooney posed the question,

Box 2.9.5 Aspects of equity in health and healthcare	
Equity	Fairness, or justice, in respect of treatment of different individuals or groups (Last 2007)
Horizontal equity	The extent to which equals are treated in proportion to their equality
Vertical equity	The extent to which unequals are treated in proportion to their inequality
Equity in financial contribution	The extent to which individual or household contributions are consistent with their capacity to pay
Equity in access to healthcare	The extent to which there is a fair distribution of access to healthcare in relation to need, including equal access for equal need (horizontal) and unequal access for unequal need (vertical)
Equity in health	The extent to which there is a fair or just distribution of health among individuals and groups in a population
Effective coverage	The proportion of the population in need of an intervention that has received an effective intervention (Shengelia et al. 2005)

'what would amount to a fair distribution of health resources, given this large difference in health status?' (Mooney 1996). There is little consensus, on how questions concerning this vertical dimension of equity should be answered (Mooney 2000). Marginalized groups such as indigenous populations, new migrants, homeless people, or prisoners may be regarded as 'hard to reach' or at least 'underserved' by standard services and there may sometimes be a case for developing targeted services. There is a concern that such targeted services may become 'poor services for poor people'. More generally, there is increasing emphasis on designing local services to meet locally expressed needs, leading to greater variation in the organization and delivery of services, in contrast to the uniform approach implied by the pursuit of horizontal equity. In the United Kingdom, the tension between these two dimensions of equity has been addressed by introducing national level service specifications, while accommodating local discretion in organizing their implementation.

Equity of access: Availability of services

There are generally substantial inequities in healthcare access among different groups in the populations of middle- and low-income countries. Gwatkin characterized health systems in middle- and low-income countries as 'consistently inequitable, providing more and higher quality services to the well-off, who need them less, than to the poor, who are unable to obtain them'. (Gwatkin *et al.* 2004) (p. 1273).

Health services in middle- and low-income countries do not usually provide full population coverage. In some of the more affluent middle-income countries, such as the small islands of the Caribbean, government services offer access to primary care services that are mainly used by the poor, while private practitioners' services are utilized by the better off. However, as national income decreases, government expenditure on healthcare as a per cent of GDP declines and population coverage by government services diminishes (Table 2.9.1). Services tend to be concentrated close to urban areas, where they may be more readily utilized by better off groups leading to a markedly pro-rich distribution of expenditure on government health services. The distribution of expenditure on primary healthcare services generally shows a lesser degree of inequity than all healthcare spending (Fig. 2.9.1). In rural areas, access to government health services may be extremely limited, with non-governmental organizations such as religious bodies and charities sometimes offering alternative sources of provision. Thus, not only is the overall supply of services in middle- and low-income countries generally limited, but also the geographical distribution of services disadvantages the poor. Geographical barriers to accessing services are important not only in terms of distance but also in terms of the difficulty and costs of travelling long distances to access services.

In China, the lack of availability of rural health services was addressed between 1965 and the early 1980s by the development of 'barefoot doctors'. These were rural farm workers who were given basic health training over several months in order to provide a combination of traditional Chinese and Western medicines to rural communities. The success of this strategy is debated. However, the barefoot doctor approach was regarded as a model for the development of community health workers in other countries and provided an important inspiration for the 1978 Alma Ata Declaration that initiated the 'Health for All' strategy. The Alma Ata Declaration promoted access to primary care, with an emphasis on community participation and universality, as a means of facilitating equity in health.

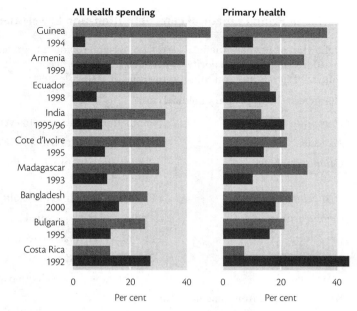

Fig. 2.9.1 Share of public spending that accrues to the richest (top bar) and poorest fifths (bottom bar) of the population.
Source: World Bank (2004).

The importance of the concept of primary healthcare was restated recently by Margaret Chan in her speech to the World Health Assembly following her election as Director General of WHO in 2006 when she said 'When we talk about capacity, we absolutely must talk about the importance of primary healthcare. It is the cornerstone of building the capacity of health systems' (Chan 2006).

Definition of primary healthcare

There are several definitions of primary healthcare. The WHO makes a distinction between primary healthcare, which encompasses public health activities directed at environmental determinants of health, and primary medical care, including first point of contact care in the community. The UK Departments of Health define primary healthcare simply as care provided outside hospitals by family health services (including family physicians, dentists, pharmacists, and opticians) and community health services (including community doctors, dentists, nurses, midwives, and health visitors and other allied professions). Other definitions characterize primary healthcare according to key attributes (Box 2.9.6). Primary care providers are community-based, easily accessible, and offer population coverage. Primary care provides the first point of contact with the health system and is comprehensive in its scope, addressing all potential health problems. Primary care also provides ongoing care over time with continuity or longitudinality representing a key element in most definitions. Primary care services are generally less costly and more affordable than specialist services. In high-income countries, primary medical care practitioners generally have a gatekeeper role in which they regulate and coordinate access to specialist care (Starfield 1992). However, specialist expertise is increasingly being embedded in primary care teams in order to improve the quality of chronic illness management (Bodenheimer *et al.* 2002).

Through its emphasis on universality, accessibility, and affordability, primary medical care generally promotes equity of access to healthcare. Through its community orientation and emphasis on

---

Box 2.9.6 Primary medical care, definition, and key elements

Definition of primary medical care: Care which provides integrated, accessible healthcare services by clinicians who are accountable for addressing a large majority of personal healthcare needs, developing a sustained partnership with patients, and practising in the context of family and community (Institute of Medicine 1994)

Characteristics of primary medical care

Universal	Population-based, open to everyone
Accessible	Enabling people to use services when they are needed
Community-based	Placing the patient within the wider familial or social context necessary for addressing multiple causes of illness
First point of contact	Providing entry into the health system
Comprehensive	Addressing most personal care needs including preventive, curative, and rehabilitative
Continuity	Providing care that is patient-focused over time
Coordination	Coordinating and regulating use of other levels of care
Affordable	Consistent with capacity to pay

Source: Modified from Macinko *et al.* (2003).

---

out-of-hospital care, primary medical care generally enhances efficiency through the application of more cost-effective and appropriate health technologies. The gatekeeper role of the primary care practitioner generally has the consequence of promoting more efficient utilization of resources compared with systems where individual patients can gain direct access to specialists.

Primary care and population health

Does the availability of primary healthcare contribute to improved population health? In general, those countries that have followed policies emphasizing universal primary healthcare coverage have achieved more favourable health outcomes. The Cuban health system is frequently cited as one that has successfully adopted the primary care approach. In 2001, life expectancy at birth in Cuba was 76.3 years compared with 77.4 years in the United States, and the infant mortality rate was 7.2 per 1000 in both countries in spite of the great disparity in economic conditions (Pan American Health Organization 2007). In Costa Rica, commitment to the development of public health services and primary care has been associated with favourable health outcomes and the second highest life expectancy in the Americas (Table 2.9.1) (Unger *et al.* 2007).

Evidence is also provided by ecological analyses from high-income countries. In the United States, states with a greater supply of family physicians have lower mortality rates after adjusting for income inequality and smoking (Shi *et al.* 1999). In the United Kingdom, districts with higher supply of family physicians have lower mortality from all causes but while this association is sensitive to adjustment for several measures of healthcare needs. Hospital utilization shows a strong negative association with the supply of primary care physicians (Gulliford 2002). In an analysis of data for eighteen Organisation for Economic Cooperation and Development (OECD) countries, Macinko and colleagues (Macinko *et al.* 2003) suggested that the strength of a country's primary healthcare system is associated with lower all-cause mortality and reduced premature years of life lost from all-causes and from respiratory and cardiac disease.

These studies provide preliminary information about the relationship between systems of organizing the delivery of healthcare and population health outcomes. Given the ecological nature of the data, and the imprecise and incomplete measurement of confounding variables, there is a risk of bias. Illich observed that 'the fact that the doctor population is higher where certain diseases have become rare has little to do with the doctors' ability to control or eliminate them. It simply means that doctors deploy themselves as they like, more so than other professionals, and that they tend to gather where the climate is healthy, water is clean and where people are employed and can pay for their services' (Illich 1976, p. 30).

Inverse care law

Inequality in the availability of health services is a concern for all countries for the reasons outlined by Illich (1976); without regulation, the supply of healthcare resources is distributed towards more affluent areas with fewer health needs. This situation was described by the British general practitioner Julian Tudor Hart as an 'inverse care law' with 'the availability of good medical care tending to vary inversely with the need for it in the population served' (Tudor Hart 1971) (p. 405).

In countries which, like the United Kingdom, have a dominant national health service funded from general taxation, this situation has been addressed through the development and application of explicit formulae linking the allocation of resources for hospital and community services in different areas to measures of population size and health needs (Smith *et al.* 1994). The number of primary care doctors in an area is also regulated. Nevertheless, historical patterns of the supply of services have been resistant to change and socioeconomically deprived areas continue to have fewer doctors and less well-developed primary care facilities (Gulliford *et al.* 2004). Similar resource allocation methods have been recommended for application to public services in some middle- and low-income countries (Laxminarayan *et al.* 2006). In countries with more pluralistic systems of providing care, or where fee-for-service payment is dominant, greater inequities in the supply of services develop. For example, in US cities, the poor are significantly 'underserved' by health services, both because of inequalities of supply and because of financial barriers to accessing care (Institute of Medicine 2003). In most countries, the rural poor are significantly disadvantaged by relative or absolute lack of availability of services.

Equity of access: Utilization of services

The availability of services does not ensure that those who need them will use them, and there may be important personal, financial, or organizational barriers to the uptake of services. The probability of an individual utilizing services depends on their perceptions of their needs, on social and cultural norms and expectations, and on previous experiences of utilizing care. Patterns of utilization may not be consistent with medically defined need, as when people do not take up preventive services, delay in presenting with serious conditions, or utilize services for apparently trivial conditions. In many health systems, the financial cost of utilizing healthcare may present a very significant barrier to utilization.

Financial barriers to access

Out-of-pocket expenditure is an important method of funding healthcare in middle- and low-income countries (Table 2.9.1) and the impact of these financial contributions is usually disproportionate for poorer groups (Pannarunothai & Mills 1997). This has the consequence that poor people may be unable to obtain needed healthcare, or may find it necessary to utilize less costly and less appropriate forms of care such as private drug vendors (Whitehead *et al.* 2001). People may delay accessing care until their illness becomes more severe, requiring more costly treatment (Whitehead *et al.* 2001). Health expenditures for serious illness may then be catastrophic leading to impoverishment of households. In Asia, illness is one of the principal reasons for households falling into poverty. Across eleven Asian countries, if household expenditures on healthcare are taken into account, then an estimated additional 2.7 per cent of the population (78 million people) live in absolute poverty with household incomes of less than US$1 per person per day when compared with conventional estimates (van Doorslaer *et al.* 2006b). Xu and colleagues (Xu *et al.* 2003) reported a multi-country study of catastrophic health expenditures, which they defined as health expenditure exceeding 40 per cent of household

income after subsistence needs were met. In household survey data, more than 2 per cent of households in 17 out of 59 countries experienced catastrophic expenditures. Based on between-country comparisons, high healthcare expenditures were more likely if health services require direct payment, if households have limited capacity to pay, and if methods to pool risks are lacking. This leads to a paradox observed by Frenk (2006) that while healthcare should be an important factor in reducing poverty, expenditure on healthcare is itself a cause of poverty. This paradox was addressed in Mexican health reforms through the introduction of a new form of health insurance (Seguro Popular) that extends coverage of the poor and provides access to a set of basic medical interventions (Frenk *et al.* 2006). Bleich *et al.* (2007) found that hypertensive subjects who were insured through Seguro Popular were more likely to have their hypertension treated and controlled, compared with sociodemographically matched but uninsured controls. However, the achievement of better hypertension treatment was also dependent on an adequate supply of health professionals in an area (Bleich *et al.* 2007). More generally, there is a lack of evidence concerning the costs, outcomes, and consequences for equity of such models of financing care (Palmer *et al.* 2004; Gwatkin *et al.* 2004).

Equity of healthcare utilization in high-income countries

Many studies have evaluated the overall impact of barriers to the utilization of medical care in high-income countries that, with the exception of the United States, offer universal healthcare coverage. In a recent study, the utilization of physician services was evaluated in relation to respondents' self-rated needs for care (van Doorslaer *et al.* 2006a). Gini-like indices of horizontal inequity were estimated to summarize the utilization of care in relation to household income level. The results showed that utilization of primary care visits was generally either equitably distributed among income groups, or showed a pro-poor distribution (Fig. 2.9.2). However, utilization of specialists' services generally showed some degree of pro-rich inequity, that is higher-income groups utilized more specialist care than lower-income groups at a given level of need. This is a consistent finding from a number of studies and suggests that higher socioeconomic position, including higher income or education, may facilitate access to specialist care through increased ability to negotiate financial or organizational barriers. These results from a range of

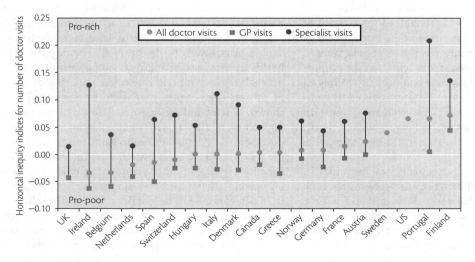

Fig. 2.9.2 Horizontal inequity (HI) indices in relation to household income for the annual mean number of visits to a doctor in 19 OECD countries.
Source: van Doorslaer *et al.* (2006a).

countries suggest that in many instances a degree of equity of access to primary care has been achieved, but inequity persists in the utilization of specialist care.

Equity of access: Relevance and effectiveness

Socio-economic groups differ not only with respect to the volume of care consumed but also with respect to the type of care utilized. There is a considerable body of evidence to show that preventive medical interventions are taken up less by lower socioeconomic groups, with a risk of increasing inequalities in health. In Belgium, for example, overall utilization of family physician services showed substantial pro-poor inequity, but there was marked pro-rich inequity in the uptake of influenza vaccination, cholesterol testing, mammography, and cervical cancer screening (Lorant *et al.* 2002). Problems of poor quality care typically vary between socioeconomic groups with disadvantaged groups receiving lower quality care. The US Institute of Medicine has reviewed a large and consistent body of evidence to show that US black and ethnic minority populations are less likely to receive needed care even after allowing for socioeconomic variables including insurance status, income, age, and severity of condition (Institute of Medicine 2003). For example, there are lower rates of utilization of appropriate cardiac treatment including coronary artery bypass surgery, lower rates of renal dialysis or transplantation, but higher rates of unfavourable events such as diabetes-related lower limb amputations.

Access to care and equity in health

In low-income countries, it is clear that lack of access to healthcare contributes to unfavourable population health outcomes. The 1993 World Development Report estimated that 32 per cent of the burden of disease in low-income countries could be avoided by extending coverage of low-cost interventions (World Bank 1993). This is recognized in the Millennium Development Goals that aim to improve the status of the world's poorest populations with specific health-related objectives of reducing child mortality, improving maternal health and combating HIV/AIDS, malaria, and other diseases. There have now been significant increases in life expectancy, leading to reduced between-country inequalities, but preventable mortality and morbidity from malaria, TB, diarrhoea, and pneumonia remain important in the poor populations of many countries (Jamison 2007). At the same time, the emergence of chronic non-communicable diseases is contributing to a 'double burden' of disease (Jamison 2007). The WHO has developed the concept of 'effective coverage' (Box 2.9.5) as a measure of the extent to which health services deliver appropriate interventions to those groups of people who need them. Effective coverage is defined as the proportion of the population in need of an intervention that receives an effective intervention. An equity dimension is introduced by comparing effective coverage in different population sub-groups. In Mexico, effective coverage was estimated to range from 52 per cent in the lowest wealth quintile to 61 per cent in the highest quintile (Lozano *et al.* 2006).

In high-income countries, the consequences of inequities in healthcare access are less easy to discern because problems resulting from inadequate healthcare are not easily distinguished from the consequences of inequalities in the wider determinants of health, often sustained over generations. Here, promoting a greater degree of equity of access to healthcare than already exists is not usually viewed as a major strategy for reducing inequalities in health. Instead, inequalities in the wider determinants must be addressed more directly (Acheson 1998). In England, among ten headline indicators on inequalities in health requiring action by local health bodies, only one, the number of primary care professionals per 10 000 population, refers to the provision of healthcare. This does not mean, however, that it is not important to ensure that all groups have equal access to the benefits offered by effective healthcare interventions.

Some indirect evidence suggests that inequity in access to specialist care may contribute to inequalities in health in high-income countries. In England and Wales, there are substantial socioeconomic inequalities in survival with cancer that have been increasing over time and are greater for treatable cancers (Coleman *et al.* 2004). For example, the difference in 5-year survival between the highest and lowest quintiles of deprivation in women is 5.8 per cent for breast cancer, 8.3 per cent for rectal cancer, and 7.3 per cent for colon cancer, compared with 0.2 per cent for oesophageal cancer, a less treatable condition. Evidence such as this has been used to advocate the routine implementation of 'equity audit' as part of routine service evaluation. In the United States, there are significant black–white inequalities in mortality, with life expectancy for black men being 6.3 years lower, and for women 4.5 years less, than for whites. Cardiovascular disease and diabetes account for 35 per cent of this difference in men and 52 per cent in women (Harper *et al.* 2007). Differential access to healthcare may contribute to these differences (Institute of Medicine 2003).

In order to promote equity in health, new policies and services have sometimes been implemented on the basis of their potential to reduce inequalities in health. In England, following a White Paper on cigarette smoking, smoking cessation services were developed in deprived areas, providing nicotine replacement therapy free of charge (Chambers 1999). Universal antenatal and newborn screening programmes for sickle cell disease and thalassaemia were implemented with specific recognition of their potential to reduce health inequalities associated with black and ethnic minority status (Sassi *et al.* 2001). At local level, outreach services have been developed to target specific groups such as homeless people with serious mental illness.

Conclusion

This chapter started by asking 'What is the role of health services in improving population health?' It went on to distinguish two separate questions: 'How can health gains be maximized?' and 'How should health gains be distributed?' The negative argument that health services have little impact on population health now seems untenable. Modern healthcare offers a wide range of interventions of proven effectiveness that when implemented widely can be shown, at least indirectly, to contribute to improving trends in population health status in countries at different levels of economic development. Population health gains can be increased by investing resources in the most cost-effective interventions, by increasing effective coverage of the population, increasing quality of care, and optimizing systems for organizing and delivering care. Inequalities in health continue to be sustained by the inequalities in distribution of the determinants of health within- and between-countries. While a degree of equity of access to primary care has been achieved in high-income countries, this is generally far from being the case in middle- and low-income countries. The challenge now is to ensure that all groups obtain a fair share of the benefits of healthcare intervention. Public health specialists should advocate principles of efficiency and equity and contribute to realizing these through participation in processes of needs assessment, health technology assessment, quality improvement, and facilitating access to needed healthcare for all groups.

References

Acheson, E.D. (1998). *Independent inquiry into inequalities in health*. The Stationery Office, London.

Allgood, P.C., Warwick, J., Warren, R.M.L. *et al.* (2008). A case-control study of the impact of the East Anglian breast cancer screening programme on breast cancer mortality. *British Journal of Cancer*, **98**, 206–9.

Ashworth, M., Charlton, J., Ballard, K. *et al.* (2005). Variations in antibiotic prescribing and consultation rates for acute respiratory infection in UK general practices 1995–2000. *British Journal of General Practice*, **55**, 603–8.

Ashworth, M., Latinovic, R., Charlton, J. *et al.* (2004). Why has antibiotic prescribing for respiratory illness declined in primary care? A longitudinal study using the General Practice Research Database. *Journal of Public Health*, **26**, 268–74.

Bhasale, A.L., Miller, G.C., Reid, S.E. *et al.* (1998). Analysing potential harm in Australian general practice: An incident-monitoring study. *The Medical Journal of Australia*, **169**, 73–6.

Blake, S.C., Thorpe, K.E., and Howell, K.G. (2003). Access to healthcare in the United States. In *Access to healthcare* (eds. M.C. Gulliford and M. Morgan), Routledge, London.

Blanks, R.G., Moss, S.M., McGahan, C.E. *et al.* (2000). Effect of NHS breast cancer screening programme on mortality from breast cancer in England and Wales, 1990–8: comparison of observed with predicted mortality. *British Medical Journal*, **321**, 665–9.

Bleich, S.N., Cutler, D.M., Adams, A.S. *et al.* (2007). Impact of insurance and supply of health professionals on coverage of treatment for hypertension in Mexico: Population-based study. *British Medical Journal*, doi:10.1136/bmj.39350.617616.BE (published 22 October 2007).

Bloom, D.E., Canning, D., and Jamison, D.T. (2004). Health, wealth and welfare. *Finance and Development*, 10–15.

Bodenheimer, T., Wagner, E.H., and Grumbach, K. (2002). Improving primary care for patients with chronic illness. *Journal of the American Medical Association*, **288**, 1775–9.

Braveman, P., Starfield, B., Geiger, H.J. *et al.* (2001). World Health Report 2000: How it removes equity from the agenda for public health monitoring and policy Commentary: Comprehensive approaches are needed for full understanding. *British Medical Journal*, **323**, 678–81.

Brennan, T.A., Leape, L.L., Laird, N.M. *et al.* (1991). Incidence of adverse events and negligence in hospitalized patients. Results of the Harvard Medical Practice Study I. *New England Journal of Medicine*, **324**, 370–6.

Bunker, J.P., Frazier, H.S., and Mosteller, F. (1994). Improving health: Measuring effects of medical care. *Milbank Quarterly*, **72**, 225–58.

Cancer Research UK (2008). *Breast cancer survival statistics*. Cancer Research UK, London. Source: http://info.cancerresearchuk.org/cancerstats/types/breast/survival/ accessed 25th January 2008.

Chambers, J. (1999). Being strategic about smoking. *British Medical Journal*, **318**, 1–2.

Chan, M. (2006). *Speech to the World Health Assembly*. World Health Organization, Geneva. Available at http://www.who.int/dg/chan/speeches/2006/wha/en/index.html accessed 21st June 2007.

Cochrane, A.L. (1972). *Effectiveness and efficiency. Random reflections on health services*. Nuffield Provincial Hospitals Trust, London.

Coleman, M.P., Rachet, B., Woods, L.M. *et al.* (2004). Trends and socioeconomic inequalities in cancer survival in England and Wales up to 2001. *British Journal of Cancer*, **90**, 1367–73.

Commission on Macroeconomics and Health (2001). *Macroeconomics and health: Investing in health for economic development*. Report of the Commission on Macroeconomics and Health. World Health Organization, Geneva.

Cutler, D.M., Rosen, A.B., and Vijan, S. (2006). The Value of Medical Spending in the United States, 1960–2000. *New England Journal of Medicine*, **355**, 920–7.

Daniels, N., Kennedy, B., and Kawachi, I. (2004). Health and inequality, or why justics is good for our health. *Public health, ethics and equity*. Oxford University Press, Oxford.

Donabedian, A. (2003). *An Introduction to quality assurance in healthcare*. Oxford University Press, Oxford, New York.

Doran, T., Fullwood, C., Gravelle, H. *et al.* (2006). Pay-for-Performance Programs in Family Practices in the United Kingdom. *New England Journal of Medicine*, **355**, 375–84.

Dworkin, R. (1977). *Taking rights seriously*. Duckworth, London.

Ebrahim, S. and Smith, G.D. (2001). Exporting failure? Coronary heart disease and stroke in developing countries. *International Journal of Epidemiology*, **30**, 201–5.

Eccles, M., Grimshaw, J., Walker, A. *et al.* (2005). Changing the behavior of healthcare professionals: The use of theory in promoting the uptake of research findings. *Journal of Clinical Epidemiology*, **58**, 107–12.

Faculty of Public Health (2007). *Three key domains of public health practice*. Faculty of Public Health, London. Available at http://www.fphm.org.uk/about_faculty/what_public_health/3key_areas_health_practice.asp accessed 21st June 2007.

Fenner, F., Henderson, D.A., Arita, I. *et al.* (1988). *Smallpox and its eradication*. World Health Organization, Geneva.

Frenk, J., Gonzalez-Pier, E., Gomez-Dantes, O. *et al.* (2006). Comprehensive reform to improve health system performance in Mexico. *Lancet*, **368**, 1524–34.

Fulop, N., Allen, P., Clarke, A. *et al.* (2003). From health technology assessment to research on the organisation and delivery of health services: Addressing the balance. *Health Policy*, **63**, 155–65.

GAVI Alliance (2007). *Global alliance on vaccines and immunisation*. Available at http://www.gavialliance.org/ accessed 21st June 2007.

Gillon, R. (2005). *Philosophical medical ethics*. John Wiley, Chichester.

Global Polio Eradication Initiative (2006). *Global Polio Eradication Initiative. 2005 Annual Report*. World Health Organization, Geneva.

Gotzsche, P.C. and Olsen, O. (2000). Is screening for breast cancer with mammography justifiable? *Lancet*, **355**, 129–34.

Gulliford, M., Figueroa-Munoz, J., Morgan, M. *et al.* (2002). What does 'access to healthcare' mean? *Journal of Health Services Research and Policy*, **7**, 186–8.

Gulliford, M.C., Jack, R.H., Adams, G. *et al.* (2004). Availability and structure of primary medical care services and population health and healthcare indicators in England. *BMC Health Services Research*, **4**, 12.

Gulliford, M.C. (2002). Availability of primary care doctors and population health in England: is there an association? *Journal of Public Health Medicine*, **24**, 252–4.

Gwatkin, D.R., Bhuiya, A., and Victora, C.G. (2004). Making health systems more equitable. *Lancet*, **364**, 1273–80.

Harper, S., Lynch, J., Burris, S. *et al.* (2007). Trends in the Black-White Life Expectancy Gap in the United States, 1983-2003. *Journal of the American Medical Association*, **297**, 1224–32.

Health Protection Agency (2007). *Health Protection Agency publishes quarterly Clostridium difficile and MRSA figures*. Available at http://www.hpa.org.uk/infections/topics_az/hai/Mandatory_Results.htm accessed 21st June 2007.

Hogerzeil, H.V. (2006). Essential medicines and human rights: What can they learn from each other? *Bulletin of the World Health Organisation*, **84**, 371–5.

Holland, W.W. (1991) *European community atlas of 'Avoidable Death'*. Second Edition. Oxford Medical Publications, Oxford.

Institute of Medicine (1994). *Defining primary care. An interim report.* National Academies Press, Washington DC. Available at http://books.nap.edu/openbook.php?record_id=9153andpage=1 accessed 21st June 2007.

Institute of Medicine (2005). *Crossing the quality chasm. A new health system for the 21st Century.* National Academy Press, Washington, DC.

Institute of Medicine (2003). *Unequal treatment: Confronting racial and ethnic disparities in healthcare.* National Academies Press, Washington DC.

Ivan Illich (1976). *Limits to medicine. Medical nemesis: The expropriation of health.* Penguin Books, Harmondsworth.

Jamison, D.T. (2006). *Investing in health.* In *Disease control priorities in developing countries.* Chapter 1 (eds. D.T. Jamison *et al.*). World Bank Group, Washington DC. Available at http://files.dcp2.org/pdf/DCP/DCP01.pdf accessed 21st June 2007.

Janjua, N.Z., Akhtar, S., and Hutin, Y.J.F. (2005). Injection use in two districts of Pakistan: Implications for disease prevention. *International Journal for Quality in Healthcare*, **17**, 401–8.

Kohn, L,T., Corrigan, J.M., and Donaldson, M.S. (2000). *To err is human; building a safer health system.* National Academy Press, Washington DC.

Laatikainen, T., Critchley, J., Vartiainen, E. *et al.* (2005). Explaining the decline in coronary heart disease mortality in Finland between 1982 and 1997. *American Journal of Epidemiology*, **162**, 764–73.

Last, J.M. (2007). *A dictionary of public health.* Oxford University Press, Oxford.

Last, J.M. (2001). *Dictionary of epidemiology.* Oxford University Press, Oxford.

Lau, J., Antman, E.M., Jimenez-Silva, J. *et al.* (1992). Cumulative meta-analysis of therapeutic trials for myocardial infarction. *New England Journal of Medicine*, **327**, 248–54.

Laxminarayan, R., Mills, A.J., Breman, J.G. *et al.* (2006) Advancement of global health: Key messages from the Disease Control Priorities Project. *Lancet*, **367**, 1193–208.

Loevinsohn, B., Aylward, B., Steinglass, R. *et al.* (2002). Impact of targeted programs on health systems: A case study of the polio eradication initiative. *American Journal of Public Health*, **92**, 19–23.

Lohse, N., Hansen, A.B.E., Pedersen, G. *et al.* (2007). Survival of persons with and without HIV infection in Denmark, 1995 to 2005. *Annals of Internal Medicine*, **146**, 87–95.

Lopez, A.D., Mathers, C.D., Ezzati, M. *et al.* (2006). Global and regional burden of disease and risk factors, 2001: Systematic analysis of population health data. *Lancet*, **367**, 1747–57.

Lorant, V., Boland, B., Humblet, P. *et al.* (2002). Equity in prevention and healthcare. *Journal of Epidemiology and Community Health*, **56**, 510–16.

Lozano, R., Soliz, P., Gakidou, E. *et al.* (2006) Benchmarking of performance of Mexican states with effective coverage. *Lancet*, **368**, 1729–41.

Macinko, J., Starfield, B., and Shi, L. (2003). The contribution of primary care systems to health outcomes within Organization for Economic Cooperation and Development (OECD) countries, 1970–1998. *Health Services Research*, **38**, 831–65.

Mackenbach, J.P. and Kunst, A.E. (1997). Measuring the magnitude of socio-economic inequalities in health: An overview of available measures illustrated with two examples from Europe. *Social Science and Medicine*, **44**, 757–71.

Mahabir, D. and Gulliford, M.C. (2005). Changing patterns of primary care for diabetes in Trinidad and Tobago over 10 years. *Diabetic Medicine*, **22**, 619–24.

Mannion, R., Davies, H.T., and Marshall, M.N. (2005). Cultural characteristics of 'high' and 'low' performing hospitals. *Journal of Health Organisation and Management*, **19**, 431–9.

Maxwell, R.J. (1984). Quality assessment in health. *British Medical Journal*, **288**, 1470–2.

Mckeown, T. (1979). *The role of medicine.* Blackwell, Oxford.

Mooney, G. (2000). Vertical equity in healthcare resource allocation. *Healthcare Analysis*, **8**, 203–15.

Mooney, G.H. (1996). And now for vertical equity? Some concerns arising from aboriginal health in Australia. *Health Economics*, **5**, 99–103.

Mossialos, E., and Thomson, S. (2003). Access to healthcare in the European Union: the impact of user charges and voluntary health insurance. In *Access to Healthcare* (eds. M.C. Gulliford and M. Morgan). Routlegde, London.

Murray, C.J. and Frenk, J. (2000). A framework for assessing the performance of health systems. *Bulletin of the World Health Organisation*, **78**, 717–31.

Nystrom, L., Andersson, I., Bjurstam, N. *et al.* (2002). Long-term effects of mammography screening: Updated overview of the Swedish randomised trials. *Lancet*, **359**, 909–19.

Office for National Statistics (1998). *DH2. Number 25.* Office for National Statistics, London.

Office of the High Commissioner for Human Rights (2007). *International covenant on economic, social and cultural rights.* Office of the High Commissioner for Human Rights, Geneva. Available at http://www.unhchr.ch/html/menu3/b/a_cescr.htm accessed 21st June 2007.

Office for National Statistics (2006). Report: Deaths involving MRSA: England and Wales, 2000-2004. *Health Statistics Quarterly*, **29**, 63–8.

Oxman, A.D., Thomson, M.A., Davis, D.A. *et al.* (1995). No magic bullets: A systematic review of 102 trials of interventions to improve professional practice. *Canadian Medical Association Journal*, **153**, 1423–31.

Palmer, N., Mueller, D.H., Gilson, L. *et al.* (2004) Health financing to promote access in low income settings—how much do we know? *Lancet*, **364**, 1365–70.

Pan American Health Organization (2007). Regional Core Health Data System. Country Profile: Cuba. Data updated for 2001.

Pannarunothai, S., and Mills, A. (1997). The poor pay more: Health-related inequality in Thailand. *Social Science and Medicine*, **44**, 1781–90.

Phillips, D. (1996). Medical professional dominance and client dissatisfaction: A study of doctor-patient interaction and reported dissatisfaction with medical care among female patients at four hospitals in Trinidad and Tobago. *Social Science and Medicine*, **42**, 1419–25.

Potter, J.E., Berquo, E., Perpetuo, I.H.O. *et al.* (2001). Unwanted caesarean sections among public and private patients in Brazil: Prospective study. *British Medical Journal*, **323**, 1155–8.

President's Commission for the Study of Ethical Problems in Medicine and Biomedical and Behavioural Research (1983). *Securing access to healthcare.* US Government Printing Office, Washington DC.

Roberts, I., Yates, D., Sandercock, P. *et al.* for CRASH trial collaborators. (2004). Effect of intravenous corticosteroids on death within 14 days in 10008 adults with clinically significant head injury (MRC CRASH trial): Randomised placebo-controlled trial. Lancet, **364**, 1321–8.

Roland, M. (2004). Linking Physicians' Pay to the Quality of Care—A Major Experiment in the United Kingdom. *New England Journal of Medicine*, **351**, 1448–54.

Sassi, F., Le Grand, J., and Archard, L. (2001). Equity versus efficiency: A dilemma for the NHS. *British Medical Journal*, **323**, 762.

Sehon, S.R. and Stanley, D.E. (2003). A philosophical analysis of the evidence-based medicine debate. *BMC Health Services Research*, **3**, 14.

Sheldon, T.A. (2001). It ain't what you do but the way that you do it. *Journal of Health Services Research and Policy*, **6**, 3–5.

Shengelia, B., Tandon, A., Adams, O.B. *et al.* (2005). Access, utilization, quality, and effective coverage: An integrated conceptual framework and measurement strategy. *Social Science and Medicine*, **61**, 97–109.

Shi, L., Starfield, B., Kennedy, B. *et al.* (1999). Income inequality, primary care, and health indicators. *Journal of Family Practice*, **48**, 275–84.

Smith, R., Beaglehole, R., Woodward, D. *et al.* (2003). *Global public goods for health. Health economic and public health perspectives.* Oxford University Press, Oxford.

Smith, P., Sheldon, T.A., Carr Hill, R.A. *et al.* (1994). Allocating resources to health authorities: Results and policy implications of analysis of use of inpatient services. *British Medical Journal*, **309**, 1050–4.

Starfield, B. (1992). *Primary care: Concept, evaluation and policy*. Oxford University Press, New York.

Starfield, B. (2000). Is US health really the best in the world? *Journal of the American Medical Association*, **284**, 483–5.

Stevens, A., Raftery, J., and Mant, J. (2004). The epidemiological approach to healthcare needs assessment. In (Eds.), *Healthcare needs assessment: the epidemiologically based needs assessment reviews* (eds. A. Stevens, J. Raftery, J. Mant, and S. Simpson), pp. 1–15. Radcliffe Medical Press, Oxford.

Taylor, C.E., Cutts, F., and Taylor, M.E. (1997). Ethical dilemmas in current planning for polio eradication. *American Journal of Public Health*, **87**, 922–5.

The Global Fund (2007). *The Global Fund to fight AIDS, Tuberculosis and Malaria*. Available at http://www.theglobalfund.org/en/ accessed 21st June 2007.

The NHS Health Technology Assessment Programme (2007). Health Technology Assessment.

Tudor Hart, J. (1971). The inverse care law. *Lancet*, **297**, 405–12.

Unal, B., Critchley, J.A., and Capewell, S. (2004). Explaining the decline in coronary heart disease mortality in England and Wales between 1981 and 2000. *Circulation*, **109**, 1101–7.

Unger, J.P., De Paepe, P., Buitron, R. *et al.* (2008). Costa Rica: Achievements of a heterodox health policy. *American Journal of Public Health*, **98**, 636–43.

United Nations (2007). Universal Declaration of Human Rights. United Nations, New York. Available at http://www.un.org/Overview/rights.html accessed 21st June 2007.

van Doorslaer, E., Masseria, C., Koolman, X. and for the OECD Health Equity Research Group (2006a). Inequalities in access to medical care by income in developed countries. *Canadian Medical Association Journal*, **174**, 177–83.

van Doorslaer, E., O'Donnell, O., Rannan-Eliya, R.P. *et al.* (2006b). Effect of payments for healthcare on poverty estimates in 11 countries in Asia: An analysis of household survey data. *Lancet*, **368**, 1357–64.

von Gottberg, A., de Gouveia. L., Madhi, S.A. *et al.* (2006). Impact of conjugate Haemophilus influenzae type b (Hib) vaccine introduction in South Africa. *Bulletin of the World Health Organisation*, **84**, 811–18.

Wagstaff, A., van Doorslaer, E., and Paci, P. (1991). On the measurement of horizontal inequity in the delivery of healthcare. *Journal of Health Economics*, **10**, 169–205.

Wald, N.J. and Law, M.R. (2003). A strategy to reduce cardiovascular disease by more than 80%. *British Medical Journal*, **326**, 1419.

Wanless, D. (2004). *Securing good health for the whole population. Final report*. HMSO, London.

Whitehead, M., Dahlgren, G., and Evans, T. (2001). Equity and health sector reforms: can low-income countries escape the medical poverty trap? *Lancet*, **358**, 833–6.

Wilkinson, R.G. and Pickett, K.E. (2006). Income inequality and population health: A review and explanation of the evidence. *Social Science and Medicine*, **62**, 1768–84.

Williams, A. (1999). Calculating the global burden of disease: Time for a strategic reappraisal? *Health Economics*, **8**, 1–8.

Wooton, D. (2006). *Bad medicine: Doctors doing harm since Hippocrates*. Oxford University Press, Oxford.

World Alliance for Patient Safety (2007). *Clean care is safer care*. World Health Organization, Geneva.

World Bank (2004). *World Development Report 2004. Making services work for poor people*. World Bank, Washington DC, Oxford University Press.

World Bank (2006). *World Development Indicators 2006*. World Bank, Washington DC.

World Bank (1993). *World Development Report 1993*. World Bank, New York, Oxford University Press.

World Health Organization (2007a). *2006 Tuberculosis facts*. Geneva, World Health Organization.

World Health Organization (2000). *The World Health Report 2000*. Geneva, World Health Organization.

World Health Organization (2007b). *WHO vaccine preventable diseases: monitoring system. 2006 global summary*. World Health Organization, Geneva.

Xu, K., Evans, D.B., Kawabata, K. *et al.* (2003). Household catastrophic health expenditure: A multicountry analysis. *Lancet*, **362**, 111–17.

2.10

Assessing health needs: The global burden of disease approach

C.J.L. Murray, A.D. Lopez, and Colin Douglas Mathers

Introduction

The epidemiological transition and rapid changes in disease patterns have posed serious challenges to health-care systems and forced difficult decisions about the allocation of scarce resources. Epidemiological information is often required at all levels of health systems, and compilations of mortality and morbidity statistics at the national and subnational levels have been published by many countries for several decades. However, prior to the first global burden of disease (GBD) study, which began in 1992, there had been no comprehensive efforts to provide comparable regional and global estimates and projections of disease and injury burden based on a common methodology and denominated in a common metric.

The first GBD study was commissioned by the World Bank in 1991 to provide a comprehensive assessment of the disease burden in 1990 for 107 diseases and injuries and 10 selected risk factors for the world and 8 major regions (Murray & Lopez 1996b, 1996c; World Bank 1993). One of the major goals of the GBD 1990 study was to facilitate the inclusion of non-fatal health outcomes into debates on international health policy, which had largely drawn on the mortality data available in countries, much of it referring to children. Second, there was a need to decouple epidemiological assessment from advocacy so that estimates of the mortality or disability from a condition are developed as objectively as possible. In addition, there was a need to quantify the burden of disease using a measure that could then be used for cost-effectiveness analysis.

The basic philosophy guiding the burden of disease approach is that best-estimates of incidence, prevalence, duration, and death can be generated through the careful analysis and correction for bias of all available sources of information in a country or region. To assess the burden of disease, a time-based metric that combined years of life lost due to premature mortality and years of life lost due to time lived in health states less than ideal health, the DALY, was developed (Murray 1996). The GBD 1990 study represented a quantum step in the global and regional quantification of the impacts of diseases, injuries, and risk factors on population health. Its results have been widely used by government and non-government agencies alike to inform debates on priorities for research, development, and policy response.

In 2000, the World Health Organization (WHO) began publishing annual updates of the GBD for the world and 14 WHO subregions as annex tables to the World Health Reports (World Health Organization 2000, 2004). These were based on an extensive analysis of mortality data for all regions of the world together with systematic reviews of epidemiological studies and population health surveys for selected causes, as well as incorporating a range of methodological improvements. Additionally, a major and expanded research programme, the Comparative Risk Assessment project, was undertaken to quantify the global and regional attributable mortality and burden for 26 major risk factors (World Health Organization 2002).

The WHO GBD analysis for the year 2001 was used as the framework for cost effectiveness and priority-setting analyses carried out for the Disease Control Priorities Project, a joint project of the World Bank, WHO, and the National Institutes of Health, funded by the Gates Foundation (Jamison et al. 2006). The GBD results were documented in detail, with information on data sources and methods as well as uncertainty and sensitivity analyses, in a book published as part of the Disease Control Priorities Project (Lopez et al. 2006).

Despite these considerable efforts to quantify the burden of disease, the WHO updates were incremental updates that did not achieve a complete systematic reassessment of the data on all diseases and injuries. Additionally, changes in methods and data with successive updates meant that results were not comparable with earlier estimates, particularly those for 1990 from the first study. The WHO revisions have continued to largely rely on the original GBD weights, although better population-based methods and data are now available to develop improved disability weights included in the GBD. For these reasons, the Bill and Melinda Gates Foundation has funded a consortium lead by the Institute for Health Metrics and Evaluation involving the WHO, University of Queensland, Johns Hopkins University, and Harvard University to undertake a complete revision of the GBD for 1990 and 2005 (known as the GBD 2005 study). This 3-year project intends to publish results in 2010.

Measuring disease burden

The incorporation of the burden of premature mortality and disability into one summary measure requires a common metric. Since the late 1940s, researchers have generally agreed that time is an appropriate currency: Time (in years) lost through premature death and time (in years) lived with a disability. A range of such time-based measures has been used in different countries, many of them variants of the so-called quality-adjusted life year. For the GBD study, an internationally standardized form of the quality-adjusted life year was developed, called the disability-adjusted life year or DALY. The DALY expresses years of life lost to premature death and years lived with a disability of specified severity and duration. Here, a premature death is defined as one that occurs before the age to which a person could have expected to survive if he or she were a member of a model population with a life expectancy at birth approximately equal to that of the world's longest-surviving population—Japan. One lost DALY can be thought of as one lost year of 'healthy' life (either through death or illness/disability), and total DALYs (the burden of disease) as a measurement of the gap between the current health of a population and an ideal situation where everyone in the population lives into old age in full health.

To calculate total DALYs for a given condition in a population, years of life lost (YLL) and years lived with disability (YLD) for that condition must each be estimated, and then summed. The YLL for deaths at a given age x are calculated from the number of deaths, d_x, at that age multiplied by a global standard life expectancy, L_x, which is a function of age x. The GBD 1990 study chose not to use an arbitrary age cut-off such as 65 or 70 years in the calculation of YLL, but rather specified the loss function L_x in terms of the life expectancies at various ages in standard life tables with life expectancy at birth fixed at 82.5 years for females and 80 years for males. YLD for a particular condition in a particular time period are calculated by multiplying the number of incident cases, i_x, at each age x in that period by the average duration of the condition for each age of incidence, l_x, and a weight factor, dw_x, that reflects the severity of the condition on a scale from 0 (full health) to 1 (dead). YLD are generally calculated either for the average incident case of a given disease, or for one or more disabling sequelae of the disease. For example, YLD for onchocerciasis are calculated by adding the YLD for the sequelae of low vision, blindness, and itchy dermatitis.

The first GBD study chose to apply a 3 per cent time discount rate to the YLL in the future to estimate the net present value of YLL in calculating DALYs, and also incorporated non-uniform age weights that gave less weight to years of healthy life lost in early childhood or at older ages. When discounting and age weighting are both applied, a death in infancy corresponds to 33 DALYs, whereas deaths at ages 5–20 equate to around 36 DALYs. A more complete account of the DALY, and the value choices it incorporates, is given elsewhere (Murray 1996; Murray *et al.* 2002). All DALY results discussed here use age-weighted and discounted DALYs, although results have also been published elsewhere using other value choices.

Summary measures of population health

Over the past thirty or so years, several indicators have been developed to adjust mortality in order to reflect the impact of morbidity or disability. These summary measures of population health fall into two basic categories: Health expectancy and health gap (Fig. 2.10.1)

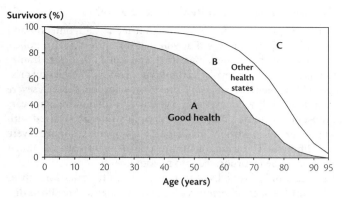

Fig. 2.10.1 The relationship between health expectancies and health gaps in a stationary population.
The health gap is area C + f(B), where f(B) is a function of B in the range 0 to area B representing the lost equivalent years of full health lived in states B. The health expectancy is the area A + g(B), where g(B) = B − f(B) represents the equivalent years of full health lived in states B.

(Murray *et al.* 2000). Within the former category, Sullivan (1971) first suggested weighting life expectancy to measure the health of a population using a single indicator, disability-free life expectancy. Disability-free life expectancy incorporates a dichotomous weighting scheme; that is, it does not account for varying levels of severity. Wilkins and Adams (1983) suggested a more sensitive weighting scheme based on functional limitations, leading to the disability-adjusted life expectancy approach.

As a summary measure of the burden of disability from all causes in a population, disability-adjusted life expectancy has two advantages over other summary measures (Murray & Lopez 1996c). The first is that it is relatively easy to explain the concept of a lifespan without disability to a non-technical audience. The increasing popularity of health expectancy indicators among policy makers has been documented (Robine *et al.* 2003). The second is that it is easy to calculate disability-adjusted life expectancy using the Sullivan method, which relies on prevalence data.

The DALY is an example of a particular type of health gap summary measure that allows the disaggregation of overall disease burden into the burden attributed to specific diseases, injuries, or exposures. In the GBD study, the aim was to develop a summary measure based on explicit and transparent value choices that may be readily debated and modified. Overall, the DALY used in the GBD study is an egalitarian measure, in that it is built on the principle that only two characteristics of individuals that are not directly related to their health, their age and their sex, should be taken into consideration when calculating the burden of a given health outcome in that individual. Other characteristics, such as socioeconomic status, race, or level of education are not considered.

Along with ongoing efforts to improve the analysis of mortality and epidemiological data for the estimation of DALYs, the WHO explored the use of health-adjusted life expectancies (HALEs) as a single summary indicator of population health (Mathers *et al.* 2004), and also extensively explored the ethical, conceptual, and philosophical underpinnings for quantifying population health as part of the overall effort to foster summary measures of population health (Murray *et al.* 2002).

Disability weights and health-state weights

In order to quantify time lived with a non-fatal health outcome and assess disabilities in a way that will help to inform health policy, disability must be defined, measured, and valued in a clear framework that inevitably involves simplifying reality. There is surprisingly wide agreement between cultures on what constitutes a severe or a mild disability. For example, a year lived with blindness appears to most people to be a more severe disability than a year lived with watery diarrhoea, whereas quadriplegia is regarded as more severe than blindness. These judgments must be made formal and explicit if they are to be incorporated into measurements of disease burden. The 'valuation' of time lived in non-fatal health states formalizes and quantifies social preferences for different states of health as disability weights (dw_x). Depending on how these weights are derived, they are variously referred to as disability weights, quality-adjusted life year (QALY) weights, health-state valuations, or health-state preferences. Because the DALY measures loss of health (unlike the QALY, which measures equivalent healthy years lived), the disability weights for DALYs are inverted, running from 0 (ideal health) to 1 (state comparable to death).

A number of methods have been developed to formalize social preferences for different states of health. Most involve asking people to make judgments about the trade-off between quantity and quality of life. This can be expressed as a trade-off in time (how many years lived with a given disability would a person trade for a fixed period of perfect health), a trade-off between persons (whether the person would prefer to save 1 life-year for 1000 perfectly healthy individuals or 1 life-year for perhaps 2000 individuals in a worse health state), or a 'standard gamble' between remaining in a certain health state or accepting a given risk of death in order to return to a state of perfect health.

The original GBD study used two forms of the person trade-off method to value health states and asked participants in weighting exercises to make a composite judgment about the severity distribution of the condition and the preference for time spent in each severity level. This was largely necessitated by the lack of population information on the severity distribution of most conditions at the global and regional levels. In a formal deliberative exercise involving small groups of health workers from all regions of the world, health-state valuations were derived for a set of 22-indicator disabling conditions—such as blindness, depression, and conditions that cause pain. Disability weights for other GBD sequelae were then derived by ranking against these conditions. Subsequent valuation exercises carried out in various cultures have closely matched the results of the original GBD exercise and suggest that cross-cultural variation in health-state preferences is less important than has been argued by some commentators (Salomon & Murray 2002a).

A Dutch disability weight study also attempted to address concerns that valuations by health professionals may differ from those of the general population (Stouthard et al. 1997). Using similar methodology to the original GBD study with three panels of public health physicians and one lay panel, this study concluded that it makes little difference whether the valuation panels comprise medical experts or lay people, as long as accurate functional health-state profiles are provided. In this study, the distribution of health states associated with each sequela was defined using the EuroQol health profile to describe the health states.

The valuation methods used in the original GBD have been criticized on the grounds that the groups used to elicit weights were not representative of the general global population, that the person trade-off method used in the GBD is unethical, in that it involves hypothetical scenarios trading off saving the lives of people in full health versus saving the lives of people with specified health conditions (Arnesen & Nord 1999), and that the inclusion of disability in the DALY implies that people with disability are less valued than people in full health (Mont 2007). In response, the conceptual basis of the DALY has been further developed to clarify that the DALY is quantifying loss of health, not broader valuations of the 'quality of life', 'wellbeing', or 'utility' associated with health states (Salomon et al. 2003). As used in the DALY, the term 'disability' is essentially a synonym for health states of less than full health. Subsequent GBD work on eliciting health-state valuations has moved away from reliance on the person trade-off method, and has also made use of large representative population surveys (Salomon et al. 2004), although a full revision of the disability weights used in the GBD is only now being undertaken as part of the GBD 2005 study.

Other social value choices incorporated in the DALY

To assess premature mortality, the GBD studies have utilized a standard life table for all populations, with life expectancies at birth fixed at 82.5 years for women and 80 years for men. A standard life expectancy allows deaths at the same age to contribute equally to the burden of disease irrespective of where the death occurs. Alternatives, such as using different life expectancies for different populations that more closely match their actual life expectancies, violate this egalitarian principle. As life expectancy is rarely equal for men and women, the GBD assigned men a lower reference life expectancy than women. However, because much of the difference between men and women is determined by men's higher exposure to various risks such as alcohol, tobacco, and occupational injury rather than purely biological differences, this choice could be modified in future revisions of the Study (Waldron 1993; Wong et al. 2006).

If individuals are forced to choose between saving a year of life for a 2-year-old and saving it for a 22-year-old, most prefer to save the 22-year-old. A range of studies confirms this broad social preference to weight the value of a year lived by a young adult more heavily than one lived by a very young child or an older adult. Adults are widely perceived to play a critical role in the family, community, and society. It was for these reasons that the GBD study incorporated age-weighting into the DALY. It was assumed that the relative value of a year of life rises rapidly from birth to a peak in the early twenties, after which it steadily declines.

Individuals commonly discount future benefits against current benefits similarly to the way that they may discount future dollars against current dollars. Whether a year of healthy life, like a dollar, is also deemed preferable now rather than later is a matter of debate among economists, medical ethicists, and public health planners, as discounting future health affects both measurements of disease burden and estimates of the cost-effectiveness of an intervention. There are arguments for and against discounting. In the GBD studies to date, future life years have been discounted by 3 per cent per year. This means that a year of healthy life bought for 10 years hence is worth around 24 per cent less than one bought for now, as discounting is represented as an exponential decay function.

As the impact of discounting is significant, GBD findings have been published for DALYs with and without discounting and age weights. Discounting future health reduces the relative impact of a child death compared with an adult death. Another effect is that it reduces the value of interventions that provide benefits largely in the future, such as vaccinating against hepatitis B, which may prevent thousands of cases of liver cancer, but some decades later. The Disease Control Priorities Project chose to use DALYs with discounting but not age weights, as have some national burden of disease studies. With the increased emphasis on DALYs as quantifying loss of health rather than the social value of health, it is likely that future revisions of the GBD will revisit the choices for discounting and age-weighting.

Sensitivity analyses

To gauge the impact of changing these social choices on the final measures of disease burden, both the GBD 1990 and the GBD 2001 assessments were recalculated with alternative age-weighting and discount rates, and with alternative methods for weighting the severity of disabilities (Murray & Lopez 1996c; Mathers et al. 2006).

Weighting the years of healthy life lost uniformly at all ages, compared to non-uniform age weights, resulted in somewhat more weight being given to the chronic diseases of older ages and somewhat less weight being given to mental disorders and injuries, which affect younger adults disproportionately. In low- and middle-income countries, people aged 60 years and older suffered 21 per cent of the total burden of disease and injury. This declined to 13 per cent when non-uniform age weights were used, increasing the weight placed on young and middle-aged life years. The rates of discounting the future stream of life have important effects on the proportion of the burden due to non-fatal outcomes (YLD), on the age distribution of disease burden, and on the distribution of the burden by broad cause group. Discounting future years of lost healthy life at 3 per cent resulted in 36–38 per cent of the burden being due to YLD, depending on whether or not age weights were also applied, compared to just over one quarter when the discount rate was set to zero. Because, for most causes, the 'duration' associated with the years lost due to premature death is longer than the duration with disability for an incident case, discounting has a greater effect on reducing YLL than on YLD. Different choices of discount rates and age weights do not cause any large changes in the rank ordering of diseases and injuries.

In addition to these sensitivity analyses, Mathers et al. (2006) attempted to estimate uncertainty ranges for the GBD results at regional level arising from data limitations. Uncertainty in estimated all-cause mortality ranged from ±1 per cent for high-income countries to ±15–20 per cent for sub-Saharan Africa, reflecting differential data availability. Uncertainty ranges were even larger for deaths from specific diseases. Uncertainty ranges for YLD assessments varied considerably, ranging from relatively certain estimates for diseases such as polio, for which intensive surveillance systems are in place, to highly uncertain estimates for those such as osteoarthritis, for which in some regions no usable data source was found, and for others the latest available data were decades old. Typical uncertainty for regional prevalence estimates ranged from ±10 per cent to ±90 per cent, with a median value of ±41 per cent, among a subset of diseases for which uncertainty analysis was carried out (Mathers et al. 2006).

The conclusion drawn from both sets of sensitivity analyses was that, in general, the accuracy of the underlying basic epidemiological data from which disease burden is calculated will influence the final results much more than the discount rate, the age weight, or the disability weighting method. If, for example, estimates of the incidence of blindness are off by a factor of 2, then the results, whatever the social value choices used in the metric, will be substantially incorrect. Thus, much more effort needs to be invested in improving the basic epidemiological data than in analysing the effects of what are eventually minor adjustments to the particular summary measure of population health employed.

Estimating mortality and disability
Classification

As many developing countries still have only limited information about the distribution of causes of death in their populations, a primary objective of the GBD study has been to develop comprehensive internally consistent mortality estimates worldwide for each major cause. Diseases and injuries that cause death and burden of disease were classified using a tree structure based on the International Classification of Diseases (Murray & Lopez 1996c). The highest level of aggregation consists of three broad cause groups: Group I (communicable, maternal, perinatal, and nutritional conditions), Group II (non-communicable diseases), and Group III (injuries). Group I causes are those conditions that occur largely in poorer populations and typically decline at a faster pace than all-cause mortality during the epidemiological transition.

Each group was then subdivided into categories; for example, cardiovascular diseases and malignant neoplasms are two subcategories of Group II. Beyond this level, there are two further disaggregation levels such that over 120 individual causes can be listed separately. The GBD cause list was slightly expanded for the WHO revisions, resulting in 135 disease and injury categories.

The basic units of analysis for the first GBD study were the eight World Bank regions defined for the 1993 World Development Report. The heterogeneity of these large regions limited their value for comparative epidemiological assessments. For the WHO updates, a more refined approach was followed. Mortality estimates by disease and injury cause, age, and sex were first developed for each of the 192 WHO member states using different methods for countries with different sources of information on mortality. Epidemiological estimates for incidence, prevalence, and YLD were developed for 17 groupings of countries, and then imputed to country populations using available country-level information and methods to ensure consistency with the country-specific mortality estimates. The resulting country-level estimates were made available by WHO at a summarized level for 14 subregions of the six WHO regions, and also facilitated the production of regional estimates for any desired regional groupings of countries (World Health Organization 2008).

Estimating regional mortality patterns

The GBD 1990 study and the WHO updates drew on four broad sources of mortality data: Death registration systems with medically certified cause-of-death information, sample death registration systems for India and China relying predominantly on verbal autopsy-based information, epidemiological assessments for specific causes, and cause-of-death models. We summarize the approach used for the GBD 2002 estimates; more detail is provided by Mathers et al. (2006).

Life tables specifying mortality rates by age and sex for 192 WHO Member States were developed for 2002 from available death registration data (112 member states), sample registration systems

(India, China) and data on child and adult mortality from censuses and surveys such as the Demographic and Health Surveys (DHSs) and UNICEF's Multiple Indicator Cluster Surveys (MICSs). For countries without useable death registration data, estimated levels of child and adult mortality were applied to a modified logit life table model, using a global standard, to estimate the full life table for 2001 (Murray *et al.* 2003). For 55 countries, 42 of them in sub-Saharan Africa, no information was available on levels of adult mortality. Based on the predicted level of child mortality in 2001, the most likely corresponding level of adult mortality (excluding HIV/AIDS deaths where necessary) was selected, along with uncertainty ranges, based on regression models of child versus adult mortality as observed in a set of almost 2000 life tables judged to be of good quality.

Death registration data containing useable information on cause-of-death distributions were available for 107 countries, the majority of these in the high-income group, Latin America and the Caribbean, and Europe and Central Asia. Population-based epidemiological studies, disease registers, and notifications systems (in excess of 2700 data sets) also contributed to the estimation of mortality due to 21 specific communicable causes of death, including HIV/AIDS, malaria, tuberculosis, childhood immunizable diseases, schistosomiasis, trypanosomiasis, and Chagas disease. Almost one third of these data sets related to sub-Saharan Africa.

In order to address information gaps relating to other causes of death for populations without useable death registration data, models for estimating broad cause-of-death patterns based on GDP and overall mortality levels were used. These are based on the fact that the broad cause structure of mortality is closely related to the level of mortality in a population. Such models estimate the distribution of deaths by cause in a population from historical studies of mortality patterns in countries with vital registration. The models developed for the initial GBD study drew on a data set of 103 observations from 67 countries between 1950 and 1991, and were used primarily to provide plausibility bounds on estimates derived from epidemiological assessments. The approach to cause-of-death modelling for the GBD 2000–2002 estimates was revised and enhanced, drawing on a substantially larger data set of 1613 country–year observations (Salomon & Murray 2002b).

Assessing disability

A disease or injury may have multiple disabling effects, or sequelae. For example, diabetes may result in diabetic vascular disease, retinopathy, or amputation. To estimate the total burden of disability, the GBD measured the amount of time lived with each of the various disabling sequelae of diseases and injuries, in both treated and untreated states, and weighted for their severity in each population. In all, 271 disabling sequelae of disease and injuries were analysed for GBD 2000–2002, for all regions and age groups, and for both sexes.

Calculating the number of years lived with a disabling condition requires information about its incidence, the average age of onset, the average duration of the disability, and the severity weight for the condition. Epidemiological experts were requested to estimate each of these variables for each condition based on an in-depth review of published and unpublished studies. For each sequela, prevalence, case-fatality, remission, and mortality were estimated. This information allowed correction of the preliminary estimates for internal consistency; that is, ensuring that the estimated prevalence

was consistent with estimated incidence and vice versa. Consistency was validated using DISMOD software specifically developed for the GBD (Fig. 2.10.2). DISMOD is a computer model (DISease MODel) that allows simultaneous estimation of age patterns of basic epidemiological parameters, such as incidence, prevalence, case-fatality, and duration, based on knowledge of a limited set of these variables (Barendregt *et al.* 2003). When inconsistencies were detected, epidemiological experts were asked to revise their initial estimates.

The number of years lived with a given disability for each individual were calculated from the incidence of the disability, with the 'stream' of disability arising from it measured from the age of onset, for the estimated duration of the disability, multiplied by the condition's severity weight. To calculate the years lived with disability due to a condition in any given population, the number of years lived with disability lost per incident case must be multiplied by the number of incident cases. A case of asthma, for example, carries a disability weight of 0.1 if untreated and 0.06 if treated. If the annual incidence of asthma in males aged 15–44 years is 1 million cases, the untreated proportion is 35 per cent, and the average duration is 7 years, then this sequela alone is estimated to cause 664 000 years lived with disability for that demographic group. Unlike the estimates of YLL, not all sequelae of all conditions could be explicitly assessed for years lived with disability. Estimates for conditions not explicitly considered were made based on information about the ratio of total premature mortality to disability for each broad cause group.

While the GBD 2000–2002 updates drew on substantially more data for both mortality and epidemiological estimates, an incremental revision strategy was followed and new systematic reviews and estimates were not completed for all causes; some such as dengue and Japanese encephalitis continued to rely on the original GBD assessments of the mid 1990s. Additionally, YLD estimates for most causes continued to be based on the disability weights estimated for the original GBD study (Murray 1996).

Data sources for YLD estimation included disease registers, epidemiological studies, health surveys, and health-facility data (where relevant). Mathers *et al.* (2006) estimated that around 8700 data sets were used to quantify the YLD estimates for GBD 2000–2002, of which more than 7000 related to Group I causes. One quarter of the data sets related to populations in sub-Saharan Africa, and around one fifth to populations in high-income countries. Together with the more than 1370 additional data sets used for the estimation of YLL, the 2000–2002 GBD study incorporated information from over 10 000 data sets relating to population health and mortality.

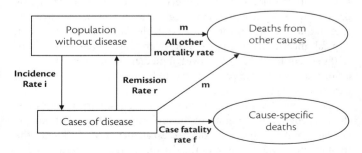

Fig. 2.10.2 The basic disease model underlying DISMOD (DISease MODel).

Global burden of disease 1990 study

Initial results of the GBD 1990 study were published in the 1993 World Development Report (World Bank 1993) and in WHO publications (Murray & Lopez 1994; Murray *et al.* 1994). After further revisions of epidemiological assessments and disability weights, the final results were published in 1996 (Murray & Lopez 1996a, 1996b, 1996c). The results of the Study demonstrated clearly that disability plays a central role in determining the overall health status of a population. Yet that role had previously been almost invisible to public health. The leading causes of disability were shown to be substantially different from the leading causes of death, which has considerable implications for the practice of judging a population's health from its mortality statistics alone.

The leading causes of disease burden in 1990 were childhood diseases (lower respiratory diseases, diarrhoeal diseases, and perinatal causes such as birth asphyxia, birth traumas, and low birth weight), in part because of the greater weight given to deaths at younger ages by the DALY. Depression ranked fourth globally, ahead of ischaemic heart disease, cerebrovascular disease, tuberculosis, and measles. Road traffic accidents also ranked in the top 10 causes of DALYs worldwide. The results of the original GBD study were surprising to many health policy makers, more familiar with the pattern of causes represented in mortality statistics. Neuropsychiatric disorders and injuries were major causes of lost years of healthy life as measured by DALYs, and were greatly undervalued when measured by mortality alone (Murray & Lopez 1996a, 1997). More broadly, non-communicable diseases, including neuropsychiatric disorders, were estimated to have caused 41 per cent of the global burden of disease in 1990, only slightly less than communicable, maternal, perinatal, and nutritional conditions combined (44 per cent), with 15 per cent due to injuries.

The methods and findings of the original (1990) GBD study were widely published, and the GBD approach was widely adopted by countries and health-development agencies alike as the standard for health accounting. The methods and findings of the original GBD study stimulated quite a number of national disease burden studies of varying scope and methodological rigour during the 1990s. The earliest comprehensive studies were for Mexico (Lozano *et al.* 1995) and Mauritius (Vos *et al.* 1995), followed by studies in the late 1990s in the Netherlands (Stouthard *et al.* 1997; Melse & Kramers 1998; Ruwaard & Kramers 1998) and Australia (Mathers *et al.* 1999). Since 2000, comprehensive national burden of disease studies have also been carried out in countries such as Brazil, Iran, Malaysia, Turkey, South Africa, Zimbabwe, Thailand, and the United States, and recently, follow-up analyses of burden of disease have been carried out for Australia (Begg *et al.* 2008) and Mexico (Mexican Ministry of Health, National Institute of Public Health, Harvard Initiative for Global Health 2008). New or follow-up studies are now underway in a number of other countries.

Disease and injury burden in 2002: An overview

A key aim of the GBD studies has been to quantify the burden of fatal and non-fatal health outcomes in a single measure, the disability-adjusted life year (DALY). This section gives an overview of the main results of the GBD update for 2002 in terms of mortality and DALYs. More details on the age–sex–cause and sequelae patterns can be found elsewhere (World Health Organization 2008; Mathers *et al.* 2006). Results are presented here in terms of World Bank geographic regions, with high-income countries aggregated as a separate group.

Global and regional mortality in 2002

Slightly over 56 million people died in 2002, 10.5 million (or nearly 20 per cent) of whom were children younger than 5 years of age. Of these child deaths, 99 per cent occurred in low- and middle-income countries. Additionally, there are a comparatively high number of deaths in low- and middle-income countries at young and middle-adult ages. In these regions, 30 per cent of all deaths occur at ages 15–59 years, compared to 15 per cent in high-income countries (Fig. 2.10.3). The causes of death at these ages, as well as in childhood, are thus important in assessing public health priorities.

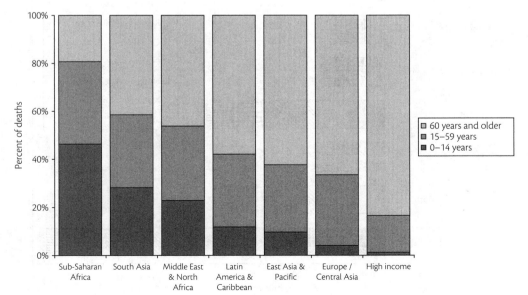

Fig. 2.10.3 Per cent distribution of deaths by age group and region, 2002.

Worldwide, one death in every three is from a Group I cause (communicable, maternal, and perinatal conditions, and nutritional deficiencies). This proportion remains almost unchanged from 1990, with one major difference: Whereas HIV/AIDS accounted for only 2 per cent of Group I deaths in 1990, it accounted for an estimated 15 per cent in 2002. This latter figure has subsequently been revised downward to around 11 per cent, as described in the following paragraphs.

The risk of a child dying before age five ranged from 17 per cent in sub-Saharan Africa to 0.7 per cent in high-income countries in 2002. Low- and middle-income countries accounted for 99 per cent of global deaths among children under the age of 5 years, and 85 per cent of these were in the low-income countries. Just five preventable conditions—pneumonia, diarrhoeal diseases, malaria, measles, and perinatal causes—are responsible for 70 per cent of all child deaths (see Fig. 2.10.4). If all countries had the Japanese rates for child mortality, the lowest in the world, the annual number of child deaths would fall by 90 per cent, to around 1 million.

In developing countries, Group II causes (non-communicable diseases) were responsible for more than 50 per cent of deaths in adults aged 15–59 in all regions except South Asia and sub-Saharan Africa, where Group I causes including HIV/AIDS remained responsible for one third and two thirds of the deaths, respectively (Fig. 2.10.5). In other words, the epidemiologic transition is already well established in most developing countries.

The leading causes of death in 2002 are shown in Table 2.10.1. The extent of epidemiological transition worldwide is reflected in the dominant role of ischaemic heart disease and stroke (cerebrovascular disease) as the leading killers, together accounting for more than 1 in 5 deaths. Major communicable diseases such as lower respiratory infections, diarrhoeal diseases, and tuberculosis are among the top ten causes of death as are road traffic accidents and lung cancer. It should be noted that since the GBD estimates for 2002

were published in the World Health Report 2004 (World Health Organization 2004), WHO and UNAIDS estimates of incidence, prevalence, and mortality for HIV have been substantially revised to take into account advances in methodology and increased data availability (UNAIDS, World Health Organization 2007). The estimated global prevalence of HIV for 2002 was revised downwards by around 16 per cent and the estimated global deaths due to HIV were revised from 2.7 to 2 million, making it the sixth rather than fourth leading cause of death globally. The single biggest reason for this reduction was the intensive exercise to assess India's HIV epidemic, which resulted in a major revision to the country's estimates, almost halving the estimated prevalence. Around 70 per cent of the reduction in HIV estimates is due to changes in India and five African countries: Angola, Kenya, Mozambique, Nigeria, and Zimbabwe.

Leading causes of disability

The original GBD study brought to the attention of health policy makers the previously largely ignored burden of non-fatal illnesses, particularly mental disorders. The findings of the GBD for 2002, based on updated data and analyses, confirm that disability and states of less than full health, caused by diseases and injuries, play a central role in determining the overall health status of populations in all regions of the world.

The overall burden of non-fatal disabling conditions is dominated by a relatively short list of causes. In all regions, neuropsychiatric conditions are the most important causes of disability, accounting for 35 per cent of YLDs among adults aged 15 years and over. The disabling burden of neuropsychiatric conditions is almost the same for males and females, but the major contributing causes are different. Whereas depression is the leading cause of disability for both males and females, the burden of depression is 50 per cent higher for females than males, and females also have higher burden

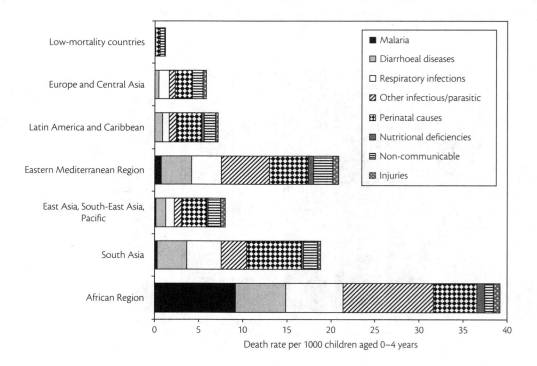

Fig. 2.10.4 Death rates by broad cause group and region, children aged 0–4, 2002.

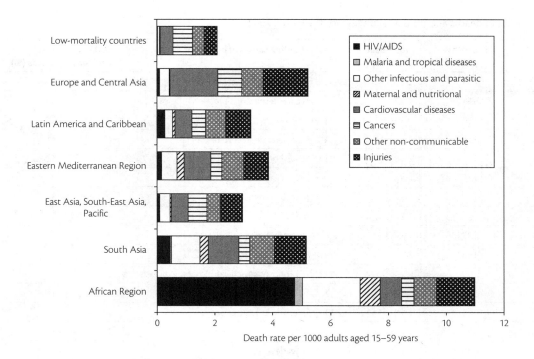

Fig. 2.10.5 Death rates by broad cause group and region, adults aged 15–59, 2002.

from anxiety disorders, migraine, and senile dementias. In contrast, the male burden for alcohol and drug use disorders is nearly six times higher than that for females, and accounts for one quarter of the male neuropsychiatric burden.

Surprisingly, more than 80 per cent of global non-fatal health outcomes occur in middle- and low-income countries. Nearly half of all YLDs arise due to diseases and injuries in the low-income countries. Although the prevalence of disabling conditions such as dementia and musculoskeletal disease is higher in countries with long life expectancies, this is offset by lower contributions to disability from conditions such as cardiovascular disease, chronic respiratory diseases, and the long-term sequelae of communicable diseases and nutritional deficiencies. In other words, people living in low-income countries not only have lower life expectancies (higher risk of premature death) than those in high-income countries, but also live a higher proportion of their lives in poor health.

The burden of diseases and injuries

The analyses presented here reinforce the conclusions of the original GBD study about the importance of including non-fatal outcomes in a comprehensive assessment of global population health. They have also confirmed the growing importance of non-communicable diseases in low- and middle-income countries. The results also highlight important changes in population health in some regions since 1990, as discussed in the following paragraphs.

The epidemiological transition in low- and middle-income countries has resulted in a 20 per cent reduction since 1990 in the per-capita disease burden due to Group I causes (communicable, maternal, perinatal, and nutritional conditions). Without the HIV/AIDS epidemic and the associated lack of decline in tuberculosis burden, this reduction would have been substantially greater, closer to 27 per cent over the period. HIV/AIDS is now among the leading cause of burden of disease globally, and the leading cause in sub-Saharan Africa, followed by malaria. Seven other Group I causes also appear in the top ten causes for this region (see Fig. 2.10.5).

The burden of non-communicable diseases is increasing, accounting for nearly half of the global burden of disease (all ages), a 10 per cent increase from estimated levels in 1990. Indeed, more than 40 per cent of the adult disease burden in low- and middle-income countries of the world is now attributable to non-communicable disease. Implementation of effective interventions for Group I diseases, coupled with population ageing and the dynamics of risk for non-communicable disease, in many developing countries are the likely causes of this shift. The burden of disease in Europe and Central Asia is dominated by ischaemic heart disease and stroke, which together account for more than 20 per cent of total disease burden. In contrast, in Latin America and Caribbean countries, these diseases account for only 6 per cent of disease burden. However, there are very high levels of diabetes and endocrine disorders in this region, compared to others.

The per-capita disease burden in Europe and Central Asia increased by nearly 20 per cent over the period since 1990, so that this region now has worse health than all other regions of the world apart from South Asia and sub-Saharan Africa. This largely reflects the substantial increases in adult male mortality and disability in the 1990s, leading to the highest male–female differential in disease burden in the world. A significant factor in this trend is thought to be increasing alcohol abuse, particularly among males, which led to high rates of accidents, violence, and cardiovascular disease (McKee & Shkolnikov 2001; Men *et al.* 2003; Shkolnikov *et al.* 2001). From 1991 to 1994, the risk of adult (15–59 years) premature death increased by 50 per cent for Russian males. It improved somewhat between 1994 and 1998, but has increased significantly again in the first few years of the twenty-first century.

Violence is the sixth leading cause of burden in Latin America and Caribbean countries: Although it is not ranked in the top ten in any other region, it is nonetheless significant. Injuries primarily affect young adults, often resulting in severe disabling sequelae. All forms of injury accounted for 14 per cent of adult burden in the world in 2002. Road traffic accidents, falls, violence, and self-inflicted

Table 2.10.1 The twenty leading causes of deaths and burden of disease for the world, 2002

	Leading causes of death	Deaths (million)	Total deaths (%)		Leading causes of burden of disease	DALYs (million)	Total DALYs (%)
1	Ischaemic heart disease	7.21	12.6	1	Perinatal conditions	97	6.5
2	Cerebrovascular disease	5.51	9.7	2	Lower respiratory infections	91	6.1
3	Lower respiratory infections	3.88	6.8	3	HIV/AIDS	84	5.7
4	HIV/AIDS	2.78	4.9	4	Unipolar depressive disorders	67	4.5
5	Chronic obstructive pulmonary disease	2.75	4.8	5	Diarrhoeal diseases	62	4.2
6	Perinatal conditions	2.46	4.3	6	Ischaemic heart disease	59	3.9
7	Diarrhoeal diseases	1.80	3.2	7	Cerebrovascular disease	49	3.3
8	Tuberculosis	1.57	2.7	8	Malaria	46	3.1
9	Malaria	1.27	2.2	9	Road traffic accidents	39	2.6
10	Trachea, bronchus, lung cancers	1.24	2.2	10	Tuberculosis	35	2.3
11	Road traffic accidents	1.19	2.1	11	Chronic obstructive pulmonary disease	28	1.9
12	Diabetes mellitus	0.99	1.7	12	Congenital anomalies	27	1.8
13	Hypertensive heart disease	0.91	1.6	13	Hearing loss, adult onset	26	1.7
14	Self-inflicted injuries	0.87	1.5	14	Cataracts	25	1.7
15	Stomach cancer	0.85	1.5	15	Measles	21	1.4
16	Cirrhosis of the liver	0.79	1.4	16	Violence	21	1.4
17	Nephritis and nephrosis	0.68	1.2	17	Self-inflicted injuries	21	1.4
18	Colon and rectum cancers	0.62	1.1	18	Alcohol use disorders	20	1.4
19	Liver cancer	0.62	1.1	19	Protein-energy malnutrition	17	1.1
20	Measles	0.61	1.1	20	Falls	16	1.1

injuries are all among the top 20 leading causes of burden. The former Soviet Union and other low- and middle-income countries of Europe have rates of injury death and disability among males similar to those in sub-Saharan Africa. In Latin America and the Caribbean, as well as the Europe and Central Asian region, and the Middle East and North Africa, more than 30 per cent of the entire disease and injury burden among male adults aged 15–44 is attributable to injuries, including road traffic accidents, violence, and self-inflicted injuries. Additionally, injury deaths are noticeably higher for women in some parts of Asia and the Middle East and North Africa, in part due to high levels of suicide and violence.

The GBD results clearly illustrate the 'double burden' of disease faced by the poorer developing countries of South Asia and Africa. Countries that are still struggling with 'old' and 'new' infectious disease epidemics must now also deal with the emerging epidemics of chronic non-communicable disease such as heart disease, stroke, diabetes, and cancer.

Regional imbalances in the burden of disease

Sub-Saharan Africa and South Asia (which includes India) together accounted for more than 53 per cent of the total global burden of disease in 2002, although they made up only 34 per cent of the world's population. In contrast, the high-income countries, with about 15 per cent of the world's population, together bore less than 8 per cent of the total disease burden. China emerged as substantially

the most 'healthy' of the low- and middle-income countries, with 15 per cent of the global disease burden and a fifth of the world's population. This means that about 546 years of healthy life were lost for every 1000 people living in sub-Saharan Africa, compared with just 127 for every 1000 people in the high-income countries, a more than fourfold differential (Fig. 2.10.6).

The global burden of risk factors in the 2000s

Perhaps the most important methodological progress since the GBD 1990 study has been with respect to quantification of disease burden caused by risk factors. In the initial study, the population health effects of ten risk factors were quantified, but there was limited emphasis on the comparability of the estimates. Different risk factors have very different epidemiological traditions, particularly with regard to defining 'hazardous' exposure, the strength of evidence on causality, and the availability of epidemiological research on exposure and outcomes. Moreover, classical risk-factor research has treated exposures as dichotomous, with individuals either exposed or non-exposed, with exposure defined according to some, often arbitrary, threshold value. Recent evidence for such continuous exposures as cholesterol, blood pressure, and body mass index (BMI) suggests that such arbitrarily defined thresholds are inappropriate, because hazard functions for these risks rise (or decline)

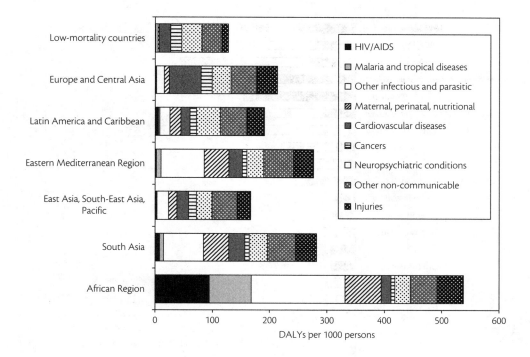

Fig. 2.10.6 The burden of disease, by broad cause group and region, 2002.

Legend:
- HIV/AIDS
- Malaria and tropical diseases
- Other infectious and parasitic
- Maternal, perinatal, nutritional
- Cardiovascular diseases
- Cancers
- Neuropsychiatric conditions
- Other non-communicable
- Injuries

Regions (top to bottom): Low-mortality countries; Europe and Central Asia; Latin America and Caribbean; Eastern Mediterranean Region; East Asia, South-East Asia, Pacific; South Asia; African Region

X-axis: DALYs per 1000 persons (0, 100, 200, 300, 400, 500, 600)

continuously across the entire range of measured exposure levels, with no obvious threshold (Eastern Stroke and Coronary Heart Disease Collaborative Research Group 1998).

For the GBD 2000 study, a new framework for quantifying risk-factor burden was defined, which measured changes in disease burden that would be expected under different population distributions of exposure (Murray & Lopez 1999). Fractions of disease burden attributable to a risk factor were then calculated based on a comparison of disease burden expected under the current (i.e. 2000) estimated distribution of exposure, by age, sex, and region, with that expected if a 'counterfactual' distribution of exposure had applied. To improve comparability across risk factors, a counterfactual distribution was defined for each risk factor as the population distribution of exposure that would lead to the lowest levels of disease burden. Thus, for example, in the case of tobacco, this theoretical-minimum-risk (counterfactual) exposure distribution would be 100 per cent of the population being life-long non-smokers; for overweight and obesity, it would be a narrow distribution of BMI centred around an optimal level (e.g. 21 [SD 1] kg/m^2), and so on. The theoretical-minimum-risk exposure distributions for the risk factors quantified in the WHO Comparative Risk Assessment (CRA) study (the risk-factor arm of the GBD 2000 study) were developed by expert groups for each risk factor, together with systematic reviews and analyses of extant sources on risk-factor exposure and hazard, using an iterative process that increased comparability across risk factors (Ezzati *et al.* 2002, 2004).

The comparative risk assessment for 26 global risk factors, carried out as part of the GBD 2000 study are summarized in Figs 2.10.7 and 2.10.8, and in Table 2.10.2. The analysis was carried out for 14 subregions of the six WHO regions; these subregions were further grouped into 'developed', 'low-mortality developing' including China and much of Latin America, and 'high-mortality developing' including sub-Saharan Africa, and many countries in Western and Southern Asia, including India, Bangladesh, and Myanmar.

These results show that risk factors for communicable, maternal, perinatal, and nutritional conditions (e.g. unsafe sex, child and maternal undernutrition, indoor air pollution from household use of solid fuels, and poor water, sanitation, and hygiene)—whose burden is primarily concentrated in the low-income regions of sub-Saharan Africa and South Asia—and risk factors for non-communicable diseases (e.g. smoking, alcohol, high blood pressure and cholesterol, and overweight and obesity) are leading causes of global disease burden, the latter being globally widespread.

These results suggest that the world is currently experiencing a 'risk-factor' transition, in developed countries characterized by high disease burden from tobacco, suboptimal blood pressure, alcohol, cholesterol, and overweight. Disease burden in the poorest countries, on the other hand, is primarily caused by underweight, unsafe sex, unsafe water and sanitation, indoor air pollution, and micronutrient deficiencies (zinc, iron, vitamin A). Interestingly, the risk factors causing, on average, the greatest disease burden among the 2.4 billion people living in low-mortality, developing countries are a mixture of both, led by alcohol, suboptimal blood pressure, and tobacco, followed by underweight and overweight. This juxtaposition of what might be termed 'new' and 'old' risk factors strongly suggests that health policy in developing countries must increasingly address risks such as tobacco and blood pressure that have often mistakenly been labelled, and treated, as conditions of affluence.

Undernutrition was the leading global cause of health loss in 2000, as it was in 1990 (the 2000 results disaggregate undernutrition into underweight and micronutrient deficiencies). Undernutrition was responsible for a lesser proportion of the global burden of disease in 2000 as compared to an estimated 15.6 per cent in 1990. Part of this reduction is due to a real decrease in levels of undernutrition, and part to the improved methods of the GBD 2000 study. Similarly, due to a mix of reduced exposure and methodological improvements, the estimated burden attributable

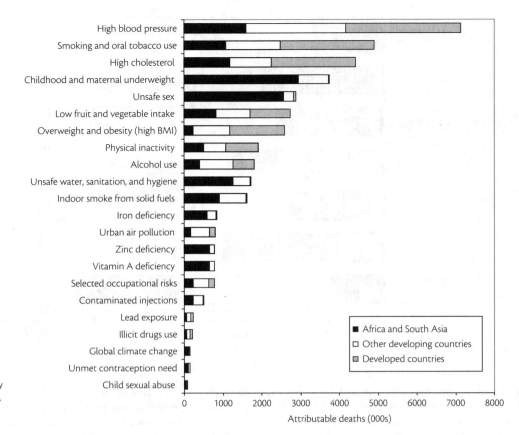

Fig. 2.10.7 Attributable mortality, by selected major risk factors and region, 2000.

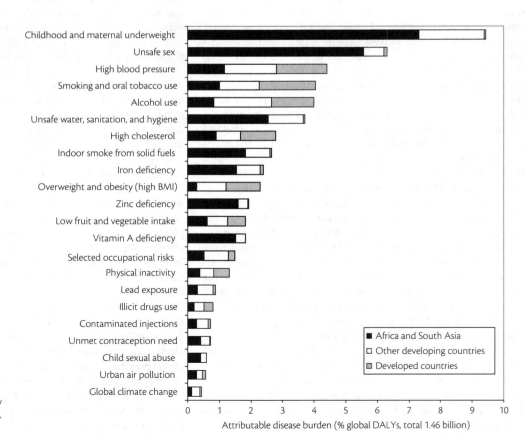

Fig. 2.10.8 The burden of disease, by selected major risk factors and region, 2000.

Table 2.10.2 The twenty leading risk factors for deaths and burden of disease, for the world, 2000

Attributable mortality				Attributable burden of disease			
	Risk factor	Deaths (million)	Total deaths (%)		Risk factor	DALYs (million)	Total DALYs (%)
1	High blood pressure	7.1	12.8	1	Childhood and maternal underweight	137.4	9.4
2	Smoking and oral tobacco use	4.9	8.8	2	Unsafe sex	91.9	6.3
3	High cholesterol	4.4	7.9	3	High blood pressure	64.3	4.4
4	Childhood and maternal underweight	3.7	6.7	4	Smoking and oral tobacco use	59.1	4.1
5	Unsafe sex	2.9	5.2	5	Alcohol use	58.3	4.0
6	Low fruit and vegetable intake	2.7	4.9	6	Unsafe water, sanitation and hygiene	54.2	3.7
7	Overweight and obesity (high BMI)	2.6	4.6	7	High cholesterol	40.4	2.8
8	Physical inactivity	1.9	3.4	8	Indoor smoke from household use of solid fuels	38.5	2.6
9	Alcohol use	1.8	3.2	9	Iron deficiency	35.1	2.4
10	Unsafe water, sanitation and hygiene	1.7	3.1	10	Overweight and obesity (high BMI)	33.4	2.3
11	Indoor smoke from household use of solid fuels	1.6	2.9	11	Zinc deficiency	28.0	1.9
12	Iron deficiency	0.8	1.5	12	Low fruit and vegetable intake	26.7	1.8
13	Urban air pollution	0.8	1.4	13	Vitamin A deficiency	26.6	1.8
14	Zinc deficiency	0.8	1.4	14	Selected occupational risks[a]	21.9	1.5
15	Vitamin A deficiency	0.8	1.4	15	Physical inactivity	19.1	1.3
16	Selected occupational risks[a]	0.8	1.4	16	Lead exposure	12.9	0.9
17	Contaminated injections in healthcare settings	0.5	0.9	17	Illicit drugs use	11.5	0.8
18	Lead exposure	0.2	0.4	18	Contaminated injections in healthcare settings	10.5	0.7
19	Illicit drugs use	0.2	0.4	19	Non-use and use of ineffective methods of contraception	8.8	0.6
20	Global climate change	0.2	0.3	20	Child sexual abuse	8.2	0.6

[a] Includes occupational risk factors for injuries, occupational carcinogens and airborne particulates, ergonomic stressors, and occupational noise.

to unsafe water and sanitation declined from 6.8 per cent in 1990 to 3.7 per cent in 2000.

The 2000 study attributed 4.4 per cent of the global burden of disease to higher than optimal blood pressure, taking into account all increased cardiovascular disease risk for systolic blood pressure distributions relative to a counterfactual distribution with mean 110 mmHg and SD 10 mmHg; on the other hand, the 1990 study attributed only 1.4 per cent of the global burden of disease to hypertension (also using a reference level of 110 mmHg). The GBD 2000 results for smoking and unsafe sex were also much higher than those estimated for 1990—4.1 per cent in 2000 versus 2.6 per cent in 1990 for smoking and 6.3 per cent in 2000 versus 3.5 per cent in 1990 for unsafe sex. Work carried out since the GBD 2000 has examined risk factors for cancers and cardiovascular disease in more detail, and has also updated the analyses of the attributable burden of child and maternal undernutrition (Danaei 2005, 2006; Black 2008).

Despite substantially improved comparability in GBD 2000, the quantification of risk-factor burden needs to expand to include a larger number of risk factors for tropical diseases, injuries, and mental health. The GBD 2005 study will examine the feasibility of including additional important public health risks.

Projections of the global burden of disease

To plan health services effectively, policy makers need to know how health needs might change in the future. To meet this need, the GBD 1990 study included projections of mortality and disability from 1990 to 2020, by cause, for all regions and both sexes. A set of relatively simple models was used to project future health trends for baseline, optimistic, and pessimistic scenarios, based largely on projections of economic and social development, and using the historically observed relationships of these with cause-specific mortality rates (Murray 1997). Updated projections of future trends for mortality and burden of disease between 2002 and 2030 have been prepared by WHO using similar methods to the GBD 1990 study and updated inputs (Mathers & Loncar 2006).

Projection methods

Rather than attempt to model the effects of the many separate direct, or proximal, determinants of disease from the limited data that are available, mortality change was modelled as a function of a limited number of socioeconomic variables: (a) income per capita; (b) the average number of years of schooling among adults, termed 'human capital'; and (c) time, a proxy measure for the secular improvement in health in the twentieth century that partly resulted from accumulating knowledge and technological development. These socioeconomic variables show clear historical relationships with mortality rates; for example, income growth is closely related to the improvement in life expectancy that many countries achieved in the twentieth century. Because of their relationships with death rates, these socioeconomic variables may be regarded as indirect, or distal, determinants of health. In addition, a fourth variable, tobacco use, was included because of its overwhelming impact on health, using information from more than four decades of research on the time lag between persistent tobacco use—measured in terms of 'smoking intensity'—and its effects on health (Peto *et al.* 1992).

Separate projection models were used for HIV and tuberculosis, with various scenarios for scale up of treatment, and with modifications for the interaction between HIV and tuberculosis. In addition to baseline projection scenarios, optimistic and pessimistic scenarios were also developed using different projections of the independent variables.

The data inputs for the projections models were updated by Mathers and Loncar (2006) to take account of the greater number of countries reporting death registration data to the WHO, particularly from developing regions, and to use the latest projections for HIV/AIDS, tuberculosis, tobacco smoking, and overweight and obesity.

Mortality projections

According to both sets of projections, overall (age-standardized) mortality rates worldwide are expected to decline by around 0.5–1 per cent per year over the next 30 years, but at two to three times this rate for most major communicable diseases. While the proportion of deaths from non-communicable diseases is expected to rise everywhere, rates of mortality from these diseases collectively are expected to decline at somewhat less than 1 per cent per year. Major failures with tobacco and obesity control efforts could dramatically alter this prediction, as was seen in several Western countries in the 1950s and 1960s.

Among young children and adolescents under the age of 15 years, the risk of death is projected to decline dramatically in all regions, falling by about two thirds in sub-Saharan Africa and India. Deaths from communicable, maternal, and perinatal conditions, and nutritional deficiencies (Group I) are expected to fall substantially in developing regions, and this projected overall reduction runs counter to the now widely accepted belief that infectious diseases are making a comeback worldwide. It partly reflects the relative contraction of the world's 'young' population, and the growth of the older adult populations. In addition, the projection reflects the observed overall decline in Group I conditions over the past four decades owing to increased income, education, and technological progress in the development of antimicrobials and vaccines.

Clearly, it should not be taken for granted that the progress of the past four decades against infectious diseases will be maintained. It is possible, for example, that antibiotic development and other control technologies will not keep pace with the emergence of drug-resistant strains of important microbes such as *Mycobacterium tuberculosis*. If such a scenario were to prove correct, and in addition, if case-fatality rates were to rise because of such drug-resistant strains, the gains of the present century could be halted or even reversed. The evidence to date nonetheless suggests that, as long as current efforts are maintained, Group I causes are likely to continue to decline.

Deaths from non-communicable diseases are projected to climb from 33 million deaths in 2002 to 51 million in 2030, a 50 per cent increase in absolute numbers. In proportionate terms, Group II deaths are expected to increase their share of the total from 59 per cent in 2002 to 69 per cent in 2030. Mortality attributable to tobacco is expected to rise from its 2002 level of 8 per cent of deaths worldwide to more than 11 per cent of deaths in 2030. Many governments have yet to confront this global health emergency.

Non-communicable diseases are projected to dominate the burden in 2030

When disability is taken into account as well as death, a different view of the future emerges—one that emphasizes adult health problems still further. By 2030, the disease burden due to communicable diseases, maternal, and perinatal conditions, and nutritional deficiencies (excluding HIV/AIDS) is expected to fall to one fifth of the total. The burden attributable to non-communicable diseases, accordingly, is expected to rise sharply, and the burden from injuries is also expected to rise to around 75 per cent of that of Group I conditions, largely from increased traffic accidents. In low- and middle-income countries as a group, deaths from non-communicable diseases are expected to rise from 47 per cent of the burden to almost 70 per cent.

The steep projected increase in the burden of non-communicable diseases worldwide is largely driven by population ageing, augmented by the large numbers of people in developing regions who are now exposed to tobacco. The projected small decrease in the age-specific rates of these diseases in low-income countries is far outweighed by the large and demographically driven increase in the absolute numbers of adults at risk for these diseases, augmented by the tobacco epidemic.

In 2002, the three leading causes of disease burden were, in descending order, conditions arising in the perinatal period, pneumonia, and HIV/AIDS. The three conditions projected to take their place by 2030 are depression, ischaemic heart disease, and road traffic accidents. Perinatal conditions is expected to fall to fourth place and pneumonia to seventh. According to latest UNAIDS projections, HIV would fall to around eleventh place by 2030. Not surprisingly, these changes are not expected to be evenly dispersed worldwide. The total number of lost years of healthy life in the high-income countries is likely to fall slightly, whereas it will increase in sub-Saharan Africa, partly due to a substantial rise in the projected burden of injuries from road accidents.

Limitations of the GBD projections

The 1990 GBD study's HIV/AIDS projections severely underestimated the spread of the epidemic in sub-Saharan Africa, particularly southern Africa; by 2000, HIV/AIDS was estimated to have killed several times more people than projected. On the other hand, the projections published by Mathers and Loncar (2006) probably severely overestimated the projected deaths due to HIV in future years.

In late 2007, UNAIDS and WHO revised estimates and projections of HIV deaths downwards from around 3 million deaths annually to 2 million deaths annually and also concluded that the epidemic had already peaked in sub-Saharan Africa. Rather than continuing to increase to 6 million deaths per annum globally in 2030, the latest projections of HIV mortality suggest that it could decline to around 1 million deaths in 2030.

Apart from the inherent difficulties in predicting the future course of epidemic diseases such as HIV, there can be considerably more confidence in the general picture provided by the projections for the future course of non-communicable disease mortality, based on the historical evidence on the epidemiological transition and on the strong influence of population ageing. However, by their very nature, projections of the future are highly uncertain and need to be interpreted with caution. The burden and mortality projections are not intended as forecasts of what will happen in the future but as projections of current and past trends, based on certain explicit assumptions and on observed historical relationships between development and mortality levels and patterns. The results also depend strongly on the assumption that future mortality trends in low-income countries will have the same relationship to economic and social development as has occurred in the higher-income countries in the recent past.

The GBD projections have not taken explicit account of trends in major risk factors apart from tobacco smoking, and in the recent update, to a limited extent overweight and obesity. If broad trends in risk factors are for worsening of risk exposures with development, rather than the improvements observed in recent decades in many high-income countries, then the GBD projections for low-income countries may be optimistic. There is a need to develop more comprehensive projection models that take explicit account of available information on trends in a wide range of risk factors.

The GBD 2005: Priorities for a new and comprehensive assessment

The Bill and Melinda Gates Foundation has provided funding for a new GBD 2005 study, to be carried out over 3 years, commencing in 2007. The study will be led by the new Health Metrics and Evaluation Institute, hosted by the University of Washington (Moszynski 2007), with key collaborating institutions including Harvard University, the WHO, Johns Hopkins University, and the University of Queensland. This study will also draw on the world's cumulative descriptive epidemiology expertise through a network of around 40 expert working groups. As well as developing new and improved methods to make full use of the increasing amount of health data, particularly from developing countries, the GBD 2005 study will include a comprehensive and consistent revision of disability weights, and assess trends from 1990 to 2005, with projections to 2010.

Several hundred collaborating experts in approximately 40 scientific working groups will conduct systematic reviews of the incidence and prevalence of disease and disabling sequelae, and of exposure and effects of risk factors. The new GBD study will attempt to make full use of new sources of primary data that have recently become available including the WHO World Health Surveys and a number of national health interview and examination surveys. New methods are under development for estimating adult mortality, analysing verbal autopsy data, modelling cause-of-death composition, computing attributable fractions for multiple risk factors, correcting for differential item functioning in health surveys, and imposing internal consistency constraint. Responding to critiques and improvements in the field, the new study will aim to make major progress in disability assessment, using new survey instruments to update disability weights and gather data on health states.

Discussion and conclusions

The GBD study has provided a bold and much needed strategy to estimate current and projected health needs. In particular, it has shown that non-communicable diseases are rapidly becoming the dominant causes of ill health in all developing regions except sub-Saharan Africa, has revealed the extent to which mental health problems have been underestimated worldwide, and has shown the significance of injuries as a problem for the health sector in all regions.

The development and widespread application of a single summary measure of population health (DALYs) has greatly facilitated scientific and political assessments of the comparative importance of various diseases, injuries, and risk factors, particularly for priority-setting in the health sector. Comparative rankings of DALYs have led to strategic decisions by some agencies, such as the WHO, to invest greater effort in programme developments in order to address priority health concerns such as tobacco control and injury prevention. The subsequent GBD 2000–2002 updates, and a plethora of country applications, have led to substantial improvements in both methods and data availability, as well as in the comparability of results. Such global comparative assessments have identified dramatic changes in global health conditions, including impressive reductions in child and adult mortality in many middle-income countries, and some low-income countries, the explosion of the HIV/AIDS epidemic during the 1990s in sub-Saharan Africa, and the dramatic adult health reversal in the former Soviet countries in the 1990s.

The comparable analyses of the GBD/CRA 2000 frameworks have confirmed the advanced epidemiological transition in most regions for both diseases and their risk factors, with the possible exception of South Asia and Africa. To the unfinished agendas of the neglected tropical diseases, malaria, tuberculosis, HIV/AIDS, child and maternal mortality have been added new agendas of non-communicable disease prevention and control, injury prevention and control, and new health threats associated with globalization and trade, particularly tobacco.

The burden of disease methodology and the DALY measure have stimulated considerable debate, particularly in the international and national health policy arenas, among the health economics and epidemiological research communities, and among disability interest groups (Fox-Rushby 2002). Criticisms of the GBD approach fall into two main groups. First, there are concerns about the desirability and implications of extrapolation of population health estimates where data are limited, uncertain, or missing (Cooper et al. 1998). Second, there has been a lively debate in the literature about the way that the DALY summarizes fatal and non-fatal health outcomes (Mont 2007; Anand & Hanson 1997; Williams 1999).

Murray and colleagues have argued that health planning, including that based on uncertain assessments of the available evidence which synthesizes the available data and information while ensuring consistency and adjustment for known biases, will almost always be more informed than planning based on ideology, special interests, or crude statistics that are often biased and inconsistent (Murray *et al.* 2003). Murray has recently clarified the roles of crude, corrected, and predicted health statistics (Murray 2007). Although we strongly advocate that corrected and predicted health statistics should be used to produce a comprehensive and unbiased picture of the global burden of disease for health policy and planning, evaluation and monitoring of health systems and interventions, on the other hand, should be based on corrected, but not predicted, statistics.

One of the major innovations of the GBD study was the attempt to measure and value states of health worse than perfect health in a comparable fashion across various societies. Self-report instruments currently in use lack cross-cultural comparability, with the result that the measurement of health in various populations is largely not comparable. The development and operation of a conceptual framework to measure and describe health in a way that improves comparability across populations is a key challenge for burden of disease research (King *et al.* 2003). The GBD 2005 study will also explicitly approach the quantification of health-state preferences as quantifying loss of health, not of broader valuations of 'quality of life' or 'well-being'.

The issue of co-morbidity is another measurement problem to emerge from the GBD which requires further methodological work. In the GBD work to date, co-morbid conditions have been valued separately and time spent in these combined states valued as the sum of the individual state valuations. This additive model is clearly problematic and more sophisticated approaches have been developed in some national studies and for the calculation of overall levels of disability in populations (Mathers *et al.* 2006; Begg *et al.* 2007). More data are required on the prevalence of major co-morbidities in order to avoid multiple attributions in health-state valuations.

Widespread use of published summary measures provides clear evidence that there is a demand for the simplification of epidemiological complexity that summary measures provide. Of course, the provision of summary measures does not preclude the full dissemination of the underlying internally consistent incidence, prevalence, and mortality estimates. In particular, there is considerable demand for a revised GBD study that reliably measures changes in global health and disease patterns over the past 15 years or so. More money is being spent on global health than ever before—by governments, private foundations, and non-governmental organizations. Donors and others in the global health community are increasingly demanding a better understanding of trends in health in order to better allocate their resources and make real progress in improving health. Critical policy questions depend upon understanding trends. The new GBD study will also revise 1990 estimates using consistent data and methods to assess trends in the global burden of diseases and injuries from 1990 to 2005.

As international programmes and policies to improve health worldwide become more widespread, so too will the need for more comprehensive, credible, and critical assessments to periodically monitor population health and the success, or otherwise, of these policies and programmes. Repeated one-off assessments of the global burden of disease do not provide comparability over time due to improvements in data and methods. There is a need to move beyond these, towards truly consistent and comparable monitoring of the world population's health over time.

References

Anand S., Hanson K. Disability-adjusted life years: a critical review. *Journal of Health Economics* 1997;**16**(6):685–702.

Arnesen T., Nord E. The value of DALY life: problems with ethics and validity of disability adjusted life years. *British Medical Journal* 1999;**319**(7222):1423–5.

Barendregt J., van Oortmarssen G.J., Vos T. *et al.* A generic model for the assessment of disease epidemiology: the computational basis of DisMod II. *Population Health Metrics* 2003;**1**:4.

Begg S.J., Vos T., Barker B. *et al.* Burden of disease and injury in Australia in the new millennium: measuring health loss from diseases, injuries and risk factors. *Medical Journal of Australia* 2008;**188**(1):36–40.

Begg S., Vos T., Barker B., Stevenson C., Stanley L., Lopez A. *The burden of disease and injury in Australia 2003.* Canberra, Australian Institute of Health and Welfare; 2007.

Cooper R.S., Osotimehin B., Kaufman J.S. *et al.* Disease burden in sub-Saharan Africa: what should we conclude in the absence of data?. *Lancet* 1998;**351**(9097):208–10.

Eastern Stroke and Coronary Heart Disease Collaborative Research Group. Blood pressure, cholesterol, and stroke in Eastern Asia. *Lancet* 1998;**352**:1801–7.

Ezzati M. *et al.*, Comparative Risk Assessment Collaborative Group. Selected major risk factors and global and regional burden of disease. *Lancet* 2002;**360**(9343):1347–60.

Ezzati M., Lopez A.D., Rodgers A. *et al. Comparative quantification of health risks: global and regional burden of disease attributable to selected major risk factors.* Geneva: World Health Organization; 2004.

Fox-Rushby J.A. *Disability adjusted life years (DALYS) for decision-making? An overview of the literature.* London: Office of Health Economics; 2002.

Jamison D.T., Breman J.G., Measham A.R. *et al. Disease control priorities in developing countries.* 2nd ed. New York (NY): Oxford University Press; 2006.

King G., Murray C.J.L., Salomon J.A. *et al.* Enhancing the validity and cross-cultural comparability of measurement in survey research. *American Political Science Review* 2003;**93**(4):567–83.

Lopez A.D., Mathers C.D., Ezzati M. *et al. Global burden of disease and risk factors.* New York (NY): Oxford University Press; 2006.

Lozano R., Murray C.J.L., Frenk J. *et al.* Burden of disease assessment and health system reform: results of a study in Mexico. *Journal for International Development* 1995;**7**(3):555–64.

Mathers C.D., Iburg K.M., Begg S. Adjusting for dependent comorbidity in the calculation of healthy life expectancy. *Population Health Metrics* 2006;**4**:4.

Mathers C.D., Iburg K., Salomon J. *et al.* Global patterns of healthy life expectancy in the year 2002. *BMC Public Health* 2004;**4**(1):66.

Mathers C.D., Loncar D. Projections of global mortality and burden of disease from 2002 to 2030. *PLoS Medicine* 2006;**3**(11):e442.

Mathers C.D., Lopez A.D., Murray C.J.L.. The burden of disease and mortality by condition: data, methods and results for 2001. In: Lopez AD *et al.*, editors. *Global burden of disease and risk factors.* New York (NY): Oxford University Press; 2006. p. 45–240.

Mathers C.D., Salomon J.A., Ezzati M. *et al.* Sensitivity and uncertainty analyses for burden of disease and risk factor estimates. In: Lopez A.D. *et al.*, editors. *Global burden of disease and risk factors.* New York (NY): Oxford University Press; 2006. p. 399–426.

Mathers C.D., Vos T., Stevenson C. *The burden of disease and injury in Australia.* Canberra: Australian Institute of Health and Welfare; 1999.

McKee M., Shkolnikov V. Understanding the toll of premature death among men in eastern Europe. *British Medical Journal* 2001;**323**(7320):1051–5.

Melse J.M., Kramers P.G.N. Berekening van de ziektelast in Nederland. Achtergronddokument bij VTV-1997; deel III, hoofdstuk 7 [Calculation of the burden of disease in the Netherlands. Background document to VTV-1997: III; chapter 7]. Bilthoven, the Netherlands: Rijksinstitut voor Volkgezondheid en Milieu [National Institute of Public Health and the Environment]; 1998.

Men T., Brennan P., Boffetta P. *et al*. Russian mortality trends for 1991–2001: analysis by cause and region. *British Medical Journal* 2003;**327**(7421):964.

Mexican Ministry of Health, National Institute of Public Health, Harvard Initiative for Global Health. *Mexico health metrics 2005 report: section 1—comparative risk assessment*. Mexico: Systema Nacional de Informacion en Salud (SINAIS); 2005. Available from: http://sinais.salud.gob.mx/metrica/areas/mcr.html [accessed 2008 Jan 15].

Mont D. Measuring health and disability. *Lancet* 2007;**369**(9573):1658–63.

Moszynski P. Gates Foundation funds new institute to evaluate global health data. *British Medical Journal* 2007;**334**(7606):1238.

Murray C.J.L., Ferguson B.D., Lopez A.D. *et al*. Modified logit life table system: principles, empirical validation and application. *Population Studies* 2003;**57**(2):1–18.

Murray C.J.L., Lopez A.D., Jamison D.T. The global burden of disease in 1990: summary results, sensitivity analysis and future directions. *Bulletin of the World Health Organization* 1994;**72**(3):495–509.

Murray C.J.L., Lopez A.D. Evidence-based health policy—lessons from the Global Burden of Disease Study. *Science* 1996a;**274**(5288):740–3.

Murray C.J.L., Lopez A.D. *Global comparative assessments in the health sector: disease burden, expenditures and intervention packages: collected reprints from the Bulletin of the World Health Organization*. Geneva: World Health Organization; 1994.

Murray C.J.L., Lopez A.D. *Global health statistics*. Cambridge (MA): Harvard University Press; 1996b.

Murray C.J.L., Lopez A.D. Global mortality, disability and the contribution of risk factors: global burden of disease study. *Lancet* 1997;**349**(9063):1436–42.

Murray C.J.L., Lopez A.D. On the comparable quantification of health risks: lessons from the global burden of disease study. *Epidemiology* 1999;**10**(5):594–605.

Murray C.J.L., Lopez A.D. *The global burden of disease: a comprehensive assessment of mortality and disability from diseases, injuries and risk factors in 1990 and projected to 2020*. Cambridge (MA): Harvard University Press; 1996c.

Murray C.J.L., Mathers C.D., Salomon J.A. Towards evidence-based public health. In: Murray C.J.L., Evans D, editors. *Health systems performance assessment: debates, methods and empiricism*. Geneva: World Health Organization: 2003. p. 715–26.

Murray C.J.L., Salomon J.A., Mathers C.D. *et al*. *Summary measures of population health: concepts, ethics, measurement and applications*. Geneva: World Health Organization; 2002.

Murray C.J.L., Salomon J.A., Mathers C.D. A critical examination of summary measures of population health. *Bulletin of the World Health Organization* 2000;**78**(8):981–94.

Murray C.J.L. Rethinking DALYs. In: Murray C.J.L., Lopez A.D., editors. *The global burden of disease*. Cambridge (MA): Harvard University Press; 1996. p. 1–98. vol 1.

Murray C.J.L. Towards good practice for health statistics: lessons from the Millennium Development Goal health indicators. *Lancet* 2007;**369**(9564):862–73.

Peto R., Lopez A.D., Boreham J. *et al*. Mortality from tobacco in developed countries: indirect estimation from National Vital Statistics. *Lancet* 1992;**339**(8804):1268–78.

Robine J.M., Jagger C., Mathers C.D. *et al*. *Determining health expectancies*. Chichester: John Wiley & Sons; 2003.

Ruwaard D., Kramers P.G.N. Public health status and forecasts. Health prevention and health care in the Netherlands until 2015. Elsevier, the Netherlands: National Institute of Public Health and Environmental Protection; 1998.

Salomon J., Mathers C.D., Chatterji S. *et al*. Quantifying individual levels of health: definitions, concepts and measurement issues. In: Murray C.J.L., Evans D., editors. *Health systems performance assessment: debate, methods and empiricism*. Geneva: World Health Organization; 2003. p. 301–18.

Salomon J.A., Murray C.J.L. Estimating health state valuations using a multiple-method protocol. In: Murray C.J.L. *et al*., editors. *Summary measures of population health: concepts, ethics, measurement and applications*. Geneva: World Health Organization; 2002a.

Salomon J.A., Murray C.J.L. The epidemiologic transition revisited: compositional models for causes of death by age and sex. *Population and Development Review* 2002b;**28**(2):205–28.

Salomon J.A., Tandon A., Murray C.J.L., World Health Survey Pilot Collaborating Group. Unpacking health perceptions: multi-country survey study using anchoring vignettes to enhance comparisons of self-rated health. *British Medical Journal* 2004;**328**(7434):258–61.

Shkolnikov V., McKee M., Leon D. Changes in life expectancy in Russia in the mid-1990s. *Lancet* 2001;**357**(9260):917–21.

Stouthard M., Essink-Bot M., Bonsel G. *et al*. *Disability weights for diseases in the Netherlands* Rotterdam, the Netherlands: Department of Public Health, Erasmus University; 1997.

Sullivan D.F. A single index of mortality and morbidity. *HSMHA Health Reports* 1971;**86**(4):347–54.

UNAIDS, World Health Organization. *AIDS epidemic update: December 2007*. Geneva: UNAIDS; 2007.

Vos T., Tobias M., Gareeboo H. *et al*. *Mauritius health sector reform, national burden of disease study*. Mauritius: Ministry of Health and Ministry of Economic Planning and Development; 1995.

Waldron I. Recent trends in sex mortality ratios for adults in developed countries. *Social Science and Medicine* 1993;**36**(4):451–62.

Wilkins R., Adams O.B. Health expectancy in Canada, late 1970s: demographic, regional and social dimensions. *American Journal of Public Health* 1983;**73**(9):1073–80.

Williams A. Calculating the global burden of disease: time for a strategic reappraisal?. *Health Economics* 1999;**8**:1–8.

Wong M.D., Chung A.K., Boscardin W.J. *et al*. The contribution of specific causes of death to sex differences in mortality. *Public Health Reports* 2006;**121**(6):746–54.

World Bank. *World development report 1993. Investing in health*. New York (NY): Oxford University Press for the World Bank; 1993.

World Health Organization. *Global burden of disease estimates*. Geneva: World Health Organization; 2008. Available from: http://www.who.int/healthinfo/bodestimates/en/index.html [accessed 2008 Feb 27].

World Health Organization. *World health report 2000. Health systems: improving performance*. Geneva: World Health Organization; 2000.

World Health Organization. *World health report 2002. Reducing risks, promoting healthy life*. Geneva: World Health Organization; 2002.

World Health Organization. *World health report 2004: changing history*. Geneva: World Health Organization; 2004.

SECTION 3

Public health policies

3.1

Overview of policies and strategies

Walter W. Holland

Introduction

The prime aim of health policies worldwide has been the maintenance and improvement of the health status of populations. This implies an understanding of human health and disease in order to determine the major biological, political, social, environmental, and lifestyle factors influencing health status and the burden of disease. The risk factors which influence health differ between countries, and the examples in this book illustrate their investigation, influence on health, and methods of control. Thus, policies for health will be influenced by different factors in each country and region. Although it may appear that the problems addressed in this chapter are mainly concerned with developed countries, it is important to emphasize that the issues are the same in all countries at all stages of development. Public health problems in the developing world may appear different and greater, but the principles are the same.

Health status

Knowledge of the health status of a population is essential in the formulation of any public health strategy. Although, in general, health has improved, variations in health status both between countries, within countries, and between different gender, social, and ethnic groups remain and, in some instances, have become more pronounced. This chapter deals with some of the changes and differences in health in different parts of the world. In developed countries the most important causes of mortality are from the chronic diseases. Infective diseases have become less important as a major cause of mortality, although with the appearance of AIDS, SARS etc. are still important. In the developing countries infectious diseases such as malaria, tuberculosis, acute respiratory infections, gastrointestinal conditions are still of great importance, although in many chronic diseases have already overtaken the toll of death from infectious diseases.

With the increase in the chronic diseases and ageing of the population the measurement of mortality has become a less important measure of the health status of any population. Morbidity and disability are an important measure of health status. The difficulty is, however, in the acceptability of measures which have been proposed. Mathers (2007) provides a succinct review and analysis of the various measures which have been proposed and are being used. For most purposes, the combination of mortality with disability would provide a good measure to describe the health status of any population group. Sullivan (1966), Sanders (1964), and Robine et al. (2003) devised a method combining such data to estimate disability-free life expectancy. However it was found that this required information based on community surveys. The problem with this is the impossibility of comparing results cross-nationally (or even within a country) because of different expectations and norms for health in different groups.

In view of these difficulties a number of other measures have been tried, such as healthy-life expectancies, potential years of life lost, and disability adjusted life years (DALY). The latter is a summary measure which combines time lost through premature death and time lived in states of less than optimal health, referred to as 'disability'. The DALY is, essentially, a measure of the potential years of life lost (PYLL) but includes lost good health. It is thus, theoretically, a better measure of the burden of disease of any population group. Mathers (2007) describes how these measures have been developed and are used. The health state measures do reflect the severity of a disease dependent on the social preference for different states of health—they can thus be used as a 'common currency' for combining mortality and non-fatal health events in the comparison of health status of different groups. They can thus also be thought of as quality adjusted life years (QALY) widely used in economic evaluations. However, it must be emphasized that all these measures depend on assessment of 'disability' by individuals responding to interviews or questionnaires. Mortality, by contrast, depends on the measurement of an event.

WHO, in its analysis of the burden of disease comparisons between communities and regions, uses the DALY approach (Murray 1996). The summary measures are thus based on a mixture of reasonably accurate, comparable data (mortality) and level and frequency of 'disability' on responses to enquiries. Although there is reasonably reproducible and comprehensive data available on the latter in many developed countries, information on this are less adequate for developing countries as they often rely on proxy replies rather than responses of individuals. Nonetheless, they may provide a rough guide to the importance of different conditions and their burden, which should assist those responsible for the development of proper public health strategies. Mathers (2007) describes the criticisms of the WHO measures and provides tables for the 'burden of disease' as measured by mortality and DALYs in both low- and middle-income versus high-income countries and the world as a whole. For both groups, ischaemic heart disease, cerebrovascular disease, and lower respiratory infections, in that order, have the highest death rates; high blood pressure, smoking, and high cholesterol are the global risk factors with the highest death rates. If DALYs are used, the order for death rates is perinatal conditions, lower respiratory infections, and ischaemic heart disease, while childhood underweight, high blood pressure, and unsafe sex are the most important risk factors. This illustrates the importance of using a variety of measures for the determination of the health status of any population, the need for public health to define precisely the method used in the description of health status, and to be clear as to the reason for which the health status measurement will be used.

Health services

As the health of most of the populations of the developed world has improved, complaints and concerns with the health services have risen. All health systems face the challenges of demographic change (ageing of the population), increasing population mobility, growing social exclusion, costly new therapeutic techniques, and rising public demands and expectations. While all these place mounting pressure on service provision at a time that public spending is under tight constraints, there are new opportunities for prevention and treatment, there is growing interest in prevention and health promotion, and the quality, as well as quantity, of life is generally improving.

The public has widely different views on the quality of health services, ranging from 95 per cent considering that health services are good in France to only 25 per cent in Greece (Ferrara 1993). All countries face similar problems as follows:

(1) Inequalities in both health status and health service provision between different geographic areas and social groups.

(2) Variations in the utilization of services for similar conditions (e.g. hysterectomy).

(3) Difficulties in the apportionment of limited resources to different strategies (e.g. prevention versus cure, or cure versus care) or between services (e.g. cardiac services versus renal services).

(4) Many of the problems are related to lifestyle behaviour and political/economic issues (e.g. cigarette smoking).

These issues have been described in detail for the countries of the European Union (Abel-Smith *et al.* 1995; Holland & Mossialos 1999).

The following chapters all illustrate the approaches adopted in individual countries to cope with these dilemmas. Most people accept that difficult choices need to be made. Most concentrate on the provision of health services, but health services in themselves do relatively little to bring about an improvement in the health status of populations. Environmental factors, such as housing, traffic, and employment, and behavioural factors, such as smoking, diet, and alcohol consumption, probably make greater contributions. Nonetheless, health services have an essential role in improving quality of life and can produce specific valuable improvements in other aspects of health status.

In its World Health Report (2000), WHO attempted to assess the performance of health systems. It considers that the key functions of health systems are 'providing services, generating the human and physical resources that make service delivery possible; raising and pooling the resources used to pay for healthcare and setting and enforcing the rules of the game and providing strategic direction for all the actors involved'. The Report assesses the performance of a country's health system on the 'basis of three overall goals: Good health, responsiveness to the expectations of the population, and fairness of financial contribution'.

The Report gives details of the measures used in its assessments. Population health, the defining objective of any health system, was assessed on the basis of the measures described above in the section on health status—mortality and DALYs. Responsiveness was assessed on the basis of responses by key informants on respect for persons, which included respect for dignity, confidentiality, and autonomy as well as client orientation which included prompt attention, quality of amenities, access to social support networks, and choice of provider.

Fair financing means 'that the risks each household faces due to the costs of the health system are distributed according to ability to pay rather than to the risk of illness: A fairly financed system ensures financial protection for everyone'. Thus, 'the way healthcare is financed is perfectly fair if the ratio of total health contributions to total non-food spending is identical for all households independently of their income, their health status or their use of the health system'. A great deal of effort was expended on developing information on expenditure on health and constructing national health accounts.

The final score on the performance of an individual country's health performance based on the above criteria was weighted as follows: Health (DALYs)—total 50 per cent, overall or average 25 per cent, distribution or equality, 25 per cent; responsiveness—total 25 per cent, overall or average 12.5 per cent, distribution or equality 12.5 per cent; fair financial contribution—distribution or equality 25 per cent.

The World Health Report (2000) gives details of the variation of each of these measures between countries as well as the total score achieved by a country on the above scale. Full statistical details are given for each of the above measures, as well as for the main causes of mortality in each country. The Report concludes by making the overall health attainment, according to the WHO index. Japan has rank 1, followed by Switzerland, Norway, and Sweden. France comes in at Number 6, the United Kingdom ninth, the United States fifteenth. Niger, Somalia, Central African Republic, and Sierra Leone are last at 188–191. In general, African countries have the lowest scores.

Not unexpectedly, this analysis has given rise to a great deal of discussion. Individual countries objected to the order in which they were placed. However for public health purposes the publication of the Report has encouraged analysis of the components of an 'ideal' health system. The individual measures included are open to a great deal of criticism—the report is transparent that many of the judgements made were subjective, based on selected respondents and not tested for reliability. But, at the very least, it opened the debate on both the adequacy of an individual country's system as well as the measures required by assessment.

Organization and financing

The promotion of services to improve health by those working in public health and the influence that can be brought to bear on the management and administration of all services are important contributions to health service planning. Most health systems in developed countries have well-developed mechanisms for funding and provision. The problems in developing and developed countries may differ widely. In the former, health services are usually well organized in the urban areas, with deficits in the rural areas. But there are also problems in the former. In many developing countries most doctors are paid by the state, and are not well paid. However, opportunities usually exist for doctors in urban areas to supplement their income by private practice, which leads to great difficulties and disparities both between different groups of practitioners as well as between different areas in a country. There are also problems relating to the distribution of health workers caused by migration to developed countries. This may have grave implications for the supply and quality of health services. Different solutions are being developed; one suggestion is that all doctors who provide clinical services should be in private practice, and only those in public health and/or health planning should be employed by the state at a reasonable salary.

Although this problem also exists in developed countries, it does not have such an impact on the delivery of basic health services. Countries differ, however, in their ability to use these structures to initiate broad policies to maximize the population's health. All health systems operate within a framework of national law. In some countries, such as the United Kingdom, the state is clearly visible as a regulator and provider of services. In others, legislation creates an environment in which doctors, hospitals, and insurance agencies operate with less visible state intervention. The ability of health services to co-operate with other agencies varies but it is less where there is little formal control beyond legislation of the health system itself. Most countries have endorsed the World Health Organization (WHO) *Health for All* charter but there is great variation in implementation in national and local policies. The state is involved in all health systems in varying degrees:

(1) As legal regulator of the arrangements for patients to receive medical care and doctors to receive remuneration

(2) As a contributor to healthcare financing, either through formal taxes or through quasi-taxes such as compulsory social insurance

(3) As a guardian, to ensure that the correct balance of resources is used to achieve optimum population health

Healthcare may be conceived in an economic framework as an exchange of goods. Patients seeking medical care are making demands while doctors are supplying services. However, there are ways other than medical treatment of using resources to improve population health and the priorities of medical practice emphasizing technical over social models of care do not always provide optimal health benefits. There is a role in all healthcare systems for an overview of resource allocation, health policy, and population health outcomes; this is the task of health commissioning. The latter is the means to secure the best value by specifying and procuring services for the population to deliver the best possible health and well-being outcomes within the best use of available resources. For example, in an area with many childhood accidents, it may be better to commission services which help to reduce road and home accidents than to improve accident and emergency services.

The problems of organization and financing are particularly great in the low- and middle-income countries. As the World Health Report demonstrates, it is in these countries that mortality and disability rates are particularly high. Not only do these countries suffer from a high burden of acute infective diseases, but also from increasing incidence of chronic diseases. It is these countries that suffer from poor environmental conditions, inadequate transport, and above all poor, inadequate education.

Many of these poor countries are the successors to a past colonial regime. In some instances, this has left a deficient system of governance and great turmoil. Hence, not only are these countries poor and unhealthy, they also have great extremes of poverty and wealth. Thus, their ability to develop fair, equitable systems of organization and financing are grossly impaired. It is these, the poorer countries and areas, that have the most health problems—and the worst health systems. This circle of inadequacy is compounded by the emigration of the educated health service workers to the wealthier nations which have needs for such trained personnel. The problem in low-income countries is compounded by their aspirations. The need in these areas is mainly for the development of public health and primary healthcare facilities. Unfortunately, few have the willingness (or ability) to restrict the development of secondary and tertiary healthcare, much more expensive in both monetary terms as well as skills required by personnel. Thus, the reduction of levels of ill-health is impeded by the desire to develop (unnecessary) secondary and tertiary facilities.

Health commissioning (in the past, the term 'health administration' subsumed 'commissioning')

Health commissioning needs to take into account the following factors:

(1) Improvement in health status (e.g. targeting smokers to reduce smoking should result in fewer cases of ischaemic heart disease)

(2) Risk reduction (e.g. as above, reducing the number of smokers in a population)

(3) Services and protection needed to achieve improvements in health and reduction of risks (e.g. product labelling)

(4) Data needs for monitoring the achievement of the tasks identified (discussed in detail by Holland (1995))

The prerequisites for achieving these goals need to be clear. The best model for this is that developed in the Netherlands (Ministry of Health, Welfare and Cultural Affairs 1993) which considers that health is seen as 'the possibility for every member of society to function normally and to participate in social life'. Thus, the need for healthcare is 'to enable an individual to share, maintain, and if possible improve his or her life together with other members of the community'. This implies that necessary healthcare is that which allows the individual to be a full participant in society. This societal perspective is a little different from the individual perspective, where health is seen as the balance between what the individual wants to do and what the individual can do, or the professional approach where health is the absence of disease. The Dutch model is the best one to follow in the arena of public health choices. It should be noted that although this is an excellent model, even in the Netherlands, changes in the structure and financing of services for health have been difficult to achieve. A recent publication,

Exter *et al.* (2004), gives an interesting chronological account of the various changes and emphasizes that there are many interested groups and powerful lobbies which slow down progress in implementing changes. Government in Holland cannot impose changes without consent. Since 1993 there have been at least 15 major reports concerned with change. Within that framework it is necessary to consider the place of public health. For that the current British definition is helpful as discussed below.

It is often considered that health commissioning is particularly suited for wealthy countries. But it is just as applicable in countries with few resources. The crucial prerequisite is for those responsible for the administration of services for health are committed to improving health status rather than only the provision of clinical (health) services. If it is accepted that a country's goal is to improve health status then, by having a robust system of health commissioning, priorities can be set to favour the development of appropriate measures to reduce risks, e.g. by smoking policies or immunization, rather than the provision of 'rescue' services such as the treatment of lung cancer or pneumonia. This is addressed in greater detail under priorities.

Role of public health

> *Public Health is the science and art of preventing disease, prolonging life, promoting health through the organised efforts of society. Public Health Medicine is that branch of medicine which specialises in public health. Its chief responsibilities are the surveillance of the health of the population, the identification of its health needs, the fostering of policies which promote health and the evaluation of health services.* (Acheson 1988)

For the proper application of these principles it is essential to appreciate the methods to be used. Epidemiology, which is the science fundamental to the study and practice of public health, increases the understanding of the determinants of health and disease and the knowledge of their occurrence in populations and groups. Such information indicates the action that can be taken to prevent disease and promote health by health education or social policies which aim to modify behaviour, prophylactic procedures like immunization, screening for identification of those at special risk or in need of special care, and protection against specific environmental hazards. Preventive programmes also need to be monitored to determine whether they are achieving their objectives, at what cost, and how they may need to be modified.

A further function is the study of the nature and extent of disease and disability in the population and how this varies with age, sex, economic, and social circumstances, occupation, and environment. Information on the patterns of disease is essential in defining health needs and tasks for health services and in setting priorities. It also allows the review of the services as they now are and the identification of those who do and do not use them so that the need for new services or the modification of the present ones can be judged. In addition, it is necessary to evaluate how effective the services are in helping the community in cure and care, in the relief of suffering, the maintenance of working capacity, rehabilitation of the disabled, and lowering of death rates. It also needs to assess how efficient the services are in using the community's resources. Both aspects are critical in ensuring value for money, and are an integral part of health service management and resource planning—the more so since technology is always offering expensive new options.

Thus, the problems for which public health action is required include:

(1) Outbreaks of disease caused by infectious or toxic agents, e.g. smallpox, typhoid, food poisoning, bovine spongiform encephalopathy, radiation, and so on;

(2) Problems arising from social and environmental issues such as inadequate housing, unemployment, poverty, abortion, fluoridation of water, and global environmental and population issues (McMichael & Powles 1999; Raleigh 1999);

(3) Behavioural concerns such as smoking, excessive consumption of alcohol, drug abuse, and insufficient exercise;

(4) Health service issues including assessment of healthcare needs and outcomes, and the effectiveness and efficiency of particular services.

Public health, as a discipline, should not become involved in the direct management of clinical services in the community or within institutions—it lacks the expertise essential for these tasks. Its prime responsibilities are to promote health and to prevent and control disease. It thus has responsibility for surveillance and for the planning and co-ordination of measures that promote and maintain health. It must be involved in the planning and distribution of clinical services in accordance with measures of need and demands and the assessment of effectiveness.

The UK Faculty of Public Health considers that public health practitioners need to have skills in nine key areas:

(1) Surveillance and assessment of the populations' health and well-being

(2) Assessing the evidence of the effectiveness of health and healthcare interventions, programmes, and services

(3) Policy and strategy development and implementation

(4) Strategic leadership and collaborative working for health

(5) Health improvement

(6) Health protection

(7) Health and social service quality

(8) Public health intelligence

(9) Academic public health

These are considered to be the main skills needed for the three main domains of public health practice—health protection, health improvement, and service quality. A number of chapters in this Textbook address these issues in much greater detail.

Assurance of appropriateness

Few countries, at present, appear to have developed an organizational framework whereby the principles and methods of determining appropriateness are systematically applied.

In considering the provision of services for health, it is important to be clear about what is to be achieved. In most countries, it is now accepted that everyone who needs healthcare must be able to obtain it. However, that is not always the rule, as is shown in the following chapters.

The form and content of the right to healthcare are the result of a series of political and social compromises. As the Dutch *Report on Choices in Health Care* emphasizes, responsibility for others, the ideal of equality, and the social benefits of good public health have encouraged the belief that people are responsible for their own health, and are free to choose how to use healthcare and which risks they are willing to take (Ministry of Health, Welfare and Cultural Affairs 1993). The fusion of such different starting points has always brought strain to the design of healthcare systems That these strains are limited in the determination of rights is partly due to a pragmatic coupling between equality and freedom of choice so that, in principle, everyone has equal rights to virtually all of the facilities of healthcare. People do not need everything they want and not all needs for healthcare are equally important. There is a need for healthcare services to maintain or restore health, for care and nursing of impaired health, or to relieve suffering. The concept of health is therefore the most appropriate standard to determine as to when there is a need for healthcare. A definition of 'health' is that it is the ability to function normally. In this definition, there will be a need for healthcare when people are restricted in their normal functioning or when there is a threat of such restriction. Such a need is more essential when the restrictions are greater or threaten to be greater. From a community-oriented view of health, this is an incomplete statement. Health has a value in itself because it allows a people to participate in social life and to develop themselves. The more the health problems restrict a person's possibilities in society, the more the need for healthcare.

As stated above, there are a variety of approaches to health. From the perspective of the individual, health is linked to self-determination or autonomy. To be healthy is to be able, as an individual, to achieve in society what one has chosen to aim for. Whether that is possible depends not only on one's physical, material, and psychological resources, but also on what one wishes to achieve. Health can be described as a balance between what people want and what they can achieve. Thus, there will be differences in how individuals express a desire for healthcare.

From the medical professional perspective, health is the absence of disease, and is seen as a deviation from normal biological function. In this definition, there is a clear distinction between healthcare for the sick and social services for people who are not sick, where healthcare must be seen as professionally given care, provided on the basis of indications defined objectively by the provider.

The effectiveness of care is also defined objectively with the most important criteria being danger to life and the extent of normal biological function. Biological functions seem ultimately to be directed at survival and reproduction. From that perspective, demands can be sorted according to gravity, and it is possible to distinguish necessary from less necessary care.

From the community-oriented approach, health is seen as the possibility of every member of the society to function normally. The choices are made at the level of society because individual health is linked to the possibility of participation in social life. Care is thus necessary when it enables an individual to share, maintain, and if possible improve his or her life together with other members of the community. Of course this question is not answered in the same way by all communities. There are three points of departure: The fundamental equality of people, the fundamental need for the protection of human life, and the principle of solidarity. Thus, the major aim of any such system is the improvement of health and the ability to participate within society. If one accepts this Dutch model, then it is possible to define the different types of care that need to be provided in a variety of ways.

The WHO (Europe) has discussed the key areas specifically for public health (WHO 1999). These can be summarized as understanding health and disease, measuring health status, appropriate disease surveillance and control, promoting health and well-being, evaluating and improving health outcomes, intersectoral and collaborative working, and advocacy and communications. These define the role of public health within a health system which includes healthcare and ensures that appropriate decisions are made.

Criteria, access, and utilization

The first criterion that needs to be established is whether care is necessary or not. The second criterion is the effectiveness of the services provided, the efficiency with which they are provided, and whether the individual could take responsibility for providing them.

These principles are established in some way or another in most health systems. They are thus concerned with improvement of health status, risk factor reduction, and improvement of services and protection.

In most developed countries, there is now a split between provision and purchasing for healthcare. The relative role of those who purchase healthcare varies between countries. In most private insurance systems, what is insured constitutes what is bought; however, in those that have managed care, or purchasing authorities, these decide what care should be purchased and where it should be obtained. It is thus feasible to introduce healthcare systems that consider the improvement of health on a societal basis. The characteristic that prevents medical care becoming an ordinary market, from an economic viewpoint, is that the receivers of services are often unable to make informed choices about care. However, it should be noted that patients do make many of the key choices over healthcare, whether their feelings and symptoms indicate that they are ill, and whether to consult a doctor.

There are wide variations between the different methods of organization and responses of individuals to healthcare. Similarly, doctors do not perform uniformly. Individual doctors vary in their action when faced with similar conditions. In both the National Health Services and social insurance systems, doctors are gate keepers to resources. They legitimize a patient's claim for services. Health systems seek to influence doctors' decisions broadly, e.g. in the level of remuneration given to a particular service.

As indicated, in all systems it is crucial that there is interaction between the different sectors of society. Health can only be improved through changes in the environment, through occupation, including agriculture as well as health services and education, and unless there is some degree of co-ordination between these activities the optimal distribution of resource will be lacking. This also has an important impact on the improvement of health which is the aim of most national health systems. Most systems have now come to terms with the fact that they cannot only treat established disease but also have to be considered with the improvements of health and the prevention of disease.

International trends in healthcare

Abel-Smith *et al.* (1995) reviewed trends in healthcare. They note that there is a worldwide trend towards giving every citizen in a country the same rights to healthcare, but not in the United States. President Clinton made proposals so that would also have been the case in America. Although there seems to be little chance of this right being available for all the citizens of the country with the largest healthcare expenditure, some US states, e.g. Massachusetts, are experimenting in providing this. There has been an increase in public financing of healthcare quantitatively whether by compulsory insurance contribution or taxation in most countries. There is some trend towards consumers making a contribution in the forms of co-payments, e.g. prescription charges. Some countries are following the trend set by the United Kingdom in 1978 (Department of Health and Social Security 1976) of distributing resources on a geographical per head of population basis.

Recent developments in the United Kingdom, as well as in some other European countries, e.g. Sweden, have been to develop quasi-markets with an increase in consumer-choice. This has been achieved by the development of privately financed healthcare facilities, mainly for simple elective procedures, e.g. cataract and hip replacement. Patients choosing these providers have the costs met by the NHS.

Some countries are encouraging people to take out private insurance or even to contract out of the public system.

Most countries are attempting to improve efficiency and effectiveness by introducing charters for waiting times. These indicated the right to be treated within a given time and reduce travel times by locating services in individual practices or locations rather than concentrated in a few large centres; however, some specialist services (e.g. cancer) are only provided in a limited number of institutions. All countries and political regions have become concerned with quality and effectiveness and a few, e.g. the European Union, have developed indices of outcome (Holland 1997).

Unfortunately, in most developed and many developing countries, the trend has been to increase expenditure on clinical services while simultaneously diminishing, or slowing the rate of growth, for public health and preventive services.

Politicians and electorates in most countries demand the development of clinical services which can demonstrate their benefit rapidly, but are much less concerned with promoting or developing public health preventive services where the benefit is far more long-term, in spite of many academic studies demonstrating the cost effectiveness of the latter.

Provider–purchaser model for both public health and personal health services

The separation of commissioning and providing services discussed above theoretically enables better decisions to be made over which services are to be provided within a limited budget. Theoretically, it should also be possible to balance preventive, curative, and rehabilitative services. For this to be effective an adequate knowledge of the epidemiology, including the natural history, of conditions is necessary. However, this is not possible for more than a small number of conditions, although a few, such as coronary heart disease, chronic obstructive lung disease, and lung cancer, may represent a large proportion of the disease burden in a particular population.

Coronary heart disease may be used as an example. The prevalence of the various stages of the disease can be ascertained in a defined population by appropriate epidemiological studies or estimated by extrapolation from studies in equivalent populations.

Incidence figures for each stage of the condition are obtained in the same way. Many of the factors responsible for the development of coronary heart disease, e.g. smoking cigarettes, blood pressure, and poor diet are known. Evidence of the effectiveness of various approaches to prevention, e.g. advise school children not to start smoking, counselling adults smokers to stop when they attend the doctor, banning cigarette advertising, and so on, is known (or required). Evidence of the effectiveness and procedures to be used for the treatment of the early stages of diseases such as angina is available.

It is thus possible to devise an appropriate model of the requirement for different treatment strategies like the use of aspirin, thrombolytics, and anticoagulants, and the need for efficient ambulance services, coronary care beds, and so on. Finally, knowledge is available of the appropriate rehabilitative services that are effective after a myocardial infarction.

From this complex model, it is thus possible to consider the balance of resources to be devoted to, or invested in, the development of effective methods to both reduce the burden of coronary heart disease as well as to improve the outcome of those who develop the condition.

Obviously, this scheme is idealistic so far, but it remains the underlying rationale for the separation of purchasing and providing health services. Managed care, now so popular in the United States, is an example of this type of separation. All these models rely on the development of knowledge of the effective methods of treatment or prevention of a condition.

The problem in all countries is that, although the effectiveness of many procedures or treatments is known, understanding of many common ailments, e.g. arthritis, is still poor. Thus, all countries are involved in a variety of schemes to identify cost-effective methods of investigation, prevention, treatment, and rehabilitation (Holland & Mossialos 1999).

It is encouraging that many countries, e.g. Ireland, England, France, and some cities in the United States, e.g. New York, have, by 2007, introduced a ban on smoking in public places—recognizing that this public health measure will have a major impact on the incidence of smoking-related diseases as it has already led to a reduction in the prevalence of smoking.

The role of public health in the determination of priorities

The role of public health is in the determination of priorities among these possibilities for improving health. Theoretically, the role of public health is clear in almost all the systems described here. It has the necessary tools to describe the problems and to devise appropriate mechanisms for their solution. In all the systems, however, the ability for public health to influence health policy is limited. Few of the countries described have effective mechanisms to influence individual health behaviours (e.g. the smoking of cigarettes) or to consider investment in non-health activities (e.g. education or employment) which are known to have more profound effects on health status than the use of medical care services (Black 1980; Acheson 1998). Nonetheless, the framework and structures currently being devised, coupled with concerns about the environment and demography, as well as increasing fiscal constraints in all systems, is forcing all countries to begin to confront these issues.

Previously, decisions on expenditure and treatment were largely controlled by those who were providing services. The treatment or service delivered to an individual or community was rarely questioned. With improvements in educational attainments and rising costs of medical procedures all societies have begun to question health expenditure. Thus, decisions on priorities have become more explicit and democratic. Most countries have begun to debate how and what should be done; e.g. should preventive services be provided to all the population or should heart transplants be available on demand (dependent on a sufficient supply). As a result, most countries have also begun to spend resources more effectively and to examine ethical issues involved in the setting of priorities and supply of services.

To address these issues, countries have developed a variety of mechanisms to involve the public more in such issues, e.g. citizen juries, opinion surveys, focus groups, and including patients or consumers in the groups which advise on priorities in an area or country. The problem is that, although the inclusion of 'consumers' is welcome, it also gives rise to problems. In public health priority setting, an attempt is made to rank the priorities by their importance in terms of impact on the health of a population. Thus, in developed western countries the most important risk factor is smoking as a cause of disease. Thus, it should rank as first priority. In a developing country, e.g. in Africa, smoking is uncommon, so the first priority might be the containment/eradication of malaria or a safe water supply. This illustrates the importance of knowledge of local conditions and is equally true for all parts of the world. Priorities for health services must be concerned with local needs.

The setting of priorities is a political process. Several chapters in this book discuss priorities in different areas of the world and for different conditions. These take into account the importance and severity of the condition and should also be concerned with the effectiveness and possibilities for intervention, such as available trained manpower, facilities, drugs, etc. All of this is fine in theory, but practice often is more murky. In many developed areas the consumer—who elects the politicians who are ultimately responsible—will be interested in the priorities for interventions likely to be of benefit to him/her. The immediate return from a clinical/curative intervention is usually more attractive than the long-term investment for a public health intervention. It must not be forgotten that, in addition, most politicians and senior administrators at the government level are not usually qualified but are no different to the average consumer. Thus, to develop and implement public health intervention priorities requires a great deal of skill by individual public health practitioners including the ability to communicate. We may have excellent technical schemes—as described above—but the main public health skill of ability to communicate is crucial. The other main contributor to the setting of priorities is also the occurrence of a scandal—e.g. an outbreak of typhoid will have/has had a dramatic effect on concern with water and food safety. All these issues are addressed in this book. But, a word of caution: In spite of the appreciation by most practitioners that alleviation of poverty is crucial for the achievement of most public health priorities, few countries have developed adequate interventions.

Conclusion

The chapters describing the policies and strategies of various countries demonstrate the progress that has been made not only in the control of disease but also in the delivery of services. Most countries demonstrate a willingness to consider a wider perspective in the provision of health services than purely concern with treatment activities. Most countries, with the notable exception of the United States, have developed mechanisms for beginning to address the problem of inequalities and deprivation. Most are facing the problem of increasing costs of medical care by rational deliberations and are beginning to consider alternative approaches, including an increased investment in public health research, in order to be able to introduce appropriate and effective preventive strategies.

References

Abel-Smith, B., Figueras, J., Holland, W. et al. (1995). Choices in health policy; an agenda for the European Union. Darmouth, Aldershot.

Acheson, E.D. (Chairman) (1988). Public health in England. Report of the Committee of Inquiry into the Future Development of the Public Health Function. HMSO, London.

Acheson, E.D. (1998). Independent inquiry into inequalities in health. HMSO, London.

Black, D. (1980). Inequalities in health. Department of Health and Social Security, London.

Department of Health and Social Security (1976). Sharing resources for health in England. Report of the Resource Allocation Working Party. HMSO, London

Exter, A., Hermans H., Dosljak M. et al. (2004). Health care systems in transition: Netherlands, Copenhagen. WHO Regional Office for Europe on behalf of the European Observatory on Health Systems and Policies.

Ferrera, M. (1993). EC citizens and social protection: main results from a Eurobarometer survey. Commission of the European Communities, Brussels.

Holland, W.W. (1995). Achieving an ethical health service: the need for information. Journal of the Royal College of Physicians, London, 29, 325–34.

Holland, W.W. (Project Director) (1997). EC atlas of 'avoidable death' (3rd edn), pp. 1–2, Oxford Medical Publications.

Holland, W. and Mossialos, E. (Ed.) (1999). Public health policies in the European Union. Ashgate, Aldershot.

Mathers, C. (2007). Epidemiology and world health. In: The Development of Modern Epidemiology, Ed. W.W. Holland, J. Olsen, C. Florey, Oxford Union Press, Chapter 5 pp. 41–60.

McMichael, A.J. and Powles, J.W. (1999). Human numbers, environment, sustainability and health. British Medical Journal, ii, 977–80.

Ministry of Health, Welfare and Cultural Affairs (1993). Report on choices in health care. Ministry of Health, Welfare and Cultural Affairs, The Hague. MUG.

Murray, C.J.L. (1996). Rethinking DALY's. In: The Global Burden of Disease, Ed. C.J.L. Murray and A.D. Lopez, Global Burden of Disease and Injury Series, Volume 1, Harvard University Press, Cambridge, MA.

Raleigh, V.S. (1999) World population and health in transition. British Medical Journal, 2, 981–4.

Robine, J.M., Jagger C., Mathers C.D. et al. (2003). Determining Health Expectancies. John Wiley & Sons, Chichester.

Sanders, B.S. (1964). Measuring community health levels. American Journal of Public Health, 54, 1063–70.

Sullivan, D.F. (1966). Conceptual problems in developing an index of health. National Centre for Health Statistics, Rockville, MD. (available at http://www.cdc.gov/nchs/data/series/sr_02/sr02_017.pdf).

WHO (World Health Organization) (1999). The changing role of public health in the European region. EUR/RC 49/10 and EUR/RC 49/Conf. Doc./6 Appendix 1. WHO, Geneva.

World Health Organization (2000). The World Health Report 2000. Health systems: improving performance. WHO, Geneva.

3.2

Public health policy in developed countries

John Powles

Persuasion requires shared standards of evidence, chains of authority, networks of trust, and accepted rules of logic and evidence. Changes in the rules of discourse and communication, no less than the knowledge unearthed by science, are the background to the changes in health and longevity that are the mark of the 'modern' age. (Mokyr 2002 p. 180)

Abstract

In the developed market economy (OECD) countries, adult mortality risks halved in the second half of the twentieth century. Trends were less favourable in Eastern Europe and were actually adverse in the Slavic and Baltic republics of the former Soviet Union.

These variable health gains cannot easily be related to explicit health policies or to organizational forms within health ministries. An alternative approach is to explore ways in which knowledge has been developed and used in response to leading adult health risks. In the last half century, there were historically unprecedented levels of investment in medical research, especially in the Scandinavian and English-speaking countries.

New knowledge has been used to protect and enhance health in a variety of ways according to the nature of the health risks being addressed. In general, knowing what to do has been powerfully permissive of it (ultimately) being done.

Linkages between the development and successful use of knowledge have not, however, been tight—in part, because openly published science is a global public good. The United States, in particular, has been more successful as a generator than as a successful user of knowledge, suggesting that health protection and enhancement are being impeded by distinctive features of its political economy.

The diverse ways in which knowledge has been used extend well beyond processes appropriately described as 'interventions'. Decentralized, informal, and 'spontaneous' uses have also played important roles.

Investments in medical research by government, civil, and commercial organizations should be sustained at high levels in expectation of continuing favourable returns to human well-being. Difficult unsolved problems—such as those related to excess adiposity and ecological disruption—are likely to require a wide repertoire of inventive responses, suggesting a need to leave space for decentralized activity and institutional creativity.

Introduction: The nature and scope of public health policy

The scope and purpose of public health policy may be seen as implicit in widely used definitions of public health. Winslow's definition, as adapted by the Acheson Report in England, is:

The science and art of preventing disease, prolonging life and promoting health through organised efforts of society (Secretary of State for Social Services 1988).

Public health policies might thus be thought of as the policies that guide these 'organized efforts' to protect and improve health. The scope of such policies depends a good deal, however, on what is considered to be entailed by 'organized efforts', and on how these 'organized efforts' are understood to be related to efforts that are less organized, more informal, more decentralized, or perhaps even 'spontaneous'.

Approaches that favour restricting the scope of public health to the more formal actions of state organizations may do so with a more or less positive attitude towards the benefits of such state action. Either way, these interpretations have the merit of identifiability and concreteness: It is not too difficult to identify the proclaimed public health policies of governments or to trace the actions of official bodies that follow their adoption.

Interpretations which emphasize the beneficent effects of state action are common in the public health literature. But the political tide in most developed countries has recently been flowing in a contrary—liberal conservative—direction and the case for governmental or other collective action now needs to be made in a more sceptical environment. Liberal opinion, both classical and 'neo', is sceptical both of the legitimacy and of the effectiveness of actions to improve well-being that are mediated by state institutions. Exponents of a strong (or 'hard') liberal viewpoint—for example, Friedrich von Hayek—emphasize that it is individuals who understand best what is needed for their own good. The knowledge needed to optimize well-being is thus essentially decentralized and it is best put to use through the mediation of institutions that facilitate the exchange of decentralized knowledge, that is, by markets. It is simply not possible, in Hayek's view, for officials in centralized institutions, even when enlightened and well-intentioned, to possess the detailed knowledge needed to act in the best interests of large, highly diverse publics. Hayek's censure fell not only on public officials but also on scientific intellectuals who dreamt of bringing social practices more in line with scientific discoveries—a tendency he called 'scientism' (Hayek 1942, 1943, 1944; Gamble 2006). In Hayek's view, this 'visible hand of human reason . . . lacked the all-important sanction of [social] evolutionary experience, and therefore risked claiming a knowledge which humans could not possess' (Gamble 2006, p. 126).

Hayek played an important role in the revival of 'hard' liberalism in the second half of the twentieth century, with politicians such as Margaret Thatcher acknowledging their debt to him (Gamble 1996, p. 151). Hayek preferred the liberal (though undemocratic) political economy of nineteenth-century Britain and regretted the expanding role of state institutions from that century's end. From a public health perspective this is rather unfortunate as this was the period when child mortality risks declined rapidly from the high levels that had persisted throughout the Victorian age. Historical analyses reveal that much of the improvement in health through the late nineteenth and early twentieth centuries was not market-mediated (Easterlin 1999; Szreter 1988; Mokyr 2002). If, counterfactually, the political economy of Hayek's golden age had been maintained, the price in child health gains foregone, may have been considerable.

Looking back from the first decade of the twenty-first century, the transformations of health during the second half of the twentieth century are more salient than the transformation of child health at its beginning. Figure 3.2.1 summarizes the reductions between 1950 and 2000 in the risks of dying before age 15 and between ages 15 and 60.

Between 1950 and 2000, the downward trajectory in the risks of dying in childhood tended, if anything, to accelerate, with those countries starting with the highest levels showing the biggest absolute gains by century's end. These may be identified by reading

from the right on the X axis of Fig. 3.2.1 (A): The points are, respectively, for Portugal, Bulgaria, Slovakia, Spain, Hungary, and Japan. Reductions in the risk of dying in childhood in Japan, Portugal, Spain, Italy, Austria, the Czech and Slovak republics, and Finland, all exceeded 90 per cent. In England and Wales, childhood mortality risks fell by 81 per cent, and in the United States, they declined by 76 per cent. Although proportional differences remained substantial by century's end, the absolute range was small: From 0.5 per cent in Sweden to 2.4 per cent in Russia, exceeding 1 per cent only in the ex-Soviet states, Hungary, Slovakia, and Bulgaria. (Among the ex-Soviet states, only the Slavic republics—Russia, Ukraine, and Belarus—and the Baltic republics—Estonia, Latvia, and Lithuania—are included in these analyses.)

Achievements in reducing mortality risks between ages 15 and 60 were much more variable, with all the ex-Soviet states included here actually experiencing higher risks in 2000 than in 1959 (when their data series commence). Risks were roughly halved in the OECD countries, with Japan, Spain, Italy, Finland, and Australia achieving the biggest proportional reductions (all above 55 per cent), and with reductions of around 50 per cent in England and Wales and 45 per cent in the United States. At the turn of the century, absolute risks in the OECD countries included here were concentrated in a narrow range, being lowest in Sweden, Japan, Italy, Switzerland, and Australia (all below 8 per cent) and highest in the United States (11.3 per cent).

Some US economists have assessed the value of that country's reductions in adult mortality risks during the second half of the twentieth century to be very substantial—bearing comparison with the value of the total increase in economic product during this period (Nordhaus 2002).

How one traces these divergent recent gains and losses in adult health via their social and institutional causes to the policies that may have helped make them possible will colour one's interpretation

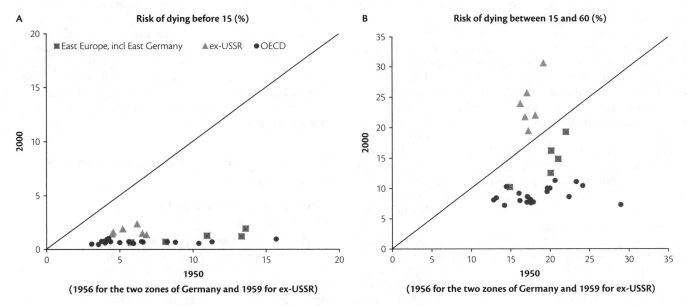

Fig. 3.2.1 Risks of dying, %, based on period mortality rates for both sexes combined, 1950 vs. 2000, developed countries: A—before 15, B—between 15 and 60 * (* Values are $_{15}q_0$ (A) and $_{45}q_{15}$ (B) for both sexes combined. Based on period mortality rates. Diagonals indicate no change. Base year for the two zones of Germany is 1956 and for the former member states of the USSR is 1959, not 1950. Data for the two zones of Germany are kept separate to 2000.
Source: Human Mortality Database (www.mortality.org).

of the role of public health policy in today's developed societies. The dramatic deterioration in the performance of the ex-Soviet states—which had been relatively impressive up to around 1960 but turned disastrous afterwards—suggests a failure of institutional adaptation as the composition of adult mortality risks came to be dominated by vascular disease and injury.

The reason for singling Hayek out above is because of the central role he accords, in his analytic approach, to the way in which societies use knowledge. This emphasis on the use (and we may add, generation) of knowledge offers a potentially fruitful approach to understanding how public policy in developed countries has served to protect and enhance health—or, alternatively, has failed to do so. Valuing Hayek's emphasis on the role of knowledge does not require agreement with his other views on political economy. We can provisionally agree that how knowledge is mobilized and used to enhance well-being is a fundamental characteristic of a country's political economy and leave open, for further consideration, the extent to which these processes are actually and properly sensitive to public policy. We have already noted how successes in reducing child mortality in the early twentieth century raise serious difficulties for those wishing to follow Hayek in deprecating 'scientism'.

The scope of this chapter can now be reconsidered. When Winslow was drawing lessons from the dramatic reduction in child mortality in the early decades of the twentieth century, he was reflecting on a period in which the scientific advances of preceding decades were put to work only after some delay. Application of the new bacteriological knowledge to control infectious disease in urban and domestic settings had been delayed by the reluctance of physicians to accept it. Time was also needed to build the institutional means for its propagation among the public (principally among mothers) (Ewbank & Preston 1989). The situation with the control of chronic disease (paradigmatically ischaemic heart disease) and injury (paradigmatically road traffic injury) in the second half of the twentieth century has been essentially different: Investments in the development of new knowledge to deal with these problems have been integral to efforts directed at their control—especially where those efforts appear to have been most successful. Furthermore, these investments have been on an entirely new scale. In the United States, President Harry Truman signed the National Heart Act in June, 1948 and between 1950 and 2000 the budget of what was to become the National Heart Lung and Blood Institute rose from US$10 million to over US$2 billion (http://www.nih.gov/about/history.htm, accessed December 18, 2007). The combined budget of the National Institutes of Health passed US$20 billion just after the turn of the century. The recent scale of scientific investigation into the causes of ill-health in developed countries is without precedent. Governments fund a large proportion of this research and state institutions play a central role—along with professional bodies and research institutions—in orchestrating and directing scientific endeavours.

A simple model now suggests itself: Countries which invest more in medical research—especially in those fields most relevant to the prevention and control of chronic disease—achieve higher levels of scientific awareness among their practising physicians and public health professionals which in turn carries through to higher levels of public awareness of the causes and preventability of chronic diseases and injuries. State-funded institutions for nurturing and guiding the scientific quest to understand and control disease have developed strongly in many OECD countries. By contrast, the

corresponding Soviet institutional response was very weak. The authoritarian political culture inhibited the use of science to address problems with a potential social or political dimension (McKee 2007; Krementsov 1997). The Soviet State may have seemed strong in its ability to control many parameters of citizens' lives, but as a collective problem-solving agency it was a timid shadow of its Western counterparts.

Figure 3.2.2 provides a convenient bibliometric index of research publications on cardiovascular disease during the 1990s. Although there may be some bias against Cyrillic language publications in this source, this is unlikely to account for the overall pattern which shows higher publication rates in the OECD countries, and extremely low publication rates in the ex-USSR countries, with the Eastern European countries generally in between. Identifying a society's mobilization of scientific endeavour towards the solution of its health problems as an important part of its public health policy response seems reasonable. But a closer look at differences between countries suggests that it is, indeed only part of the picture. The United States, for example, appears to have been much more proficient as a contributor to the advancement of knowledge relevant to disease prevention than it has been as a successful user of such knowledge. Portugal, on the other hand, has shown dramatic reductions in adult mortality risks despite its low publication rate. To the extent that gains in countries such as Portugal have been built on the advancing global stock of knowledge they will have benefited from the character of openly published scientific knowledge as a 'global public good': No one may be excluded from using it and use by one party does not diminish the opportunity for others to use it (technically, goods are 'public' when 'consumption' is 'non-excludable' and 'non-rival').

It is also clear that there are important determinants of adult mortality levels and trends that are independent of deliberate efforts to control disease—countries with Mediterranean or East Asian food cultures, for example, have enjoyed some protection against the epidemic waves of ischaemic heart disease, that was independent of deliberate efforts to achieve this result. Observations such as this also make it unlikely that there will be a simple correlation between the scale of scientific endeavour and the magnitude of health gains.

The next section of this chapter shall examine some examples of policies to protect and enhance health. The intention is partly to explore the range of policy responses that have been evoked by different kinds of public health challenges. Special attention will be paid throughout to the role of knowledge. The examples to be reviewed are set out in Table 3.2.1.

Policies to protect and improve health: Some examples

Fluoridation of water supplies (and toothpaste)

Fluoridation of water supplies introduces to this discussion the idea of preventing disease by administrative means. In 1929, a dentist in Colorado, USA, observed that mottled tooth enamel (which he suspected was associated with the water supply) was associated with fewer dental caries. The factor in the water supply was soon identified as fluoride. During the 1930s, inverse associations between fluoride concentrations in 21 cities' water supplies and a newly developed quantitative index of dental caries (DMFT, decayed, missing, and filled teeth) were reported. Caries prevalence

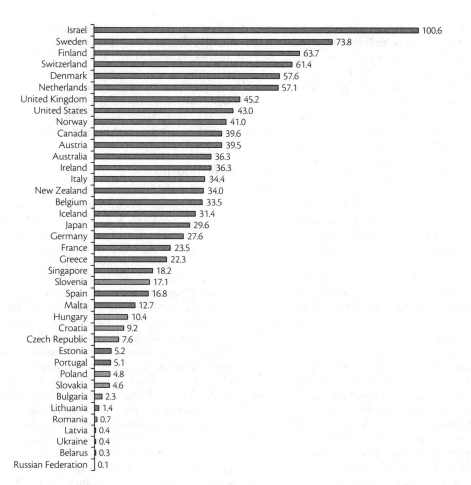

Israel 100.6
Sweden 73.8
Finland 63.7
Switzerland 61.4
Denmark 57.6
Netherlands 57.1
United Kingdom 45.2
United States 43.0
Norway 41.0
Canada 39.6
Austria 39.5
Australia 36.3
Ireland 36.3
Italy 34.4
New Zealand 34.0
Belgium 33.5
Iceland 31.4
Japan 29.6
Germany 27.6
France 23.5
Greece 22.3
Singapore 18.2
Slovenia 17.1
Spain 16.8
Malta 12.7
Hungary 10.4
Croatia 9.2
Czech Republic 7.6
Estonia 5.2
Portugal 5.1
Poland 4.8
Slovakia 4.6
Bulgaria 2.3
Lithuania 1.4
Romania 0.7
Latvia 0.4
Ukraine 0.4
Belarus 0.3
Russian Federation 0.1

Fig. 3.2.2 Publications on cardiovascular disease indexed in Medline, 1991–2001, per million population.
Source: MacKay and Mensah 2004.

Table 3.2.1 Some types of public health policy responses with illustrative examples

Type of policy response	Nature of problem addressed	Examples (those in italics are discussed further in the text)
Administrative measures applied to whole populations	Problems amenable to specific measures administered by public agencies and requiring little public involvement for their effect	Regulation of the sale and of use of hazardous chemicals; Regulation of occupational hazards. (Discussed elsewhere in this textbook.)
Combinations of administrative measures and mass behaviour change	Problems addressed by combinations of regulation and mass behaviour change	*Fluoridation (of water supplies and of toothpaste (1))*; *Control of road traffic injury* (including changes in the design of roads and of motor vehicles) (2).
Large-scale change in behaviour	Problems whose solution requires large-scale behavioural change, typically requiring supporting institutional changes	*HIV infection and sudden infant death syndrome (3)*; *Disease attributable to smoking (4)*; Disease attributable to non-optimal dietary composition
Enhanced use of clinical procedures applied to individuals (for prevention)	Problems where 'organized efforts' are used to enhance population coverage by clinical procedures of defined efficacy and feasibility	Immunization; *Enhanced clinical management of vascular risk (especially from raised blood pressure) (5)* Cancer screening
Unsolved	Problems without clearly defined solutions with current knowledge and within current institutional arrangements	*Disease attributable to declining physical activity and excess adiposity (6)*; Asthma and allergic diseases; *Effects of large-scale ecological disruption (7)*.

was reported to decline as concentrations of natural fluoride in the water supply approached 1 part per million, with little additional benefit at higher concentrations. In 1945, community intervention trials of the effects of adjusting fluoride levels to 1–1.2 parts per million began in four pairs of cities, one pair in Canada. After 13–15 years caries was reported to be reduced by 50–70 per cent in the experimental cities compared to the controls. Official recommendations for the fluoridation of community water supplies were formalized in the United States in 1962, and the proportion of the population receiving fluoridated water from community supplies rose from 40 per cent in the mid-1960s to around 56 per cent in 1992. Over this same period, the mean DMFT among all 12-year-olds fell dramatically from around 4 to just over 1. With time, the potential benefits of water fluoridation have lessened as those without such supplies get fluoride from other sources, including toothpaste and drinks and foods manufactured in fluoridated areas (Division of Oral Health 1999).

In both the United States and the United Kingdom, fluoridation enjoys the support of around 70–75 per cent of respondents to national opinion surveys (American Dental Association 1999; British Dental Association 1999). However, implementation requires local decisions, and these have frequently been blocked by opponents. In the United States, local referenda have been lost because opponents have been more committed and better organized than proponents. Legal challenges in the lower courts have also blocked adoption, though the highest courts have upheld none.

Proposals to flouridate water supplies rested on quantitative research in populations. The development of a simple index of tooth decay was important as were experiments conducted on whole communities. However, with time methodological knowledge has advanced and evidence that seemed convincing at the time may seem less robust when set against today's standards. Scientific reviewers in the United Kingdom have recently 'been surprised by the poor quality of the evidence and the uncertainty surrounding the beneficial and adverse effects of flouridation' (Cheng et al. 2007 p. 699). The best estimate (by these reviewers) of the increase, in flouridated areas, in the proportion of children free of caries, was a median of 15 per cent with an interquartile range of 5–22 per cent. Even this wide range understated the uncertainty because 'potential confounders were poorly adjusted for' (NHS Centre for Reviews and Dissemination 2000). Evidence for the effectiveness of flouridated toothpastes is much more certain, being based on some 70 randomized controlled trials (preventive fraction 24 per cent, 95 per cent confidence interval 21–28 per cent) (Marinho et al. 2003).

Opponents of flouridation have claimed harmful effects. There is now a much more adequate understanding of how difficult it is to exclude harms of potential public health importance—say increases of 20 per cent for non-trivial conditions with relatively low background risks. It is now understood that studies of sufficient size and duration to detect such effects have not been done.

One of the most interesting observations from the recent reviews has been the marked secular declines in caries prevalence in EU member states, reflecting the declines, noted above, in the United States. These declines bear little obvious relationship to the prevalence of water flouridation (Cheng et al. 2007). It is plausible that the widespread use of flouridated toothpastes deserves a substantial part of the credit. If true it could mean that the main benefits of the flouride hypothesis are being realized through the decentralized purchase decisions of parents and that what seemed at first to be a means of improving health by administrative means turns out to be both more complicated and more interesting. What remains central is the role of knowledge—the quantitative methodologies which were initially used to support advocacy of water fluoridation are now being marshalled in support of a more sceptical stance. Meanwhile the universal availability of flouridated toothpaste attests to the diffusion amongst parents of the belief that flouride does indeed prevent tooth decay.

Road traffic injuries

Traffic injuries ranked tenth in their contribution to the burden of disease and injury in developed countries in 2002 (http://www.who.int/healthinfo/bodgbd2002revised/en/index.html, accessed December 18, 2007). Because of the short time lags between control measures and their expected effects, traffic injuries also provide a sensitive field in which to explore the relationship between policies, programmes, and effects. Also of interest is the relative contributions of 'passive' measures, largely independent of driver behaviour—for example redesign of roads and vehicles to make them safer—and measures aimed at changing road user behaviour.

Deaths from traffic crashes in relation to the number of registered vehicles follow a general, and pronounced, downward trend as the number of motor vehicles increases in relation to population (Smeed's Law: Deaths/vehicle = 0.0003(vehicles/population)$^{-0.66}$) (Smeed 1972). In the mid-1960s, two-thirds of 70 populations analysed by Smeed had rates within 40 per cent of his prediction. This implies that societies generally learn how to use motor vehicles more safely as familiarity with them and the resources available for safety measures both increase. Because the overall tendency is general, it is unlikely to depend on the specifics of policies variably adopted—although it may be contributed to by the 'public good' character of enhanced vehicle crashworthiness (all tend to benefit from design changes introduced in large demanding markets). But it is also the case, that around the general trends, some societies have performed better than others.

Figure 3.2.3 shows the decline in Victoria, Australia, in deaths per 10 000 vehicles as the number of vehicles increased in relation to population. Over 80 per cent of the reduction in fatalities per 10 000 vehicles that occurred between 1920 and 2005 happened before 1970. During these five early decades, Victoria generally had ratios in excess of Smeed's prediction. Then, in a little more than two decades from 1970, it changed from being a relatively poor performer in this domain to being one of the best (Fig. 3.2.4).

During the 1960s, there had been a growing political consensus in Victoria that the loss of so many lives on the roads was no longer tolerable. In December 1970, it became the first jurisdiction in the world to make the wearing of seat belts compulsory. A string of legislative measures followed, including random testing of the breath alcohol concentrations of drivers in 1977. After the decline in fatality rates faltered in the late 1980s, a very strong 'social marketing' campaign was launched in combination with intensive policing (Powles & Gifford 1993). The number of speed camera checks per year rose to 8 per licensed driver and the proportion of vehicles recorded as speeding fell from 20 to 3 per cent. In 1994, 1.6 million random breath tests were performed, a number equal to about half of the driving age population (Hendrie & Ryan 1995, p. xi–xii). Fatality rates fell sharply and have stayed down. Since the early 1990s, the Transport Accident Commission (TAC), which carries all

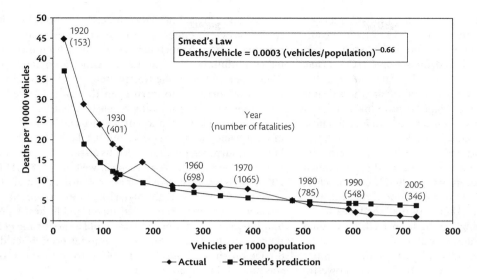

Fig. 3.2.3 The actual versus predicted decline in traffic fatalities per 10 000 vehicles with increasing motorization, State of Victoria, Australia, 1920–2005. *Sources*: Hawthorne (1991); Smeed (1972); Australian Transport Safety Bureau (2007).

compulsory traffic injury insurance and makes 'no-fault' compensation payments to victims, has spent significantly on traffic accident prevention programmes, including intensive use of paid television advertising. Ten per cent of the spend has been allocated to evaluation, from which the TAC has been able to conclude that its benefits-to-costs ratio, from reduced injury claims, has been very favourable (Cameron & Newstead 1996). By 2005, the fall in deaths per 10 000 vehicles relative to the level in 1960 was around tenfold.

Several points can be made about this spectacular public health success: (1) Most of the very large secular declines in traffic injury deaths per unit vehicles (or distance travelled) observed around the world are likely to have occurred with a substantial degree of independence from the specific policies and programmes adopted in different political jurisdictions; (2) Against this broad background trend, a second order, but never-the-less important degree of variation seems attributable to the intensity and nature of the specific control measures taken locally; (3) In the relatively compact political environment of an Australian state, it was possible to build support for the escalation of control measures as less forceful measures proved inadequate to achieve widely desired goals—notwithstanding a

political culture that valued personal independence; (4) The comparative trend line for Britain (in Fig. 3.2.4), ending with rates among the lowest in Europe, shows that Victoria does not differ so much in the level it has attained as in the distance it has travelled (so to speak) over four decades of intensive political attention; (5) Success has depended on knowing what to do—guided by research bodies such as the Monash University Accident Research Centre (in Victoria), the Insurance Institute for Highway Safety (in the United States), and the Transport Research Laboratory (in the United Kingdom); (6) Although not easy to identify in the illustrated data for Victoria, improved vehicle crashworthiness is likely to have also been a major contributor to mortality decline. Robertson (2001) allocates 90 per cent of US vehicle occupant mortality decline between 1964 and 1990 to this source.

This example also illustrates the powerful social benefits of having single, substantial 'pots of gold' for dealing with leading sources of disease or injury. By linking the size of the 'pot' to the scale of the problem—in this case by the level of compensation payments for traffic injuries—a resource is created that bears some commensurability with the public health challenge faced. The custodians

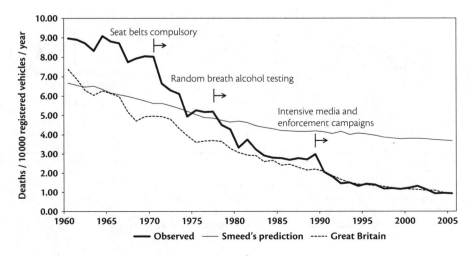

Fig. 3.2.4 Decline in traffic fatalities per 10 000 vehicles, 1960–2005, State of Victoria, Australia and Great Britain (with predicted trend using Smeed's Law). *Source*: Smeed (1972); Australian Transport Safety Bureau (2007); Department for Transport (2007).

of this fund can then gain social approbation both by reducing a recognized evil and by reducing the financial levy needed to compensate for it. (Anti-smoking programmes funded by hypothecated tobacco taxes, as also exist in Victoria and, for example in California, exploit an analogous linkage.)

As a contrast, one may note the situation in Russia where deaths per 10 000 vehicles are over 10 times higher than in low risk jurisdictions (OECD 2007, p. 236). Russia appears to have invested little in the science needed for traffic injury control. There were 14 publications in the last 10 years indexed in Medline on 'Accidents/traffic' combined with 'Russia', compared to 236 when combined with 'Australia' (searched on December 14, 2007). On March 7, 2007, Deputy Prime Minister Medvedev announced that the government was responding to the 35 000 annual road deaths by 'examining the issue of equipping reanimation facilities located throughout the road network' (Medvedev 2007).

In addition to the measures considered here for reducing injury risks per unit of exposure to car usage, there are other powerful health and environmental considerations favouring a reduction in car use itself (Woodcock *et al.* 2007).

Human immunodeficiency virus (HIV) and sudden infant death syndrome (SIDS)

The epidemic of HIV infection in Europe followed that of the United States. The time course of the epidemic through the population of homosexual and bisexual males in England and Wales has been reconstructed by 'back projection' from the subsequent epidemic of AIDS (de Angelis *et al.* 1998). The incidence of HIV infection appears to have peaked in 1983 and then to have fallen sharply (Fig. 3.2.5).

Against the time course of the infection rate can be set the timing of the formal control measures. Intensive 'social marketing' campaigns to promote changes to safer sexual practices were not launched by the UK government until March 1986 (Acheson 1993). It is thus likely that most of the change in sexual practices responsible for the sudden turnaround and decline in HIV incidence after 1983 had occurred before the formal programme began. How is this to be explained? New knowledge about the dire consequences

of HIV and (mostly indirect) indications about how it might be spread passed through both the general news media and through communication channels used especially by homosexual and bisexual communities. Because the epidemic in England substantially lagged behind that in the United States (perhaps by 3 years), there was an opportunity to learn from the United States where suspected modes of transmission had been identified as early as 1982, well before the identification of the virus in 1984 (US Department of Health and Human Services and Batelle 1995, p. 29). There was, however, surprisingly little direct discussion of sexual transmission in British newspaper accounts until well into 1983 (Hilliard *et al.* 2007). This suggests a prominent role for informal, 'horizontal' communication among the high risk group. In cases like this where sensitive behaviours are involved, formal public health programmes may be delayed by the need to first build a supporting political consensus. In the United States, a national household drop of an 8-page brochure, *Understanding Aids*, from the Surgeon General was not conducted until 1988.

The decline in Sudden Infant Death Syndrome (SIDS) in England (also shown in Fig. 3.2.5) illustrates apparently similar communication processes. In August 1988, a letter from an Adelaide paediatrician was published in *The Lancet* in which results from several small studies were pooled. It showed that front sleeping had a statistically significant association with increased risk (Beal 1988). Death rates from SIDS fell by more than a third in the next 3 years before the UK government's formal public health programme ('Back to sleep') began in December 1991 (OPCS 1988 and 1995; Hiley & Morley 1994), suggesting that mass behaviour change began well in advance of the formal programme. Why it did so is something of a mystery. Coverage of SIDs in British newspapers during this period increasingly emphasized that scientists were busy on the case and that a wide range of hypotheses was under investigation. No special salience was given to the role of sleeping position (Hilliard *et al.* 2007). The rate of decline in SIDS did, however, accelerate sharply after the national 'Back to sleep' programme began, with incidence halving in the subsequent 12 months. Official advice on sleeping position changed in the Netherlands before it did in the United Kingdom, and in the United Kingdom before the

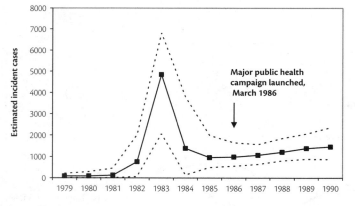

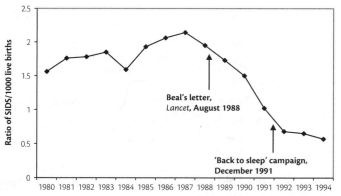

Fig. 3.2.5 Left: HIV incidence in homosexual and bisexual males, England and Wales, estimates by back-projection for 1979–90 (with 95 per cent credible interval) and timing of main public health campaign; Right: Ratio of deaths attributed to SIDS per 1000 live births, England and Wales, 1980 to 1984, with timing of major public health campaign.
Sources: HIV: De Angelis, personal communication, Acheson (1993); SIDS: Office of Population, Censuses and Statistics (1988, 1995).

United States. Gilbert and colleagues have gathered evidence on the sleeping positions of control infants in epidemiological studies showing that the prevalence of the hazardous front sleeping position fell first in the Netherlands, then in the United Kingdom, and finally in the United States (Gilbert *et al.* 2005, Fig. 3.2.4). The national declines in SIDS occurred in the same sequence.

These two examples—of HIV and of SIDS—show how, in highly literate and health-conscious populations, much of the benefit from new knowledge may flow more or less automatically from its dissemination through channels other than formal public health programmes. In these circumstances, it is the advance of science, perhaps even more than the strength of public health programmes, that sets the pace for health improvement (Dwyer & Ponsonby 1996). This is not to claim that the incremental gain from formal programmes is typically negligible; it may still be very worthwhile relative to their typically modest resource requirements.

In these two examples, informed publics seem to have made their own good use of new knowledge, without the necessity of professional or administrative mediation. This casts doubt on the helpfulness of the widespread practice of equating of 'medicine' with the knowledge held by and acted on by physicians. On the basis of this equation, one might conclude that the decline in the HIV epidemic in England in the early 1980s (for example) was due to 'non-medical measures'. A semantic sleight of hand of this kind led Thomas McKeown astray in his attempts to explain earlier falls in mortality. (McKeown 1976) The reality is that the lay public and physicians draw on the same stocks of knowledge: Conflating medicine as a social institution with its professional practice is an avoidable source of confusion.

In relation to the decline in SIDS, Gilbert and colleagues' demonstration that if, counterfactually, current methods of evidence synthesis had been available in 1970 and used to pool data from the two case control studies published by then, the cumulated odds ratio for front versus back sleeping would have been determined to be 2.9 (95 per cent CI 1.15–7.47). They estimate that over 50 000 excess infant deaths occurred in North America, Europe, and Australasia because of the delay in advocating back sleeping (Gilbert *et al.* 2005, p. 883). This example shows how capacities to protect and improve health may owe as much to advances in methodological knowledge (in this case, knowing how to make the best use of what is known) as to advances in substantive knowledge.

Tobacco smoking

It is ironic that medicine provided a 'cultural bridge' across which tobacco was transferred from the exotic rituals of the Amerindian cultures to the everyday life of seventeenth-century Europe. By explaining tobacco's properties within the contemporary humoral theories of well-being, physicians such as the Sevillian Nicolas Monades provided what was to be the main, medical, justification for tobacco use until into the nineteenth century, when 'recreational' justifications came to the fore (Goodman 1993). With the advent of manufactured cigarettes in the late nineteenth century, tobacco use was made more convenient and more deadly. In the twentieth century, increased purchasing power resulting from economic development has been almost universally accompanied by widespread adoption of cigarette smoking (Tobacco Advisory Group 2000). These epidemics of nicotine addiction can, on the experience of 'early adopters' such as England, be expected to last at least a century (Lopez *et al.* 1994). As a public health problem, cigarette smoking is thus distinguished not only by the great quantity of disease attributable to it—accounting at its peak, in the United Kingdom, for almost a half of male and a quarter of female deaths between 35 and 69 (Peto & Lopez 1994, p. 206)—but also by the protracted time scale over which it evolves. It will, for example, be half a century before the full health effects of onsets of nicotine addiction in today's adolescents become fully manifest. Tobacco smoking is, in addition, a form of addiction that is both legal and extremely profitable.

Although earlier studies were published in Nazi Germany, for readers of the English-language literature the health effects of cigarette smoking were mostly revealed to by epidemiological studies conducted between the late 1940s and the mid-1960s. A question of interest is how this new knowledge (since much strengthened) has influenced the course of the smoking 'epidemic' and the epidemics of disease that have followed in its train.

From around 1950 to the mid-1960s, it was the general news media that conveyed new knowledge of the health effects of smoking to the public. The Royal College of Physicians report in the United Kingdom in 1962 (Royal College of Physicians 1962) and the Surgeon General's report in the United States in 1964 (which it stimulated) (United States Public Health Service 1964) were 'organized efforts' that, nevertheless depended for their effects on such news coverage. A study of this process in the United States showed that the intensity of print media discussion of the risks of smoking was closely mirrored in adult smoking cessation rates through the 1950s and 1960s (Pierce & Gilpin 2001).

The intensification of 'organized efforts' to discourage tobacco smoking dates mainly from the 1970s. The main measures have included price increases (by specific taxes), bans on advertising and other forms of promotion, requirements for warning labels on tobacco products and on advertisements, restrictions on smoking in public places, health education in schools, mass education and persuasion, enhanced advice, and assistance with cessation.

Attempts to assess the contribution of these measures to national trends in smoking prevalence (and with appropriate lags, to national trends in attributable mortality) needs to take account of the variation in the time of onset of the smoking epidemics, before its health effects were understood. In Europe, UK males and females and Finnish males (but not females) were 'early adopters' of cigarette smoking (Lopez 1996). A general pattern of 'first in, first out' of the smoking epidemic might have been expected, to some extent independently of the timing and strength of national counter measures. Lung cancer mortality in early middle-aged males (ages 35–54) peaked in the 1950s in United Kingdom, in the 1960s in Finland, and in the 1970s in the United States. Falls since these peaks have exceeded 70 per cent in the United Kingdom and Finland and been around 50 per cent in the United States. Rates in 2000 were respectively: 15.4, 13, and 23 per 100 000 person-years (age standardized using equal weights, Peto *et al.* 1994, 2003).

It also happens that Finland (which banned tobacco advertising in 1978) (Harkin *et al.* 1997, p. 29) and the United Kingdom have been among the leaders in efforts to reduce smoking. Finnish females, whose delayed smoking epidemic came to maturity during a period of tobacco control activity, have experienced a lung cancer mortality peak (at about 7/100 000 for 45–54-year-olds in 1990) less than one-third as great as that experienced by UK females (about 27/100 000 for 45–54-year-olds in 1975) (Peto & Lopez 1994): The size of the smoking epidemic in UK females was largely determined in the pre-control period (Lopez 1996). This pattern—of smoking epidemics having lower amplitudes when maturing in an environment of tobacco control activity—suggests that control measures are effective.

Although trends in adult smoking prevalences in developed countries have generally been favourable, trends since the early 1990s in smoking uptake by adolescents have been mixed. In many European countries 30-day smoking prevalences in 15–16-year-olds have been in the range of between 20 and 40 per cent between 1995 and 2003 (Hibbel *et al.* 2003). In the United States, the remarkable California Tobacco Control Program appears to have succeeded with adolescents where many others have failed. In 2004, 30-day smoking prevalences for 9th–12th graders (roughly 15–17-year-olds) were only 13 per cent, compared to a US national average of 22 per cent (California Department of Health Services 2007).

To summarize: Cigarette smoking remains the leading public health problem in developed countries. As a specific behaviour it is without rival in the disease burden it generates. It illustrates well how the evolution of some public health problems may need to be viewed within a very prolonged time frame. Peak smoking prevalences appear to have been lower in the higher educated strata in 'late uptake' countries—where knowledge of health effects has had more opportunity to influence behaviour—there are notable exceptions, such as the high smoking prevalences among Spanish physicians as recently as the 1990s (Harkin 1997, p. 10). Reductions in attributable mortality within the next half century will need to mainly come from encouraging and supporting cessation in current smokers. But if the course of the epidemic of nicotine addiction is to be curtailed, inter-generational transmission must also be minimized. This will be helped if there are declines in parental smoking whilst their children are at the ages most sensitive to their influence. The relevant parental ages will presumptively be before 40 or so. This keeps the reduction of smoking uptake in adolescence, and an increase in quitting in the early adult years both in the frame as important objectives.

The history of efforts to reduce health losses from tobacco also illustrates how the development of quantitative methods has supported appropriate policy responses. It is striking that high level policy debates in the United Kingdom during the 1950s and 1960s revolved around a largely illusory search for 'proof of causation' rather than quantifying how much was at stake (Pollock 1999). Artificial stimulation of this controversy over causation was also a deliberate strategy of commercially powerful tobacco companies. With increased acceptance of epidemiological reasoning and its transmission to political and wider publics (for example Peto & Lopez 1994), quantitative assessments have become much more central to policy deliberations. Changes, like this, in the rules of discourse, have enhanced the propensity to act on new knowledge (as noted by Mokyr in quote at start of chapter).

Enhanced clinical management of vascular risk

Half a century of epidemiological research on ischaemic heart disease and stroke has progressively clarified the quantitative relationships between the three main risk factors—usual blood pressure, usual blood cholesterol concentration, and smoking—and the risk of heart attack and stroke. Even measurements made on a single occasion—which capture usual values only with some error—are sufficient to stratify individuals into groups at vastly differing levels of vascular risk (Stamler *et al.* 1986).

For persons in their 60s, risk of heart attack is lower by 25 per cent and risk of stroke by 35 per cent for each 10 mmHg reduction in usual systolic blood pressure (Lawes *et al.* 2004a, p. 325, 326) and the risk of heart attack is lower by 30 per cent for each 1 mmol/l reduction in usual cholesterol concentration (Lawes *et al.* 2004b, p. 428). All of the excess stroke risk appears to be reversible if blood pressure is lowered to target levels by medication and about two-thirds of the excess risk of heart attack may be reversible.

This predictability and demonstrated reversibility of vascular risk in individuals has provided the basis for the prevention of heart attack and stroke by the clinical management of risk factors—especially blood pressure and blood cholesterol concentration. The United States has national programmes for each—The National High Blood Pressure Education Program (NHBPEP), established in 1972 and the National Cholesterol Education Program, established in 1985. The former has been running for longer, and it will be explored a little further here.

The NHBPEP has aimed to make case-finding more complete and control more effective. National progress in blood pressure control is monitored through the National Health and Nutrition Examination Survey (NHANES) (Table 3.2.2). Despite the limitations of these data on the proportions of 'hypertensives' 'aware, treated, and controlled', they suggest a substantial improvement in case-finding and control between the late 1970s and the turn of the century. The proportion of those defined as hypertensive who were taking medication doubled from 31 per cent in 1976–80 to 61 per cent in 1999–2004. Proportions controlled rose from 10 to 35 per cent over the same period (National Heart Lung and Blood Institute 2007).

The Framingham Study cohorts have provided the opportunity to track changes over a longer time span, though in a population that is likely to be more health conscious than average. The proportion of those aged 45–74 who reported antihypertensive medication increased from 2 per cent in the 1950s to 25 per cent in the 1980s in males and from 6 to 28 per cent in females. Those with blood pressures above 160/100 measured on a single occasion (and irrespective of treatment status) fell from 19 to 9 per cent in the case of males and from 28 to 8 per cent in the case of females. Bigger proportionate declines occurred in progressively higher blood

Table 3.2.2 United States: Trends in awareness, treatment, and control of high blood pressure in persons 18–74, 1976 to 1994

	Per cent of those either above 140/90 at time of survey or reporting antihypertensive medication			
	1976–80	1988–91*	1991–1994*	1999–2004
Aware that they have high blood pressure	51	73	68	72
Report taking anti-hyptertensive medication	31	55	53	61
Controlled (below 140/90 at time of survey)	10	29	27	35

* These estimates are based on NHANES III in which blood pressure was measured on 2 occasions.

Source: Joint National Committee 1997, p. 3; National Heart Lung and Blood Institute 2007.

pressure strata and the prevalence of left ventricular hypertrophy fell markedly. These findings are consistent with other data pointing to substantial secular declines, especially in severe hypertension (Mosterd *et al.* 1999).

In assessing the National High Blood Pressure Education Program and other formal public health programmes seeking to enhance control of blood pressure, three questions need to be addressed: (1) To what extent has the improvement in case-finding and management for high blood pressure been attributable to the 'organized effort' of programmes such as the NHBPEP? (2) How much effect has improved treatment had on the numbers at risk because of raised blood pressures? And (3) How much of the observed decline in vascular risk is likely to be attributable to the reduction of blood pressures by clinical means?

Studies designed to answer the first two questions appear to have been very limited. In rural Kentucky a community high blood pressure control programme was run in two counties between 1979 and 1984, with a third county serving as control. In the intervention counties, the percentage of 'hypertensives' whose blood pressure was controlled to below 140/90 rose from 37 to 53 per cent, with no change in the control county. Cardiovascular mortality fell in the intervention counties, while remaining constant in the control (Kotchen *et al.* 1986).

Some US observers believed, in the early 1980s, that '. . . the documented improvements in hypertension control since the beginning of the NHBPEP must be considered a major contribution . . .' to the decline in cardiovascular mortality rates' (Lenfant & Roccella 1984). Over the longer period from 1963 to 2004 in the United States, age-adjusted death certification rates for heart attack and stroke each fell by around 70 per cent (National Heart Lung and Blood Institute 2007). There is a good deal of credit waiting to be attributed somewhere.

For persons aged 60–74, data from the US national health surveys show a substantial shift downwards in blood pressure distributions from the early 1960s to the most recent survey period around 2000. Because nearly all treated persons stay above the median, reductions in the median provides a more robust measure of shifts in the central tendency due to causes other than treatment. Median systolic pressures at ages 60–74 fell over this period by about 16 mmHg, from 148 to 132 mmHg. The fall had actually occurred by the early 1990s and there is little evidence of further reduction since. The reduction in the upper tail of the distribution was more marked, with 90th centiles falling by about 30 mmHg— from around 191 mmHg to 160 mmHg (estimates from smoothed distributions in Fig. 3.2.1 of Burt *et al.* 1995 and analyses of data from NHANES IV (http://www.cdc.gov/nchs/nhanes.htm)). Some of the credit for these improvements should go to enhanced clinical control of blood pressure.

Rose coined the term 'prevention paradox' to describe how, when risk is related monotonically to a quantitative attribute such as blood pressure, the interventions which offer most to the individuals at high risk contribute less to reducing the population burden of the disease than do small downward shifts in the whole distribution (Rose 1985). Strachan and Rose reworked these analyses taking account of the misclassification of risk status when blood pressure is only measured on a single occasion. Assuming a reliability coefficient of 0.5, over 50 per cent of the population risk of fatal stroke attributable to true (usual) blood pressures higher than those in the lowest decile, was to be found in those whose true pressures were in the top decile. Yet, even in these apparently promising circumstances, a 'high risk' case-finding strategy that correctly identified all in the true top decile and that achieved an average reduction of 7.5 mmHg diastolic in all those offered treatment, would reduce stroke mortality only by about the same amount as would result from a 3 mmHg reduction in diastolic blood pressures across the whole distribution (Strachan & Rose 1991). Thus, although classification on the basis of usual blood pressures enhances the relative effectiveness of the 'high risk' strategy in relation to stroke, it still remains modest when compared to downward shifts in the whole distribution of blood pressures. Earlier analyses of the contribution of hypertension treatment to the decline in stroke mortality between 1970 and 1980 placed it in the range of 6–25 per cent (Bonita & Beaglehole 1989).

Rose expounded his 'prevention paradox' by considering one risk factor at a time. Optimal strategies for risk reduction in multicausal diseases like ischaemic heart disease have since been further clarified. Law and Wald showed that the important thing was to identify persons whose absolute vascular risk was high—whether from modifiable or non-modifiable causes—because the absolute benefit from risk lowering therapy is directly proportional to the absolute risk. Preventive efforts should therefore be calibrated against absolute risk and not against the levels of individual modifiable risk factors (Law & Wald 2002). This approach is now incorporated in guidelines for prescribing expensive statin drugs in the UK National Health Service.

To conclude this example: The 'organized efforts' of the NHBPEP and other similar programmes will account for part of the improved case-finding and management for persons with usual blood pressures above treatment thresholds. This improved management will account for part of the decline in the prevalence of persons above treatment thresholds. The decline in the prevalence of persons above treatment thresholds will account for part of the decline in stroke and ischaemic heart disease mortality attributable to raised blood pressures.

Despite this cumulative diminution of the contribution of the NHBPEP that contribution is still likely to have been very worthwhile because even small reductions in the heavy burdens imposed by heart attack and stroke will add up to a big benefit in absolute terms. Furthermore, the gains attributable to the NHBPEP are notable for having been achieved within a pluralistic and organizationally diverse system of medical care.

The relatively limited likely contributions of clinical control to substantial secular declines in blood pressure and blood cholesterol concentrations leaves open the attribution of much of the credit for large declines in death from vascular causes attributable to favourable shifts in risk factor distributions. Between 1970 and 2000, the death certification rates for coronary heart disease at ages 35–74 fell by about two-thirds in the United States and by almost four-fifths in Australia (National Heart Lung and Blood Institute 2007). For the United States, it has been estimated that risk factor changes contributed about half the fall in deaths from coronary disease 'prevented or deferred' between 1980 and 2000 (Ford *et al.* 2007). The proportional contribution of risk factor change to life years gained will have been greater because deaths averted by risk factor changes, yield, on average, longer streams of life. The diffusion of knowledge about risk factors to the general public is likely to have made a substantial contribution to these declines. In societies that have been less successful in reducing vascular risk, popular knowledge of risk factors may be very much lower (Dokova *et al.* 2005).

> *Unless Prudence be a constant attendant on Opulence . . . tis better living on a slender fortune.* Richard Mead (1673–1754)

Unsolved problems: Physical inactivity and adiposity

The material basis of modernization lies in the replacement of muscle, wind, and water power by energy carried by steam, electricity, and liquid hydrocarbons. Of the main adverse consequences for health, two—air pollution and transport injuries—have been largely brought under control. The third—the physiological consequences of declining energy expenditure—remains unsolved.

Data, of known validity, on time trends in energy expenditure is generally unavailable for developed populations. Because of the technical difficulties involved, the measurement of total energy turnover in representative free-living individuals is a major challenge for contemporary public health surveillance. The 'doubly labelled water' technique provides a gold standard but is too expensive for large-scale use. Individually calibrated heart rate monitoring is the next best but so far only one study has reported findings from a broadly representative study population (Wareham *et al.* 1997).

In the absence of data on trends in energy expenditure over time, data on recorded energy consumption may be used as a proxy, bearing in mind that such records tend to underestimate true intake and that an assumption of a roughly constant under-reporting bias over time is required. Data for English adults show substantial declines since the first 7-day-weighed dietary intakes of the 1930s (Widdowson 1936; Widdowson & McCance 1936; Bingham *et al.* 1981; Prentice & Jebb 1995). Data abstracted from a large series of dietary studies in the United States show falls of around 17 per cent in recorded energy consumption of US adults (without adjustment for increasing body weight) between the 1940s and the early 1980s (Stephen & Wald 1990).

The Physical Activity Level (PAL) is the ratio of total energy expenditure to basal metabolic rate (James & Schofield 1990). It is an important determinant of public health via two types of effects. First, activity is directly protective of health (independently of its effects on body composition and of its contribution to aerobic fitness) (US Department of Health and Human Services 1996, Wareham *et al.* 2000). Second, as activity levels decline, the prevalence of obesity increases (Prentice & Jebb 1995).

Tentative suggestions are that mean PALs of the order of 1.75 may be needed to help prevent mass obesity. This compares with current average values for developed countries of around 1.55–1.60. To close the gap would require the addition of around 1 h of moderately intensive activity to the average citizen's daily routine (Saris *et al.* 2003). The effect of the decline in physical activity levels over past decades is compounded by the increased availability and declining real prices of energy dense foods, which some analysts see as the more important contributor to the rise in adiposity (Bleich *et al.* 2008).

The widespread rise of obesity in developed countries is visible to all. Recent declines in adult mortality in rich countries have, in most cases, been occurring in spite of adverse trends in two related health determinants—physical activity and adiposity. What might be required to reverse these trends?

The difficulty faced may be compared with that of changing the composition of the diet in order to favour health. Although there are hedonic attractions in unhealthy dietary compositions—chocolate, ice cream!—attractive alternatives that favour health are also available—for example, Mediterranean diets. But exertion is, alas, not as attractive as indolence. During our evolutionary past, there was unlikely to have been a survival advantage in exertion in the absence of hunger or other immediate need. In this light, the origins of our problems with obesity and inactivity are profoundly social: They are a consequence not so much of individual misbehaviour as of our collective transformation of the way we provision society and the resulting marked reduction in the need for muscular exertion.

Investment in new knowledge is a clear priority. Strategic importance, and the indications that solutions will not be easy, both point to the need to establish physical activity and energy balance as high priorities in public health research. Given the rapid advances in identifying genetic susceptibility, preventive strategies will be needed at all levels—universal (for the whole population), selective (for the susceptible), and targeted (for those already affected) (World Health Organization 1998, p. 168). Assuming further research confirms the fundamental importance of low physical activity levels, the most feasible and attractive ways of increasing such activity will need to be found. These are likely to entail significant and pervasive institutional change.

Unsolved problems: Sustainability

Averting harm to health from the disruption of the ecological systems on which human well-being depends is unlike other public health challenges. The need for action cannot be inferred from empirical observations of previous harm from this source, but rather is to be inferred from highly uncertain models of what may happen in the future. Those averse to 'speculation' might be inclined to defer judgement until there has been time for the relevant models to be more thoroughly challenged, and the contributory evidence better marshalled. The argument against delay is that the interacting momenta of population increase and economic development are likely to result in 'overshoot and collapse' unless corrective action begins now. If attempts to extend the current pattern of energy and resource-intensive industrialism to the whole of an increasing human population are likely to come seriously unstuck, then the sooner the transition to more sustainable material culture is begun the better. This topic is too vast to be properly addressed here—beyond noting that transitions to durable solutions (if made in time) are likely to require fundamental institutional changes. Many of the needed changes could also bring 'health dividends', for example via increased energy expenditure in moving around and reduced consumption of red meat (McMichael *et al.* 2007).

Some reflections on the examples considered

The topic of public health policy in developed countries is a vast one. I have sought to approach it by asking first whether knowledge plays a more important role than is implied by its relative neglect in commonly invoked models of the 'wider determinants of health'.

Several conclusions can be drawn from the examples considered.

1. Knowing what to do—to protect and enhance health—is powerfully permissive of it (ultimately) being done. This emerges clearly from all the examples where substantial gains in health

have been achieved (1 to 5 above). The relationship is not one to one. Health protective changes may occur for other reasons and knowing may not lead to doing because of the difficulties involved (adiposity provides the obvious example).

2. Because openly published science is a global public good, the proximity between the generation of new knowledge and the capacity to use it need not be close. The United States, for example, ranks more highly as a generator of knowledge than it does as a successful user. Generation and use are not too disjoint however, because a high investment in research relevant to public health is associated with a diffusion of the relevant 'rules of discourse'. Publics familiar with 'risk' and 'risk factors' will more readily assimilate new knowledge expressed in this way.

3. New knowledge may flow to its ultimate users through a variety of channels, ranging from formal health education programmes (sleeping position and SIDS in the United Kingdom, from December 1991) to highly informal, horizontal channels (sexual practices and HIV).

4. Advances in methodological knowledge—knowing better how we can know and how to make the best use of what we do know—have in some cases been as important as advances in substantive knowledge.

5. 'Interventions' that tell people what to do have often been found to be ineffective. These null results have often occurred against a background of favourable, and presumably knowledge-based, changes in the relevant behaviours in the host population. This apparent paradox—of interventions without success against a background of success without interventions—is discussed further below.

Restoring knowledge to a central role in recent health trends in developed countries has an additional merit: It provides a common theme with explanations of trends in other times and in other populations. In the early twentieth century, the decline of childhood mortality was powerfully determined by the propagation to parents of new bacteriological knowledge (Ewbank & Preston 1989). For last decades of the twentieth century in low- and middle-income countries, Jamison and colleagues have concluded that:

Increased access to knowledge and technology has accounted for perhaps as much as two-thirds of the impressive 2 per cent per year rate of decline in under five mortality rates (Jamison 2006, p. 4).

Liberalism and knowledge: Standing Hayek on his head

Liberalism tends to view politics as artificial (Zvesper 1987) and emphasizes the decentralized use of knowledge. Hayek's 'hard liberalism' sees the way knowledge is used as a central characteristic of political economy and deprecates centralized uses of knowledge.

The examples I have reviewed reinforce the central role of knowledge in the protection and enhancement of health in developed countries over the last half century. Some also demonstrate the importance of diffuse and decentralized processes in the successful use of knowledge. But the centrality of politics (think of the protracted tobacco wars) and the role of state and other centralized institutions—professions, scientific institutions, research

'charities'—in these processes, can neither be denied as a reality nor valued negatively. Massive state investments in medical research—most notable, ironically, in countries espousing economic liberalism and most deficient in the former communist states make the case. We can therefore accept Hayek's proposition that how knowledge is used is a fundamental characteristic of a society then turn him on his head and view positively rather than negatively the political and often centralized processes that have made the generation and diffusion of knowledge about how to protect and enhance health so fruitful of human well-being over the last half century.

Interventions without success and success without interventions

The idea of an intervention—defined by the *Oxford English Dictionary* as 'The action of intervening, "stepping in", or interfering in any affair, so as to affect its course or issue' (http://dictionary.oed.com)—has become pervasive in medicine and public health. Interventions clearly need intervenors: Professionals, programme administrators, or others. Recent medical usage links the idea to actions that can be subject to tests of effectiveness by a randomized control trial (RCT)—the most potent known salve for cognitive insecurity. Being testable in an RCT in turn implies actions that can be objectively pre-specified. This would seem to rule out actions that are informal, spontaneous, contingent, or 'one off'.

We have seen above how many of the processes leading to the turnaround in the HIV epidemic and to the reduction in SIDS (up to the formal programme at the end of 1991) appear to have been of an informal kind, making them, to a large degree 'successes without interventions'. There is only space here to add a couple of examples from the field of tobacco control, namely 'George Godber's lunch' and The California Tobacco Control Program.

In the late 1950s, George Godber was Deputy Chief Medical Officer in Britain and was very keen to act on the increasing knowledge of the harmful effects of smoking. But the Chief Medical Officer did not want to take the matter forward with the Minister of Health. Godber visited Charles Fletcher, a respiratory physician, at a London teaching hospital and invited him to his club for lunch so that they could discuss strategies. They decided on working through the Royal College of Physicians in order to by-pass the Chief Medical Officer. The College took up the matter energetically and decided to produce a report aimed at a large audience. In 1962, *Smoking and Health* appeared and quickly sold out (Pollock 1999; Lock *et al.* 1998). The United States was stimulated to follow suit and in 1964 the Surgeon General's report on *The Health Effects of Smoking* appeared. News media coverage of smoking and health was responsive to these reports and Pierce and colleagues have shown that smoking cessation rates in US middle-aged adults were, in turn, responsive to the extent of news coverage. (Pierce & Gilpin 2001) The point of this story is that all these processes are knowledge-based without qualifying as interventions.

Only a compulsive sceptic could doubt that the California Tobacco Control Program has contributed importantly to the reduction of tobacco smoking in that state. Since it achieved dedicated funding it has included many activities that would qualify as interventions. But the programme itself was created and sustained by a protracted political process—beginning with an 'indoor air ordinance' in Berkeley in April 1977 and reaching a decisive step with the passage of Proposition 99 in a statewide referendum in November 1988. This placed a tax of 25 cents on each pack of cigarettes that was hypothecated to the Program. The first city to make its restaurants 100 per cent smoke-free was Lodi in June 1990, and in January 1998 bars were made smoke free statewide. (Glantz & Balbach 2000). The proportion of households reporting themselves smoke free rose from 51 per cent in 1993 to 77 per cent in 2002. 'It is likely that the emphasis placed on the dangers of secondhand smoke by the California Tobacco Control Program media campaign, led to the adoption of home smoking restrictions'. (California Department of Health Services 2003, pp. 6–9.) (Such restrictions were not initially promoted by the Program.) Complex dynamics of this kind, including protracted political contests and 'spontaneous' household behaviour changes are not well captured in the idea of 'interventions'. But these elements are very likely to have contributed to the success of the Program.

Knowledge may thus be acted on in many ways in order to protect and enhance health, only some of which are appropriately described as 'interventions'.

Public health problems and public health investments

One reason why it is not always easy to see in health levels the short- to medium-term effects of public health programmes is that the causal path may go in the opposite direction: The nature and magnitude of health problems experienced may determine the strength of the public health response. Finland and Australia provide cases in point.

In the late 1960s, mortality from vascular disease in middle-aged males in the Finnish province of North Karelia was far above levels in other developed countries and the risk of dying before 65 approached 50 per cent. These risks were perceived, by the local people, as unacceptable and so they petitioned the national government to mount a preventive programme. From this the North Karelia Project was born and it in turn, stimulated investment in public health institutions (Vartiainen *et al.* 1994). Despite its modest

population, Finland now has over 1000 staff in its National Institute of Public Health, and it ranks at the top in its rate of publication in leading international epidemiological journals (Fig. 3.2.6). Proportional mortality reductions in Finland have been amongst the biggest in the developed countries. Evaluative studies of the North Karelia project itself suggest it was effective. Lung cancer mortality fell sooner and further there consistent with early results for changes in smoking prevalence (Puska *et al.* 1993).

Australia, like Finland, faced adverse mortality trends in the sixth and seventh decades of the twentieth century with male life expectancy at birth falling during the seventh decade. Rising death rates from coronary heart disease, car crashes, and suicide were responsible. A country which had been notable for its favourable mortality levels at the beginning of the century, that had experienced a long post-war economic boom and that thought of its way of life as being especially favourable to health had to come to terms with a serious loss of rank in international health comparisons. Strong institutional responses evolved in relation to traffic injuries, heart disease, and tobacco control (Powles & Gifford 1993). These institutional developments have plausibly contributed to Australia's recent ranking as a relatively good performer in reducing overall mortality.

The strong development of public health institutions oriented towards chronic disease control in countries such as Finland and Australia may be contrasted with experience in countries such as France, Italy, and Spain where the evolving nature of public health challenges has been different. Vascular mortality in these countries did not persist at high levels, but tended to fall, often rapidly: This brought down all-cause mortality rates and made the case for re-invigorating public health institutions to prevent chronic disease less pressing. In these countries, traffic injuries, HIV, tobacco control, and the reduction of harm from alcohol use are among the most salient challenges.

The challenge of inequality

Recent favourable trends in overall adult mortality have been accompanied by growing inequalities in countries across Western

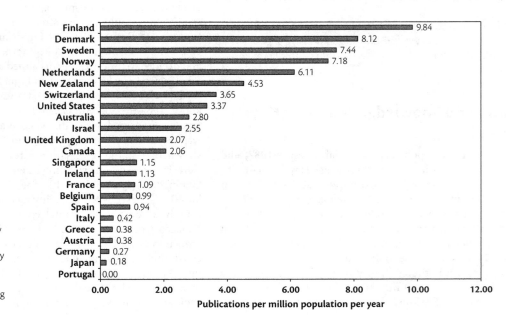

Fig. 3.2.6 Publications in the *American Journal of Epidemiology* plus the *International Journal of Epidemiology* classified by country of author's address, per million population, average for 1995–98. *Source*: Author's calculations using Medline records.

Europe because mortality declines have been proportionally greater in more favoured strata. Increasing inequalities in vascular mortality has been an important contributor (Mackenbach 2003). The causes of, and appropriate remedies for, these inequalities in health have been a major pre-occupation in policy discussions in the United Kingdom (Black *et al.* 1980; Acheson 1998). There is no tendency for mortality inequalities to be lesser in countries with higher income equality. The causes of death contributing most to these differences do, however, vary markedly between countries: '. . . mortality from ischaemic heart disease was strongly related to occupational class in England and Wales, Ireland, Finland, Sweden, Norway, and Denmark, but not in France, Switzerland, and Mediterranean countries. In the latter countries, cancers other than lung cancer and gastrointestinal diseases made a large contribution to class differences in total mortality. Inequalities in lung cancer, cerebrovascular disease, and external causes of death also varied greatly between countries' (Kunst *et al.* 1998b).

Black and colleagues have articulated a 'materialist' interpretation of the cause of inequalities in the United Kingdom. This gives primacy to 'material deprivation' (both absolute and relative) and draws attention to the marked increase in income inequalities there between 1979 and 1995/96—for example, over this period, the number of persons living in households with less than half the national average income increased from 4.5 to 12.2 million persons (Black *et al.* 1999). However, the finding of Kunst and colleagues that relative mortality inequalities are not less in countries with more equal income distributions does not support this interpretation. Furthermore, constrained consumption opportunities are not everywhere associated with high mortality levels: Cretan villagers observed in the 1960s and 1970s in the Seven Countries study had favourable mortality levels, despite their extremely frugal circumstances (Keys 1980). Thus, within some material cultures (all of which seem to have warm-ish climates!), it has become possible to attain low mortality on low incomes. The health effects of limited consumption opportunities therefore appear to depend strongly on the context in which consumption choices are made. Materialist explanations, if they are to be persuasive, need either to acknowledge their limited sphere of applicability ('northern commodity-intensive cultures'?) or, more informatively, to incorporate explicit reference to the kinds of differences between life in a Cretan village in the 1960s and life on housing estate in a British industrial city in the 1990s that are likely to be most important for health: Dietary traditions (related also to local food producing possibilities), norms governing alcohol and tobacco use (and purchasing power for cigarettes), and obligatory daily energy expenditure might be starters. Given that the relative importance of causes contributing to mortality inequalities varies by country, responses should also differ. In France, where inequalities in males appear to be amongst the largest within Western Europe, chronic diseases related to the volume of alcohol consumed make a major contribution; policies to reduce consumption will therefore be important. In Finland, injuries related to drunkenness are more salient, pointing to the need both for 'harm reduction' policies (such as control of drunk driving), and for programmes to encourage a change away from the traditional 'peak drinking' pattern. Measures to counter smoking are of primary importance in countries where a mature smoking epidemic is combined with a high background risk of vascular disease (roughly the 'northern' countries). (In countries at earlier stages in their smoking epidemics, programmes to encourage quitting may

have the effect of increasing mortality inequalities. This does not, of course, mean that they should not be implemented.)

Jarvis and colleagues have shown for the United Kingdom that the current social gradient in smoking prevalence has been mainly created by greater rates of smoking cessation in the upper social strata: 'What we need to explain above all is not so much why poor people start smoking, but why they do not give it up' (Jarvis & Wardle 1999). Plasma cotinine levels among smokers show that nicotine dependence increases systematically with deprivation and that poor smokers obtain more nicotine per cigarette smoked. Using the indirect method of Peto, Lopez, and others (1992) (in which lung cancer mortality is used as a measure of tobacco exposure to estimate the proportion of other deaths attributable to smoking), it is estimated that, in the United Kingdom, smoking attributable deaths contribute about two-thirds of the excess mortality in the less favoured groups. The most obvious short-term policy response is to greatly strengthen assistance for quitting. In the long term, all measures that contribute to making tobacco use uncommon will have helped to reduce a major actual or potential cause of health inequality.

Making progress safe

Material progress—understood as the intensification of commodity production—both favours and harms health. One of the continuing challenges for public health institutions is to help resolve this ambivalence by countering the manifest and potential harms to health arising from material progress. This enables the net effect of affluence on health to approximate more closely towards those effects which are intrinsically beneficial. In nineteenth century Britain, industrialism did not impress as 'progress' until ways had been found to control the increase of fatal infection in the new industrial towns (Szreter 1997). In the twentieth century, the increased consumption opportunities generated by economic development has permitted a global epidemic of nicotine addiction which, especially when combined, in susceptible food cultures, with 'early dietary affluence' resulted in epidemic waves of tobacco-caused cancer and tobacco-amplified vascular disease. These epidemics were sometimes big enough, at least in males, to substantially nullify beneficial effects of economic development on traditional infective killers of adults such as tuberculosis and pneumonia. Now, as we have noted these two related epidemics are generally in retreat in developed countries. But history has not ended. Challenges and unsolved problems are ever renewed. As noted above, the uptake of tobacco smoking by young people has ceased declining in many developed countries and there is no plausible solution to the rising prevalence of obesity in sight. Industrialism in its current form is now known not to be generalizable to the whole human population without serious damage to planetary systems. Although we cannot predict the exact ways in which the cumulative disruption of major ecological processes will rebound on our health, the likelihood of serious harm from this source is now substantial. Public health endeavour will continue to be an important determinant of what we are able to mean by 'progress' and of whether we shall be able to make it safe.

Acknowledgements

I am grateful to Nick Day for the examples relating to HIV transmission and the decline in SIDS, to Daniela de Angelis for the

model data on HIV in England, and to Christine Lim for help with
Fig. 3.2.1.

Key points

◆ Adult mortality risks in established market economies and in
European communist countries diverged markedly during the
last four decades of the twentieth century.

◆ A fruitful approach to understanding these processes is to examine
how knowledge has been developed and used in response to
leading adult health risks.

◆ Knowing what to do has been powerfully permissive of it
(ultimately) being done.

◆ The ways in which knowledge is used to protect and enhance
health extend beyond formal 'interventions' to informal, decentralized, and 'spontaneous' processes.

◆ Creative institutional responses in areas such as heart disease
prevention, tobacco control, and traffic injury control have
extended the boundaries of what is achievable with given stocks
of knowledge.

◆ So far, there has been little success in preventing the rise of excess
adiposity, or in achieving transitions to sustainable productive
systems. These provide current tests for the capacity of states to
act as stewards over society's problem-solving capacities.

References

Acheson, E.D. (1993). Behold a pale horse: A view from Whitehall. *PHLS Microbiology Digest*, **10**, 133–40.

Acheson, E.D. (1998). *Independent inquiry into inequalities in health*. The Stationery Office, London.

American Dental Association (1999). *Fluoridation facts (revised)*. American Dental Association, Chicago (http://www.ada.org/consumer/facts/ff-menu.html, accessed November 12, 1999).

Australian Transport Safety Bureau (2007). *Road deaths Australia 2006 Statistical summary*. Australian Transport Safety Bureau, Canberra.

Beal, S. (1988). Sleeping position and SIDS [letter]. *Lancet*, **2**, 512.

Berry, C.J. (1994). *The idea of luxury: A conceptual and historical investigation*. Cambridge University Press, Cambridge.

Bingham, S.A., McNeil, N.I., and Cummings, J. H. (1981). The diet of individuals: A study of a randomly chosen cross section of British adults. *British Journal of Nutrition*, **45**, 23–35.

Black, D., Morris, J.N., Smith, C., and Townsend, P. (1980). *Inequalities in health: Report of a research working group*. Department of Health and Social Security, London.

Black, D., Morris, J.N., Smith, C. *et al.* (1999). Better benefits for health: Plan to implement the central recommendation of the Acheson report. *British Medical Journal*, **318**, 724–7.

Bleich, S., Cutler, D., Murray, C. *et al.* (2008). Why is the developed world obese? *Annual Review of Public Health*, **29**, 273–95.

Bonita, R. and Beaglehole, R. (1989). Increased treatment of hypertension does not explain the decline in stroke mortality in the United States, 1970–1980. *Hypertension*, **13**, I69–73.

Breslow, L. (1996). Social ecological strategies for promoting healthy lifestyles. *American Journal of Health Promotion*, **10**, 253–7.

British Dental Association (1996). *Oral health, tooth decay and the need for water fluoridation (Parliamentary Briefing)*. British Dental Association, London (http://www.derweb.ac.uk/bfs/bdaparli.html, accessed November 12, 1999).

Bunker, J.P. (2000). Medicine matters after all. *Journal of the Royal College of Physicians of London*, **29**, 105–12.

Burt, V.L., Culter, J.A., Higgins, M. *et al.* (1995). Trends in the prevalence, awareness, treatment, and control of hypertension in the adult US population. Data from the health examination surveys, 1960 to 1991 [published erratum appears in Hypertension 1996 May; 27(5):1192]. *Hypertension*, **26**, 60–9.

California Department of Health Services, Tobacco Control Section (2003). Tobacco control successes in California: A focus on young people, results from the California Tobacco Surveys, 1990–2002 (http://www.dhs.ca.gov/tobacco, accessed December 18, 2007).

California Department of Health Services, Tobacco Control Section. (2007) Prevalence: Youth smoking (http://www.dhs.ca.gov/tobacco, accessed December 18, 2007).

Cameron, M. and Newstead, S. (1996). *Mass media publicity supporting police enforcement and its economic value*. Monash University Accident Research Centre, Melbourne (www.general.monash.edu.au/muarc/media/media.htm, accessed October 20, 1999).

Cheng, K.K., Chalmers, I., and Sheldon, T.A. (2007). Adding fluoride to water supplies. *BMJ*, **335**, 699–702.

De Angelis, D., Gilks, W.R., and Day, N.E. (1998). Bayesian projection of the acquired immune deficiency syndrome epidemic. *Applied Statistics*, **47**, 449–98.

Department for Transport (2007). *Road casualties Great Britain: 2006*. Department for Transport, London.

Division of Oral Health, Centers for Disease Control (1999). Fluoridation of drinking water to prevent dental caries. *Morbidity and Mortality Weekly Report*, **48**, 933–40.

Dokova, K.G., Stoeva, K.J., Kirov, P.I. *et al.*(2005). Public understanding of the causes of high stroke risk in northeast Bulgaria. *The European Journal of Public Health*, **15**, 313–16.

Dwyer, T. and Ponsonby, A.L. (1996). The decline of SIDS - a success story for epidemiology. *Epidemiology*, **7**, 323–5.

Easterlin, R.A. (1999). How beneficent is the market? A look at the modern history of mortality. *European Review of Economic History*, **3**, 257–94.

Ewbank, D.C. and Preston, S.H. (1989). Personal health behaviour and the decline in infant and child mortality: the United States, 1900–1930. In *What we know about health transition; The cultural, social and behavioural determinants of health: Proceedings of an international workshop,Canberra, May 1989* (ed. J.C. Caldwell *et al.*), pp. 116–49. Australian National University, Canberra.

Ford, E.S., Ajani, U.A., Croft, J.B. *et al.* (2007). Explaining the decrease in U.S. deaths from coronary disease, 1980–2000. *The New England Journal of Medicine*, **356**, 2388–98.

Gamble, A. (1996). *Hayek: The iron cage of liberty*. Polity Press, Cambridge.

Gamble, A. (2006). Hayek on knowledge, economics, and society. In *The Cambridge companion to Hayek* (ed. E. Feser), pp. 111–31. Cambridge University Press, Cambridge.

Gilbert, R., Salanti, G., Harden, M. *et al.* (2005). Infant sleeping position and the sudden infant death syndrome: systematic review of observational studies and historical review of recommendations from 1940 to 2002. *International Journal of Epidemiology*, **34**, 874–87.

Glantz, S.A. and Balbach, E.D. (2000). *Tobacco war: Inside the California battles*. University of California Press, Berkeley.

Goodman, J. (1993). *Tobacco in history: The cultures of dependence*. Routledge, London and New York.

Harkin, A.M., Anderson, P., and Goos, C. (1997). *Smoking, drinking and drug taking in the European Region*. WHO Regional Office for Europe, Copenhagen.

Hawthorne, G. (1991). *Pre-driver education: An evaluation of a traffic safety education program for senior students in Victorian post-primary schools*. PhD thesis submitted to Monash University 1991. Monash University, Melbourne, Australia.

Hayek, F.A. (1942). Scientism and the Study of Society, Part I. *Economica*, **9**, 267–91.

Hayek, F.A. (1943). Scientism and the Study of Society, Part II. *Economica*, **10**, 34–63.

Hayek, F.A. (1944). Scientism and the Study of Society, Part III. *Economica*, **11**, 27–39.

Hendrie, D. and Ryan, G.A. (1995). *Review of road safety practices in Australia and recommendations for Western Australia*. Road Accident Prevention Research Unit, Department of Public Health, University of Western Australia, Perth.

Hibell, B., Andersson, B., Bjarnason, T. et al. (2003). *The ESPAD Report: Alcohol and other drug use among students in 35 European countries*. The Swedish Council for Information on Alcohol and Other Drugs, Stockholm.

Hiley, C.M.H. and Morley, C.J. (1994). Evaluation of government's campaign to reduce risk of cot death. *British Medical Journal*, **309**, 703–4.

Hilliard, N., Jenkins, R., Pashayan, N. et al. (2007). Informal knowledge transfer in the period before formal health education programmes: Case studies of mass media coverage of HIV and SIDs in England and Wales. *BMC Public Health*, **7**, 293.

James, W.P.T. and Schofield, C. (1990). *Human energy requirements*. Oxford University Press, Oxford.

Jamison, D.T. (2006). Investing in Health. In *Disease control priorities in developing countries* (2nd edn.), (ed. D.T. Jamison et al.), pp. 3–36.

Jarvis, L. (1997). *Smoking among secondary school children in 1996: England*. The Stationery Office, London.

Jarvis, M.J. and Wardle, J. (1999). Social patterning of individual health behaviours: The case of cigarette smoking. In *Social determinants of health* (eds. M.G. Marmot and R.G. Wilkinson), pp. 240–55. Oxford University Press, Oxford.

Joint National Committee (1997). The sixth report of the Joint National Committee on prevention, detection, evaluation, and treatment of high blood pressure [published erratum appears in Arch Intern Med 1998 Mar 23;**158**(6):573]. *Archives of Internal Medicine*, **157**, 2413–46.

Keys, A. (1980). *Seven countries: A multivariate analysis of death and coronary heart disease*. Harvard University Press, Cambridge.

Kotchen, J.M., McKean, H.E., Jackson-Thayer, S. et al. (1986). Impact of a rural high blood pressure control program on hypertension control and cardiovascular disease mortality. *Journal of the American Medical Association*, **255**, 2177–82.

Krementsov, N.L. (1997). *Stalinist science*. Princeton University Press, Princeton, NJ.

Kunst, A.E., Groenhof, F., and Mackenbach, J.P. (1998a). Mortality by occupational class among men 30–64 years in 11 European countries. EU Working Group on socioeconomic inequalities in health. *Social Science and Medicine*, **46**, 1459–76.

Kunst, A.E., Groenhof, F., Mackenbach, J.P., and EU working group on socioeconomic inequalities in health (1998b). Occupational class and cause specific mortality in middle aged men in 11 European countries: Comparison of population based studies. *British Medical Journal*, **316**, 1636–42.

Law, M.R. and Wald, N.J. (2002). Risk factor thresholds: Their existence under scrutiny. *BMJ*, **324**, 1570–6.

Lawes, C.M.M., Vander Hoorn, S., Law, M.R. et al. (2004a). High blood pressure. In *Comparative quantification of health risks: Global and regional burden of diseases attributable to selected major risk factors*, Vol. 1 (eds. M. Ezzati et al.), pp. 281–390. World Health Organization, Geneva.

Lawes, C.M.M., Vander Hoorn, S., Law, M.R. et al. (2004b). High cholesterol. In *Comparative quantification of health risks: Global and regional burden of diseases attributable to selected major risk factors* (eds. M. Ezzati et al.), pp. 391–496. World Health Organization, Geneva.

Lenfant, C. and Roccella, E.J. (1984). Trends in hypertension control in the United States. *Chest*, **86**, 459–62.

Lock, S., Reynolds, L.A., and Tansey, E.M. (1998). *Ashes to ashes: The history of smoking and health*. Rodopi, Amsterdam.

Lopez, A. (1996). The lung cancer epidemic in developed countries. In *Adult mortality in developed countries* (ed. A. Lopez), pp. 111–34. Oxford University Press, Oxford.

Lopez, A.D., Collishaw, N.E., and Piha, T. (1994). A descriptive model of the cigarette epidemic in developed countries. *Tobacco Control*, **3**, 242–7.

Mackay, J. and Mensah, G. (eds.) (2004). *The atlas of heart disease and stroke*. World Health Organization, Geneva.

Mackenbach, J.P., Bos, V., Andersen, O. et al. (2003). Widening socioeconomic inequalities in mortality in six Western European countries. *International Journal of Epidemiology*, **32**, 830–7.

Marinho, V.C., Higgins, J.P., Sheiham, A. et al. (2003). Fluoride toothpastes for preventing dental caries in children and adolescents. *Cochrane Database of Systematic Reviews*, CD002278.

McKee, M. (2007). Cochrane on Communism: The influence of ideology on the search for evidence. *International Journal of Epidemiology*, **36**, 269–73.

McKeown, T. (1976). *The modern rise of population*. Arnold, London.

McMichael, A.J., Powles, J.W., Butler, C.D. et al. (2007). Food, livestock production, energy, climate change, and health. *Lancet*, **370**, 1253–63.

Mead, R. (1775). *The medical works of Richard Mead, M.D.* Alexander Donaldson & Charles Elliot, Edinburgh (reprint by AMS Press, New York, 1978), p. 438.

Medvedev, D. (2007). Excerpts from the transcript of the session of the Presidential Council for Implementing Priority National Projects and Demographic Policy. Kremlin, Moscow (http://www.kremlin.ru/eng/text/speeches/2007/03/07/1944_type82913type82917_119295.shtml, accessed December 18, 2007).

Mokyr, J. (2002). *The gifts of Athena: Historical origins of the knowledge economy*. Princeton University Press, Princeton, N.J.

Mosterd, A., D'Agostino, R.B., Silbershatz, H. et al. (1999). Trends in the prevalence of hypertension, antihypertensive therapy, and left ventricular hypertrophy from 1950 to 1989. *New England Journal of Medicine*, **340**, 1221–7.

National Heart Lung and Blood Institute (2007). Factbook. (http://www.nhlbi.nih.gov/about/factbook/chapter4data, accessed December 18, 2007)

NHS Centre for Reviews and Dissemination (2000). *A systematic review of public water fluoridation*. NHS CRD, York.

Nordhaus, W. D. (2002). *The health of nations: The contribution of improved health to living standards*. Working Paper 8818. National Bureau of Economic Research, Boston.

OECD (2007). *Factbook 2007*. OECD, Paris.

Office of Population, Censuses and Statistics (1988, 1995). *OPCS Monitor, Series DH3 Sudden Infant Deaths*. OPCS, London.

Peto, R., Lopez, A.D., Boreham, J. et al.(1994). *Mortality from smoking in developed countries, 1950–2000: Indirect estimates from national vital statistics*. Oxford University Press, Oxford.

Peto, R., Lopez, A.D., Boreham, J. et al. (1992). Mortality from tobacco in developed countries: Indirect estimation from national vital statistics. *Lancet*, **339**, 1268–78.

Peto, R., Lopez, A.D., Boreham, J. et al. (2003). *Mortality from smoking in developed countries, 1950–2000* (2nd edn.). Clinical Trials Service Unit, Oxford University (web based update of first edition), Oxford. (http://www.ctsu.ox.ac.uk/~tobacco, accessed December 18, 2007).

Pierce, J.P. and Gilpin, E.A. (2001). News media coverage of smoking and health is associated with changes in population rates of smoking cessation but not initiation. *Tobacco Control*, **10**, 145–53.

Pollock, D. (1999). *Denial and delay: The political history of smoking and health, 1951–1964*. Action on Smoking and Health, London.

Powles, J.W. and Gifford, S. (1993). Health of nations: Lessons from Victoria, Australia. *British Medical Journal*, **306**, 125–7.

Prentice, A.M. and Jebb, S.A. (1995). Obesity in Britain: Gluttony or sloth? *British Medical Journal*, **311**, 437–9 (and response to correspondence in **311**, 1568–9).

Puska, P., Korhonen, H.J., Torppa, J. *et al.* (1993). Does community-wide prevention of cardiovascular diseases influence cancer mortality? *European Journal of Cancer Prevention*, **2**, 457–60.

Robertson, L.S. (2001). Groundless attack on an uncommon man: William Haddon, Jr, MD. *Injury Prevention*, **7**, 260–2.

Rose, G. (1985). Sick individuals and sick populations. *International Journal of Epidemiology*, **14**, 32–8.

Royal College of Physicians (1962). *Smoking and health*. Pitman Medical, London.

Saris, W.H., Blair, S.N., van Baak, M.A. *et al.* (2003). How much physical activity is enough to prevent unhealthy weight gain? Outcome of the IASO 1st Stock Conference and consensus statement. *Obesity Reviews*, **4**, 101–14.

Secretary of State for Social Services (1988). *Public health in England: The report of the Committee of Inquiry into the future development of the Public Health Function* (D. Acheson, Chairman). HMSO, London.

Smeed, R.J. (1972). The usefulness of formulae in traffic engineering and road safety. *Accident Analysis and Prevention*, **4**, 303–12.

Stamler, J., Wentworth, D., and Neaton, J.D. (1986). Is relationship between serum cholesterol and risk of premature death from coronary heart disease continuous and graded? Findings in 356,222 primary screenees of the Multiple Risk Factor Intervention Trial (MRFIT). *JAMA*, **256**, 2823–8.

Stephen, A.M. and Wald, N.J. (1990). Trends in individual consumption of dietary fat in the United States, 1920–1984. *American Journal of Clinical Nutrition*, **52**, 457–69.

Strachan, D. and Rose, G. (1991). Strategies of prevention revisited: effects of imprecise measurement of risk factors on the evaluation of "high-risk" and "population-based" approaches to prevention of cardiovascular disease. *Journal of Clinical Epidemiology*, **44**, 1187–96.

Szreter, S. (1988). The importance of social intervention in Britain's mortality decline c.1850–1914: A re-interpretation of the role of public health. *Journal of the Society for the Social History of Medicine*, **1**, 1–37.

Szreter, S. (1997). Economic growth, disruption, deprivation, disease, and death: on the importance of the politics of public health for development. *Population and Development Review*, **23**, 693–728, 929,931.

Tobacco Advisory Group, Royal College of Physicians (2000). *Nicotine addiction in Britain*. Royal College of Physicians, London.

United States Public Health Service (1964). *Smoking and health: Report of the advisory committee to the Surgeon General of the Public Health Service*. US Department of Health, Education and Welfare, Washington.

US Department of Health and Human Services and Batelle (1995). *For a healthy nation: Returns on investment in public health*. US Government Printing Office, Washington.

US Department of Health and Human Services (1996). *Physical activity and health: A report of the Surgeon General*. US Department of Health and Human Services, Centers for Disease Control and Prevention, Atlanta, GA.

Vartiainen, E., Puska, P., Jousilahti, P. *et al.* (1994). Twenty-year trends in coronary risk factors in North Karelia and in other areas of Finland. *International Journal of Epidemiology*, **23**, 495–504.

Wareham, N.J., Hennings, S J., Prentice, A.M. *et al.* (1997). Feasibility of heart-rate monitoring to estimate total level and pattern of energy expenditure in a population-based epidemiological study: the Ely Young Cohort Feasibility Study 1994–5. *British Journal of Nutrition*, **78**, 889–900.

Wareham, N.J., Wong, M.Y., and Day, N.E. (2000). Glucose intolerance and physical inactivity: The relative importance of low habitual energy expenditure and cardiorespiratory fitness. *American Journal of Epidemiology*, **152**, 132–9.

Widdowson, E.M. (1936). A study of English diets by the individual method, part I. Men. *Journal of Hygiene*, **36**, 269–92.

Widdowson, E.M. and McCance, R.A. (1936). A study of English diets by the individual method, part II. Women. *Journal of Hygiene*, **36**, 293–309.

Woodcock, J., Banister, D., Edwards, P. *et al.* (2007). Energy and transport. *Lancet*, **370**, 1078–88.

World Health Organization (1998). *Obesity: Preventing and managing the global epidemic. Report of a WHO Consultation on obesity, Geneva 2–5 June 1997*. World Health Organization, Geneva.

Zvesper, J. (1987). Liberalism. In *The Blackwell encyclopaedia of political thought* (ed. D. Miller), pp. 285–89. Blackwell, Oxford.

3.3

Health policy in developing countries

Miguel Angel González-Block,
Adetokunbo Lucas,
Octavio Gómez-Dantés,
and Julio Frenk

Abstract

Health policy making in developing countries is increasingly being envisaged as a stewardship process concerned with attaining trust and legitimacy between a government and its people towards the improvement of the welfare of populations. Health policy today involves multiple actors and an increased role by global and international agencies. Increased investment in the context of the Millennium Development Goals is also placing greater attention on good national and international governance. Particular attention is being paid to governance of the new breed of vertical programmes. This approach has demonstrated benefits for the specific diseases being tackled, yet it threatens other programmes and the capacity of local authorities to meet broad health needs. Developing country governments should set clear priorities on the basis of health needs and infrastructure capacity as well as on sound ethical guidance that help achieve maximum improvement in health in return for minimum expenditure.

Comprehensive national health accounts is an important policy tool to track health spending from all sources. Performance assessment can support policy making in monitoring and evaluating attainment of critical outcomes and the efficiency of the health system in a way that allows comparison over time and across systems. Particular attention is being given to financing healthcare for the more than 1.3 billion rural poor and informal sector workers in developing countries without financial protection against the catastrophic costs of healthcare. Success with these and other innovations will depend on solving the multiple challenges facing the health workforce. Relying on public–private mix of services to address health infrastructure faces the question of the capacity by government to develop contracts, set prices, and monitor and supervise private providers.

It is not always easy to reconcile efficiency and equity in health policy. Equity should be a primary concern for sustainable policy making, and tools are available to trace the extent to which investments at national levels benefit the poor and needy. In many respects, health policy in developing countries is all about the encouragement of innovation and the scaling-up of life-saving technologies and systems. Access to knowledge and technology has accounted for a high proportion in the decline in mortality rates. New strategies for organizing health research systems can contribute to make evidence-based policy a reality in developing countries.

Introduction

Most developing nations are making important strides towards better health and universal health service coverage through policies that are increasingly influenced by international experience. The flow of financial resources is also rapidly increasing thanks to the role that health investments are playing in the wider strategy towards democracy, economic growth, and global security (Frenk & Gómez-Dantés 2007; Hecht & Shah 2006; Brown et al. 2001). Health policy in the South is thus increasingly being influenced by globalization, both by responding to global threats and by doing so through extensive use of the pool of global experiences.

Health policy has been critical for the diffusion of life-saving technologies and knowledge that are behind the drop in disparities in life expectancy across rich and poor countries at least since the middle of the last century. Taken as a group, the poorer countries have seen gains of about 5 years on average per decade since 1960, against half this much by the better-off. Critically, the pace of technology diffusion has been more influential for health than changes in the levels of income. Increased access to knowledge and technology thanks to appropriate health policies has accounted for perhaps as much as two-thirds of the 2 per cent per year rate of decline in under-5 mortality rates (Jamison 2006).

However, health policy still has important challenges in a world saddled with conflict, poverty, and the pandemic of HIV/AIDS. In some African countries, the trend in the mortality rate for children under 5 has been reversed. While, between 1960 and 1990, African countries made substantial progress in reducing this rate, in many countries this effort was slowed down considerably, and in some others mortality even rose between 1990 and 2002 (UNICEF 2004).

In this chapter, we review the context in which health policies are being developed in low- and middle-income countries. We discuss several key concepts associated with health policy; and we describe some of the tools available for policy making. In the first part, we discuss the role of health policy as a stewardship instrument and the general context in which health policies are being designed and implemented in developing nations. In the second part, we describe some of the novel tools available for policy making, including burden of disease, national health accounts, and health system performance assessment. We discuss the increasing international financing for healthcare and the alternatives for providing financial protection against catastrophic costs of healthcare to the rural and urban poor. We then analyse the search for equity in health and discuss the role of international agencies and health research in the design and implementation of health policies. The main messages of the chapter are the following:

1. Health policy is being called not only to address the pressing needs of infectious diseases and malnutrition and the emerging problems of non-communicable diseases and injuries, but also the new challenges related to globalization.

2. Sound health policy making can contribute to the consolidation of democracy, to economic growth, and to global security. The broad consensus generated around this issue has helped to mobilize **more money for health** in developing nations.

3. Policy-making should be evidence-based, and also results-oriented. Careful planning and skilled management can achieve good results and allow developing countries to deliver **more health for the money**.

Health policy as stewardship

Health policy making in developing countries is seeking a new model of action to increase health and welfare, largely based on the separation of health system stewardship from service delivery through various forms of decentralization (Murray & Frenk 2000; Bossert 1998). Policy making is increasingly being envisaged as a stewardship process concerned with attaining trust and legitimacy between a government and its people towards the improvement of the welfare of populations (Londoño & Frenk 1997; Gilson

2003; Bankauskaite *et al.* 2007; Garret 2007). The *World Health Report 2000* defined stewardship of the health system by national governments as a critical function to realign incentives and to mobilize and allocate resources to achieve the final goals of health gain, financial protection, and responsiveness. Stewardship has also been defined as a function of international agencies to enable co-ordination of health systems at the global level (WHO 2000).

Stewardship is an ethically based, outcome-oriented policy approach and as such it is more interventionist than the economically driven agency approach to state regulation (Fig. 3.3.1). The notion of stewardship, if properly developed, is also consistent with an evidence-based health policy framework (Saltman 2000). A national health strategy based on stewardship can marshal the available evidence to support population-based measures that can improve overall health status. Stewardship capacity is synonymous with the quality of governing institutions within countries, and with the trust that societies place in their governments. In a global climate of increased support for public investments in health, increasing attention is being paid to differentiate countries with 'good' and 'stressed' governance in order to marshal international aid support for policy making.

The process of policy making for the health sector has become increasingly intricate. Health practitioners, policy makers, and planners have to contend with three main issues: **Diversity, complexity, and change**.

There is often great **diversity** within developing countries, as well as between and within different geographical areas. Ecological and geographical factors are recognized as important determinants of health conditions. Economic, social, and cultural determinants also contribute to diversity. The association of poverty, exclusion, and discrimination with poor health status is a consistent finding in both developed and developing countries and has a long research tradition (Evans *et al.* 1994). In general, policy making fails to systematically recognize and act on these determinants. The WHO Commission on Social Determinants of Health is attempting to redress this shortcoming by creating awareness of such determinants among political leaders and stakeholders, and helping countries adopt comprehensive health and development policies oriented towards them (Irwin *et al.* 2006).

Complexity in health needs of populations is another challenge. In contrast with rich countries that experienced a substitution of old for new patterns of disease, developing nations are facing

Characteristic	Agency theory	Stewardship theory

1. Model of man
   Behaviour
	Economic man
	   Self-serving
		Self-actualizing man
		   collective serving

2. Psychological mechanisms
   Motivation
	Lower order/econimic needs
	   (physiological, security, economic)
		Higher order needs (growth,
		   achievement, self-actualization)

Social comparison
   Identification
   Power
	Extrinsic
	   Other managers
	   Low value commitment
	   Institutional (legitimate,
	   coercive, reward)
		Intrinsic
		   Stakeholders
		   High value commitment
		   Personal (expert, referent)

3. Situation mechanisms	Control-oriented	Involvement-oriented

4. Management philosophy
   Risk orientation
   Time frame
   Objective
	Control mechanisms
	   Short-term
	   Cost control
	   Individualism
		Trust
		   Long-term
		   Performance enhancement
		   Collectivism

5. Cultural differences	High-power distance	Low-power distance

Fig. 3.3.1 Comparison of agency theory and stewardship theory. *Source:* Armstrong (1997), adapted from Davis *et al.* (1997).

a triple burden of ill health: First, the unfinished agenda of infections, malnutrition, and reproductive health problems; second, the emerging challenges represented by non-communicable diseases and injuries, which already comprise half the disease burden in low- and middle-income countries; third, the health risks associated with globalization, including the threat of pandemics like AIDS and influenza, the trade in harmful products like tobacco, and other drugs, the health consequences of climate change, and the dissemination of harmful lifestyles.

Annual changes in mortality projections between 2002 and 2020 suggest decreases in tuberculosis of over 5 per cent yet increases of between 2.1 and 3 per cent for HIV/AIDS. Diabetes mellitus and road traffic mortality are projected to increase over 1 per cent per year, an alarming rate (Table 3.3.1). In projections to 2030 (Table 3.3.2), cardiovascular disease will account for 13.4 per cent of the total world mortality and will rank as the first or second cause of mortality in all income regions. Tobacco consumption is largely responsible for many disease trends, and particularly ischaemic heart disease. This is a product of relentless push of industry into new, unregulated contexts susceptible to lifestyle changes.

While knowledge and innovative health technologies have been critical in healthcare in developing countries, the explosion of new technologies designed for rich countries as well as innovations of critical importance to the South such as ARV and IMCI have markedly increased the **complexity of healthcare**. The expanding scope of prophylactic, diagnostic, and therapeutic options demands an increasing range of specific programmes with the associated need for specialist personnel, new categories of support staff, high-technology equipment, and infrastructure. Figure 3.3.2 illustrates the complex interaction of medical and non-medical factors that are involved in perpetuating the high maternal mortality rates occurring in the developing world. It also offers clues as to the package of interventions that are required to reduce maternal mortality (McCarthy & Maine 1992). A particular challenge is a renewed tendency to deliver new technologies through vertical programmes that may fail to support the health system while weakening existing programmes (WHO 1996; Molineaux & Nantulya 2004; Unger et al. 2003; Garret 2006).

The interaction of medical and non-medical factors in the dynamics of health and disease calls for a critical analysis of needs and opportunities as a basis of designing and managing health programmes. Rather than blindly attempting to deliver standardized, pre-packaged, stereotyped interventions, policy makers should try to match the services to suit local needs. Because of the important influence of non-medical factors on health, it is necessary to mobilize inter-sectoral action to complement strictly medical inputs from the health sector. However, policy makers in developing countries should measure their capacity and ensure they first reap their benefits of interventions they can directly control within their health systems (Jamison 2006).

Policy making in developing countries also has to be fluid and dynamic to adapt strategies and programmes to the many **changes** that are occurring in the environment. Two critical changes are accountability and socioeconomic change.

Global as well as national influences are leading towards greater **accountability** of policy makers to parliaments, provincial stakeholders, as well as to donors, clients, and populations. Decentralization has continued its pace giving provincial authorities and

Table 3.3.1 Projected average annual rates of change in age-standardized death rates for selected causes: World 2002–2020

Group	Cause	Average annual change (per cent) in age-standardized death rate	
		Males	Females
All Causes		−0.8	−1.1
Group I		−1.4	−5.3
	Tuberculosis	−5.4	−5.3
	HIV/AIDS	3.0	2.1
	Malaria	−1.3	−1.5
	Other infectious diseases	−3.4	−3.3
	Respiratory infections	−2.7	−3.4
	Perinatal conditions*	−1.7	−1.9
	Other Group I	−3.0	−3.6
Group II		0.0	−0.8
	Cancer	−0.2	−0.4
	Lung cancer	0.1	0.3
	Diabetes mellitus	1.1	−1.3
	Cardiovascular diseases	−1.1	−1.2
	Respiratory diseases	0.3	−0.1
	Digestive diseases	−1.3	−1.7
	Other Group II	−0.7	−1.1
Group III		0.0	−0.2
	Unintentional injuries	−0.2	−0.2
	Road traffic accidents	1.1	1.1
	Intentional injuries	0.2	−0.2
	Self-inflicted injuries	−0.3	−0.4
	Violence	0.4	0.2

[a] Causes adding in the perinatal period as defined in the ICD, principally prematurity and birth asphyxia, and does not include all deaths occurring in the neonatal period (under 1 mol)

Source: Mathers & Loncar (2006).

local officials greater autonomy for innovations but also increased responsibility (Hutton 2002; Bossert 1998). Policy making in the health sector is thus moving from a technical and highly hierarchical approach towards recognizing the role of new actors and processes set in a political and participatory environment.

Changes in the economic and social situation in the country may have a profound effect on the health sector. Health policies have had to be modified in the light of rapid development in some countries and economic recession in others. In the immediate post-World War II era, macroeconomic policies emphasizing central planning and welfare programmes gained popularity. During the 1980s and 1990s, this trend was reversed, with national policies increasingly favouring free market economy in place of welfare programmes and central control. These changes brought about a slow-down in public health sector investments and the introduction of user fees, without visible improvements (Alliance HPSR 2004). Today, international agencies such as the IMF and the World Bank have reversed their policies (WB IMF Development Committee 2003), and funding has been substantially increased aiming to double the level of international aid to support the

Table 3.3.2 Mortality rate rank and percentage of total deaths projected to 2030. World and income regions

Income group	Rank	Disease or injury	Per cent of total deaths
World	1	Ischaemic heart disease	13.4
	2	Cerebrovascular disease	10.6
	3	HIV/AIDS	8.9
	4	COPD	7.8
	5	Lower respiratory infections	3.5
	6	Trachea bronchus, lung cancers	3.1
	7	Diabetes mellitus	3.0
	8	Road traffic accidents	2.9
	9	Perinatal conditions	2.2
	10	Stomach cancer	1.9
High-income countries	1	Ischaemic heart diseases	15.8
	2	Cerebrovascular disease	9.0
	3	Trachea, bronchus, lung cancers	5.1
	4	Diabetes mellitus	4.8
	5	COPD	4.1
	6	Lower respiratory infections	3.6
	7	Alzheimer and other dementias	3.6
	8	Colon and rectum cancers	3.3
	9	Stomach cancer	1.9
	10	Prostate cancer	1.8
Middle-income countries	1	Cerebrovascular disease	14.4
	2	Ischaemic heart disease	12.7
	3	COPD	12.0
	4	HIV/AIDS	6.2
	5	Trachea, bronchus, lung cancers	4.3
	6	Diabetes mellitus	3.7
	7	Stomach cancer	3.4
	8	Hypertensive heart disease	2.7
	9	Road traffic accidents	2.5
	10	Liver cancer	2.2
Low-income countries	1	Ischaemic heart disease	13.4
	2	HIV/AIDS	13.2
	3	Cerebrovascular disease	8.2
	4	COPD	5.5
	5	Lower respiratory infections	5.1
	6	Perinatal conditions	3.9
	7	Road traffic accidents	3.7
	8	Diarrhoeal disease	2.3
	9	Diabetes mellitus	2.1
	10	Malaria	1.8

Source: Mathers & Loncar (2006).

Millennium Development Goals. Government capacity is being revamped to ensure efficiency and equity in investments.

Countries face different degrees of resource development, of government control, and of public and private investment. These dimensions define a spectrum of country situations that goes from the accumulated conditions of poverty and underdevelopment seen in low-income countries, to the emerging conditions most notably seen in middle-income countries (Fig. 3.3.3). This chapter focuses on eight critical issues along this spectrum:

1. Health reform with special emphasis on structural reform and decentralization

2. Tools for policy making—burden of disease, national health accounts, and performance assessment

3. Financing healthcare—SWAPs and health insurance

4. Human resources for health

5. Public–private contracting

6. Equity in health

7. International agencies and public–private partnerships

8. Health research

Health reform

The rapid advances in health technologies, the increasing demands and expectations of populations, and the escalating costs of healthcare are challenging governments both in developed and developing countries. Governments are responding to these changes and the associated challenges by undertaking reforms of the health sector.

Structural reform

Health sector reform has been defined as the sustained and purposeful change to improve efficiency, equity, and effectiveness of the health sector (Berman & Bossert 2000; Roberts *et al.* 2003). Reforms have also been equated with comprehensive and integral change at the structural, programmatic, organizational, and instrumental levels of the health system (Frenk 1994; Gonzalez Block 1997).

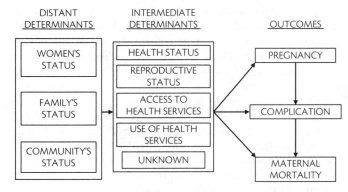

Fig. 3.3.2 Interaction of factors involved in the epidemiology of maternal mortality.
Source: McCarthy & Maine (1992).

COMPONENT	TYPE OF CHALLENGE	
	Accumulated	Emerging
Population	◆ **Epidemiological backlog** 　◆ Common infections 　◆ Malnutrition 　◆ Reproductive health 　　problems ◆ **Health gap** ◆ **Inequity**	◆ **New pressure** 　◆ Non-communicable diseases 　◆ Injuries 　◆ Emerging infections ◆ **Changes in demand patterns** ◆ **Political pressures**
Institutions	◆ **Insufficient coverage** ◆ **Poor technical quality** ◆ **Allocational inefficiency** ◆ **Inadequate patient 　referral** ◆ **Deficient management 　of institutions**	◆ **Cost escalation** ◆ **Inadequate incentives** ◆ **Financial insecurity** ◆ **Patient dissatisfaction** ◆ **Technological expansion** ◆ **Deficient management 　of the system**

Fig. 3.3.3 Challenges facing health systems in developing countries, by population and institutional components.
Source: Londoño & Frenk (1997).

At the **structural** level, changes such as the universalization of access to services, new financing arrangements and the separation of stewardship and delivery functions have been critical. In turn, reforms at the **programmatic** level may include the definition of specific service rights and predefined packages of interventions through explicit choices based on a calculus of benefits and costs. Changes at the **organizational** level may involve increasing provider choice and introducing provider payment mechanisms to promote quality and efficiency. At the **instrumental** level, reforms may imply increasing reliance on research, evaluation, and monitoring mechanisms, as well as incentives for human resource and technology development.

Health reforms require the development of monitoring mechanisms to ensure the attainment of objectives in the mid to long term. Such mechanisms should pay attention both to the technical and the ethical components of health reforms. A number of technical areas for monitoring and decision making have been identified. These areas include effective coverage; general level and distribution of health conditions; general level and distribution of responsiveness; and fair financing (see below under Performance Assessment) (WHO 2000). This framework was successfully used for monitoring and evaluation purposes at the subnational level in the recent reform experience of the Mexican health system (Frenk *et al.* 2006).

The ethical monitoring of health sector reforms has been enabled through a set of benchmarks of fairness (Daniels *et al.* 1996). These benchmarks identify and measure the degree of fairness of health systems and of the different objectives pursued by health reforms. While this approach was developed to assess reforms brought about by managed care in the United States, it has been tested in several developing countries with some success (Daniels *et al.* 2005).

Decentralization

The decentralization of the planning and management of health services from national authorities to provincial governments is a common feature of structural reforms. However, we are witnessing new trends towards recentralizing services, due both to an assessment

of past strategies but more importantly as a result of scaling-up efforts for disease control.

Especially in large countries with dispersed populations, governments cannot efficiently manage the delivery of healthcare from their central offices. In a decentralized system, the central Ministry of Health can set national goals and targets, whilst devolving the responsibility for detailed management of the services to local authorities. Such arrangements promise improved allocative and technical efficiency, organizational innovation to meet local needs, improved service quality as well as greater equity together with transparency, accountability, and legitimacy for the health sector as a whole. Three questions are critical to assess the effectiveness of decentralization: (a) The amount of choice that is transferred from central institutions to institutions at the periphery of health systems, (b) what choices local officials make with their increased discretion, and (c) what effect these choices have on the performance of the health system; see Fig. 3.3.4 and Table 3.3.3 (Bossert 1998).

Beyond the administrative form that decentralization takes (deconcentration, delegation, or devolution), policy making depends on the relationships established between diverse actors and on the various influences they can exert on each other.

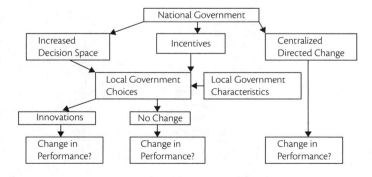

Fig. 3.3.4 Decision space and changes in performance in a decentralized healthcare system.
Source: Bossert (1998).

Decentralization entails the establishment of principal–agent relationships, whereby the principal transfers responsibilities but tries to maintain overall control, for example, on the kind of services provided, their quality and the equity attained (Bossert 1998). Information, assessment, and monitoring instruments are therefore critical for the success of decentralization reforms. Economic theories based on the choice that consumers have on the consumption of public resources have been useful to understand decentralization in developed countries. However, under conditions of meagre resources there is less local political and economic competition. More importantly perhaps is the reliance on trusted institutions at the local level and the strengthening of their capacity to ensure common interests across the multiple actors and often multiple principals that exert influence on health service providers (Gilson 2003).

Decentralization has not been without its critics, arguing that it has been often imposed upon local governments as a means of reducing central government obligations (Ugalde & Homedes 2006). The assessment of the effects of decentralization is now leading to recentralize a number of health functions in both rich and poor countries. This is the case of hospital administration in Norway (Bankauskite *et al.* 2007) and of public health surveillance in Mexico. Of greater significance for recentralization, however, is the increased funding by global health initiatives for disease control programmes such as malaria and HIV/AIDS. A new breed of vertical programmes is thus emerging, with forceful central funding, planning, and supervision yet relying on often decentralized primary healthcare services for their implementation. This approach has demonstrated benefits for the specific diseases being tackled, yet it threatens other programmes and the capacity of local authorities to meet broad health needs (Garrett 2007).

Tools for policy making

Policy making in developing countries has not always been guided by the best available evidence. In the immediate post-independence period, some developing countries copied models of health services in developed countries with particular emphasis on specialized curative care and the construction of large tertiary hospitals. The high cost of maintaining such establishments often distorted the national health budget, leaving very little resources for supporting less expensive but highly effective community-based services. Because of severe resource constraints, developing countries should set clear priorities and adopt policies that help achieve maximum improvement in health in return for minimum expenditure.

The establishment of priority lists of disease conditions and interventions was relatively easy in the traditional epidemiological situation where a few major conditions, mainly acute infectious diseases, accounted for a high proportion of deaths. In such situations one could rank priorities by considering the mortality rates from specific acute infectious diseases or the prevalence of chronic disabling diseases like onchocerciasis, a blinding disease. The process of priority setting has become more complex with the epidemiological transition and the increasing differentiation of health systems.

Efficient decision making for the allocation of scarce resources for health interventions requires setting priorities in terms of a

Table 3.3.3 Comparing the decision space in Ghana, Philippines, Uganda, and Zambia

Functions	Range of choice		
	Narrow	**Moderate**	**Wide**
Financing			
Source of revenue	Zambia	Ghana, Uganda	Philippines
Expenditures		All four	
Income from fees		Ghana, Zambia, Uganda	Philippines
Service organization			
Hospital autonomy	Ghana, Zambia	Uganda	Philippines
Insurance plans	Ghana, Uganda		Zambia, Philippines
Payment mechanisms	Ghana, Uganda	Philippines	Zambia
Contracts with private providers		Ghana, Zambia, Philippines	Uganda
Human resources			
Salaries	All four		
Contracts	Ghana,	Philippines	Zambia, Uganda
Civil service	Ghana	Zambia, Uganda, Philippines	
Access rules	Ghana	Zambia, Uganda, Philippines	
Governance			
Local government	Ghana, Zambia		Uganda, Philippines
Facility boards	All four		
Health offices	Ghana, Philippines	Zambia, Uganda	
Community participation	Ghana, Uganda	Zambia Philippines	
Country totals			
Ghana	11	4	0
Zambia	5	7	3
Uganda	5	7	3
Philippines	3	7	5

Source: Bosser & Buveais (2000).

wide range of considerations (Musgrove 1999, Gericke *et al.* 2005), to include: (i) The potential health impact and cost of interventions; (ii) the 'public good' character of interventions as well as their externalities and their consequence for catastrophic expenditure in the absence of public interventions; (iii) anti-poverty and equity considerations; and (iv) the capacity of health systems to implement new interventions

Burden of disease and priority setting

Health measures are critical for policy making, in general, and for priority setting, in particular. One of the most widely applied indexes used to measure health needs is disability adjusted life years (DALYs), which combines losses from premature death and from disability (Murray 1994 a,c).

The most common use of the DALY is simply to rank diseases and conditions by the burden of disease that they contribute, thus highlighting their relative importance for population health. The DALY is also being used to measure the burden of disease attributable to specific risk factors such as tobacco and obesity. On the basis of such measures, DALYs have been used to assess the impact of major control programmes and to estimate cost-effectiveness of interventions by comparing the cost of averting a DALY across them. In its 2000 World Health Report, WHO published data on Healthy Life Expectancy (HALE), which is defined as the average number of years that a person can expect to live in 'full health' by taking into account years lived in less than full health due to disease and/or injury.

The DALY approach has been critiqued by several authors with respect to technical, methodological and conceptual issues (Schneider 2001). The data required to estimate the DALY is extensive and is not always available to the extent necessary or with the required quality in developing countries. This has led to the use of questionable assumptions, such as the use of data for non-representative population segments. Another difficulty with the DALY is the combination of death and disability measures under the assumption that these phenomena lie on the same continuum along time (Anand & Hanson 1997).

Most critique of the DALY has centred on the large number of value-based judgements necessary to assign unequal age weights, to estimate the discounting of future health years, as well as to establish the disability weights (Anand & Hanson 1997). Furthermore, disability is quantified with respect to the limitation that diseases impose on individual functionality and does not consider pain and suffering.

The DALY is proving a useful tool but more work is required to refine and simplify it. Under the guidance of WHO, low- and middle-income countries are striving to improve the quality of data collection so as to improve the accuracy of national estimates of burden of disease. Some middle-income countries like Sri Lanka, Mexico, and Brazil are already making effective use of these tools (Morrow & Bryant 1995; Hyder *et al.* 1998). In Tanzania, the burden disease approach was adapted to prioritize interventions in the rural districts of Morogoro and Rufiji. After a 5-year period of offering a package of essential health services, under-5 mortality rates had declined by 40 per cent, to less than 100 deaths per 1000 live births, in contrast with the child mortality rate for the country as a whole which remained in 160 deaths during the period of the intervention (deSavigny *et al.* 2004).

The public good character of interventions offers another criterion for priority setting. Public investment will be justified if the interventions do not have sufficient supply or demand. Such is the case for vector control or environmental risk surveillance. However, even if there is some private supply and demand, the public intervention would be justified if it can be demonstrated that enlarging services would benefit an even wider population beyond that which is consuming the service directly. Such is the case of immunizations, where individual consumption offers herd immunity to populations at large.

The risk by the poor or the near-poor of incurring catastrophic expenditures when seeking healthcare or as a result of disability to work is in itself a reason to invest public resources. Indeed, in Mexico, around 3 million households suffer impoverishing or catastrophic health expenditures annually, a situation that led the government to implement the programme Seguro Popular de Salud (Popular Health Insurance) as a means of universalizing public insurance (Knaul & Frenk 2005).

The condition of poverty of specific population groups is in itself an important criterion to consider for allocating resources on a priority basis. However, poverty in itself is not a reason to provide services indiscriminately, as scarce resources would not be used efficiently in the fight against poverty. This is why it is ethically acceptable to provide a package of highly cost-effective services for the poor, so long as the package is also acceptable to the poor themselves.

The criteria thus far considered for prioritizing public investments in health interventions can be summarized in Fig. 3.3.5, which suggests that investments should be spent on public goods only when they are cost-effective and when they have inadequate private supply and demand. Interventions that particularly benefit the poor should also be prioritized, as are those threatening with catastrophic health expenditure. Vertical and horizontal equity will not always be compatible with cost-effectiveness, leaving decision making open to political criteria (Musgrove 1999).

The setting of priorities to invest in specific interventions should also consider the capacity of the health systems to formulate appropriate programmes and to deliver on the ground. Assessing health system capacity is today paramount, as new interventions are being scaled-up for the control of malaria, TB, and HIV/AIDS, among other diseases. These interventions require human, technical, and material resources that are often lacking. Four dimensions have been proposed for the assessment of the organizational and economic context (Gericke *et al.* 2005): (i) Technical characteristics of interventions; (ii) the logistical and delivery requirements; (iii) the requirements stemming from governmental regulation; and (iv) the characteristics of demand and utilization.

Technical characteristics of interventions include the basic design of products and technologies, such as stability and shelf-life. Product standardization is critical as similar interventions will be more easily implemented. Costs that are incurred during implementation but that may not have been considered in cost-effectiveness analysis include safety monitoring, supervision, storage and regular, on-time delivery. Regulatory costs can be considerable, such as accreditation of health providers and facilities to ensure service quality as well as measures to curb corruption. Often the costs necessary to ensure compliance and coercion are not considered when formulating new programmes, leading to low enforcement of measures to increase quality and efficiency. Finally, priority setting should consider the ease of use of technologies by the population at large, including the extent to which health education is required to ensure demand and compliance. Ease of use may also be related

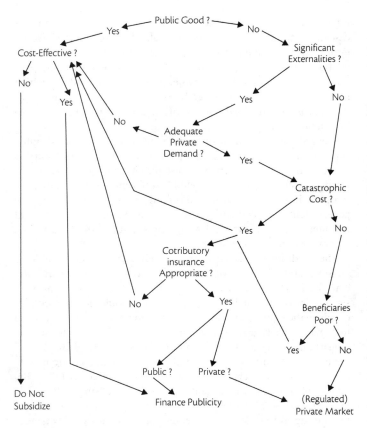

Fig. 3.3.5 Decision tree for assessing public investments in health.
Source: Musgrove (1999).

to the proliferation of black markets and forgery for which countermeasures should be implemented.

National health accounts

In the past, policy makers concentrated mainly on spending within the public sector, ignoring private spending through insurance, corporate arrangements, and employees' schemes, and out-of-pocket spending. Furthermore, spending within the public sector lacked clear indicators on resource flows, thus contributing to growing inequity and inefficiency. Policy makers now obtain a more comprehensive view of health expenditures thanks to the use of national health accounts developed through a uniform methodology. These analyses integrate health spending from all sources—public and private, corporate, and personal—within comprehensive accounts. National health accounts can affect the choices made within the public sector but also influence the role of public agencies in providing guidelines to the private sector and to communities regarding the most cost-effective uses of their investments and expenditures.

Health accounts consist of a basic matrix, where the columns list all sources of health spending—public (taxation and national social insurance), and private sources including employment-based schemes, privately financed insurance, and out-of-pocket expenditure. The rows of the matrix show the distribution of expenditure for personal healthcare, public health, and environmental sanitation services, and administration. Disaggregating the items in the columns and rows generates more elaborate analyses, providing more detailed information about sources and spending. Thus, the analyses could show variations over time, by geography, by population

sub-groups, or any other variable that is relevant to policy making (Berman 1997; WHO 2003). Today, health accounts are being prepared not only at the national level but also by specific programmes such as HIV/AIDS and reproductive health.

Health system performance assessment

The *World Health Report 2000* offered a comprehensive methodology and reported results to assess the overall performance of health systems in terms of health gain, responsiveness to the legitimate expectations of the population, and fairness of financing (WHO 2000). These outcomes are conceived as the direct consequence of the health system functions of stewardship, financing, resource generation, and service provision (Fig. 3.3.6). The three health system outcomes were assessed in terms of equity and efficiency, except financial fairness for which only equity is appropriate. Health gain was measured through healthy life expectancy, already described under the priority setting section above. The methodology enabled the measurement of each health system goal separately as well as through a combined indicator. All WHO member countries were then ranked as a means of highlighting the benefits and limitations of health system designs as well as to promote analysis and improvements.

Performance assessment can support policy making in monitoring and evaluating attainment of critical outcomes and the efficiency of the health system in a way that allows comparison overtime and across systems. Performance assessment enables to measure the relationship between design of health systems and outcomes and to disseminate evidence on the benefits of diverse health system designs and reforms. The use of a widely accepted, comparative method was intended to feedback the policy debate as well as to empower the public with information relevant to their well-being (Murray & Evans 2003).

The methodology for performance assessment was widely debated by academics and governments. It was argued that intersectoral action for health was not subject to monitoring, focusing only on those functions and outcomes that are more directly under the control of ministries of health. Given that health sector policy making may be the result of actions taken in an indefinite past, it will not be clear whose actions are being assessed at any given point in time.

Perhaps most controversial was the lack of consensus on the weighting that was given to each of the three separate dimensions of performance, where following a Web survey, health gain was assigned 50 per cent and responsiveness and financial protection 25 per cent each. Data used for the 2000 report was also faulted for excessive use and lack of clarity of the estimations that were necessary, given poor data quality and availability in many countries.

Performance assessment has been widely endorsed as a tool for policy making for developing countries and, as mentioned above, was the basis for the monitoring of health sector reform in Mexico. However, improvements need to be made. Greater attention should be placed to the broader health system as well as to the relationship between measured outcomes and health system functions. Inequality should be more broadly measured, to include both health as well as socioeconomic inequality. Sub-national analyses should be carried out to identify success and limitations that can be more easily disseminated at the national level. Furthermore, national health information systems need to be strengthened as tools for performance assessment through the development of a broad range of health metrics (WHO 2007).

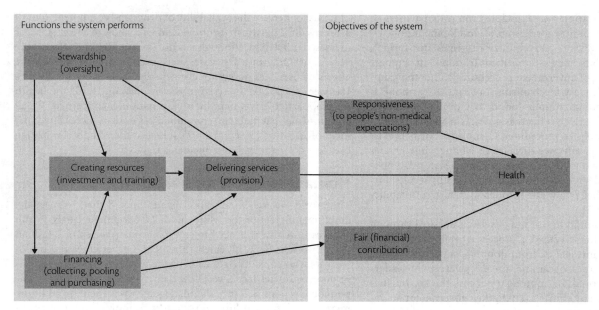

Fig. 3.3.6 Functions and objectives for the measurement of health system performance.
Source: WHO (2000), Fig. 2.1.

Mexico demonstrates how middle-income countries with reasonably developed information systems can make use of data for health system performance assessment. From 2000 to 2006, a set of health conditions and service benchmarks were systematically measured at state level and disseminated at yearly intervals. Evidence indicates that state authorities agreed on the quality and relevance of these measures and have accepted on this basis to be systematically monitored by federal health authorities and interested actors. Systematic monitoring has also led to the development of effective coverage measures, defined as the proportion of potential health gain that could be delivered by the health system to that which is actually delivered (Lozano *et al.* 2006). A total of 14 health interventions have been monitored and overall effective coverage assessed through a comprehensive indicator. Overall coverage ranged from 54 per cent in Chiapas, a poor state, to 65.1 per cent in Mexico's capital. These findings suggest that basic health interventions are much more equitably distributed in Mexico with respect to other health indicators.

Financing and contracting for healthcare

During the 1980s, international financing agencies restrained public investments in health as part of structural adjustment programmes with negative consequences for health systems. These policies have now been reversed as the UN enshrined the Millennium Development Goals (MDGs) with important health targets for maternal and child health as well as HIV/AIDS, TB, and malaria among other epidemic diseases. MDGs served as a basis on which to mobilize national and international resources (WB IMF Development Committee 2003). Also, the Commission on Macroeconomics and Health, convened by WHO under the leadership of Jeffrey Sachs, produced analytical data advocating massive investments in health as a means of spurring economic growth (Commission on Macroeconomics and Health 2001). The Monterrey Consensus agreed at the 2002 UN Financing for Development Conference intends to double the level of international aid through

an additional US$20 billion per annum to enable poor countries to achieve the MDGs (Sachs 2004).

Scaling up health financing in poor countries

Government capacity is now being revamped in many countries to ensure that massive scaling-up of health interventions can be undertaken under conditions of efficiency and equity. However, before interventions can be scaled up, low-income countries under stress—essentially countries with low governance—will have to strengthen their institutional capacity to ensure efficient and equitable resource allocation. It has also been recommended that resources be allocated to interventions whose delivery is least covered by the market so as to increase the impact of government services (Filmer *et al.* 2000).

The IMF and World Bank estimate that large increases in aid (a doubling or more of current flows) could be used effectively in countries with good governance such as Bangladesh, India, Indonesia, Pakistan, and Vietnam, and in some sub-Saharan African countries, such as Ethiopia. These countries have a combination of good policies and prospects for further improvement, large unmet needs relative to the MDG targets, and relatively low levels of aid dependence. Sub-Saharan African countries considered to have good governance such as Burkina Faso, Mozambique, Tanzania, and Uganda could also use additional aid productively to supplement the sizable flows they already receive—an increase of about 60 per cent on average in the medium-term.

Evidence suggests that international short-term health aid is indeed supporting economic growth, regardless of the strength of governments (Clemens *et al.* 2004). Effective low-cost health interventions have also been effectively put in place and sustained in countries with weak governments or even under conflict situations (Medlin *et al.* 2006; Center for Global Development 2007).

Aid harmonization and sector-wide approaches

Donors and recipient countries have achieved a high degree of consensus regarding the provision of international aid. The Paris Aid

Harmonization Declaration and Principles commits partners to recognize developing country ownership of development policies, and the alignment of donors with country strategies, institutions, and procedures. This implies a commitment by donors to support capacity strengthening of government procedures, rather than supporting specific aid delivery mechanisms. In terms of harmonization, the Paris declarations commit donors to a more harmonized, transparent, and collectively effective giving through common arrangements and simplified procedures. Complementarity is to be sought through a more effective division of labour while greater attention should be paid to aid provision in fragile states. Aid policies should be devised so that they can be managed by results, furthering collaborative behaviour and through mutual accountability (Paris Declaration 2005).

Donor harmonization in health has also been pursued through Sector Wide Approaches (SWAps), a process whereby funding for the sector—whether internal or from donors—supports a single policy and expenditure programme, under government leadership, and adopting common approaches across the sector. It is generally accompanied by efforts to strengthen government procedures for disbursement and accountability. A SWAp should ideally involve broad stakeholder consultation in the design of a coherent sector programme at micro, meso, and macro levels, and strong co-ordination among donors and between donors and government. (Brown *et al.* 2001).

Health insurance and financial protection

Attention is increasingly being paid on how to finance healthcare for the more than 1.3 billion rural poor and informal sector workers in low- and middle-income countries without financial protection against the catastrophic costs of healthcare. Community health insurance has been proposed to improve access by rural and informal sector workers to needed heath care. Macro-level cross-country analyses give empirical support to the hypothesis that risk-sharing in health financing matters in terms of its impact on both the level and distribution of health, financial fairness, and responsiveness indicators (Preker *et al.* 2003; Alliance HPSR 2004).

Five key policies are available to governments to improve the effectiveness and sustainability of community financing schemes:

◆ Increased and well-targeted subsidies to pay for the premiums of low-income populations

◆ Insurance to protect against expenditure fluctuations and re-insurance to enlarge the effective size of small risk pools

◆ Effective prevention and case management techniques to limit expenditure fluctuations

◆ Technical support to strengthen the management capacity of local schemes

◆ Establishment and strengthening of links with the formal financing and provider networks

Middle-income countries with segmented health systems face particular challenges to extend insurance coverage to a rising population employed in the informal sector. New schemes have been implemented aiming at universal access to care through voluntary, government-subsidized schemes. Short-term assessments point to success (Gaikidou *et al.* 2006).

It is clear now that where user fees are established, critical factors for success in utilization are exemptions for the poor and the retention of funds to increase the availability of drugs and equipment. Out of a review of 22 African countries, only 8 showed clear signs of increased utilization, although it is not known how fees affected the very poor. Only in a few cases were exemptions instituted. The effects of user fees on equity are negative (Alliance HPSR 2004). User fees should be analysed in the overall context of the health system, particularly where their elimination is concerned. Illegal and informal payments in the public system are increasingly the focus of attention (Savedoff 2007). It is clear that simply eliminating user fees does not lead to reducing charges.

Human resources for health

The World Health Organization has estimated that, to meet the ambitious targets of the Millennium Development Goals, health services in Africa will need to train and retain an extra 1 million health workers by 2010, chiefly nurses and other classes of health workers who constitute the bulk of the workforce. Health systems in poor countries face a very low density health workforce, compounded by poor skill mix and inadequate investment. In addition, migration of trained human resources to more developed countries is becoming an ever more important issue.

Mass migration of health personnel is often a symptom of the 'sick system syndrome', in which many essential components of healthcare services are malfunctioning and mismanaged. Policies on migration must tackle the 'pull factors', which induce trained personnel to seek better living conditions abroad, as well as the 'push factors', which make disaffected and frustrated health workers seek employment elsewhere. Health challenges, such as the HIV/AIDS epidemic, impose additional pressures on health workers in their workplaces and at home, exposing them to contagious hazards, which adversely affect the morbidity and mortality of the workforce. The 'anchor factors' which encourage workers to remain in public service are important too. These should include financial incentives as well as well designed training programmes, that increase workers' skill and competence, boost their morale, increase their job satisfaction, and improve the performance of services (Lucas 2005).

Effective policy making for human resources has to overcome the low attention that is given by both national governments and international agencies. Fiscal discipline depends on restriction of staff numbers and compensation levels, with staff salaries now consuming 60–80 per cent of diminished public budgets in the health sector. There is also a lack of coherent and integrated investment strategies to strengthen the workforce, resulting in an over-emphasis on workshops and training sessions that have an unclear effect. Such constraints operate in a context of health-sector and civil-service reforms that have altered the work environment through expansion of the private sector, downsizing, and decentralization in the public sector. Public–private contracting has thus been increasingly sought after as a means of addressing multiple constraints.

An informal global network of health leaders supported by the Rockefeller Foundation's Joint Learning Initiative has proposed four immediate steps towards a reinvigorated human resources for health policy (Joint Learning Initiative 2004):

◆ Large-scale advocacy to achieve heightened political awareness within countries and globally, leading to a social mobilization to respond to the crisis in the short term.

♦ Improve information and develop a commonly accepted framework of ideas, terms, and relations to guide analysis for policy formulation, particularly on the mobility of health professionals and the relations between health equity and human resources.

♦ Learn from history and identify success stories demonstrating the goodwill and commitment of health workers in spite of adverse conditions. Lessons from BRAC in Bangladesh are highlighted, employing over 30 000 village health workers to raise awareness of health issues among the rural poor.

♦ Address the supply, demand, and mobility of personnel, linking across training and education, health systems, and labour markets to develop a system that ensures continuity of policies over time. This includes a process of addressing low wages, as well as creating an incentive structure that supports providers over the course of their working lives.

International debate around the responsibilities of all actors has also produced an interesting range of proposals, including ethical recruitment guidelines and financial compensation for exporting countries. (Brush *et al.* 2004). Diagnostic approaches are required to inform evidence-based action: Identify signs and causes of the 'sick system syndrome'. These should lead to develop and adopt policies on human resources which are relevant, affordable, and sustainable, and are realistic about migration of trained staff (Lucas 2005).

Policy making and the public–private mix

The private health sector may be defined as comprising all providers who exist outside the public sector, whether their orientation is philanthropic or commercial, and whose aim is to treat illness or prevent disease (Mills *et al.* 2002). However, the public and private sectors are highly related as public sector workers often have a private practice and many public facilities offer private wards or services or operate in such a manner that they are indistinguishable from profit-seeking private providers (Meng *et al.* 2004).

As stated previously, even in developing countries with a widespread public system such as Mexico, catastrophic or impoverishing out-of-pocket health expenditures, which imply an extensive use of private medical services, affect a large proportion of the population (Knaul & Frenk 2005). In these contexts, it is vital to support consumers in their use of health services. Such efforts could stimulate appropriate demand through improving consumer information or could make services or products more affordable. Efforts can also influence the supply of services through creating institutions that give consumers greater authority to challenge care of poor quality (Mills *et al.* 2002, Soderlund *et al.* 2003).

Social marketing is an approach to stimulate demand of cost-effective interventions by increasing consumer information and subsidizing access to services. This approach has been particularly used to demand services within the private sector for reproductive health and basic sanitation. Limitations have been identified with regard to the extent to which social marketing stimulates or rather limits the private sector, the targeting of the poor, and leakage of benefits to the better-off who could afford to pay full-price for health services and commodities.

The use of vouchers has been tested on a limited scale as a means of targeting the poor without having to provide a generic subsidy. Protection of patients has also been pursued through the establishment of specialized government agencies to facilitate the settlement

of malpractice and negligence, attempting to reduce the costs and negative consequences of litigation (Tena & Sotelo 2005).

Efforts on the supply side to improve the quality and value of private providers have included the promotion of professional training and accreditation as well as giving access to their patients to a limited range of public goods or services as for the treatment of TB (Marek *et al.* 1999). However, the most important efforts have been in the area of purchasing or contracting of a full range of primary or hospital services for specific population groups. These functions involve the separation of purchasing and provision at the government level and exercising stewardship functions, as already noted at the beginning of this chapter. The main challenge with these approaches lies in the capacity by government to develop contracts, set prices, and monitor and supervise private providers (Slack & Savedoff 2001; Palmer *et al.* 2003).

Equity in health

Policy makers in most developing countries are aware that poverty and ill health are intertwined and that important differences in health exist both across countries and provinces and across socio-economic groups (Figs 3.3.7 and 3.3.8). It is now accepted that poverty breeds ill health and that ill health keeps poor people poor (Fig. 3.3.7). The concept of equity in health is based on a fundamental principle: That differences in health that are the result either of the exposure to unhealthy life or working conditions or limited access to essential health services are morally unacceptable (Whitehead 1990; Dahlgren & Whitehead 1991).

Inequality in the health status of individuals and communities is a global phenomenon. Such disparities have been observed even in the most affluent countries but are most striking in developing countries where the poorest citizens often lack access to the most basic healthcare. Efforts to reduce such disparities have only been partially successful and too little is known on the reasons behind failure (Wagstaff 2002).

Equity can be assessed in three complementary dimensions: In health status of families, communities, and population groups; in allocation of financial, technical, and material resources and, in access to and utilization of high-quality services. Attention must be paid to political commitment towards equity and to equitable policy formulation To this end, information, monitoring, and evaluation for equity should be in place. Each of these dimensions of equity and of their political and policy dimensions are now considered.

The basic dimensions of health equity

Gross inequality in health status is regarded as prima facie evidence of inequities in the healthcare system. Significant inequalities in health status are found even in the most affluent developed countries, with long traditions of national health services that are designed to provide universal coverage (Black *et al.* 1998; Pollock 1999). A consistent finding is the strong association between poverty and poor health as defined by such indicators as the expectation of life, the incidence of acute diseases and injuries, the prevalence of chronic diseases and disabilities, and low access to services (Gwatkin 2000; Wagstaff 2002).

This consistent association of poverty with ill health makes it necessary for health systems to address the needs of the poor, and it strengthens the case in favour of programmes for the alleviation of poverty as important strategies for health promotion. It also draws

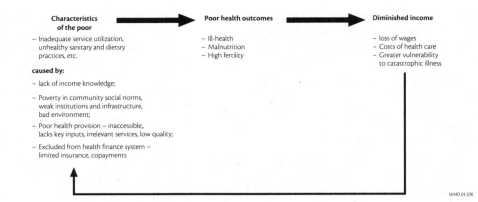

Fig. 3.3.7 The cycle of health and poverty.
Source: Wagstaff (2002).

attention to the influence of factors outside the health sector on health development: Education especially of girls, access to adequate quantity of safe water, environmental sanitation; as well as food and nutrition. Lifestyle and human behaviour, including such personal choices like smoking, use of alcohol, sexual behaviour, and physical exercise, also have important effects on health outcomes (Gwatkin 2003).

Equity is also examined in terms of the allocation of resources to different sections of the population. On moral and ethical grounds, the objective of allocative equity is for public resources to be shared out in a fair manner (Taipale 1999). The simplest formula would be a uniform per capita allocation. However, if large differences in health status already exist, an equal allocation would tend to perpetuate the inequalities. It can be argued that it is the responsibility of governments to perform a re-distributive function by allocating resources from the more affluent sector of society to meet the needs of lower-income individuals and families, the so-called vertical equity already mentioned when addressing priority setting, above.

Another view of equity is that everyone should have an equal opportunity of receiving care. This so-called horizontal equity proposes that individuals in like situations should be treated in like manner. Access is often defined in terms of the availability of services and its geographical coverage but experience has shown that the potential access, i.e. the services are within geographical range, does not necessarily correspond to real access as measured by the utilization of services (Jacobs & Price 2006).

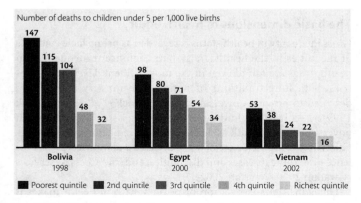

Fig. 3.3.8 Inequalities in under-5 mortality rates within socioeconomic groups of selected developing countries. 1998–2002.
Source: Gwatkin *et al.* (2003).

Marked disparities are often found in the geographical distribution of health facilities: Between regions, between urban and rural areas, between rural areas and within urban areas. (Phillips 1990). The differential ratios of persons per facility—hospital beds, nurses, and doctors—are used to measure the disparities. The distribution of health centres and other institutions in relation to the population—how far people have to travel to reach such facilities—are also used to indicate the uneven distribution of resources.

Political commitment for equity and equitable policy formulation

The political commitment of the government is the essential basis for promoting equity in health (Feacham 2000). The objective of equity in health fits well with the political philosophy in welfare states that have the clear goal of providing universal coverage of comprehensive healthcare for the entire population 'from the womb to the tomb'. In such countries, the question is not whether the State should embrace equity in health but how to achieve this goal in practice. Many developing countries have adopted more limited but realistic goals of providing universal access to a cost-effective package of services, together with universal financial protection through social health insurance (Frenk *et al.* 2006). In Mexico, a package of essential health services was devised using cost-effectiveness criteria as a priority-setting tool. However, the package was also a means to ensure that all citizens, regardless of their labour or socioeconomic status, have the right to universal access to healthcare. The Mexican model may be seen as reconciling two extremes: The selective, technocratic approach to the distribution of healthcare, which provides practical alternatives but is usually morally neutral, and the rights-based approach, which has a strong value foundation but has lacked operational support (Frenk & Gómez-Dantés 2007).

Political commitment for equity is also required to correct the inequities that result from discrimination on the basis of gender, race, ethnic group, and religion. Often, inequalities in health status reflect the marginalization of disadvantaged groups (Brockerhoff & Hewett 2000). The plight of indigenous populations in the Americas and Australasia is a special case.

In weighing policy options, a good guideline would be to examine critically the expected impact of the selected option on equity. The formulation of health policies has to contend with a variety of pressures including the increasing demands of populations for more services, the desire to achieve maximal improvement in health of the populations served, and the need to contain costs. Reforms of the health sector aim at improving efficiency, effectiveness, cost-effectiveness, and equity. It is not always easy to reconcile these goals. For example, the delivery of care to the populations in remote areas is relatively expensive and less cost-effective than services to dense urban areas. However, in the interest of equity, health services should reach the underserved populations even in remote settings.

The impact of macroeconomic policies on health also deserves attention. For example, under pressure from the international finance agencies, some developing countries undertook Structural Adjustment Programmes (SAP) and markedly reduced public investment in health and other social sectors. UNICEF (2004) and other agencies drew attention to negative impact of SAP on the health of children. In future, careful analysis and relevant research would be used to design macroeconomic policies that would not harm the health of vulnerable groups. The international community has responded to this problem by adopting policies for alleviating poverty. Debt relief for the poorest nations has been one of the major mechanisms for alleviating poverty.

One aspect of equity is that the government should allocate financial resources fairly to the entire population. A simple demographic formula that allocates funds simply on population size may need to be adjusted to take note of special needs of particular regions; otherwise, the uniform allocation may tend to perpetuate inequalities. Another source of inequity is the degree to which local authorities can raise additional funds through taxation and by retaining user fees (Brikci & Phillips 2007). Again, the fact that the more affluent areas are able to raise much larger funds than the poorer areas may tend to widen the gap in the quantity and quality of healthcare.

Within the health budget, there is the difficult task of allocating resources to the needs of the various groups within the community. (Castro-Leal et al. 2000; Makinen et al. 2000) With finite resources, even the most affluent nations have to accept limits to the services that the public sector can provide. Hence, rationing is an inevitable feature of health planning. In the interests of equity and social justice, if economies have to be made, the burden should be fairly shared among various sectors of the community. Quantitative estimates of burden of disease and of the cost-effectiveness of various interventions help to rationalize the selection of priorities (Murray 1994a,b,c; Hyder 1998). But a point is reached at which hard choices cannot be made solely on the basis of objective measurements. At this stage, the debate must include philosophical and ethical considerations about the value of human life (Morrow & Bryant 1995).

The Poverty Reduction Strategy Papers (PRSPs) are a promising avenue to focus policy making on the poor, although much needs to be done to influence health policy making through this strategy (Laterveer et al. 2003). The majority of PRSPs lack country-specific data on the distribution and composition of the burden of disease, a clear identification of health system constraints and an assessment of the impact of health services on the population. More importantly, they make little effort to analyse these issues in relation to the poor. Furthermore, only a small group explicitly includes the interests of the poor in health policy design. Attention to policies aiming at enhancing equity in public health spending is even more limited. Few papers that include expenditure proposals also show pro-poor focused health budgets.

Tools are available to trace the extent to which investments at national levels benefit the poor and needy, taking into consideration the effects on income and health and considering the relative size of benefits given the levels of health and income (Gwatkin 2000, 2003). The better-off in Africa and in India benefit far more than the poor from public spending (Castro Leal et al. 2000). Recent analyses in Mexico suggest that the incidence of health benefits is improving for the poor thanks to financial reforms, although still inequitable (Frenk et al. 2006). However, analysis of a wide range of evidence suggests that tax-based funding distributes health benefits more evenly and targets the poor more effectively than social health insurance (Wagstaff 2007).

New tools are also being developed to forecast demand for global health funding of programmes benefiting the poor (Sekhri 2006). These efforts stem from the realization that the lack of accurate and credible information about the demand for essential health products costs lives. Gaps and weaknesses in demand forecasting result in a mismatch between supply and demand—which in turn leads to both unnecessarily high prices and supply shortages.

Equity information, monitoring, and evaluation

In order to design services that are equitable and to monitor performance of health services, each health authority needs an appropriate management information system which must include measuring inequalities in health status and inequities in access to healthcare. The data collecting instruments must be designed to take note of groups and sub-groups especially vulnerable groups whose access to services is restricted by geographical, economic, social, and cultural factors. It should include the usual demographic indicators—age, sex, and marital status, as well as socioeconomic indicators—race, ethnic origin, occupation, residence, and other social variables (Rosen 1999).

The health system should include mechanisms for monitoring equity objectively. Interest in measuring equity has generated some useful tools and some valuable experience is accumulating. In the first instance, monitoring equity is the responsibility of health authorities at each level of care. They must build into their service, sensitive indicators that would inform them of their performance with regard to equity and access to care.

In addition to such internal processes, it would be valuable to commission independent reviews of equity within the health system by groups outside the health departments. Another option would be to assign responsibility for a national equity watch to a local non-governmental organization.

International organizations

International organizations are influential in developing country policy in many conditions. A new breed of agencies, the Global Health Programs and the Public–Private Partnerships (PPPs) are also increasing their influence, particularly through financing health interventions.

UN agencies

The World Health Organization is the lead agency for health within the United Nations system. In recent years, other international agencies have increased their involvement in the health sector. The United Nations Children's Fund (UNICEF) through its child survival programme, provides massive input into the health sector often in collaboration with WHO. Other UN agencies like the United Nations Fund for Population Action (UNFPA), the International Labour

Organisation (ILO), and the Food and Agricultural Organisation (FAO) have relevant programmes involving specific aspects of the health sector. Through its lending programme, the World Bank represents an important source of external finance for the health sector and has stimulated countries to develop more efficient and cost-effective health programmes.

Generally, these external agencies operate independently of each other at country level but there have been some attempts at co-ordination and collaboration. UNICEF and WHO have established mechanisms of collaboration including such formal mechanism as the Task Force for Child Survival. WHO also sometimes executes health programmes on behalf of other external agencies. A more ambitious attempt at inter-agency collaboration is the UNAIDS programme; six UN agencies jointly manage this programme for the global control of HIV/AIDS epidemic.

Global Health Programmes and public–private partnerships

There has been a proliferation of Global Health Programmes (GHPs) and public–private partnerships, with more than 70 in existence. They account for close to 20 per cent of international aid for health. Examples include Roll Back Malaria (RBM); the Global Alliance on Vaccines and Immunization (GAVI), the International AIDS Vaccine Initiative. (IAVI) and the Global Fund for AIDS, TB and Malaria (GFATM). The vast majority focus on communicable diseases—60 per cent of identified GHPs target the big three diseases—HIV/AIDS, TB, and malaria—with HIV/AIDS attracting the most GHPs by some margin. However, almost all the 'most neglected' diseases (such as lymphatic filariasis and leishmaniasis) are now supported by at least one GHP, many of which have been established in recent years. No GHPs address non-communicable diseases, or health systems per se.

Africa has the highest number of GHPs per country, followed by Asia (East, Southeast, and Central). GHPs vary substantially in scale, cost, operational structure, and impact on systems at country level, including research and development as well as technical assistance and service support. GHPs which support improved service access may provide discounted or donated drugs, and give technical assistance. Some GHPs are dedicated to advocacy for increased international and/or national response and resource mobilization. The Global Fund is dedicated to financing for specific disease programmes.

GHPs are generally considered to deliver positive results in the following areas: Leverage of additional funds (including from private sector); promotion of global public goods; raising profile of neglected issues; more inclusive governance; enhanced aid effectiveness through pooling of resources, and reduced commodity prices. On the other hand, common criticisms levelled at GHPs are the creation of additional complexity in an international aid system that is already overloaded. For certain GHPs, poorer countries do not meet eligibility criteria or have the capacity to frame successful proposals. Other limitations include the distortion of national priorities; the provision of international aid made ad hoc and less predictable; dysfunctional national coordination mechanisms; the establishment of parallel structures or additional burden on existing national systems; displacement of existing government services; disproportionate demands on time of Ministers and senior officials; national strategic planning and budgeting processes

undermined, and diminished political accountability (Buse & Wasxman 2001; Widdus 2003).

Health research

In many respects, health policy in developing countries is all about the encouragement of innovation and the scaling-up of life-saving technologies and system processes. As highlighted previously, increased access to knowledge and technology has accounted for perhaps as much as two-thirds of the 2 per cent per year rate of decline in under-5 mortality rate (Jamison 2006). Furthermore, there is increasing realization that research and evaluation can play a valuable role for shared learning from health sector reforms (González Block 1997).

The case has been made that it is as unethical to introduce health reforms that have not been previously validated or thoroughly analysed as it is to introduce untested medical technology into healthcare. Indeed, both can have important health consequences, even more so population interventions that are adopted on a massive scale (Daniels 2006). WHO has recognized that 'Ignoring research evidence is harmful to individuals and populations, and wastes resources' (WHO 2004).

Health research—including health policy and systems research—thus plays a double role in policy making. As a core function of health systems, research contributes knowledge as one of the most critical resources for healthcare. Formulating and implementing health research policy is therefore a key component of health policy overall. On the other hand, research on health policy and systems contributes knowledge and applications to improve the way that societies organize themselves to respond to health problems and challenges (Alliance HPSR 2004). Such knowledge is today one of the scarce resources limiting health system performance.

Health research systems and policy

WHO together with the Council on Health Research for Development and the Global Forum for Health Research advocating health research policy through the development of health research systems at national level and through a well- structured international architecture (Pang *et al.* 2003). Health research systems should be strengthened by building relevant capacity, developing capable leadership, providing essential monitoring and evaluation tools, improving capacity for ethical review of research, and putting in place necessary ethical standards and regulations for population health, health services, and clinical research. Health systems should further promote access to reliable, relevant, and up-to-date evidence on the effects of interventions, based on systematic reviews of the totality of available research findings (WHO 2004).

Health research systems provide a promising opportunity to link knowledge generation with practical concerns to improve health and health equity. Pioneer health research systems from Canada and the UK show that academic centres and service agencies can be related in ways that encourage the utilization of research (Lomas 2000; Henkel *et al.* 2006), such as networking between existing stakeholders (Department of Health 2006). A key issue is the balance between funding research through independent research councils that have science-led priorities and funding research in response to the priorities of healthcare systems.

New science frameworks are solving these dilemmas through positing a move from the traditional discipline-centred mode of knowledge production (characterized as Mode 1), towards a broader conception (Mode 2) where knowledge is generated through a context of application and thus addresses problems identified through continual negotiation between actors from a variety of settings (Gibbons *et al.* 1994). Another conceptualization, Pasteur's Quadrant, suggests how types of research can be considered according to two dimensions, a quest for understanding and considerations of use. This gives rise to three categories of research depending on the extent to which general understanding arises in the process of solving specific problems, or whether only pure knowledge or pure application is generated (Stokes 1997).

Evidence-based policy making

The new science frameworks are being applied to policy making though novel strategies such as the interfaces and receptor model (Hanney *et al.* 2003) or the 'linkage and exchange' model proposed by the Canadian Health Services Research Foundation (Lomas 2000). Such strategies are promoting collaborative approaches to organizing health research systems. It has also promoted the use of knowledge brokers between researchers and policy makers. In the end, demonstrating the benefits or research for policy making and for population health and national well-being will be critical (Hanney & Gonzalez Block 2006).

Evidence-based policy making can be made a reality if research and analysis is carefully introduced along the critical steps of issue identification, policy development, implementation, monitoring, evaluation, and feedback. Evidence can provide the rationale for an initial policy direction; it can set out the nature and extent of the problem, suggest possible solutions, look to the likely impacts in the future, and evidence from piloting and evaluation can provide motivation for adjustments to a policy or the way it is to be implemented (Campbell *et al.* 2007).

Conclusion

Policy making for the design, implementation, and management of effective, efficient, and equitable health systems is today more critical than ever to address the developing country health challenges. Health policy is being called not only to address the pressing needs of infectious diseases and malnutrition and the emerging problems of violence, lesions, tobacco, and obesity. New challenges are being addressed, including the fight against poverty and the increasing global threats. The belief that sound health policy making can contribute to democracy, economic growth, and global security has influenced the availability of greater financial resources for health. However, relaxing this constraint has now brought much greater awareness to needs in key areas such as human resources and health system strengthening and research.

The information now being produced can provide valuable guidance to policy makers, although it also threatens to overpower capacities in poor countries. Not only must policy making be knowledge-based—it must also be result-oriented. Careful planning and skilled management can achieve good results even where financial resources are limited. The countries that have achieved good health at low cost challenge other countries to adapt and adopt relevant aspects of their policies.

Policy makers must give high priority to strategies that will eliminate the major items of the unfinished agenda that still plague many developing countries. Many lives can be saved and much

disability prevented by measures like boosting immunization programmes, ensuring access to adequate supplies of safe water and good sanitation, by providing effective treatment for common childhood ailments, and ensuring skilled care during childbirth including emergency obstetric care (Center for Global Development 2007). More daunting tasks include the pandemic of HIV/AIDS and the emerging non-communicable challenges, which may require complex and expensive care. Experience has shown that some progress can be made through the application of social and behavioural interventions, that can act on those risks that are responsible for the increasing burden of disease associated to chronic ailments and injuries in the developing world.

Key points

◆ Health policy making in developing countries is intricately related to global health policies and actors.

◆ Health financing is increasing, thanks to policy advocacy, but more resources and improved governance are required to meet the Millennium Development Goals.

◆ Policy tools are available to support decision making at national and global levels.

◆ Equity and efficiency trade-offs should be addressed on the basis of sound research and health research systems.

References

Alliance AHPSR (2004). *Strengthening health systems: The role and promise of policy and systems research*. Alliance AHPSR, Geneva, Switzerland.

Ameratunga, S., Hijar, M., and Norton, R. (2006). Road-traffic injuries: Confronting disparities to address a global-health problem. *Lancet*, **367**, 1533–40.

Armstrong, J.L. (1997) Stewardship and public service. Ottawa, Canadian Public Service Commission, (discussion paper).

Anand, S. and Hanson. K. (1997). Disability-adjusted life years: A critical review. *Journal of Health Economics*. Dec; **16**(6), 685–702.

Bankauskaite, V., Dubois, H.F.W., and Saltman, R. (2007). Patterns of decentralization across European health systems. In *Decentralization in health care* (eds. R. Saltman *et al.*), pp. 22–43. WHO, UK.

Berman, P.A. (1997). National health accounts in developing countries: Appropriate methods and recent applications. *Health Economics*, **6**, 11–30.

Berman, T.J. and Bossert, T. (2000). *A decade of health sector reform in developing countries: What have we learned?* Data for Decision Making Project. IHSG. Harvard School of Public Health.

Black, D., Morris, J.N., Smith, C. *et al.* (1998). Better benefits for health: plan to implement the central recommendation of the Acheson report. *British Medical Journal*, **318**, 724–7.

Bossert, T. and Beauvais, J.C. (2002). Decentralization of health systems in Ghana, Zambia, Uganda and the Philippines: A comparative analysis of decision space. *Health Policy and Planning*, **17**, 14–31.

Bossert, T., Larrañaga, O., Giedion, U. *et al.* (2003). Decentralization and equity of resource allocation: Evidence from Colombia and Chile. *Bulletin of the World Health Organization*, **91**, 95–100.

Bossert, T. (1998). Analyzing the decentralization of health systems in developing countries: Decision space, innovation and performance. *Social science & medicine*, **47**, 1513–27.

Brikci, N., Philips, M. (2007). User fees or equity funds in low-income countries. *Lancet*, **369**(9555), 10–11.

Brockerhoff, M. and Hewett, P.C. (2000). Inequality of child mortality among ethnic groups in sub-Saharan Africa. *Bulletin of the World Health Organization*, **78**, 30–41.

Brown, A.M. Foster, A., Norton, A. et al. (2001). *The status of sector-wide approaches*. Working Paper 142. ODI, London.

Brush, B., Sochalski, J., and Berger, A. (2004). Imported care: Recruiting foreign nurses to US health care facilities. *Health Affairs*, **23**(5).

Buse, K. and Waxman, A. (2001). Public–private health partnerships: A strategy for WHO. *Bulletin of the World Health Organization*, **79**(8).

Campbell, S., Benita, S., Coates, E. et al. (2007). *Analysis for policy: Evidence-based policy in practice*. Government Social Research Unit, HM Treasury, London.

Castro-Leal, F., Dayton, J., Demery, L. et al. (2000). Public spending on health care in Africa: Do the poor benefit? *Bulletin of the World Health Organization*, **78**(1), 66–74.

Centre for Global Development (2007). *Millions saved: Proven successes in global health*. 2007 Edition. CGD, Washington.

Cleland, J. and Van Ginneken, J. (1989). Maternal schooling and childhood mortality. *Journal of biosocial science*, **10**(Suppl.), 13–34.

Clements, M., Radelet, S., and Bhavnani, R. (2004). *Counting chickens when they hatch: The short-term effect of aid on growth*. Working Paper 44, Center for Global Development, Washington DC.

Commission on Macroeconomics and Health (2001). *Macroeconomics and Health: Investing in Health for Economic Development—Report of the Commission on Macroeconomics and Health*. December 20, World Health Organization, Geneva.

Dahlgren, G. and Whitehead, M. (1991). *Policies and strategies to promote equity in health*. WHO Regional Office, Copenhagen.

Daniels, N. (2006). Toward ethical review of health system transformations. *American Journal of Public Health*, **96**, 3.

Daniels, N., Flores, W., Pannarunotha, S. et al. (2005). An evidence-based approach to benchmarking the fairness of health-sector reform in developing countries. *Bulletin of the World Health Organization*, **83**(7), 534–539.

Daniels, N., Light, D.W., and Caplan, R.L. (1996). *Benchmarks of fairness for health care reform*. Oxford University Press, New York.

Dare, L. and Reeler, A. (2005). Health systems financing: Putting together the 'back office'. *British Medical Journal*, **331**, 759–62.

De Savigny, D., Kasale, H., Mbuya, C. et al. (2004). *Fixing health systems*. IDRC, Ottawa.

Denis, J. and Lomas, J. (2003). Convergent evolution: The academic and policy roots of collaborative research. *Journal of Health Services Research & Policy*, **8**, 1–6.

Department of Health (2006). *Best research for best health: A new national health research strategy*. London.

Davis, J., Donaldson, L., Schoorman, D. (1997) Towards a stewardship theory of management. Academy of Management Review, **22**(1), 20–47.

Evans, R., Barer, M., and Marmor, T. (1994). Why are some people healthy and others not? The determinants of health of populations. Aldine de Gruyter, Hawthorne (NY).

Feacham, R.G.A. (2000). Poverty and inequity: A proper focus for the new century. *Bulletin of World Health Organization*, **78**(1), 1.

Filmer, D., Hammer, J.S., and Pritchett, L.S. (2000). Weak links in the chain: A diagnosis of health policy in poor countries. *World Bank Research Observer*, **15**(2), 199–224.

Frenk, J. and Gómez-Dantés, O. (2007). La globalización y la nueva salud pública. *Salud publica de Mexico*, **49**(2), 156–164.

Frenk, J. (1994). Dimensions of health system reform. *Health Policy*, **27**(1), 19–34.

Frenk, J., Bobadilla, J., Sepúlveda, J. et al. (1989). Health transition in middle-income countries: New challenges for health care. *Health Policy and Planning*, **4**(1), 29–39.

Frenk, J., Gonzalez-Pier, E., Gómez-Dantes, O. et al.(2006). Comprehensive reform to improve health system performance in Mexico. *Lancet*, **368**, 1524–34.

Frenk, J., Lozano, R., and Gonzalez Block, M.A. (1994). *Economía y salud: propuestas para el avance del sistema de salud en México*. Fundación Mexicana para la Salud, 1994, Mexico, DF.

Gakidou, E., Lozano, R., González-Pier, E. et al.(2006). Assessing the effect of the 2001–06 Mexican health reform: An interim report card. *The Lancet*, **368**(9550), 1920–35 E.

Garret, L. (2007). The challenge of global health. *Foreign Affairs*, **86**, 14–38.

Gericke, C.A., Kurowski, C., Ranson, M.K. et al. (2005). Intervention complexity – a conceptual framework to inform priority-setting in health. *Bulletin of the World Health Organization*, **83**, 285–293.

Gibbons, M., Limoges, C., Nowotny, H. et al. (1994). *The new production of knowledge: The dynamics of science and research in contemporary societies*. Sage, London.

Gilson, L. (2003). Trust and the development of health care as a social institution. *Social Science & Medicine*, **56**, 1453–68.

Gonzalez-Block, M.A. (1997). Comparative research and analysis methods for shared learning from health system reforms. *Health Policy*, **42**, 187–209.

Gwatkin, D.R. (2000). Critical reflection: Health inequalities and the health of the poor: What do we know? What can we do? *Bulletin of the World Health Organization*, **78**(1), 3–18.

Gwatkin, D.R. (2003). How well do health programmes reach the poor? *Lancet*, **361**, 540–1.

Hanney, S. and González-Block, M.A. (2006). Building health research systems to achieve better health. *Health Research Policy and Systems*, **4**, 1–6. www.health-policy-systems.com/content/4/1/10

Hanney, S.R., Gonzalez-Block, M.A., Buxton, M.J. et al. (2003). The utilisation of health research in policy-making: Concepts, examples and methods of assessment. *Health Research Policy and Systems*, **1**: 2.

Harrison, K. (1997). The importance of the educated healthy woman in Africa. *Lancet*, **349**, 588.

Hecht, R.M. and Shah, R. (2006). Recent trends and innovations in development assistance for health. In *Disease Control Priorities in Developing Countries* (eds. D.T. Jamison, J.G. Breman, A.R. Measham, G. Alleyne, M. Claeson, D.B. Evans et al.), 2nd edition, pp. 3–34. Oxford University Press for The World Bank, 2006, Washington, DC.

Hutton, G. (2002). *Decentralization and the sector-wide approach in the health sector*. SDS, Basel.

Hyder, A.A., Rotllant, G., and Morrow, R.H. (1998). Measuring the burden of disease: Healthy life-years. *American Journal of Public Health*, **88**, 196–202.

Irwin, A., Valentine, N., Brown, C. et al. (2006). The Commission on social determinants of health: Tackling the social roots of health inequities. *PLoS medicine*, **3**(6), e106. doi:10.1371/journal.pmed.0030106.

Jacobs, B. and Price, N. (2006). Improving access for the poorest to public sector health services: Insights from Kirivong Operational Health District in Cambodia. *Health Policy Plan*, Jan, **21**(1), 27–39.

Jamison, D.T. (2006). Investing in Health. In *Disease control priorities in developing countries* (eds. D.T. Jamison, J.G. Breman, A.R. Measham, G. Alleyne, M. Claeson, D.B. Evans et al.), 2nd edition, pp. 3–34. Oxford University Press for The World Bank, 2006, Washington, DC.

Joint Learning Initiative (2004). *Human resources for health. Overcoming the crisis*. Harvard University Press, Cambridge.

Knaul and Frenk (2005). Health insurance in Mexico: Achieving universal coverage through structural reform. *Health Affairs*, **24**, 1467–76.

Kogan, M., Henkel, M., and Hanney, S. (2006). *Government and research: Thirty Years of evolution*, 2nd edition. Springer, Dordrecht.

Laterveer, L., Niessen, L.W., and Yazbeck, A.S. (2003). Pro-poor health policies in poverty reduction strategies. *Health Policy Plan*, **18**, 138–45.

Lavorack, G. and Labonte, R. (2000). A planning framework for community empowerment goals within health promotion. *Health Policy and Planning*, **15**(3), 255–62.

Lomas, J. (2000). Using 'linkage and exchange' to move research into policy at a Canadian Foundation. *Health Affairs*, **19**, 236–40.

Londono, J. and Frenk, J. (1997). Structured pluralism: Towards an innovative model for health system reform in Latin America. *Health Policy*, **41**(1), 1–36.

Lopez, A.D., Mathers, C.D., Ezzati, M. *et al.* (2006). Global and regional burden of disease and risk factors, 2001: Systematic analysis of population health data. *Lancet*. Jul 29; **368**(9533), 365.

Lozano, R., Soliz, P., Gakidou, E. *et al.* (2006). Benchmarking of performance of Mexican states with effective coverage. *The Lancet*, **368** (9548), 1729–41.

Lucas, A.O. (2005). Human resources for health in Africa. Better training and firm national policies might manage the brain drain. *British Medical Journal*, 5 November, **331**, 1037–8.

Lucas, A.O. (1992). Public access to health information as a human right. *Proceedings of the International Symposium on Public Health Surveillance. Morbidity & Mortality Weekly Report*, **41**, 77–8.

Makinen, M., Waters, H., Rauch, M. *et al.* (2000). Inequalities in health care use and expenditures: Empirical data from eight developing countries and countries in transition. *Bulletin of the World Health Organization*, **78**, 55–65.

Marek, T., Diallo, I., Ndiaye, B. *et al.* (1999). Successful contracting of prevention services: Fighting malnutrition in Senegal and Madagascar. *Health Policy and Planning*, **14**(4), 382–9.

Mathers, C.D. and Loncar, D. (2006). Projections of global mortality and burden of disease from 2002 to 2030. *PLoS Medicine*, **3**(11), e442. doi:10.1371/journal.pmed.0030442

McCarthy, J. and Maine, D. (1992). A framework for analyzing the determinants of maternal mortality. *Studies in family planning*, **23**, 23–33.

Medlin, C.A., Chowdhury, M., Jamison, D.T. *et al.* (2006). Improving the health of populations: Lessons of experience. In *Disease control priorities in developing countries* (eds. D. Jamison *et al.*), The World Bank, Washington DC.

Meessen, B., Van Damme, W., Kirunga Tashobya, C. *et al.* (2006). Poverty and user fees for public health care in low-income countries: lessons from Uganda and Cambodia. *The Lancet*, **368**, 2253–7.

Meng, Q., Shi, G., Yang, H. *et al.* (2004). *Health policy and systems research in China*. UNICEF/UNDP/World Bank/WHO. Special Programme for Research and Training in Tropical Diseases (TDR), Geneva.

Mills, A., Brugha, R., Hanson, K. *et al.* (2002). What can be done about the private health sector in low-income countries? *Bulletin of the World Health Organization*, **80**, 325–30.

Molineux, D. and Nantulya, V. (2004). Linking disease control programmes in rural Africa: A pro-poor strategy to reach Abuja targets and Millennium Development Goals. *British Medical Journal*, **328**(7448), 1129–32.

Morrow, R.H. and Bryant, J. (1995). Health policy approaches to measuring and valuing human life: Conceptual and ethical issues. *American journal of public health*, **85**, 1356–60.

Murray, C.J. (1994a). Quantifying the burden of disease: The technical basis for disability-adjusted life years. *Bulletin of the World Health Organization*, **72**, 429–45.

Murray, C.J. (1994b). National health expenditures: A global analysis. *Bulletin of the World Health Organization*, **72**, 623–37.

Murray, C.J. (1994c). Cost-effectiveness analysis and policy choices: Investing in health systems. *Bulletin of the World Health Organization*, **72**, 663–74.

Murray, C.J.L. and Evans, D.B. (eds.)(2003). *Health systems performance assessment: Debates, methods and empiricism*. WHO, Geneva.

Musgrove, P. (1999). Public spending on health care: How are different criteria related? *Health Policy*, 47.

Narasimhan, V., Brown, H., Pablos-Mendez, A. *et al.* (2004). Responding to the global human resources crisis. *Lancet*, **363**(9419), 1469–72.

Palmer, N., Mills, A., Wadee, H. *et al.* (2003). A new face for private providers in developing countries: What implications for public health? *Bulletin of the World Health Organization*, **81**(4), 292–7.

Pang, T., Sadana, R., Hanney, S. *et al.* (2003). Knowledge for better health—a conceptual framework and foundation for health research systems. *Bulletin of the World Health Organization*, **81**(11).

Paris declaration on AID effectiveness Ownership, Harmonisation Alignment Results and Mutual Accountability Paris, 2 March 2005.

Phillips, D.R. (1990) '*Health and health care in the third world*. Chapter 4. Longmans, UK.

Population Reference Bureau (2004). *Improving the health of the world's poorest people*. Population Reference Bureau, Washington.

Pollock, A.M. (1999). '*Devolution and health: challenges to Scotland and Wales*'. *British Medical Journal*, **319**, 94–8.

Preker, A.S., Carrin, G., Dror, D. *et al.* (2002). Effectiveness of community health financing in meeting the cost of illness. *Bulletin of the World Heaflth Organization*, **80**(2), 143–50.

Preker, A.S., Suzuki, E., Bustero, F. *et al.* (2003). *Costing the Millennium Development Goals*. Background paper to The Millennium Development Goals for Health: Rising to the Challenges, World Bank, Washington, DC.

Roberts, M.J., Hsiao, W., Berman, P., Reich, M.R. (2004). Getting Health Reform Right: A guide to Improving Performance and Equity. Oxford University Press, New York.

Rosen, M. (1999). Data needs in studies on equity in health and access to care—ethical considerations. *Acta Oncologica*, **38**, 71–5.

Sachs, J. (2004). Health in the developing world: Achieving the Millennium Development Goals. *Bulletin of the World Health Organization*, Dec; **82**(12) 947–952.

Saltman, B. and Ferroussier-Davis, O. (2000). On the concept of stewardship in health policy. *Bulletin of the World Health Organization*, **78**(6), 732–9.

Savedoff, W.D. (2007). *Transparency and corruption in the health sector: A conceptual framework and ideas for action in Latin America and the Caribbean*. Inter-American Development Bank, Health Technical Note 03/2007, Washington, DC.

Schneider, M. (2001). *The setting of health research priorities in South Africa*. South African Medical Research Council, Burden of Disease Research Unit, Johannesburg.

Sekhri, N. (2006). *Forecasting for global health: New money, new products & new markets*. Background Paper for the Forecasting Working Group. Center for Global Development, Washington.

Slack, K., Savedoff, W.D. (2001). '*Public purchaser-private provider contracting for health services: Examples from Latin America and the Caribbean*'. Sustainable Development Department Technical Paper 111, Inter-American Development Bank, Washington, DC.

Söderlund, N., Mendoza-Arana, P., and Goudge, J. (2003). *The new public/ private mix in health: Exploring the changing landscape*. Alliance for Health policy and Systems Research, Geneva.

Spiegel, J.M. and Yassi, A. (2004). Lessons from the margins of globalization: Appreciating the Cuban health paradox. *Journal of public health policy*, **25**(1), 85–110(26).

Stokes, D.E. (1997). *Pasteur's quadrant: Basic science and technological innovation*. Brookings Institute, Washington DC.

Taipale, V. (1999). 'Ethics and allocation of health resources—the influence of poverty on health'. *Acta Oncologica*, **38**(1), 51–5.

Tena–Tamayo, C. and Sotelo, J. (2005). Malpractice in Mexico: Arbitration not litigation. *British Medical Journal*, 20 August; **331**, 448–51.

Unger, J.P., De Paepe, P., and Green, A. (2003). A code of best practice for disease control Programmes to avoid damaging health care services in developing countries. International *Journal of Health Planning and Management*, **18**, S27–S39.

Ugalde, A. and Homedes, N. (2006). Decentralization: The long road from theory to practice. In *Health services decentralization in Mexico. A case study in state reform* (eds. A. Ugalde and N. Homedes). Center for US-Mexico Studies, La Jolla.

UNICEF (2004). *Progress for children. A child survival report card: Number 1*.

Whitehead, M. (1990). The concepts and principles of equity and health. WHO Regional Office, Copenhagen.

Wagstaff, A. (2002). Poverty and health sector inequalities. *Bulletin of the World Health Organization*, **80**(2), 97–105.

Wagstaff, A. (2007). *Social health insurance reexamined*. World Bank Policy Research Working Paper 4111, January.

WHO (2000). 'Health systems: Improving performance'. World Health Report 2000, WHO, Geneva.

WHO (2003). *Guide to producing national health accounts with special applications for low-income and middle-income countries*. WHO, 2003, Geneva.

WHO (2004). *Knowledge for better health: Strengthening health systems*. The Mexico Statement on Health Research from the Ministerial Summit on Health Research. Mexico City, November 16–20.

WHO (2004). Ministerial Summit (Web). World Health Organization. World Health Report 2004. *Changing history*. WHO, 2004, Ginebra.

WHO (2005). *Preventing chronic diseases: A vital investment*. WHO, Geneva.

WHO (2006) Human resources for health: The World Health Report 2006, Working Together for Health. WHO, 2006, Geneva.

WHO (2006) *Investing in Health Research and Development. Report of the Ad Hoc Committee on Health Research Relating to Future Intervention Options*. WHO, Geneva.

WHO (2007). Health Metrics Network Biennial Report 2005/2006. WHO, Geneva.Widdus, R. (2003). Public–private partnerships for health require thoughtful evaluation. *Bulletin of the World Health Organization*, **81**(4), 235.

World Bank–IMF Development Committee (2003). *Supporting sound policies with adequate and appropriate financing*. Discussion paper, World Bank, Washington DC.

3.4

Leadership in public health

Manuel M. Dayrit and Maia Ambegaokar

Introduction

Imagine that tomorrow you were suddenly appointed into a prominent health leader position in your country—as a Director of Department or perhaps even Minister of Health. Upon taking office, you are presented with the following urgent dilemmas by your chief advisers:

◆ We are suffering perennial outbreaks of water-borne diarrhoea in the urban slums of our largest city, caused by the illegal tapping of water lines. How can we prevent this in both the short and long terms?

◆ Other departments are preventing us enacting any measures to stop smoking in public places. How can we convince them to collaborate on this critical health issue?

◆ How can we take steps to provide anti-retrovirals for the tens of thousands of our citizens suffering from HIV/AIDS?

◆ Our government is in moral opposition to abortion, despite scientific evidence showing that decriminalizing abortion prevents maternal deaths from sepsis. Illegal abortion is high in our country. What action should we take?

How would you proceed to address these issues? Would you be able to think on your feet and respond promptly and effectively to the health needs of your populace? In other words, are you capable of being a public health leader?

These questions are examined below as we explore the nature of leadership and the possibility of learning it.

Chapter overview

There is growing recognition of the importance of leadership in public health. This is reflected in recent domestic and international initiatives to train or 'develop' leaders in the health sector (Cardenas *et al.* 2002; Saleh *et al.* 2004; Umble *et al.* 2005; Wright *et al.* 2001), to identify the skills and personal qualities of leaders (NHS Leadership Centre 2006; Wright *et al.* 2000), and to assess the effect of different types of leadership on outcomes (Firth-Cozens & Mowbray 2001; Xirasagar *et al.* 2005). In this chapter, we examine what is involved in public health leadership and illustrate our themes with experiences from the working lives of some contemporary health sector leaders. We set four tasks: To define the difference

between management and leadership; to describe the core competencies and personal characteristics of leaders; to discuss whether leadership can be taught; and to demonstrate why leadership is so important in public health. We argue that it is the complex, multi-organizational, and team-based nature of health work that necessitates leadership at many levels in order to result in success.

The broader goal in this chapter is to present the reader with the information required to forge a personal 'path to leadership'. There is an urgent need around the world for strong public health leaders to promote the health of populations, particularly the poor and vulnerable. Unfortunately, calls for stronger and better leadership are often taken as imprecise and unachievable demands. In this chapter, we attempt to circumvent that accusation by demonstrating that effective leaders have existed and continue to exist in health, and that strong leadership can be encouraged and developed. In addition, we have built the chapter on findings from interviews with individual health sector leaders.

We look in detail at the way in which the perception of leadership has evolved over the years. Having established the important distinction between 'management' and 'leadership', we explore three different aspects of leadership: the competencies of leadership; the personal characteristics of recognized leaders; and the broad division of leadership styles into either transactional or transformational. We then look to the question of whether leadership can be taught, examining existing methods and frameworks for leadership instruction and development, and we investigate how to measure leadership ability and assess the impact made by individual leaders. Finally, we compare the more theoretical findings of our chapter with public health leadership in practice, discovering the complex nature of the reality faced by public health leaders today.

At the end of the chapter, we turn to the targeted reader of this book—an early-to-mid-career public health worker—and suggest ways to develop his or her own 'path to leadership'. We urge the aspiring health leader not to forget the inseparable link between what is needed for leadership to occur and the kind of principled leadership most required in global health today.

Among the chapter's most important points:

◆ There is a distinction between leadership and management. Leadership has to do with the visionary activities of setting direction, while management has to do with the controlling tasks associated with implementation.

◆ Public health leaders need to be able to imagine and create evidence-based change. They need to be able to influence and lobby key actors for support of their public health agenda. They must operate across disciplinary and organizational boundaries, and they must be skilled at developing and working through diverse teams.

◆ Leaders are not simply born. Public health leaders can be developed by means of team-based training, mentoring and repeated practice of leadership skills at all levels and all types of public health organization. The aspiring health leader can create her or his path to leadership.

◆ Public health challenges are often politically and procedurally complex and do not lend themselves to simple medical or technical solutions. A set of guiding principles will help the leader to define appropriate actions.

Evolution of thinking about leadership

A century or so ago, thinking about leadership focused on the inherent personality of the individual and 'his or her characteristics and traits . . . were thought to be hereditary' (*Turning Point* 2001, p. 14).

*This 'Great Man Theory' approached leadership capacities as innate, fixed and cross-contextual. Skills and competencies as learned activities were disregarded. Instead, they were thought to be anchored in some internal personality or genetic set with which one was born. . . .[T]his earlier understanding of leadership [also] focused on the leader as solitary actor, as if the followers or context had no role in the leadership situation. (*Turning Point* 2001, p. 14)*

This 'great leader' theory has certainly been invoked in the health sector. For example, Halfdan Mahler, a former head of the World Health Organization, and James Grant, a former head of UNICEF, were widely thought to have innate leadership qualities that largely explained the success of their agendas. It is true, as the experiences described in our interviews demonstrate, that leaders are often people who are willing to take risks and to do things that defy convention. However, research and thinking on the question of leadership moved on in the middle of the twentieth century to consider the skills and competencies that anyone in a leadership position, regardless of personality, might develop in order to influence followers to take desired actions.

More recently, the focus has been on leaders as those who can see the way forward in the context of complexity and constant change. For a leader, achieving results in such a context requires not just the use of skills that will enable individuals to get things done, but also the ability to facilitate disparate group efforts by collaborating and sharing the leadership task:

*. . . [W]e have shifted from a view of leader as sole or unitary actor to a team or community centred view of leadership, . . .[and] the social and economic times of most organizations have produced a demand for skills and abilities that are as complex as the situations in which they are found. The rapid change has moved leadership from a hierarchical model of leadership into collaborative models. (*Turning Point* 2001, p. 15)*

In public health, the collaborative approach may be a necessity, as discussed in a later section of this chapter dealing with the complexity inherent in public health practice. This shift in the way of thinking about leadership—from a top-down model to a participatory one—has been similar to that in the way of thinking about organizational management. So what is the relationship between management and leadership?

Leadership is not the same as management

Much literature and research conflate leadership and management, but the two are not identical.

'Management' derives from the Latin word 'manus' (meaning hand) and the subsequent Italian word 'maneggiare' (to control, often horses). In effect, the origin of 'management' is manifest in Ben Hur's epic chariot races—it concerns the control of unruly beasts. 'Leadership', however, is from the Old German word 'Lidan' and the Old English derivation 'lithan' (to travel, to show the way, to guide). (Grint 2002, p. 248)

This distinction between the controlling tasks associated with implementation and the visionary activities associated with setting a direction is a useful, if simplified, way of defining management as compared to leadership. In practice, the two are often linked, in a single individual or in a particular job description. As a result, separating the characteristics of good leadership from those of good management is not straightforward.

To a certain extent, the confusion arises because historical reviews of research on leadership often begin with the early research on what makes a good manager. For example, Stone and Patterson (2005) begin with Max Weber's interest in bureaucratic hierarchies as an efficient solution to getting things done in the workplace. This led to Classical Management Theory, with its emphasis on using the bureaucracy to achieve objectives, and Scientific Management theories with their focus on 'control, ruthless efficiency, quantification, predictability, and de-skilled jobs' (Stone & Patterson 2005, p. 2). In this context, managers who could organize and direct workers below them in the hierarchy were crucial. There was little emphasis, during this period in the early part of the twentieth century, on the behavioural aspects of organizations. Instead, workers were seen as machine-like, and managers needed only to establish and oversee the correct procedures. By the middle of the twentieth century, management theorists shifted their focus to the factors that motivate people at work and the ways in which managers could harness motivation to achieve results. 'A new theory of organizations and leadership began to emerge based on the idea that individuals operate most effectively when their needs are satisfied' (Stone & Patterson 2005, p. 3). In this context, good managers were perceived as those who could do more than structure the work and give orders. They also needed to inspire their workers to lead them.

The tendency to link the characteristics of good managers with those of leaders is thus partly the result of changes in the understanding of the role of a manager. Still, the distinction between the leadership role and the managerial role is widely perceived as the difference between vision and implementation. Table 3.4.1, for example, shows one typical set of divisions.

These distinctions between leaders and managers apply as well in the health sector. For example, the director of a health district might choose to have an operations director who manages the finances and daily implementation, thus allowing her/himself the freedom

Table 3.4.1 Leadership vs. management functions

	Leadership functions	**Management functions**
Creating an agenda	*Establishing direction*: Vision of the future, develop strategies for change to achieve goals	*Plans and budgets*: Decide actions and timetable, allocate resources
Developing people	*Aligning people*: Communicate vision and strategy, influence creation of teams which accept validity of goals	*Organizing and staffing*: Decide structure and allocate staff, develop policies, procedures, and monitoring
Execution	*Motivating and inspiring*: Energize people to overcome obstacles, satisfy human needs	*Controlling, problem solving*: Monitor results against plan and take corrective action
Outcomes	Produces positive and sometimes dramatic change	Produces order, consistency, and predictability

Source: Huczynski & Buchanan, 2007, p. 698; based on John P. Kotter (1990) *A Force for Change: How Leadership Differs from Management*, Free Press, New York.

to develop strategies and engage diverse actors in a shared vision of the district's health goals. A hospital, to give another example, needs a manager who with limited finances can organize and implement a detailed schedule of surgeries involving people, equipment, and other resources. However, a hospital also needs a leader who can motivate staff to provide high-quality work in the context of budget restrictions. Sometimes these skills and job responsibilities may exist in the same person, but the nature of management tasks differ from leadership tasks.

In this chapter, we are particularly interested in leadership, rather than management. We do not mean to imply that competent management is not important. On the contrary, the ability to take care of the controlling tasks associated with implementation is crucial to the delivery of programmes and services in public health, and there is a great deal of research and funding targeting the improvement of management in order to strengthen the functioning of health systems (see, for example, Egger *et al.* 2005). However, the current interest in public health leadership is in itself worth exploring. Public health requires people who can move the agenda in a world dominated by the politics of vested interest groups. It requires individuals who can take scientific evidence and use it to change the direction of policy. This calls for 'big picture' skills and the ability to influence people both inside and outside the public health field.

What do these leaders do, exactly? We consider this question next, looking at critical competencies, personal characteristics, and the difference between transactional and transformational leadership.

Leadership competencies and personal qualities

The literature on leadership is replete with definitions and lists of leadership characteristics. In this section, we present two that are particularly thorough and intuitively useful in public health.

However, we do so with a couple of caveats. First, research on leadership has not yet presented definitive descriptions, much less definitive prescriptions. As Grint (2002, p. 249) says: 'a science of leadership . . . has proved incredibly elusive . . . [and yet] there are indeed plenty of leadership recipes on the market'. In the health sector, this is as true as in other sectors.

Second, there is reason to be concerned that some of the elements of these lists may be 'culture-bound' and thus more accurate in the North American and European settings in which they were developed. Some research has identified culture-specific differences in observed leadership traits. For example, 'participatory' working behaviour may be more relevant in some cultural contexts than others (Flahault & Roemer 1986). Having said this, there is no harm in advocating the leadership behaviours presented in the two lists below—such as acting with high ethical integrity, developing an evidence-based vision of the future, and empowering others to work towards public health goals—whatever the cultural context.

Competencies of leaders in health

What do we expect leaders in public health to be able to do? One comprehensive list (Wright *et al.* 2000) defines the following core competencies of public health leaders:

1. Transformation—Public health needs and priorities require leaders to engage in systems thinking, including analytical and critical thinking processes, envisioning of potential futures, strategic and tactical assessment, and communication and change dynamics.

2. Legislation and politics—The field of public health requires leaders to have the competence to facilitate, negotiate, and collaborate in an increasingly competitive and contentious political environment.

3. Transorganization—The complexity of major public health problems extends beyond the scope of any single stakeholder group, community unit, profession or discipline, organization or government unit, thus requiring leaders with the skills to be effective beyond their organizational boundaries.

4. Team and group dynamics—Effective communication and practice are accomplished by leaders through building team and work group capacity and capability (Wright *et al.* 2000, p. 1204).

In other words, public health leaders need to be able to imagine and create evidence-based change; they need to be able to influence and lobby politicians for support of their public health agenda; they must operate across disciplinary and organizational boundaries; and they must be skilled at developing and working through diverse teams. The authors go on to give more detail about each competency area (Wright *et al.* 2000). We present a summary in Table 3.4.2. In a practical way, the information in this table answers the question: What do public health leaders do?

Interviews with public health leaders suggest that this is an appropriate list of the types of skills public health leaders need and use in varying degrees. All the leaders interviewed for this chapter had some vision of an alternate future to which they are committed. Whether it was to improve the health services in a remote location of Uganda, strengthen the performance of an international public health bureaucracy, or lead research towards better understanding of breast cancer, each had a vision of contributing towards improving

Table 3.4.2 Competencies needed by leaders in public health

Creating change	Influencing politics	Working trans-organizationally	Building teams
Visionary leadership Be able to articulate an evidence-based vision of the future and incorporate it into strategy.	*Political processes* Determine appropriate actions on policy and political issues, organize key actors to cooperate for regulatory and legislative changes, and translate policies into programmes and services.	*Understanding of organizational dynamics* Assess and develop systems structures based on an understanding of culture and organizational behaviour.	*Develop team-oriented structures and systems* Change system infrastructure to encourage innovative, learning teams.
Sense of mission Facilitate the development of a mission, communicate it, and 'model' it through personal behaviour.	*Negotiation* Mediate potential crises, bargain, and coordinate with key stakeholders.	*Inter-organizational collaborating mechanisms* Involve key actors and networks across a broad range of organizations and groups in collaborative coalitions.	*Facilitate development of teams* Empower, motivate, and reward teams.
Effective change agent Think creatively and analytically about systems and change strategies, and facilitate dialogue and empowerment of others to take action.	*Ethics and power* Identify and use alliances based on ethical principles.	*Social forecasting* Analyse trends and communicate predictions to consortium partners.	*Serve in facilitation and mediation roles* Negotiate and intervene to help teams function.
	Marketing and education Use social marketing and health education to influence key audiences.		*Serve as an effective team member* Through own behaviour, 'model' the key characteristics of listening, encouraging and motivating while displaying integrity, commitment, and honesty.

Source: Adapted from Wright *et al.* 2000.

the people's health and well-being. Interviewees acknowledged the necessity of working in the political arena, although the extent of political engagement much depended on whether their job allowed them the opportunity to do so. The frustration of not being able to effectively exert influence beyond the health sector was a frequent observation. This confirmed the importance of working trans-organizationally as well as trans-sectorally. Working with ministries of finance was a frequently cited example of doing so. The interviewees acknowledged the critical importance of collaborative work, of building and working in teams. However, it was also suggested by some interviewees that the conventional way in which medical doctors were trained did not necessarily provide them with the skills to work collaboratively in public health teams.

Personal characteristics of leaders

The ability to conduct the change-related, trans-organizational, political, and team-building activities associated with public health leadership seems to rely on a core set of personal qualities. One particularly useful summary argues for a framework of 15 qualities important in a public health leader, broken down into three groups: Personal, cognitive, and social qualities (NHS Leadership Centre 2006).

As Fig. 3.4.1 demonstrates, at the core are the five personal qualities of self-belief, self-awareness, self-management, drive for improvement, and personal integrity. The five cognitive qualities at the top make possible the necessary analytical and procedural skills: Seizing the future, intellectual flexibility, broad scanning, political astuteness, and drive for results. These are then rounded off by five social qualities at the bottom: Leading change through people, holding to account, empowering others, effective and strategic influencing, and collaborative working.

The ten qualities associated with 'setting the direction' and 'delivering the service' shown as the outer ring of the doughnut in Fig. 3.4.1 can be viewed as another way of presenting the same basic material we have illustrated in Table 3.4.2. But the core personal qualities presented at the centre of the doughnut are worth emphasizing because they represent the personal behaviour

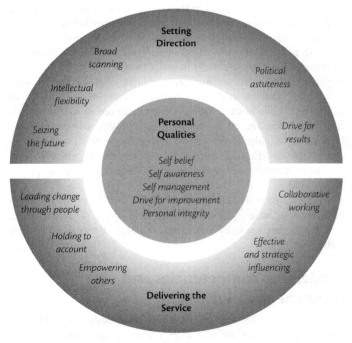

Fig. 3.4.1 NHS Leadership qualities framework.

of a leader. These core personal characteristics explain *how* leaders are able to do what they do. Self-belief, for example, is a 'positive "can do" sense of confidence which enables [outstanding leaders] to be shapers rather than followers, even in the face of opposition' (NHS Leadership Centre 2006, p. 4). Leaders are also self-aware. They know their own emotions and learn from mistakes (NHS Leadership Centre 2006, p. 13). Leaders demonstrate self-management. They are 'tenacious and resilient' in complex and difficult working environments (NHS Leadership Centre 2006, p. 5). They do not lose control, but manage their emotions (NHS Leadership Centre 2006, p. 14). Public health leaders have a vocation that feeds a 'drive for improvement': 'Outstanding leaders are motivated by wanting to make a real difference to people's health . . . [by] investing their energy in bringing about health improvements—even to the extent of wanting to leave a legacy which is about effective partnerships, inter-agency working and community involvement [rather than their own reputation]. . .' (NHS Leadership Centre 2006, p. 5). And finally, leaders demonstrate personal integrity: 'a strongly held sense of commitment to openness, honesty, inclusiveness and high [ethical and performance] standards . . .' (NHS Leadership Centre 2006, p. 16).

Transactional versus transformational leadership

In addition to their personal qualities, leaders tend to behave in one of two ways when seeking to accomplish something: They may be 'transactional' or 'transformational' in their approach (Avolio & Bass 1999). Transactional leaders are explicitly instrumental, for example by complimenting a junior for work well done or by arranging a *quid pro quo* ('you do something for me and I will do something for you'). Transactional leaders use rewards and punishments deliberately. In contrast, transformational leaders are more likely to present a co-worker with a vision of how things could be done differently. Transformational leaders give lots of personal attention to the people they work with, providing stimulation and inspiration to those around them.

Research on leaders in the public sector (including health workers) suggests they are more likely to be transformational in their approach (Alban-Metcalfe & Alimo-Metcalfe 2000). Research on the leadership styles of doctors also indicates that those with transformational behaviours are perceived as more effective leaders and are able to deliver better healthcare results (Xirasagar *et al.* 2005). Some may argue that this is likely to be true generally of health sector leaders, but the importance of the distinction could depend on context. Perhaps transactional leaders are needed in certain urgent settings (such as emergency epidemic responses or operating theatres) while transformational leaders are needed in the more operationally complex domains (such as influencing changes in health policy). However, it is worth noting that '[T]ransformational leadership has been documented to enable superior organizational performance in almost all settings that it has been tested' (Xirasagar *et al.* 2006, p. 105).

That said, a cautionary view has also been expressed by other researchers that the notion of transformational leadership must not trap the leader into thinking that he/she must have all the answers, that 'they have to do it all on their own, standing apart and moulding their organizations into shape'. The leader must be able to find the right balance that works for the specific situation at hand and must be aware of his/her personal limitations so that they can seek and receive help from colleagues (Binney *et al.* 2005, p. 104–5).

Emphasizing the special qualities of public health leaders, as we have done in this section, seems to imply that leaders are somehow born exceptional. As Firth-Cozens and Mowbray (2001) say:

It seems clear that certain traits such as arrogance, authoritarianism, and strong competitiveness may be prejudicial to good leadership, and that sociable, confident people who work well under stress have a head start in making good leaders.

Nonetheless, the personal qualities and competencies cited above, such as self-knowledge and political skill, might also result from a maturity of experience. Similarly, transformational or transactional behaviour might be picked up by people as they progress through their careers. Thus, it seems likely that leadership can be learned, at least in part. But can it be taught? We turn next to that question.

Training and assessing leaders

Training leaders

Around the world, initiatives to train health sector leaders are being developed and implemented. Some training efforts are focused on the traditional attempt to ensure that public health leaders have the epidemiological and statistical skills to understand—if not necessarily to implement—research and evaluation of interventions and outcomes. For example, the Training Programmes in Epidemiology and Public Health Interventions Network (TEPHINET), in association with the World Health Organization, has been part of training public health personnel around the world.

There is a growing interest among ministries of health in establishing new TEPHINET programmes. These programmes are becoming increasingly recognized as catalysts for strengthening the scientific basis of policy-making through the continuous examination of data. . . . (Cardenas *et al.* 2002, p. 196)

In order to be able to analyse trends and articulate a vision of the future, public health leaders clearly need to be able to assess and use the available research evidence. This skill is conventionally believed to be one that can be taught. What about skills like transorganizational work and team-building? Can these be conferred on a potential leader by means of a training programme? Some recent, interesting evaluations suggest they can.

Saleh *et al.* (2004) evaluated training provided by the Northeast Public Health Leadership Institute (NEPHLI) in the US. Issues covered in the year-long programme include such slightly nebulous topics as building collaborative relationships, group problem solving, and dealing with cultural diversity. The evaluation results show that the participants clearly believe their abilities were enhanced in the 15 competency areas assessed. In addition, those who had reason to use certain particular skills as part of their work were more likely to perceive an improvement in their competence as a result of training. A key aspect of this training was, thus, the relevance of the topics to the participants' daily work. There may be, of course, a distinction between the participants' perception that the training improved their skills and the reality when they apply these skills. Nevertheless, it seems reasonable that those (such as doctors and nurses) whose basic training and earlier work skills are technical medical ones would benefit from training that emphasizes a very different set of procedural skills. For example, in this case, the '[t]opics covered included influencing others, measuring and improving public health performance, developing collaborative relationships and partnerships, risk communication, team building, group problem solving, responding to the needs for cultural diversity and competence, and emergency preparedness training' (Saleh *et al.* 2004, p. 1245).

Another training programme evaluation sheds some light on the mechanism by which these behavioural skills are transferred to the participants. Umble *et al.* (2005) assessed a leadership training programme in which all the members of a public health team participated together in the training. In addition, the training was based on the participants' real work and on typical projects. The results showed improved outcomes with regard to collaborating and networking, key aspects of leadership.

As Fig. 3.4.2 illustrates, the training approach seems to have improved the participants' confidence to work collaboratively and to lead a team, as well as improving their practice of these behaviours. The authors conclude from this evaluation that 'networks and collaborative leaders can be developed through education, and that groups thus created can improve services and programmes'

(Umble *et al.* 2005, p. 642). This approach to bringing together, as a team, leaders who will have to work together to solve public health problems, has the potential to work elsewhere. See, for example, a story from the Philippines presented in Box 3.4.1.

In addition to formal training programmes, the development of leaders has also been promoted by means of 'mentoring', 'shadowing', or 'coaching' (*Turning Point* 2001, p. 51). Mentoring is the process by which a more experienced person guides a more junior person with regard to various work- and career-related decisions. It may involve helping the junior person solve problems at work by empathetic listening and feedback. Mentoring may also involve the experienced person giving career advice to the junior.

Shadowing can work with a more senior person either being shadowed or doing the shadowing. In the former approach, a more junior person follows the senior one in his or her job over several months. In this way, learning takes place by observing and participating in the work of an established leader. The latter approach involves a more experienced person shadowing a junior over a shorter period of a day or few days, and then giving constructive feedback on the junior's behaviour and activities at work.

Coaching does not necessarily involve a senior and junior person. A coach can provide assessment and feedback of skills and

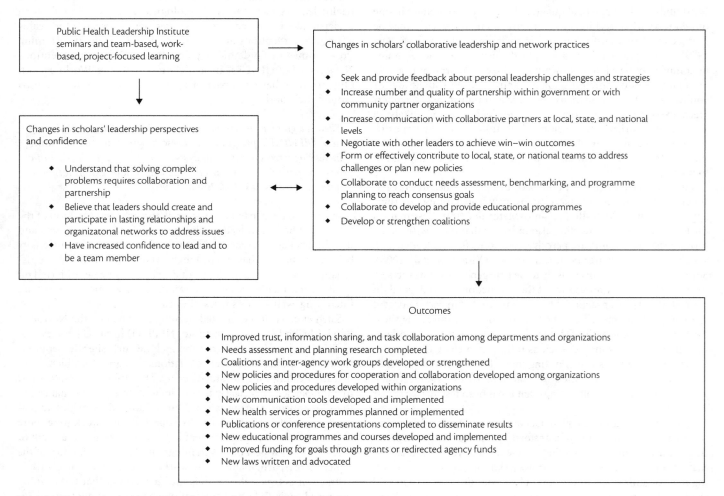

Fig. 3.4.2 Changing leadership practices through collaborative team training.
Source: Umble *et al.* (2005).

Box 3.4.1 Training local teams to be health leaders in poor communities: A case from the Philippines

The Philippines provides the story of an innovative approach to the need for leadership to address the health needs of the most deprived and vulnerable populations. Begun in 2002, the Leaders for Health Program (LHP) was predicated on the understanding that health professionals must work in concert with political and community actors if basic health problems are to be addressed in low-income communities. This 'Tri-Leader' approach brought together the community doctor, the mayor, and a local community leader and trained them, both individually and as a team.

To address the need that medical leaders understand and are able to use evidence to inform policy, doctors received postgraduate training resulting in a Master in Community Health Management. Recognizing that the local political and community leaders often did not have an advanced level of education, the programme created a certificate course in community health management tailored to them, but paralleling the master's training provided to doctors. Joint workshops and training sessions were also held for the tri-leaders together. In addition, all three benefited from coaching and mentoring from a more experienced leader of their own category in another part of the country. Once this team began to identify priorities in its locality, the LHP provided assistance in identifying donors for specific interventions. For example, some communities invested in sanitation and clean water systems. One community established a local pharmacy; another invested in a boat for emergency transport of patients.

By taking this innovative approach to leadership—one that recognizes the importance of joint leadership in the medical, political, and local communities in order to address public health needs—the LHP has been able to demonstrate greater success than other initiatives that focus only on placing trained doctors in low-income areas. Its success would seem to be due to the programme's understanding of the complexity of health systems. For example, addressing water-borne diseases properly requires sanitation systems, and sanitation systems cannot be built without political support. In addition, the programme's training of doctors together with mayors and community leaders helps doctors to see beyond the narrowly bio-medical domain to the broader political and sociological setting in which public health problems must be tackled. One mayor reported that earlier attempts to post doctors to his village were unsuccessful because the doctor was perceived to be making demands arrogantly of a resource-poor community, rather than working with the community to reach a common understanding.

Similar team-based approaches to training public health leaders have shown success elsewhere. (For an example from the United States, see our discussion in Umble *et al.* [2005].) Training medical, political, and community leaders together fosters the networking skills and builds the very communication links needed to address public health priorities. The evidence suggests that this is an approach that might reasonably be tried elsewhere.

Source: Baquiran *et al.* 2006; Leaders for Health Program 2005.

practice with a leader or someone wishing to develop leadership skills. Coaches may set goals and tasks for the subject, followed by discussion sessions designed to help him or her learn from the experience. Peers may sometimes coach one another, although this may be more successful when the peers not in direct competition with one another (*Turning Point* 2001, p. 52).

Among the leaders we interviewed, mentoring and shadowing experiences occupied a prominent place in their development. Many cited their mentors with great fondness and appreciation. And there were instances when more than one mentor was acknowledged by a leader.

It appears, then, that the training and development of leaders is possible. The former assumption that leaders are born with innate skills that cannot be taught, no longer seems true. Waiting for great leaders to emerge is not necessary. Instead, the health sector can seek to train, develop, and promote leaders. But, how do we discern which individuals exhibit leadership traits and which ones are performing well as leaders? There must be some mechanism for assessing leaders, and we turn next to that problem.

Measuring leadership ability

There are many leadership assessment tools, but three are based on empirical research. The Leadership Practices Inventory (Kouzes & Posner 1997) measures leaders on five dimensions: Challenging the process; inspiring a shared vision; enabling others to act; modelling the way; and encouraging the heart. The Multifactor Leadership Questionnaire (Avolio & Bass 1999) measures characteristics associated with transformational leadership, transactional leadership, and the absence of leadership (*laissez-faire* way of working in a leadership position). The Transformational Leadership Questionnaire (Alban-Metcalfe & Alimo-Metcalfe 2000) measures nine factors:

◆ Genuine concern for others

◆ Political sensitivity and skills

◆ Decisiveness, determination, self-confidence

◆ Integrity, trustworthy, honest, and open

◆ Empowers, develops potential

◆ Inspirational networker and promoter

◆ Accessible, approachable

◆ Clarifies boundaries, involves others in decisions

◆ Encourages critical and strategic thinking.

All three of these leadership tools are applied by asking someone other than the leader (sometimes a superior, sometimes a subordinate) to assess the leader's performance on each element along a scale. Each of the three has been applied in various settings and found to be useful in distinguishing high-performing leaders from those who demonstrate weaker leadership skills despite being in a job requiring leadership.

There are two uses for these types of tests. The first is to help individuals identify their own areas of strength and weakness in order to develop as leaders. The second is to select people for leadership positions. Neither of these is being implemented to any great extent in health sectors around the world, although richer countries probably do so more. The use of such tools could help health-sector managers to improve the leadership profile of their workforce. However, as has been noted about all attempts to list leadership characteristics, more work needs to be done to identify tools that work well across different cultures.

In this chapter so far, we have looked at the theory and thought behind leadership studies and research. We have also seen how various approaches to train and develop leaders have been implemented. But, beyond this, how does leadership work in the gritty, very real world of day-to-day public health work?

Leadership in health today

Acknowledging and addressing complexity—putting theory into practice

Health systems are complex. In all countries, health systems are broad and multi-sectoral. They involve complicated interactions among politics and policy-making, financing, training and education, and public and private organizations. It is not easy to define where public health activities end: A large manufacturing company may employ someone to conduct health education with its staff, just as the government might engage outreach workers to do the same with villagers. In the context of a very complex system that extends far beyond the boundaries of any one organization, it is not possible to 'manage' things in a mechanical way (Plsek & Wilson 2001). It is not possible to impose simple managerial or technical solutions to a public health problem and thus solve it.

Indeed, if technical and mechanistic solutions were all that were needed to address public health problems, we would not need leaders. Instead, the complex, multi-organizational, and team-based nature of public health work requires people who can inspire others to achieve results working through the complexity. And leaders are not needed just at the top of the pyramid. Increasingly, as solutions require collective action, leadership in public health is needed at all levels (Grint 2002). The 'command and control' approach will not serve to address the myriad and varied issues faced in national health sectors around the world, not to mention internationally.

Public health leaders must exercise their leadership in a complex environment. What does this mean, exactly? The leaders we interviewed voiced both enthusiasm and frustration with the work they were engaged in. While they spoke of positive gains in their work, they also spoke of conditions beyond their sphere of influence, and of existing economic and political forces far beyond their personal or their organization's capacities to change. Despite these difficulties, hardly any interviewee suggested that they should give up. The following quote from *Living Leadership: A Practical Guide for Ordinary Heroes* may be helpful in providing perspective on how leaders might conduct themselves in the face of complexity:

> *Coming alive is when leaders are able to use all their intelligence, senses and experience to connect with others and make sense of the context. They don't forget their life experience. They are able to acknowledge when a situation is different from ones they have experienced before and they need to pause and think again. They are able to tolerate the complexity of events and people and not rush to simple-minded solutions that don't make sense. Their focus is on both long- and short-term issues. They can ask for and receive help.* (Binney et al. 2005, p. 93)

We observed that the fundamental premise that keeps public health leaders going despite the difficulties is this: That a public health leader is there to serve people. And the goal of service is to improve the quality of life of people by preventing, treating, and even eliminating disease wherever possible.

This imperative to serve has to be expressed concretely. The public health leader quickly finds that his or her mission of service will lead to problems and dilemmas inherent to this complex world. Let us look at some examples of how this complexity manifests itself in the challenges that leaders face.

Consider the relationship between disease and poverty manifest in epidemics. In Manila, there are perennial outbreaks of diarrhoea in the urban slums because residents illegally tap water lines causing contamination of water. When such a water-borne outbreak occurs, the water company needs to step in. It removes the illegal connections, repairs leaks, flushes out the contamination, and increases the chlorination levels in the affected water lines. Public health authorities undertake epidemic investigations and related measures to treat the sick and prevent the infection from spreading in households.

While appearing to be a local issue, this phenomenon is a microcosm of a global problem described in the text of a WHO poster that reads: 'For the first time in history, more than half of the world's population lives in urban settings. Three billion people live in cities. One billion people live without access to safe drinking water'.

What can be done to prevent perennial outbreaks of water-borne diarrhoea in the urban slums of Manila caused by the illegal tapping of water lines? How would the public health leader deal with this situation in order to find a longer term answer to it?

The relationship between disease and people's lifestyles presents many interesting challenges. The association between smoking cigarettes and cancer is now well established. In 2003, the World Health Assembly ratified the Framework Convention on Tobacco Control, which urged member states to undertake a variety of actions in order to reduce smoking among their populations. Despite scientific advances leading to a better understanding of the ill effects of smoking and the aforementioned landmark global agreement, the prevalence of smoking among youth and women is on the rise in many countries. And while some countries have set forth legislation to ban smoking in public places, governments in many countries seem not to be doing enough to discourage and reduce smoking among their constituents.

How would the public health leader, such as a city health officer, deal with a situation where the city mayor or the city council have not enacted any measures to stop smoking in public places?

Consider the relationship between a disease, the necessary medicines for its treatment, and the commercial interests involved in making those medicines accessible to the people who need them. HIV/AIDS has become a determinant of social and economic development. Life expectancies have been shortened drastically in many African countries because thousands of people succumb to AIDS at an early age. Large numbers of AIDS orphans are overwhelming the capacities of families and societies to provide and care for them. Anti-retrovirals exist, but they are expensive and still inaccessible to millions of infected people.

How would a public health leader, such as a Minister of Health in a country with a large burden of HIV/AIDS, take steps to provide anti-retrovirals for thousands of citizens with the disease?

And what does a public health leader do when people's choices come into direct confrontation with tradition, and prevailing moral views and teachings of religious institutions? It is now commonplace for women to seek abortions in order to terminate unwanted pregnancies. Often, these abortions are conducted under surreptitious and illegal conditions, placing women at high risk of life-threatening bleeding and infection. There is ongoing debate that legalizing abortions will result in better regulation of the practice of abortion, thereby making the procedure less risky.

How does a public health leader deal with a situation where the scientific evidence shows that decriminalizing abortion prevents maternal deaths from sepsis, but where his moral beliefs run counter to implementing such a change?

The above examples are only a few of the many complex issues that public health leaders face. As they bring themselves to lead under these challenging circumstances, their aforementioned personal qualities, technical and social competencies will be tested. It can be overwhelming to lead in such complex situations, and leaders must be realistic about what they and their organizations can accomplish.

Principled leadership

In the face of such challenges, leaders need more than the attributes described above to help them succeed. Also vitally important is a set of principles that can serve as a guide to thought and action. Where would public health leaders derive such a set of principles? We offer five principles derived from the WHO Constitution (see Box 3.4.2):

1. Commitment to the vision of total human development

2. Commitment to empowering the poor and the vulnerable with knowledge and opportunity

3. Pursuit of evidence and truth

4. Commitment to fairness and equity in the provision of adequate health and social measures

5. Trustworthiness and public accountability

Applied singly or in varying combinations, we submit that these principles provide the foundation and inspiration to public healthwork.

In the first challenge discussed above, public health leaders are asked to find a longer-term solution to control water-borne outbreaks of diarrhoea in the urban slums of Manila. Principle 1, which calls for commitment to total human development, urges these leaders to think beyond epidemic control. It challenges them to address the problem of urban slums to tackle the social determinants of water-borne outbreaks. This is exceedingly complex and difficult. However, where Principle 1 is combined with Principle 2, more durable solutions have been found. The experience of Gawad Kalinga in the Philippines demonstrates how a movement to eradicate urban slums has improved the health of people in such communities and in the process has prevented the perennial occurrence of outbreaks there (see Box 3.4.3). By addressing the land and housing issues at the root of urban slum communities, Gawad Kalinga was able to build low-cost houses and proper water supplies for the families previously dwelling in slums.

Principle 5, trustworthiness and public accountability, is applicable to the second challenge. The campaign against smoking is another complex issue. There are big business interests that protect and promote the sale of cigarettes. Some of these business interests may even have philanthropic projects which benefit the public, such as grants to educational institutions or youth scholarships.

Box 3.4.2 WHO constitution

THE STATES Parties to this Constitution declare, in conformity with the Charter of the United Nations, that the following principles are basic to the happiness, harmonious relations and security of all peoples:

- Health is a state of complete physical, mental, and social well-being and not merely the absence of disease or infirmity.

- The enjoyment of the highest attainable standard of health is one of the fundamental rights of every human being without distinction of race, religion, political belief, economic or social condition.

- The health of all peoples is fundamental to the attainment of peace and security and is dependent upon the fullest co-operation of individuals and States.

- The achievement of any State in the promotion and protection of health is of value to all.

- Unequal development in different countries in the promotion of health and control of disease, especially communicable disease, is a common danger.

- Healthy development of the child is of basic importance; the ability to live harmoniously in a changing total environment is essential to such development.

- The extension to all peoples of the benefits of medical, psychological and related knowledge is essential to the fullest attainment of health.

- Informed opinion and active co-operation on the part of the public are of the utmost importance in the improvement of the health of the people.

- Governments have a responsibility for the health of their peoples, which can be fulfilled only by the provision of adequate health and social measures.

ACCEPTING THESE PRINCIPLES, and for the purpose of co-operation among themselves and with others to promote and protect the health of all peoples, the Contracting Parties agree to the present Constitution and hereby establish the World Health Organization as a specialized agency within the terms of Article 57 of the Charter of the United Nations.

Source: WHO Constitution was adopted by the International Health Conference held in New York from 19 June to 22 July 1946 (Reference: WHO Basic Documents, 2007).

It can be convenient for public health leaders to take the path of least resistance and not call for a ban of cigarettes in public places. Principle 5 calls on public health leaders to be faithful to their calling of safeguarding public health despite the odds against them. In this respect, they are trustworthy and accountable to the public for their actions, even if some of their actions may be politically unpopular. There are public health leaders who have unstintingly used the built-up scientific evidence on the ill effects of smoking to persist in the campaign to ban smoking in public places. To them, the public owes a debt of gratitude for their courage and persistence.

Box 3.4.3 Gawad Kalinga: Improving well-being by empowering the poor

Gawad Kalinga (GK) translated in English means to Guardian of care. GK is a non-profit foundation whose vision for the Philippines is a slum-free, squatter-free nation through a simple strategy of providing land for the landless, homes for the homeless, and food for the hungry in order to attain dignity and peace in poor Filipino communities.

What started in 1995 as a daring initiative by a faith-based organization to rehabilitate juvenile gang members and help out-of-school youth in a large squatters' relocation area in Metro Manila, has now evolved into a movement for nation-building. Local and multinational corporations have engaged with GK as part of their programmes for corporate social responsibility. Together with its partners, Gawad Kalinga is now in the process of transforming slum communities with the goal of building 700 000 homes in 7000 communities in 7 years (2003–2010). At the time of writing, Gawad Kalinga is in over 900 communities all over the Philippines. GK villages have also been recently introduced in Papua New Guinea, East Timor, Cambodia, and Indonesia.

As a growing multi-sectoral movement, GK works actively in the poorest urban areas and aims to improve the quality of life of its residents by providing decent homes and the resources necessary for self-sufficiency. It seeks a holistic approach to poverty alleviation which includes various components: The provision of basic healthcare, community organization, livelihood programmes, and values formation. GK has extended its activities to include poor Muslim communities in its Highway of Peace campaign where Muslim and Christians together build GK homes. In some outstanding cases of inter-community bridge building, long-standing family feuds have been reversed by one community building a house for a rival community

Even before a GK house is built in a slum community, issues of land ownership, capital for house materials, participation of the residents in the construction of the houses, eventual ownership of the built houses, and community building are considered and dealt with. Complex social dynamics are involved in dealing with these varied issues.

In 2006, GK launched its 'One Million Heroes' campaign, designed to encourage intensified volunteerism in the GK communities. Part of the current success of GK is attributed to this stewardship component which integrates leadership building into the GK communities. Every GK village has a Caretaker Team comprised mainly of resident volunteers who undertake specific responsibilities like assisting in resolving conflicts, ensuring the proper management of the resources for constructing the houses, and seeing to it that the GK standards for a well-organized community are maintained.

Principle 4, commitment to fairness and equity, may be applicable in the third challenge. In the face of the complex issues concerning the way in which pharmaceuticals are produced, sold, and distributed, answers must be found to address the lack of access to medicines by millions of people. The solutions to these imbalances are not straightforward. They involve the dynamics of the domestic and international market for medicines. Where patent issues for new medicines are involved, there are international agreements that govern the production and marketing of generic copies during the patent term. Notwithstanding these complexities, public health leaders, seeking to broaden their populations' access to medicines, have persevered to find ways to accomplish this goal. At the Sixtieth World Health Assembly in May 2007, public health leaders from around the world tackled this very issue and produced resolution WHA60.30, initially proposed by Brazil. The way this resolution was debated and eventually passed by the World Health Assembly is an example of how public health leaders from different countries can come together to agree on an exceedingly complex public health issue.

The final example focuses on the issue of abortion. The application of Principle 3—the pursuit of evidence and truth—may guide an advocate for the legalization of abortion to argue that this policy significantly decreases maternal deaths. But those against abortion will resist this evidence, taking the view that no law can justify terminating the foetus in early pregnancy. People's beliefs and values vary. In the Philippines, while there are data showing that septic abortions happen in the thousands, legalization of abortion would be unacceptable as public policy. In contrast, in Iran, abortion was made legal to address mothers' health risk in certain pregnancies (Reproductive Health Matters 2005). So, even as public health leaders pursue the evidence to justify health interventions, there may be other, historical and social considerations that override it. Public health leaders, whatever their moral beliefs, will have to respect those realities.

It is indeed exciting and challenging for the public health leader to bring together personal qualities, technical and social competencies, and principles to the job at hand.

Effective leadership

There are a variety of public health sector jobs that will allow leaders to exercise their full range of talents. At the national level, leading a public health organization (or certain programmes within the organization) is one such job. Ensuring that the bureaucracy delivers the services that the public expects of it will require the leader to exercise competencies such as empowering others, driving for results, and being held to account. Providing immunization services to millions of children every year in order to protect them from vaccine-immunizable disease is a good example of this. The leader has to keep the programme on track in the face of many competing priorities, ensuring that the right people are in place to run the programme. The leader must see to it that funds are available to procure the vaccines, and that the vaccines are delivered and used properly at the points of service throughout the country. The leader relies on a well-functioning organization to do this. Immunization targets have to be set and results achieved; and the leader must hold his/her people to account for their performance, even as he/she is held to account by his/her superiors and the public.

Where one sees an immunization programme with high immunization coverage rates, one can find examples of successful public health leadership. While the immunization example above discusses leadership at the national level, there are additional levels of leadership necessary to the programme. At the international level, global immunization strategies and targets are set in consultation with experts and various stakeholders, including Member States, international development agencies, and non-governmental organizations. At a sub-national level, leadership undertakes the planning and implementation of all the details of the programme.

This includes ensuring that the staff members are properly trained, motivated, and supervised, that vaccines and supplies are available, and that the health facilities are organized and well-prepared to deliver the service. Furthermore, there is leadership at the various levels of the service delivery chain to see to it that the children in the communities and households actually get immunized. Even at the community level, village health-workers and volunteers may play leadership roles in providing information to parents, encouraging them to ensure their children are vaccinated.

The results of effective leadership in a national immunization programme are profound in terms of preventing life-threatening illnesses in children. High-coverage rates of measles immunization have significantly reduced illness and deaths among children from pneumonia, diarrhoea, and malnutrition that are the sequelae of severe measles infection.

In times of organizational change, public health leaders will need to exercise other competencies such as seizing the future, intellectual flexibility, and broad scanning. For example, when the Philippine Department of Health decentralized its services in 1992, it devolved all provincial hospitals and municipal health centres to local governments. More than 500 hospitals, 1000 health centres, and 35 000 staff were devolved. It was a huge change, and public health leaders at all levels faced the challenge of continuing to provide services, while adapting to new organizational relationships.

The onus on the top leadership of the Department of Health was tremendous in terms of managing the transition. The devolved parts of the organization resisted the change and while they were legally bound to implement, performance dipped. The non-devolved half of the organization found itself having to implement programmes through lower levels of the organization, which were no longer under their direct administrative control.

What was once an unbroken chain of command from national to municipal level was cut in two places: The provincial and municipal levels now reported to their respective local executives.

The devolution of health services was part of an administrative re-structuring of government. It was driven by the principle of increasing the powers and responsibilities of local government, particularly in the administration of public services. Public health leaders had to manage this change as best as they could and work with local governments, many of which were unready to take over the responsibility of managing health services. During such a critical transition, public health leaders needed to provide visionary guidance and practical savvy to calm the organizational turmoil, deal with the anger of devolved staff, and the haplessness of local governments, and provide a steady and reassuring presence in what was a very trying time.

Public health leaders are not immune to political battles and on many occasions they will have to decide whether or not to engage in the fight. It is not an easy decision to take. Engagement is costly in terms of personal time and energy, as well as organizational resources. Some of the fiercest political battles involve the business sector. Regulating the sales and marketing of infant formulas in developing countries is one example of a thorny issue. Government regulates the aggressive marketing practices of the milk companies, which are known to run counter to breastfeeding promotion among mothers. In the Philippines, milk companies have filed suits against the Department of Health to challenge government regulation of these marketing practices. In instances like this, public health leaders must stand firm in the face of litigation.

Public health leaders are found not just in the state or government sector. They also work in non-governmental organizations, academia, and the private commercial sector. Activities of non-state-sector organizations do affect public health. For instance, the marketing behaviour of pharmaceutical companies affects patterns of public consumption. Non-governmental organizations' activities during disasters and natural calamities contribute to public health. The research done in academic institutions helps inform public health policy. Health leadership can thus be considered a shared responsibility. It is, therefore, critical for the leaders of the various sectors to engage in honest and effective dialogue to attain synergy of purpose and action.

Have public health leaders made a difference in this complex world? Where is the evidence that they have changed the lives of their constituents for the better? Assessing leadership is by nature a retrospective activity. It is, therefore, always difficult to know for sure whether in any particular context another leader in the same position would have acted differently, and more important, whether there would have been a different outcome had someone else been making the decisions. Furthermore, would a leader who was successful in dilemma 'X' have shone equally had he/she instead been placed into dilemma 'Y'? It is evident that in a complex reality, a leader and his/her context are in fact inseparable: Put the right person in the right place at the right time, and leadership happens. Beyond this, instinct and personal experience tells us that public health leaders *do* make a difference, and they can be responsible for collective success or failure. We can look to historical examples as further evidence.

We can look first to the 1854 cholera outbreak in Soho, London, and the famous demonstration of leadership that in many ways marked the beginning of modern epidemiological public health as a discipline. Supported by his exceptional technical, medical, and scientific skills, John Snow exhibited several of the characteristics of leadership covered in this chapter. In particular, his self-belief and confidence, and vision and belief in a better state of affairs were all monumentally demonstrated.

The historical context must especially be appreciated: Snow was active prior to the formulation of the germ theory—the theory that proposes that microorganisms are the cause of many diseases—a cornerstone of modern medicine and medical microbiology. At the time, the predominant scientific belief concerning the mechanism of spreading disease was that expounded in the Miasma theory: That diseases such as cholera and the plague were spread by poisonous air. For some years, Snow argued that this theory was mistaken, and he became convinced from his research upon various outbreaks in London that cholera was in fact spread by water.

Battling scientific convention was only a part of the struggle for what Snow thought would save lives. Implementing his theory led to another difficult conflict. When Snow postulated that the source outbreak at the time appeared to be a water pump and consequently recommended that it be blocked, there was understandable resistance from the inhabitants of the area who depended on the pump for their daily drinking water. With both science and the affected population against him, it is an extraordinary feat of negotiation that Snow eventually succeeded in convincing the local authorities to remove the handle from the pump, bringing an end to the incidence of infection and no doubt saving many lives. Snow's actions also led directly to a new understanding of how disease can spread.

Snow's leadership continued after the outbreak was under control, when he demonstrated the utmost integrity in doubting his own conclusion—pondering whether the fact that the outbreak was already on decline prior to the handle removal meant that he had been mistaken. Hence, he persevered in mapping out each cholera case in the context of its proximity to the well. In doing so, he not only consolidated the correctness of his decision, but also gave birth to what we now call epidemiology.

John Snow did not seek to be a leader. Neither was he appointed into his position as local health hero and scientific pioneer. It is clear from the story that his technical skills were secondary to his leadership qualities. His knowledge of himself, belief and vision in an improved understanding of health, personal integrity, perseverance, and a desire to serve people regardless of their social class, pushed him to succeed in the situation he found himself in the middle of.

In contrast to this first evidential example of public health leadership—historical, local, and focused on an individual—as a second example we can examine a case typical of the complex modern reality and necessary leadership of today. The successful containment of SARS in 2003 involved multi-level, multidisciplinary, collective international leadership and would not have been possible without it. One might be tempted to point to WHO and other coordinating bodies at the time as the self-appointed 'leader', but in reality a 'network of leadership' was crucial to the urgent halting of the new disease.

Originating in a Hong Kong hotel, but rapidly spreading globally via the fast-moving web of international transport, SARS proved the cliché that disease recognizes no national boundaries and does not discriminate between types of people. With such a highly contagious, little-understood, deadly respiratory disease, every human life was under threat. On the other hand, human reality *does* recognize national boundaries and so a successful public health response to SARS relied on strong leadership at the national and local levels, which simultaneously cooperated internationally. Furthermore, the impact of SARS reached far beyond the health sphere: Mass hysteria surrounding the emerging disease damaged tourism and economies, costing Asian businesses alone around US$60 billion in lost revenue (Dayrit 2004). All sectors needed to work together to minimize the human cost incurred by SARS. Given these facts, what exactly was required of national public health leadership—particularly in the more affected countries?

A typical national public health strategy to fight the disease can be considered as having rested upon five pillars:

- Minimizing the entry of imported cases through monitoring and screening of passengers in seaports and airports

- Averting local transmission of cases through contact tracing, quarantining of suspected carriers, and isolation of cases

- Preventing SARS deaths with supportive hospital treatment

- Disseminating information and health advisories to the public to control fear and panic

- Mitigating the non-health consequences of SARS

It is worth noting that of these public health responsibilities, only the third point—hospital treatment—is a purely health-oriented task. The other pillars all required public health leadership in multi-sector responses to a health threat. In many cases, national leaders had to make brave and controversial decisions in the interest of the health of their people, such as implementing new quarantine laws necessary for the protection of the population but risked being seen as limitations on civil liberties or human rights. Leaders needed to be communicative and bold, demonstrating integrity and acting with the best interests of the people at heart. Underlying their actions were not only their own guiding principles, but globalized principles of human well-being and equity, which are increasingly shared across all boundaries.

All considered, and given the immediacy and gravity of the situation, this was a massive responsibility for national health leaders and their colleagues. With the support of international bodies such as WHO, however, in winning the fight against SARS the multi-country leadership set a precedent for dealing with future international health threats, strengthening global preparedness in the process. Without that collaborative leadership, SARS would almost definitely have taken countless more lives, cost billions more to the global economy, and could still be very much at large.

We have seen a classic example of individual, localized, public health leadership in the exceptional efforts of John Snow and a contemporary, complex, international, collaborative leadership example in the multi-leader response to SARS. Both undoubtedly made an impermeable difference to the health and well-being of the world today.

Examples of leadership are multiple and varied, and yet there are common elements that can be found in them all. It is by embracing these elements that, regardless of the plethora of leadership examples, a personal 'path to leadership' can be forged.

The path to leadership

You too can become a public health leader—but how can you develop the personal qualities and competencies needed to do so?

The public health leaders we interviewed first entered the profession with a strong desire to serve. Through the course of their careers, they were exposed to circumstances that deepened their commitment. Frequently, they sought out challenging circumstances in which to gain much needed experience. They travelled, engaged in development work, often involving poor countries and communities. In the course of this exposure, they took up more advanced public health studies, perhaps did some research, wrote articles in scientific journals, or managed a healthcare facility. Some had long periods of service in their own country before being exposed to international work. For others, international exposure came early, usually through some clinical- or public health training abroad.

There are several paths to leadership. Some moved into public health after years of working in the clinics, practising a speciality like paediatrics, obstetrics, or surgery. Others came into positions of leadership through the field services, rising through a public health organization, or a non-governmental organization. Others were involved in academia, teaching and research, consulting, or working with a development agency. Public health leaders could also have been involved in politics. Or they could once have been cause-oriented activists, involved in issues such as HIV prevention and primary healthcare.

Mentors play a significant role in the development of the public health leader. Nearly everyone we interviewed cited people significant to their career at various stages.

One public health leader we spoke to for this chapter put it this way: 'A leader creates a path for others to succeed'. Another interviewee mentioned how his boss and mentor encouraged him and other young people in the organization to think up and explore new ideas. These contemporary nuggets of advice are reminiscent of a gem of wisdom found in the ancient text of the *Tao Te Ching*:

> Go to the people. Live with them. Learn from them. Love them. Start with what they know. Build with what they have. But with the best leaders, when the work is done, the task accomplished, the people will say 'We have done this ourselves'.

Many public health leaders of the last generation lived by this maxim. Similar expressions paraphrasing this attitude were made by several of the leaders we interviewed.

Central to the growth and development of the public health leader are the years when he/she developed the personal qualities of self-awareness, self-belief, and self-management. In many, there was the strong conviction that their involvement in public health was imbued with higher purpose and that they were instruments of a higher power to do good work. Certainly, the sense of 'other-orientedness' was quite a major motivation infusing the leaders' sense of service. Among those interviewed, none said that money was a strong motivating factor for the choice of a public health career. A desire to continue learning new things was often mentioned as a source of great satisfaction. One public health leader emphasized the necessity to listen and learn from others before making decisions.

Personal integrity is another of the personal qualities greatly valued by public health leaders. It is the inner core of public credibility. Trustworthiness, transparency on the job, and incorruptibility are among the attributes that they strive to maintain in themselves and look for in their colleagues. When leaders lose personal integrity—as when they fall into the trap of self-serving personal agendas, unethical conflicts of interest, or even bribe-taking—their loss of public credibility will eventually occur, just as death follows disease. Since we do not live in a perfect world, it is not unknown for public health leaders to fall from grace and lose their integrity and credibility. It is a sad day when a person in a position of public health leadership is found to have betrayed the public trust one way or the other. The path to public health leadership must strengthen and ennoble both mind and heart.

When does one know that one is ready to lead? The opportunity to lead may be sought, but very often it is given, when the higher authority deems that the individual is ready to exercise leadership. The opportunity to lead is a gift. But just as the public health leader has been selected to lead, so too is it his/her job to select others to take up positions of leadership. Leaders should nurture future leaders. Selecting a person for a leadership position is often one of the biggest decisions that a public health leader can make.

The potential health leaders of tomorrow are encouraged to forge their 'path to leadership' on three fronts:

1. Know your guiding principles.

2. Seek mentors and aim to learn from every situation you face.

3. Pursue leadership, not the leadership position.

Know your guiding principles

The WHO constitution—drawn up in a fertile climate of unprecedented hope by international leaders in every field—can be distilled into fundamental guiding principles that are central to a public health leader's work. In reality, individual context, culture, and background dictate that each leader will interpret these principles slightly differently and will complement them with principles derived from additional underlying foundations that constitute their personal philosophy of life. Together, this collection of principles will serve to give focus and meaning to the health leader's work.

Nonetheless, these principles must be embedded firmly in the mind. Leaders need to think and act on their feet. Unless one is sure of one's principles, in a time of crisis—with perhaps many lives at stake—panic and uncertainty might take over. There will not be time to think—about remembering your principles when the need to make a decision is immediate. For this reason, taking the time to understand what guides you—to 'know thyself'—is invaluable. Take time to think about what it is that guides you, or what you would like to guide you. Find your principles. Write them down. Read them out aloud. Explain and discuss them with a close friend or mentor. Take regular moments to revisit them so that they are forever under your skin, in your subconscious, never far from the surface. Together, they will serve as your guiding beacon during times that test your leadership.

Seek mentors and aim to learn from every situation you face

Both the literature on leadership and the practical experience of today's health leaders underline the crucial importance of mentorship in the development of the complete public health leader. To achieve self-improvement, being prepared to learn from superiors, fellow colleagues, friends, and public figures is essential. But how does one 'obtain' a mentor?

There is no fixed prescription for mentorship. By its very nature, it is a personal arrangement between two parties, and sometimes one of the parties (the mentor) does not even need to be aware of the fact. Some programmes encourage their participants to go out and seek a mentor other than their direct supervisor—someone they admire, probably working in their vicinity—and to invite them to act as a mentor. Following this, an arrangement can be struck that is convenient and suitable to the mentor and the mentee. The mentoring relationship could be formal and structured, with regular meetings and log book entries; or it could be more informal and sporadic, with the occasional chat over coffee or e-mail correspondence.

In whatever case best suits the people involved, the opportunity should be taken for the mentor to impart advice, the mentee to report on recent events, and for both to share thoughts on work and even wider aspects of life, particularly if relevant to a career in health and leadership. Ideally, a mentoring relationship should be mutually beneficial, with both parties learning from one another, enriching their understanding of their work and purpose.

For of course, a mentor can gain much from a mentee. One can learn as much from subordinates or peers as one learns from superiors. In this sense, mentors surround us, wherever we are. Rarely is one person not able to learn something from another. A mentor does not need to (and rarely does) exhibit all the aspects of leadership covered in this chapter. More often, elements of leadership can be found in part in various people met in the course of a career. The challenge is to identify the skills and to attempt to understand how to integrate them into one's own work and behaviour. This form of fragmented menteeship does not need to take the form of the more contractual approach mentioned above. It is up to the mentees to observe and learn by themselves—a kind of secret mentorship.

Pursue leadership, not the leadership position

Looking back to the beginning of this chapter, at the distinction between leadership and management (Tables 3.4.1 and 3.4.2 and Fig. 3.4.1), it is clear that whereas to exercise management it is necessary to be in a management position, the skills, characteristics, and competencies of leadership can more or less be practised regardless of one's position in a hierarchy. One pursues leadership by steadily inculcating in oneself the personal qualities, competencies, and principles that make up a true leader. One does not acquire these necessary attributes and skills simply by ascending to a leadership position, often via political patronage, especially if one lacks adequate preparation. Study, training, reflection, exposure, and experience are all elements of this preparation. Thus, as one's leadership traits flourish, the time will come when one is ready to assume a leadership position. Leadership should be sought in this way from day one of any career and hence, any strong public health organization should encourage leadership development at all levels.

When does one know that he/she is ready to take up a position of leadership?

The trajectory of an individual's path to leadership can rise steeply or gently. It is one's willingness to step forward, given one's self-awareness and knowledge of the prospective job, however incomplete, which might mark a person's readiness to lead. A potential leader will almost always be selected by having already demonstrated leadership and by showing readiness to lead. In deciding if one is ready to assume the responsibility of a public health leader, it of course helps to discuss the opportunity with mentors, co-workers, and family members.

Once in a leadership position, the leader must keep learning. Mistakes will be made, disappointments and conflicts will occur. The strong face of leadership is well-observed, but how do top health leaders deal with themselves during the dark hours, when the tasks seem overwhelming and when results fall short of expectations? It is often said that in these situations, leaders dig deep into themselves to find internal resources of strength. The capacity to affirm self-belief and overcome self-doubt is an important ingredient in surviving the difficult times; but it is also true that the leader turns outward to others for strength. One leader from Kenya whom we interviewed emphasized that she turned to her community for rejuvenation and inspiration. 'We hold on to each other', she said. Others turn to family members or colleagues for support. And there are many who through prayer and meditation, turn to their faith or guiding principles to find inner strength.

It is hoped that the above will help to direct the interested and motivated reader in tracing his/her own 'path to leadership'—imparting some of the information and advice needed to one day lead within the area of public health. Before bringing this chapter to a close, and as a final pointer for those wishing to serve the needy through public health leadership, we might want look at things from another perspective. Instead of asking 'What do I need in order to become a health leader?' perhaps we should ask 'What kind of leader does the world need?'

Getting the public health leaders the world needs

We need public health leaders everywhere and at every level of the health system. However, good leaders are most needed in places where people are poor and suffering simply because there is such a scarcity of them there. Committed and effective leaders often provide the vision and impetus to mobilize people and resources in needy areas (see Box 3.4.3).

How can the international health community help developing countries develop the needed leaders? A good starting point is to aim at strengthening educational institutions, which can provide relevant, team-based training, and at providing support towards helping governments and their partners to improve workplace conditions, including financial and non-financial incentives. From an international perspective we can work towards empowering nations to do this self-sufficiently, strengthening their own frameworks for leadership. Health leaders have used the term 'capacity release' in reference to this kind of endeavour (Chan 2007). It must be stressed that training programmes are only one component of a comprehensive approach that should include strategies to retain promising public health workers and sustain the idealism of leaders who are prepared to venture forth to places of hardship. We must encourage and support them to stay where they are most needed. Examples of work being done on this include the WHO framework on training leaders and managers (Egger et al. 2005) and related work to strengthen leadership at all levels of the health system.

Conclusion

As we come to the end of this chapter, let us summarize its most important points:

◆ The literature makes an academic distinction between leadership and management. Leadership has more to do with the visionary activities of setting direction, while management leans towards the controlling tasks associated with implementation. In practice, the two are often linked in the job description and work of an individual;

◆ Leaders possess certain personal qualities, skills, and principles that enable them to do what they need to do. These attributes are acquired through a variety of ways. The constant manifestation and practice of these attributes, skills, and principles is a continuing challenge in a leader's job and career;

◆ In the face of ever-increasing complexity in the world around us, public health leadership is needed to prevent, treat, and eliminate disease and promote the health of people. This capability to lead should be developed and nurtured in prospective individuals in varying social and cultural contexts and at all levels and types of public health organizations;

◆ Each 'path to leadership' is unique and very personal. However, exposure, training, mentors, and guiding principles all help in the development of leadership qualities in individuals who aspire to lead. They should be sought by anyone interested in serving as a public health leader.

In closing, the pursuit of leadership must ennoble the mind and the heart of those who aspire to it. It is a noble and never-ending quest. We bid the reader all success.

Notes

1 Leaders we spoke to were chosen from among current and former work colleagues. Information was derived from direct interviews or informal conversations. In some instances, speeches and curriculum vitae were referred to. Where interviews were made, there was no standard structure. Informants were told in advance that the purpose of the interview was to learn about their experiences as a leader in public health. They were asked simply to talk about their background and to tell stories from their experience. Follow-up questions focused on some of the broad themes arising from the literature.

Acknowledgements

The authors would like to thank Amimo Agola, Anand Kurup, Chadia Wannous, Christine Lamoureux, Claudia Vivas, Delanyo Dovlo, Dick Chamla, Francis Omaswa, Guangyuan Liu, Helen Robinson, Lealou Reballos, Maria Eufemia Yap, and Miriam Were, among others, for their insights into the issues of leadership in public health.

We would also like to acknowledge the contributions of Daniel Shaw for editing the text and providing useful material for the text and boxes. Thanks also to Carmen Dolea for her valuable comments on the manuscript and to Joanne McManus for polishing the final draft.

References

Alban-Metcalfe, Robert, J., and Alimo-Metcalfe, B. (2000). An analysis of the convergent and discriminant validity of the transformational leadership questionnaire. *International Journal of Selection and Assessment*, **8**(3), 158–75.

Avolio, B.J. and Bass, B.M. (1999). Re-examining the components of transformational and transactional leadership using the multifactor leadership questionnaire. *Journal of Occupational & Organizational Psychology*, **72**(4), 441–62.

Baquiran, R., Yap, M.E., and Bengzon, A.R.A. (2006). *Terminal grant report: Leaders for Health Program 2002–2006.* Pfizer Philippines Foundation Inc., Manila.

Binney, G., Wilke G., and Williams, C. (2005). *Living leadership, a practical guide for ordinary heroes.* Pearson Education Limited, England.

Bonita, R., Beaglehole, R., and Kjellström, T. (1993). *Basic Epidemiology.* WHO, Geneva.

Cardenas, V.M., Roces, M.C., Wattanasri, S. *et al.* (2002). Improving global public health leadership through training in epidemiology and public health: The experience of TEPHINET. Training Programs in Epidemiology and Public Health Interventions Network. *American Journal of Public Health*, **92**(2), 196–7.

Chan, M. (2007). Address to WHO staff. 4 Jan 2007. World Health Organization, Geneva.

Dayrit, M.M. (2004). *Health and population. The Macapagal–Arroyo presidency and administration – Record and legacy (2001–2004).* University of the Philippines Press, Quezon City, Philippines.

Dickinson, H., Peck, E., and Smith, J. (2006). *Leadership in organisational transition – what can we learn from research evidence?* March 2006. National Health Service Institute for Innovation and Improvement Health Services Management Centre, United Kingdom.

Dweggah, M. (2007). *Managment of Staff.* Interview with Dr Margaret Chan, Director-General, WHO; May 2007 UN Special, Geneva.

Egger, D., Travis, P., Dovlo, D. *et al.* (2005). *Strengthening management in low-income countries.* Making Health Systems Work: Working Paper Series Number 1. World Health Organization, Geneva.

Firth-Cozens, J. and Mowbray, D. (2001). Leadership and the quality of care. *Quality in Health Care*, **10** (Suppl 2), ii3–7.

Flahault, D. and Roemer, M.I. (1986). *Leadership for primary health care.* World Health Organization, Geneva.

Gawad Kalinga. Main site. http://www.gawadkalinga.org/. Accessed 10 July 2007.

Grint, K. (2002). Management or leadership? *Journal of Health Services Research & Policy*, **7**(4), 248–51.

Huczynski A.A. and Buchanan D.A. (2007). *Organizational Behaviour, an Introductory Text*, 6th edition. Pearson Education Limited, England.

Kouzes, J.M. and Posner, B.Z. (1997). *Leadership practices inventory (LPI): Facilitators Guide*, 2nd edition. Jossey-Bass, San Francisco.

Leaders for Health Program (2005). *The LHP experience: 5 stories of hope and transformation in municipal health practices (Program Document).* Ateneo Professional Schools, Makati, Philippines. www.leadersforhealth.ph.

McGrew, R.E. (1985). *Encyclopedia of Medical History.* The MacMillan Press, London.

NHS Leadership Centre (2006). *NHS leadership qualities framework.* National Health Service Institute for Innovation and Improvement, United Kingdom.

Plsek, P.E. and Wilson, T. (2001). Complexity, leadership, and management in healthcare organisations. *British Medical Journal*, **323**(7315), 746–9.

Reproductive Health Matters (2005). 'Round Up – law and Policy'. *Reproductive Health Matters*, **13**(6), 180–6.

Saleh, S. S., Williams, D., and Balougan, M. (2004). Evaluating the effectiveness of public health leadership training: The NEPHLI experience. *American Journal of Public Health*, **94**(7), 1245–9.

Stone, A.G. and Patterson, K. (2005). *The history of leadership focus.* Servant Leadership Research Roundtable – August 2005. School of Leadership Studies, Regent University.

Thomas, J.C. (2005). Ethics in public health: Skills for the ethical practice of public health. *Journal of Public Health Management Practice*, **11**(3), 260–1.

Turning Point Program. (2001). *Collaborative leadership and health: A review of the literature*, 80 pages. Leadership Development National Excellence Collaborative, Turning Point Program, Seattle, WA.

Umble, K., Steffen, D., Porter, J. *et al.* (2005). The National Public Health Leadership Institute: Evaluation of a team-based approach to developing collaborative public health leaders. *American Journal of Public Health*, **95**(4), 641–4.

Wikipedia contributors, 'Gawad Kalinga', *Wikipedia, The Free Encyclopedia.* http://en.wikipedia.org/wiki/Gawad_Kalinga_777. Accessed 10 July 2007.

World Health Organization. *Knowledge network on urban settings* (Poster). WHO Commission on Social Determinants of Health, WHO Centre for Health Development, Kobe, Japan.

World Health Organization. *The health leadership service.* World Health Organization, Geneva, Switzerland. http://www.who.int/health_leadership/en/. Accessed on 11 July 2007.

World Health Organization (2003). *WHO Framework Convention on Tobacco Control.* World Health Organization, Geneva, Switzerland. http://www.who.int/tobacco/framework/WHO_FCTC_english.pdf. Accessed on 9 July 2007.

World Health Organization (2007). *Managing the health millennium development goals – the challenge of management strengthening: Lessons from three countries.* World Health Organization, Geneva, Switzerland.

World Health Organization. (2007). *Public health, innovation and intellectual property.* 60th World Health Assembly Resolution WHA60.30, May 2007. World Health Organization, Geneva, Switzerland. http://www.who.int/gb/ebwha/pdf_files/WHA60/A60_R30-en.pdf. Accessed on 9 July 2007.

Wright, K., Rowitz, L., and Merkle, A. (2001). A conceptual model for leadership development. *Journal of Public Health Management and Practice*, **7**(4), 60–6.

Wright, K., Rowitz, L., Merkle, A. *et al.* (2000). Competency development in public health leadership. *American Journal of Public Health*, **90**(8), 1202–7.

Xirasagar, S., Samuels, M.E., and Curtin, T.F. (2006). Management training of physician executives, their leadership style, and care management performance: An empirical study. *The American Journal of Managed Care*, **12**(2), 101–8.

Xirasagar, S., Samuels, M.E., and Stoskopf, C.H. (2005). Physician leadership styles and effectiveness: An empirical study. *Medical Care Research & Review*, **62**(6), 720–40

SECTION 4

Public health law and ethics

4.1

The right to the highest attainable standard of health[1]

Paul Hunt, Gunilla Backman, Judith Bueno de Mesquita, Louise Finer, Rajat Khosla, Dragana Korljan, and Lisa Oldring

Abstract

This chapter introduces the right to the highest attainable standard of health, which is enshrined in several legally binding international treaties, as well as numerous national constitutions. It outlines the complementary relationship between public health and the right to the highest attainable standard of health, and provides a framework for analysing this human right. This analytical framework is then applied, by way of illustration, to neglected diseases, mental disability, sexual and reproductive health, and water and sanitation. The conclusion identifies the key features of a health system from the perspective of the right to the highest attainable standard of health.

Human rights

What are human rights?

Human rights are freedoms and entitlements concerned with the protection of the inherent dignity and equality of every human being. They include civil, political, economic, social, and cultural rights. The international community has accepted the position that all human rights are universal, indivisible, interdependent, and interrelated (UN 1993).

Although inspired by moral values, such as dignity and equality, human rights are more than moral entitlements: They are legally guaranteed through national and international legal obligations on duty bearers. They are enshrined, for example, in various international treaties and declarations.

International human rights treaties (often called covenants or conventions), such as the International Covenant on Economic, Social and Cultural Rights (ICESCR), are legally binding on the States that ratify them ('States parties'). In contrast, human rights declarations, such as the Universal Declaration of Human Rights, are non-binding, although many of them do include norms and principles that reflect obligations that are binding under customary international law.

Human rights have traditionally been concerned with the relationship between the State, on one hand, and individuals and groups on the other. By ratifying international human rights treaties, States assume binding legal obligations to give effect to the human rights enumerated within them.

Additionally, all States have national laws that protect some human rights. Moreover, some States have enshrined human rights—civil, political, economic, social, and cultural—in their constitutions.

Historic neglect of economic, social, and cultural rights, such as the rights to health and shelter, is gradually being overcome, thanks in part to civil society organizations across the world that have campaigned for their equal representation and advocated for specific mechanisms for their enforcement.

Who has human rights duties?

Although only States are parties to international and regional human rights treaties, and are thus fully accountable for compliance with their provisions, all members of society have responsibilities regarding the realization of human rights, including the right to the highest attainable standard of health (UN 1948, preamble; UNCESCR 2000, para. 42). This includes health workers,[2] families, communities, inter- and non-governmental organizations, civil society groups, as well as the private business sector: These so-called 'non-State actors' all have responsibilities regarding the realization of the right to health. States, as parties to international treaties, have a duty to provide an environment in which all of these individuals and groups can discharge their human rights responsibilities.

---

[1] The 'right to health' or the 'right to the highest attainable standard of health' are used as shorthand for 'the right of everyone to the enjoyment of the highest attainable standard of physical and mental health', the full title envisaged in Article 12 of the International Covenant on Economic, Social and Cultural Rights (ICESCR).

[2] A generic term encompassing doctors, nurses, midwives, public health professionals, managers/administrators, traditional health workers, as well as those working in particular contexts or specializations, such as prison health or obstetrics and gynaecology. According to the WHO definition, health workers are 'all people engaged in actions whose primary intent is to enhance health' (WHO 2006a).

Approaches to human rights

One approach to the vindication of human rights is via the courts, tribunals, and other judicial and quasi-judicial processes (the 'judicial' approach). Another approach, however, brings human rights to bear upon policy-making processes so that policies and programmes that promote and protect human rights are put in place (the 'policy' approach). Although the two approaches are intimately related and mutually reinforcing, the distinction between them is important because the 'policy' approach opens up challenging new interdisciplinary possibilities for the operationalization of human rights.

Lawyers have played an indispensable role in developing the norms and standards that today constitute international human rights law. Naturally, when it comes to the 'judicial' and 'policy' approaches, some lawyers are professionally drawn to the former. Indeed, in the context of the right to health, despite some suggestions to the contrary, this approach has a vital role to play and many courts have demonstrated that they have a crucial contribution to make.[3] It is important that this judicial contribution deepens and becomes more widespread.

In addition to this approach, however, it is vital that the right to health is brought to bear upon all relevant local, national and international policy-making processes This 'policy' approach depends upon techniques and tools—indicators, benchmarks, impact assessments, and so on—that demand close cooperation across a range of disciplines. Given its historic role and traditional expertise, public health has an indispensable contribution to make to the 'policy' approach. The Section 'New tools and techniques' below briefly introduces some of these techniques and tools in the specific context of the right to the highest attainable standard of health.

What is the right to health?

Sources of the right to health[4]

The origins of the international right to the highest attainable standard of health can be traced back over 50 years. Adopted in 1946, the World Health Organization's Constitution States: 'The enjoyment of the highest attainable standard of health is one of the fundamental rights of every human being without distinction of race, religion, political belief, economic or social condition'. Two years later, article 25(1) of the Universal Declaration of Human Rights laid the foundations for the international legal framework for the right to health. Since then, the right to health has been codified in numerous legally binding international and regional human rights treaties, and enshrined in many national laws, some of which are signalled in the following paragraphs. This gives rise to one of the most important and distinctive characteristics of human rights, including the right to the highest attainable standard of health. Human rights place legally binding obligations on States.

International human rights law

Concrete legal duties are conferred upon States when they ratify international treaties; they must ensure that all individuals within their jurisdiction can enjoy the rights envisaged within them. The cornerstone protection of the right to health in international law is found in Article 12 of ICESCR. Over 155 States have legally bound themselves, through ratification of this treaty, to its implementation.

Additional right to health protections are contained in international treaties that address issues specific to marginalized groups, such as the International Convention for the Elimination of All Forms of Racial Discrimination (ICERD);[5] the International Convention on the Elimination of All Forms of Discrimination Against Women (CEDAW);[6] and the Convention on the Rights of the Child (CRC).[7]

Authoritative and interpretive guiding principles of several of these treaty provisions on the right to health—called General Comments or General Recommendations—shed further light on the parameters and content of the right to health generally, and in relation to the application of the right to specific groups. In 2000, for example, the United Nations (UN) treaty-body responsible for monitoring ICESCR adopted General Comment 14 on the right to the highest attainable standard of health.

Moreover, some UN treaty-bodies have decided cases that shed light on the scope of health-related rights. Recently, for example, the Human Rights Committee considered the case of a 17-year old Peruvian who was denied a therapeutic abortion. When K.L was 14 weeks pregnant, doctors at a public hospital in Lima diagnosed the foetus with an abnormality that would endanger K.L's health if pregnancy continued. However, K.L. was denied a therapeutic abortion by the hospital's director. In *K.L. v Peru*, the Human Rights Committee decided that by denying the young woman's request to undergo an abortion in accordance with Peruvian law, the Government was in breach of its right-to-life obligations under the International Covenant on Civil and Political Rights (UNHRCttee 2003).

Further standards relating to specific groups are set out in non-binding legal instruments, such as the Declaration on the Elimination of Violence against Women. Additional international human rights instruments contain protections relevant to the right to health in various situations, environments and processes, including armed conflict, development, the workplace, and detention (UNCHR 2003a, Annex I).

Significantly, resolutions of the UN Commission on Human Rights, including those on disabilities and access to medication (UNCHR 2002a, b), have articulated the right to the highest attainable standard of health; while other important resolutions contain provisions that bear closely upon the right (UNCHR 2003a, Annex II).

Far-reaching commitments relating to the right to health have been made in the outcome documents of numerous UN world conferences, such as the International Conference on Population and Development (UN 1994), the Fourth World Conference on Women (UN 1995), and the Millennium Declaration (UNGA 2000). These conferences have helped to place international problems, including health issues such as HIV/AIDS, at the top of the global agenda and their outcome documents influence international and national

---

[3] For an overview of jurisprudence on the right to health, see UNHRC (2007, paras 55–89).

[4] The 'right to health' or the 'right to the highest attainable standard of health' is employed as shorthand for the full title which is 'the right of everyone to the enjoyment of the highest attainable standard of physical and mental health'.

[5] ICERD provides protection for racial and ethnic groups in relation to 'the right to public health (and) medical care' (Article 5 (e) (iv)).

[6] CEDAW provides several provisions for the protection of women's right to health (Articles 11 (1) f, 12 and 14 (2) b).

[7] CRC contains extensive and elaborate provisions on the child's right to health, including one which is fully dedicated to the right to the health of the child (Article 24), and others containing protections for especially vulnerable groups of children (articles 3 (3), 17, 23, 25, 32, and 28).

policy-making. Several refer to the right to health and health-related rights.

Regional human rights law

The right to health is recognized in human rights treaties drafted and monitored by the different regional human rights systems. These have effect only in their respective regions and include: The African Charter on Human and Peoples' Rights (Article 16); the African Charter on the Rights and Welfare of the Child (Article 14); the Additional Protocol to the American Convention on Human Rights in the Area of Economic, Social and Cultural Rights, known as the 'Protocol of San Salvador' (Article 10); and the European Social Charter (Article 11). Other regional instruments provide, through health-related rights, indirect protection of the right to health.[8]

At regional level there are also judicial and other mechanisms that adjudicate cases involving the right to health. A notable case in 2002 was the finding by the African Commission on Human and Peoples' Rights of a violation of the right to health by the Federal Republic of Nigeria, on account of violations against the Ogoni people in relation to the activities of oil companies in the Niger Delta (ACHPR 2001).

Significantly, regional mechanisms have also found breaches of other health-related rights, including the violation of the right to a home and family and private life, arising from environmental harm to human health in *López Ostra v. Spain* (ECtHR 1994), as well as the negative consequences on children's health stemming from the occurrence of child labour in *ICJ v. Portugal* (ECSR 1998).

Another important development has come from the Inter-American Commission on Human Rights, which expressed its willingness to 'take into account' provisions of the regional treaty (the Protocol of San Salvador) related to the right to health when analysing the merits of a case, even though it lacked competence to determine violations under them (IACHR 2000).

National law

A study has shown that 67.5 per cent of the constitutions of all nations have provisions regarding health and healthcare (Kinney & Clark 2004). In addition, a large number of constitutions set out States' duties in relation to health, such as the duty to develop health services, from which it is possible to infer health entitlements.

In some jurisdictions these constitutional provisions have generated significant jurisprudence, such as the decision of the Constitutional Court of South Africa in *Minister for Health v. Treatment Action Campaign*. In this case, the Court held that the Constitution required the Government 'to devise and implement a comprehensive and coordinated programme to realize progressively the right of pregnant women and their newborn children to have access to health services to combat mother-to-child transmission of HIV' (CCSA 2002, para. 135 (2) (a)). This case—and numerous other laws and decisions at the international, regional, and national levels—confirms that the courts have an important role to play in the protection of the right to the highest attainable standard of health.

---

[8] These include the American Declaration on the Rights and Duties of Man, the American Convention on Human Rights, the Inter-American Convention on the Prevention, Punishment and Eradication of Violence against Women, and the European Convention for the Protection of Human Rights and Fundamental Freedoms and its protocols.

Right to health in the context of other human rights

As already indicated, the right to health is closely related to and dependent upon the realization of other fundamental human rights contained within international law. These include the rights to life, food, housing, work, and education, as well as rights based on the freedom not to be tortured or discriminated against. Similarly, the rights to privacy, equality, access to information, and freedom of association, as well as other rights and freedoms, relate to and address integral components of the right to health.

The right to health—like other economic, social, and cultural rights—does not escape controversy and ideological objections. Some States are still reluctant to see it as a right of similar weight to others, such as the right to a fair trial. However, under international law, the right to the highest attainable standard of health is an integral part of the international code of human rights and must be given equal treatment and attention. Importantly, the interdependence and equal footing of all human rights was reaffirmed in the Vienna Declaration (UN 1993, para. 5). Furthermore, jurisprudence and international standards are gradually clarifying the mutually reinforcing relationship between the right to health and other health-related rights, such as the right to life (UNCESCR 2000, para. 3).

The complementary relationship between public health and the right to health

With a few exceptions, the relationship between health and human rights was not subject to close examination until the 1990s. Of course, the Constitution of WHO (WHO 1946) affirms the right to health and so does the Declaration of Alma-Ata (WHO 1978a). Also, some of those who were struggling against HIV/AIDS in the 1980s recognized the crucial importance of human rights. But, for the most part, these important developments were not accompanied by a detailed examination of the substantive relationship between health and human rights. That had to wait until the early 1990s. A great debt is owed to the late Jonathan Mann and his colleagues at the Harvard School of Public Health and the Francois-Xavier Bagnoud Center for Health and Human Rights for their pioneering work on the relationship between health and human rights, especially in the context of HIV/AIDS.

In the 1990s, however, Dr. Mann and others suffered from a serious limitation that does not apply today. At that time, although there was a widespread and detailed understanding of many human rights, there was no comparable understanding of the right to the highest attainable standard of health, even though this human right is the cornerstone of the relationship between health and human rights.

Today, however, the situation is significantly different. In 2000, an authoritative understanding of the right to health emerged when the UN Committee on Economic, Social and Cultural Rights, working in close collaboration with WHO and many others, adopted General Comment 14 (UNCESCR 2000). Also, some international bodies like WHO, UNFPA, UNICEF, and UNAIDS, as well as civil society organizations, have begun to give more careful attention to health-related rights, including the right to the highest attainable standard of health. These and other developments have deepened understanding of the right to health, enabling linkages to be made between public health and human rights, a process that continues to accelerate through good practice, the academic literature and widening jurisprudence.

Although in some quarters there is a presumption that the right to health relates to medical care, such a narrow definition is in fact inconsistent with international human rights law, which encompasses both medicine and public health, as confirmed by Article 12 of ICESCR and Article 24 of CRC. As well as access to medical care, the right to health encompasses the social, cultural, economic, political, and other conditions that make people need medical care in the first place (WHO 1948, preamble; Beaglehole 2002), as well as other determinants of health such as access to water, sanitation, nutrition, housing, and education. This wider perspective underscores the very extensive common ground between public health and the right to the highest attainable standard of health.

The right to the highest attainable standard of health depends upon public health measures, such as immunization programmes, the provision of adequate sanitation systems and clean drinking water, health promotion (e.g. regarding domestic violence, healthy eating, and taking exercise), road safety campaigns, nutrition programmes, the promotion of indoor stoves that reduce respiratory diseases, and so on. Also, however, the classic, long-established public health objectives can benefit from the newer, dynamic discipline of human rights. In other words, just as public health programmes are essential to the realization of the right to health, so too can human rights help to reinforce existing, good, health programmes and identify new, equitable, health policies. This chapter focuses on the relevance of the right to the highest attainable standard of health to public health. However, the indispensable contribution of public health to the right to the highest attainable standard of health also deserves careful study.

Both public health and human rights advocates wish to establish effective, integrated, responsive health systems that are accessible to all. Both stress the importance not only of access to healthcare, but also to water, sanitation, health information, and education. Both understand that good health is not the sole responsibility of the Ministry of Health, but belongs to a wide range of public and private actors. Both prioritize the struggle against discrimination and disadvantage, and both stress cultural respect. At root, those working in health and human rights are both animated by a similar concern: The well-being of individuals and populations.

Health workers—defined in the World Health Report of 2006 (WHO 2006a) as 'all people engaged in actions whose primary intent is to enhance health'—can use health-related rights to help them devise more equitable policies and programmes; to place important health issues higher up national and international agendas; to secure better coordination across health-related sectors, as well as between services within the health sector; to raise more funds from the treasury; to leverage more funds from developed countries to developing countries; in some countries, to improve the terms and conditions of those working in the health sector; and so on. The right to the highest attainable standard of health is not just a rhetorical device, but also a tool that can save lives and reduce suffering, especially among the most disadvantaged.

The following sections provide examples that illustrate the resonance between public health and the right to the highest attainable standard of health.

Although these two disciplines are, in many ways, complementary, in practice public health has been used by some States as a ground for limiting the exercise of some human rights. Indeed, under international law, States are allowed to impose some limitations on human rights, in some circumstances, for the protection of public health, an issue briefly revisited in the following section.

The contours and content of the right to health

The right to health is not a right to be healthy. It is a right to facilities, goods, services, and conditions that are conducive to the realization of the highest attainable standard of physical and mental health. Understanding of the content of the right has evolved considerably over the last 50 years, with jurisprudence, international standards, and practical implementation of the right all contributing to this process.

As we have seen, an inclusive approach to implementing the right to the highest attainable standard of health calls for its reach to extend not only to timely and appropriate medical care, but also to the underlying determinants of health, such as access to safe and potable water and adequate sanitation, healthy occupational and environmental conditions, and access to health-related education and information (UNCESCR 2000, para. 8).

The right to health can also be broken down into more specific entitlements, such as the rights to: Maternal, child, and reproductive health; healthy workplace and natural environments; the prevention, treatment and control of diseases, including access to essential medicines; and access to safe and potable water.

In times of emergency, States have a joint and individual responsibility to cooperate in providing disaster relief and humanitarian assistance, including medical aid and potable water as well as assistance to refugees and internally displaced persons (UNCESCR 2000, para. 40).

Certain limitations on the right to health do exist, as issues of public health are sometimes used by States as grounds for limiting the exercise of other fundamental rights. For such limitations to be implemented legitimately, they must be in accordance with the law and international human rights standards. In particular, they should be strictly necessary for the promotion of the general welfare in a democratic society, proportional, subject to review, and of limited duration (UNCESCR 2000, paras. 28–9; UN ECOSOC 1985, Annex).

The right to health analytical framework

In recent years, the Committee on Economic, Social and Cultural Rights, WHO, the Special Rapporteur on the right of everyone to the enjoyment of the highest attainable standard of physical and mental health, civil society organizations, academics, and many others, have developed a way of 'unpacking' or analysing the right to health with a view to making it easier to understand and apply to health-related policies, programmes, and projects in practice. The analytical framework that has been developed is made up of 10 key elements and has general application to all aspects of the right to health, including the underlying determinants of health: This has been demonstrated by the Special Rapporteur in his use of the framework throughout his work.

◆ *National and international human rights laws, norms and standards*

The relevant laws, norms, and standards relevant to the particular issue, programme, or policy must be identified. These will include both general provisions and standards relating to the right to health, in addition to international instruments that relate to specific groups and contexts (see the Section 'What is the right to health?' above) (UNCHR 2003a, Annex 1).

◆ *Resource constraints and progressive realization*

International human rights law recognizes that the realization of the right to health is subject to resource availability. Thus, what is required of a developed State today is of a higher standard than what is required of a developing State. However, a State is obliged—whatever its resource constraints and level of economic development—to realize progressively the right to the highest attainable standard of health (UN 1966b, Art. 2(1)). In essence, this means that a State is required to be doing better in 2 years time than it is doing today. In order to measure progress (or the lack of it) over time, indicators and benchmarks must be identified (see the Section 'New tools and techniques).

◆ *Obligations of immediate effect*

Despite resource constraints and progressive realization, the right to health also gives rise to some obligations of immediate effect, such as the duty to avoid discrimination (UNCESCR 2000, para. 43). These are obligations without which the right would be deprived of its raison d'être and as such they are not subject to progressive realization, even in the presence of resource constraints. (UNCESCR 1990, para.10). The precise scope of these immediate obligations has not yet been clearly defined; for the health and human rights communities, this remains important work-in-progress.

◆ *Freedoms and entitlements*

The right to health includes both freedoms (for example, the freedom from discrimination or non-consensual medical treatment and experimentation) and entitlements (for example, the provision of a system of health protection that includes minimum essential levels of water and sanitation). For the most part, freedoms do not have budgetary implications, while entitlements do.

◆ *Available, accessible, acceptable and good quality*

All health services, goods, and facilities should comply with each of these four requirements. An essential medicine, for example, should be *available* within the country. Additionally, the medicine should be *accessible*. Accessibility has four dimensions: Accessible without discrimination, physically accessible, economically accessible (i.e. affordable), and accessible health-related information. As well as being available and accessible, health services should be provided in a culturally *acceptable* manner. This requires, for example, effective coordination and referral with traditional health systems. Lastly, all health services, goods, and services should be of *good quality*; a medicine, for example, must not be beyond its expiry date. These four requirements are further explored and applied in Section 'Right to health issues through the analytical framework'.

Note the similarity between these requirements and the four 'As' of public healthcare envisaged since the 1978 Alma Ata Declaration: Geographical accessibility; financial accessibility; cultural accessibility; and functional accessibility (WHO 1978b).

◆ *Respect, protect, fulfil*

This subsidiary framework relates to the tripartite obligations of States to respect, protect, and fulfil the right to the highest attainable standard of health, as explained and used by CESCR, the Committee on the Elimination of Discrimination Against Women (CEDAW) and the Sub-Commission on the Promotion and Protection of Human Rights. A version of this subsidiary framework is also enshrined in the Constitution of South Africa.

For example, the obligation to *respect* places a duty on States to refrain from interfering directly or indirectly with the enjoyment of the right to health. The obligation to *protect* means that States must prevent third parties from interfering with the enjoyment of the right to health. The obligation to *fulfil* requires States to adopt necessary measures, including legislative, administrative and budgetary measures, to ensure the full realization of human rights, including the right to the highest attainable standard of health.

◆ *Non-discrimination, equality and vulnerability*

Because of their crucial importance, the analytical framework demands that special attention be given to issues of non-discrimination, equality, and vulnerability in relation to all elements of the right to the highest attainable standard of health.

◆ *Active and informed participation*

Participation is grounded in internationally recognized human rights, such as the rights to participate in the formulation and implementation of government policy, to take part in the conduct of public affairs, and to freedom of expression and association.[9] The right to health requires that there be an opportunity for individuals and groups to participate actively and in an informed manner in health policy-making processes that affect them (UNCESCR 2000, para. 54).

◆ *International assistance and cooperation*

In line with obligations envisaged in the UN Charter and some human rights treaties,[10] developing countries have a responsibility to seek international assistance and cooperation, while developed States have some responsibilities towards the realization of the right to health in developing countries.

◆ *Monitoring and accountability*

The right to health introduces globally legitimized norms or standards from which obligations or responsibilities arise. These obligations have to be monitored and those responsible held to account. Without monitoring and accountability, the norms and obligations are likely to become empty promises. Accountability mechanisms provide rights-holders (e.g. individuals and groups) with an opportunity to understand how duty-bearers have discharged their obligations, and it also provides duty-bearers (e.g. ministers and officials) with an opportunity to explain their conduct. In this way, accountability mechanisms help to identify when—and what—policy adjustments are necessary. Accountability tends to encourage the most effective use of limited resources, as well as a shared responsibility among all parties. Transparent, effective, and accessible accountability mechanisms are among the most crucial characteristics of the right to the highest attainable standard of health.

These 10 key elements of the right-to-health analytical framework underscore what the right to health contributes to public health. For example, the pre-occupation with non-discrimination, equality, and vulnerability requires a State to take effective measures to address the health inequities that characterize some populations. The focus on active and informed participation requires a State to adopt, so far

---

9 For example, *International Covenant on Civil and Political Rights* (ICCPR), articles 19, 22, 25; *International Covenant on Economic, Social and Cultural Rights* (ICESCR), article 13; *Convention on the Elimination of All Forms of Discrimination Against Women* (CEDAW): articles 7, 8.
10 UN Charter; ICESCR (Article 2); CRC (Article 4).

as possible, a 'bottom-up' participatory approach in health-related sectors. The requirement of monitoring and accountability can help to ensure that health policies, programmes, and practices are meaningful to those living in poverty.

Crucially, the key elements of the right-to-health analytical framework are not merely to be followed because they accord with sound management, ethics, social justice, or humanitarianism. States are required to conform to the key features *as a matter of binding law*. Moreover, they are to be held to account for the discharge of their right-to-health responsibilities arising from these legal obligations.

Right to health issues through the analytical framework

In this section, elements of the analytical framework signalled in Section 'The contours and content of the right to health' are applied to a selection of health issues. While space does not permit all of the elements to be applied to all of the selected issues, each element is applied to at least one of them.

The selected health issues are: Neglected diseases; mental disability; sexual and reproductive health, including maternal mortality; and water and sanitation. The right to health is among the most extensive and complex in the international lexicon of human rights. As already signalled, it extends much further than these four issues which are simply provided as an illustration of how the right-to-health analytical framework applies to this selection of important health issues.

Neglected diseases[11]

Although there is no standard global definition of 'neglected diseases', nor are they homogenous, they tend to share some common features. For example, they typically affect neglected populations, those least able to demand services. They are a symptom of poverty and disadvantage. Fear and stigma are attached to some neglected diseases, leading to delays in seeking treatment and to discrimination against those afflicted.

Neglected diseases include lymphatic filariasis, schistosomiasis, onchoocerciasis (river blindness), trachoma, buruli ulcer, soil-transmitted helminths, leishmaniasis, leprosy, and human African trypanosomiasis (sleeping sickness). According to WHO, 'the health impact of . . . neglected diseases is measured by severe and permanent disabilities and deformities in almost 1 billion people' (WHO 2002).

Where curative interventions for neglected diseases exist, they have generally failed to reach populations early enough to prevent impairment. Furthermore, the development of new tools to diagnose and treat them has been underfunded, largely because there has been little or no market incentive (WHO 2004a, p. 22).

◆ *Non-discrimination, equality and vulnerability*

Discrimination and social stigma can be both causes and consequences of certain neglected diseases. As non-discrimination and equal treatment are cornerstone principles in international human rights law, a rights-based approach to neglected diseases pays particular attention to policies, programmes, and projects that impair the equal enjoyment of the human rights of people suffering from these diseases.

Stigmatization and discrimination heighten people's vulnerability to ill health. Often, stigmatization is based on myths, misconceptions, and fears, including those related to certain diseases or health conditions. In turn, fear of stigmatization can lead people living with neglected diseases to avoid diagnosis, delay seeking treatment and hide the diseases from family, employers, and the community at large.

Discrimination involves acts or omissions which may be directed towards stigmatized individuals on account of their health status and/or related disabilities. For example, leprosy, lymphatic filariasis and leishmaniasis may cause severe physical disabilities, including deformities and scarring, giving rise to discrimination in the workplace, and access to healthcare and education.

The socioeconomic consequences of stigmatization and discrimination associated with neglected diseases can have devastating consequences for individuals and groups that are already marginalized, leading to further vulnerability to neglected diseases. For example, stigma related to tuberculosis can be greater for women: It may lead to ostracism, rejection, and abandonment by family and friends, as well as loss of social and economic support and other problems (WHO 2001, p. 12). Social and behavioural research on stigma and neglected diseases suggests that women also may experience more social disadvantages than men, in particular from physically disfiguring conditions like lymphatic filariasis (Coreil *et al.* 2003, p. 42).

The guarantee of non-discrimination and equal treatment enshrined under national and international human rights law requires the government to adopt wide-ranging measures, including through the implementation of health-related laws and policies, which confront discrimination in the public and private sector.

◆ *Active and informed participation*

A human rights approach not only attaches importance to reducing the incidence and burden of neglected diseases, but also to the democratic and inclusive processes by which these objectives are achieved. Such processes require the active, informed, and meaningful participation of communities affected by neglected diseases.

Affected communities have sometimes participated in aspects of prevention, treatment, and control of neglected diseases. For example, they are sometimes involved in vector control programmes, such as bed net impregnation to combat malaria, or housing improvements to combat Chagas disease, which is caused by parasites living in cracks in housing. Communities have also been involved in treatment strategies, for example, through community health workers who have been selected and trained to administer vaccinations and treatment (Espino *et al.* 2004).

However, the human rights approach means that affected communities should participate in a range of contexts, not just in implementing programmes. They should be actively involved in setting local, national, and international public health agendas; decision-making processes; identifying disease control strategies and other relevant policies; and holding duty bearers to account. While it is not suggested that affected communities should participate in all the technical deliberations that underlie policy formulation, their participation can help to avoid some of the top-down, technocratic tendencies often associated with old-style development plans and policy implementation.

Although effective participation is not straightforward, and takes time to generate, it is nonetheless an important means by which to empower and build capacity in affected communities, enhance accountability, and improve the effectiveness of interventions.

---

[11] See WHO and TDR (2007).

Therefore, as demonstrated in the following examples, participation has a positive impact on the enjoyment of the right to health.

In Peru in the 1980s, patients' associations, spontaneously set up in response to the government's failure to provide drugs and financial compensation for people who had suffered from leishmaniasis, were eventually successful in securing support from the regional and national health authorities. They became forums for discussions of wide-ranging social and political issues. This movement, which became more structured and organized over time, provided local institutions with detailed knowledge and made links with local populations so that it became possible to determine the best control and intervention strategies, and implement them successfully (Guthman *et al.* 1997).

In Uganda, Village Health Teams are able to help dispel the neglect that characterizes certain diseases and populations, ensuring that local needs are clearly identified, understood, and addressed. Moreover, the Teams can provide the crucial grassroots delivery mechanisms for community interventions in relation to neglected diseases, and health protection generally.

Vehicles for community participation such as these require adequate resources, training, and support. They must be listened to and used strategically as delivery mechanisms in relation to neglected diseases, with smooth and effective coordination, cooperation, and collaboration between them and the local political structure and health centres. For this reason, government, development actors, and others should sustain and foster vital community-based initiatives to ensure that full and effective participation can support the realization of the right to health.

◆ *Monitoring and accountability*

In practice, few accountability mechanisms give sufficient attention to neglected diseases, and often prove inaccessible to impoverished members of neglected communities. Within a national jurisdiction, parliamentarians might hold the Minister of Health to account in relation to the discharge of his or her responsibilities, yet the ability of these and other general mechanisms (such as judicial processes) to provide adequate accountability in relation to neglected diseases and the right to health is doubtful.

The right to the highest attainable standard of health demands accessible, transparent, and effective monitoring and accountability mechanisms that are meaningful to neglected communities. These could include independent national human rights institutions that monitor the incidence of neglected diseases and the initiatives taken to address them. Adopting an evidence-based approach, the institution could scrutinize who is doing what and whether or not they are doing all that can reasonably be expected of them to realize the right to health of those concerned. Whenever possible, the institution should identify realistic and practical recommendations for all those involved.

International human rights machinery can also draw attention to the issue of neglected diseases and neglected populations. For example, when a relevant State presents its periodic reports to CESCR, both the Government's reports and the human rights body's examination of them, should give careful attention to the issue of neglected diseases and neglected populations, in accordance with the national and international right to health standards to which the Government is bound.

◆ *International assistance and cooperation*

This feature of the right to health requires that donors and the international community pay particular attention to the health problems of the most vulnerable and disadvantaged individuals and communities in developing countries. For example, donors and the international community have a duty to help developing countries enhance their capacity so they can determine their own national and local health research and development priorities, such as neglected diseases.

Mental disabilities[12]

Too often, disability issues do not attract the attention they demand and deserve. This is especially true in the context of mental disabilities. The right to the highest attainable standard of health demands that due attention is given to both physical and mental disabilities.

A significant development in the field of disability was achieved with the adoption of a new international human rights treaty in 2006, the Convention on the Rights of Persons with Disabilities. Alongside this important new treaty, which will enter into force once ratified by 20 States, there are many important provisions contained in non-binding principles that have profound connections to the right to health, even if some elements are inadequate and need revisiting.[13] Where appropriate, these specialized instruments should be used as interpretive guides in relation to the right to health as it is enshrined in international law.

International human rights treaties and specialized international instruments relating to mental disabilities are mutually reinforcing, even if, as the UN Secretary General recently put it, 'a more detailed analysis of the implementation of State human rights obligations in the context of mental health institutions would be desirable' (UNGA 2003, para. 43). Inadequate attention has been given to the implementation of these obligations to date. In this context it is heartening that the new UN Convention received the highest number of signatories of any such Convention on its opening day.[14]

◆ *Freedoms and entitlements*

Freedoms
Freedoms of particular relevance to the experience of individuals with mental disabilities include the right to control one's health and body. Forced sterilizations, rape, and other forms of sexual violence, to which women with mental disabilities are particularly vulnerable, are inherently inconsistent with their sexual and reproductive health rights and freedoms, are psychologically and physically traumatic, and thus jeopardize mental health even further.

Several international human rights instruments allow for exceptional circumstances in which persons with mental disabilities can be involuntarily admitted to a hospital or another designated

---

[12] Noting the wide range of terminology available, the generic term 'mental disability' has been adopted for efficiency as an umbrella term, though it is recognized that it encompasses many profoundly different conditions. These include all major and minor mental illness and psychiatric disorders, as well as intellectual disabilities. 'Disability' refers to a range of impairments, activity limitations, and participation restrictions, whether permanent or transitory.

[13] See, for example, the *UN Principles for the protection of persons with mental illness and the improvement of mental health care*, ('UN Mental Illness Principles') (1991) (UNGA 1991).

[14] 82 countries signed the Convention on the day it opened to signature, 30 March 2007.

institution (ECHR, Article 5 (1) (e); UN Mental Illness Principles, Principle 16). However, because involuntary detention is an extremely serious interference with the freedom of persons with disabilities, in particular their right to liberty and security, international and national human rights law attaches numerous procedural safeguards to involuntary detention cases. Moreover, these safeguards are generating a significant jurisprudence, most notably in regional human rights commissions and courts (ECtHR 1979; Gostin & Gable 2004; Gostin 2000; Lewis 2002).

Entitlements

The right to health includes an entitlement to a system of health protection which provides equality of opportunity for all people to enjoy the highest attainable standard of health through access to both healthcare and the underlying determinants of health, all of which play a vital role in ensuring the health and dignity of persons with mental disabilities (UNGA 1993, Rules 2–4).

States are required to take steps to ensure a full package of community-based mental healthcare and support services conducive to health, dignity, and inclusion. These should include medication, psychotherapy, ambulatory services, hospital care for acute admissions, residential facilities, rehabilitation for persons with psychiatric disabilities, programmes to maximize the independence and skills of persons with intellectual disabilities, supported housing and employment, income support, inclusive and appropriate education for children with intellectual disabilities, and respite care for families looking after a person with a mental disability 24 h a day. In this way, unnecessary institutionalization can be avoided.

Scaling up interventions to ensure equality of opportunity for the enjoyment of the right to health requires that adequate numbers of appropriate professionals be trained. Similarly, primary care providers should be provided with essential mental healthcare and disability sensitization training to enable them to provide front-line mental and physical healthcare to persons with mental disabilities.

Underlying determinants of health that are particularly relevant to persons with mental disabilities, who are disproportionately affected by poverty and as such often deprived of important entitlements, include adequate sanitation, safe water, and adequate food and shelter (UNCESCR 2000, para. 4). The conditions in psychiatric hospitals, as well as other institutions used by persons with mental disabilities, are often grossly inadequate from this point of view.

◆ Obligations of immediate effect and progressive realization

It is reasonable to expect that countries, even those with very limited resources, undertake to implement certain measures towards realization of the right to health for people with disabilities. For example they can be expected to: Include the recognition, care, and treatment of mental disabilities in training curricula of all health personnel; promote public campaigns against stigma and discrimination of persons with mental disabilities; support the formation of civil society groups that are representative of mental healthcare users and their families; formulate modern policies and programmes on mental disabilities; downsize psychiatric hospitals and, as far as possible, extend community care; in relation to persons with mental disabilities, actively seek assistance and cooperation

from donors and international organizations (WHO 2001b, pp. 112–15).

◆ Respect, protect, fulfil

Specifically in relation to mental disabilities, the obligation to *respect* requires States to refrain from denying or limiting equal access to healthcare services and underlying determinants of health, for persons with mental disabilities. They are also required to ensure that persons with mental disabilities in public institutions are not denied access to healthcare and related support services, or underlying determinants of health, including water and sanitation (IACHR 1997).

The obligation to *protect* means that States are required to take actions to ensure that third parties do not harm the right to health of persons with mental disabilities. For example, States should take measures to protect persons with mental disabilities from violence and other right to health-related abuses occurring in private healthcare or support services.

The obligation to *fulfil* requires States to recognize the right to health, including the right to health of persons with mental disabilities, in national political and legal systems, with a view to ensuring its implementation. States should adopt appropriate legislative, administrative, budgetary, judicial, promotional, and other measures towards this end (ICESCR Article 2(1); UNCESCR 2000, para. 36). For example, States should ensure that the right to health of persons with mental disabilities is adequately reflected in their national health strategy and plan of action, as well as other relevant policies, such as national poverty reduction strategies, and the national budget (WHO 2004c). Mental health laws, policies, programmes, and projects should embody human rights and empower people with mental disabilities to make choices about their lives; give legal protections relating to the establishment of (and access to) quality mental health facilities, as well as care and support services; establish robust procedural mechanisms for the protection of those with mental disabilities; ensure the integration of persons with mental disabilities into the community; and promote mental health throughout society (WHO 2005a). Patients' rights charters should encompass the human rights of persons with mental disabilities. States should also ensure that access to information about their human rights is provided to persons with mental disabilities and their guardians, as well as others who may be institutionalized in psychiatric hospitals.

◆ International assistance and cooperation

The record shows that mental healthcare and support services are not a priority health area for donors. Furthermore, donors have sometimes supported inappropriate programmes, such as the rebuilding of a damaged psychiatric institution constructed many years ago on the basis of conceptions of mental disability that have since been discredited. In so doing, the donor inadvertently prolongs, for many years, seriously inappropriate approaches to mental disability.

It is unacceptable for a donor to fund a programme that, in moving a psychiatric institution to an isolated location, makes it impossible for its users to sustain or develop their links with the community (MDRI 2002). If a donor wishes to assist children with intellectual disabilities, it might wish to fund community-based services to support children and their parents, enabling the children to remain at home, instead of funding new facilities in a remote institution that the parents can only afford to visit once a month, if at all (Rosenthal 2000).

Donors have a right to health duty to consider more—and better quality—support in the area of mental disability. In accordance with their responsibility of international assistance and cooperation, they are required to consider adopting measures such as: Supporting the development of appropriate community-based care and support services; supporting advocacy by persons with mental disabilities, their families and representative organizations; and providing policy and technical expertise. Furthermore, donors should ensure that all their programmes promote equality and non-discrimination for persons with mental disabilities, while international agencies fulfil the role that corresponds to them by providing technical support.

◆ *Monitoring and accountability*

The right to health requires that States have in place effective, transparent, and accessible monitoring and accountability mechanisms in relation to the health of persons with mental disabilities.
In many countries, there is an absence of sustained and independent monitoring of mental healthcare, resulting in frequent abuses in large psychiatric hospitals and community-based settings going unnoticed. The Mental Illness Principles emphasize the importance of inspecting mental health facilities, as well as investigating and resolving complaints where an alleged violation of the rights of a patient is concerned (UN Mental Illness Principle 22).

Lack of surveillance is doubly problematic because persons with mental disabilities, especially those who are institutionalized, are often unable to access independent and effective accountability mechanisms when their human rights have been violated. Where accountability mechanisms do exist, the severity of their condition may render them unable to protect their interests independently through legal proceedings, to demand effective procedural safeguards where these may be lacking, or to access legal aid.

For example, the right to health requires that an independent review body must be made accessible to persons with mental disabilities, or other appropriate persons, to review cases of involuntary admission and treatment periodically (UN Mental Illness Principle 17).

Although there is a range of detailed international standards concerning the human rights of persons with mental disabilities, and procedural safeguards to protect them (UN Mental Illness Principles 11, 18), their lack of implementation poses a real challenge. The new Convention on the Rights of Persons with Disabilities will be crucial to international monitoring and accountability, especially if its Optional Protocol, which introduces a procedure under which individuals and groups can lodge complaints, were to come into force. Significantly, this mechanism strengthens the existing standards relating to the right to health of persons with mental disabilities that do not establish specific monitoring or accountability mechanisms.

Alongside this Convention, other international human rights treaties (including ICESCR, CRC, CEDAW and CERD, and ICCPR,) extend protections to persons with mental disabilities. For this reason, States should pay greater attention to them in their State party reports, and examination of these reports by the human rights treaty bodies should, in turn, give a greater focus to these issues through their discussions with States parties, concluding observations, and general comments or recommendations. Relevant civil society organizations, including representatives of persons with mental disabilities, play an important role by engaging with UN treaty bodies and special procedures.

Sexual and reproductive health, including maternal mortality

The Commission on Human Rights confirmed in 2003 that 'sexual and reproductive health are integral elements of the right of everyone to the enjoyment of the highest attainable standard of physical and mental health' (UNCHR 2003b, preamble and para. 6). The outcomes of world conferences, in particular the International Conference on Population and Development (UN 1994), the Fourth World Conference on Women (UN 1995), and their respective 5-year reviews, confirm that human rights have an indispensable role to play in relation to sexual and reproductive health issues.

More recently, there has been a deepening conceptual understanding of maternal mortality as a human rights issue (Cook *et al.* 2006; Freedman 2003). Although the issue is connected to a number of human rights, the right to the highest attainable standard of health is of particular relevance, and is the focus of the following remarks.

◆ *Freedoms and entitlements*

Freedoms
In the context of sexual and reproductive health, freedoms include a right to control one's health and body. Rape and other forms of sexual violence, including forced pregnancy, non-consensual contraceptive methods (e.g. forced sterilization and forced abortion), female genital mutilation/cutting (FGM/C), and forced marriage all represent serious breaches of sexual and reproductive freedoms, and are therefore fundamentally and inherently inconsistent with the right to health. In the specific context of maternal mortality, relevant freedoms include freedom from discrimination; harmful traditional practices, such as early marriage and violence.

For example, some cultural practices, including FGM/C, carry a high risk of disability and death. This means that where the practice exists, States should take appropriate and effective measures to eradicate it, in accordance with their obligations under the Convention on the Rights of the Child. Early marriage, which disproportionately affects girls, is predominantly found in South Asia and sub-Saharan Africa, where over 50 per cent of girls are married by the age of 18. Among other problems, early marriage is linked to health risks including those arising from premature pregnancy. Finally, in the context of adolescent health, States are obliged to set minimum ages for sexual consent and marriage (UNCRC 2003, paras. 9, 19).

Entitlements

Entitlements that form part of the rights to reproductive and sexual health include equal access, in law and fact, to reproductive and child health services, as well as information about sexual and reproductive health issues.

Specifically, States are required to provide a wide range of appropriate and, where necessary, free sexual and reproductive health services, including access to family planning, pre- and post-natal care, emergency obstetric services, and access to information. They should also ensure access to such essential health services as voluntary testing, counselling, and treatment for sexually transmitted infections, including HIV/AIDS, and breast and reproductive system cancers, as well as infertility treatment.

Unsafe abortions kill some 68 000 women each year, and thus constitute a right to life and right to health issue of enormous proportions. They also give rise to high rates of morbidity.

Women with unwanted pregnancies should be offered reliable information and compassionate counselling, including information on where and when a pregnancy may be terminated legally. Where abortions are legal, they must be safe: Public health systems should train and equip health service providers and take other measures to ensure that such abortions are not only safe but accessible (WHO 2003). In all cases, women should have access to quality services for the management of complications arising from abortion. Punitive provisions against women who undergo abortions are inconsistent with the right to the highest attainable standard of health.

Certain entitlements envisaged in international law are directly relevant to reducing maternal mortality (CEDAW Article 12 (2); UNCESCR 2000, para. 14) and, if fulfilled, would reduce its incidence. For example, an equitable, well-resourced, accessible, and integrated health system—a crucial entitlement arising from the right to health—is widely accepted as a vital pre-condition for guaranteeing women's access to the interventions that can prevent or treat the causes of maternal deaths (Freedman 2005). Other entitlements include education and information on sexual and reproductive health (UNCEDAW 1999a, para.18), safe abortion services where not against the law,[15] and primary healthcare services (UNCESCR 2000, paras. 14, 21; UNCEDAW 1999a para. 27; UN 1994, para. 8.25) especially universal access to reproductive healthcare (UNMP 2005b).

The entitlement to specific underlying determinants of health relevant to maternal mortality must also be guaranteed. The failure to safeguard women's rights is often manifested in low status of women, poor access to information and care, early age of marriage, and restricted mobility, among other problems (DFID 2005). Specifically, gender equality[16] has an important role to play in preventing maternal mortality as alongside empowerment it can lead to greater demand by women for family planning services, antenatal care, and safe delivery. Another relevant determinant of health and element of the right to health that must be ensured in order to address problems of maternal mortality is water and sanitation, which are vital to the provision of prenatal care and emergency obstetric care.

◆ *Available, accessible, acceptable and good quality*

In many countries, information on sexual and reproductive health is not readily available and, if it is, it is not accessible to all, in particular women and adolescents. Sexual and reproductive health services are often geographically inaccessible to communities living in rural areas, or provided in a form that is not culturally acceptable to indigenous peoples and other non-dominant groups. Similarly, services, and relevant underlying determinants of health, such as education, are often of substandard quality.

In order to address the problem of maternal mortality, the concept of availability calls for collective action to enhance care and improve human resource strategies, including increasing the number and quality of health professionals and improving terms and conditions (UNMP 2005c). Accessibility considers whether physical access and the cost of health services influence women's ability to seek care (UNMP 2005c). Furthermore, discriminatory laws, policies, practices, and gender inequalities prevent women and adolescents from accessing good quality services or information on sexual and reproductive health, and have a direct impact on maternal mortality (Cook *et al.* 2006). To prevent maternal mortality, scaling up technical interventions, or making the interventions affordable is insufficient: Strategies ensuring the *acceptability* of services through their sensitivity to the rights, cultures and needs of pregnant women, including those from indigenous peoples and other minority groups, are also vital (Shiffman 2006). Quality of care will influence both a woman's decision whether or not to seek care, as well as the outcome of interventions, and so is key to tackling maternal mortality through the provision of maternal healthcare services.

◆ *Discrimination, vulnerability and stigma*

Discrimination and stigma continue to pose a serious threat to sexual and reproductive health for many groups, including women, sexual minorities, refugees, people with disabilities, rural communities, indigenous persons, people living with HIV/AIDS, sex workers, and people held in detention. Some individuals suffer discrimination on several grounds, e.g. gender, race, poverty, and health status (UNCHR 2003a, para. 62).

Discrimination based on gender hinders the ability of many women to protect themselves from HIV infection and to respond to the consequences of HIV infection. Women and girls' vulnerability to HIV and AIDS is compounded by other human rights issues including inadequate access to information, education, and services necessary to ensure sexual health; sexual violence; harmful traditional or customary practices affecting the health of women and children (such as early and forced marriage); and lack of legal capacity and equality in areas such as marriage and divorce.

Stigma and discrimination associated with HIV/AIDS may also reinforce other prejudices, discrimination, and inequalities related to gender and sexuality. The result is that those affected may be reluctant to seek health and social services, information, education, and counselling, even when those services are available. This, in turn, will contribute to the vulnerability of others to HIV infection.

Vulnerability in the context of sexual and reproductive health is particularly relevant to adolescents and young people, who find themselves lacking access to relevant information and services during a period characterized by sexual and reproductive maturation. Important protections for adolescents are enshrined in CRC, which includes a number of cross-cutting principles which have an important bearing on adolescent's sexual and reproductive health, namely: The survival and development of the child, the best interests

---

[15] UN human rights bodies have also held that absolute legal prohibitions on abortion can violate the rights to life and health where they contribute to maternal mortality. For example, in its Concluding Observations on Colombia, CEDAW noted, with great concern: 'That abortion, which is the second cause of maternal deaths in Colombia, is punishable as an illegal act. No exceptions are made to that prohibition, including where the mother's life is in danger or to safeguard her physical or mental health or in cases where the mother has been raped. . . . The Committee believes that legal provisions on abortion constitute a violation of the rights of women to health and life and of article 12 of the Convention' (UN CEDAW 1999b, para. 393).

[16] States should 'take all appropriate measures to eliminate discrimination against women in the field of healthcare in order to ensure, on a basis of equality of men and women, access to healthcare services, including those related to family planning' (CEDAW, article 12.1).

of the child, non-discrimination, and respect for the views of the child (CRC Articles 2,3,5,6,12; UNCRC 2003, para.12).

Discrimination on the grounds of sexual orientation is impermissible under international human rights law. The legal prohibition of same-sex relations in many countries, in conjunction with a widespread lack of support or protection for sexual minorities against violence and discrimination, impedes the enjoyment of sexual and reproductive health by many people with lesbian, gay, bisexual, and transgender identities or conduct.[17] Similarly, criminalization can impede programmes which are essential to promoting the right to health and other human rights.[18]

Arising from their obligations to combat discrimination, States have a duty to ensure that health information and services are made available to vulnerable groups. For example, they must take steps to empower women to make decisions in relation to their sexual and reproductive health, free of coercion, violence and discrimination. They must take action to redress gender-based violence and ensure that there are sensitive and compassionate services available for the survivors of gender-based violence, including rape and incest. States should ensure that adolescents are able to receive information, including on family planning and contraceptives, the dangers of early pregnancy, and the prevention of sexually transmitted infections including HIV/AIDS, as well as appropriate services for sexual and reproductive health. Consistent with *Toonen v. Australia* and numerous other international and national decisions, they should ensure that sexual and other health services are available for men who have sex with men, lesbians, and transsexual and bisexual people. It is also important to ensure that voluntary counselling, testing, and treatment of sexually transmitted infections are available for sex workers (UNHRCttee 1994).

Finally, in the context of sexual and reproductive health, breaches of medical confidentiality may occur. Sometimes these breaches, when accompanied by stigmatization, lead to unlawful dismissal from employment, expulsion from families and communities, physical assault, and other abuse. Also, a lack of confidentiality may deter individuals from seeking advice and treatment, thereby jeopardizing their health and well-being. States are obliged to take effective measures to ensure medical confidentiality and privacy.

Water and sanitation

Healthcare attracts a disproportionate amount of attention and resources. Yet access to water and sanitation, as well as other underlying determinants of health, are integral features of the right to the highest attainable standard of health.

♦ *Available, accessible, acceptable and quality*

Available
The right to health requires a State to do all it can to ensure that safe water and adequate sanitation is available to everyone in its jurisdiction. The quantity of water available for each person should correspond to the quantity specified by WHO (Howard & Bartram 2002), though some individuals and groups may require additional

water due to health, climate, and work conditions, and the State should therefore ensure that this is also available. The right to health stipulates that States must ensure the availability of safe water for personal and domestic uses such as 'drinking, personal sanitation, washing of clothes, food preparation, personal and household hygiene' (UNCESCR 2003 para 12 (a)).

Accessible
The right to health also requires that water and sanitation be accessible to everyone without discrimination. In this context, accessibility has four dimensions:

First, water and sanitation must be within safe physical reach for all sections of the population, in all parts of the country. Water and sanitation therefore should be *physically accessible* within, or in the immediate vicinity of, the household, educational institution, workplace, and health or other institution (UN 2005, guideline 1.3). The inaccessibility of water within safe physical reach can seriously impair health, including the health of women and children responsible for carrying water. Carrying heavy water containers for long distances can cause fatigue, pain, and spinal and pelvic injuries, which may lead to problems during pregnancy and childbirth. Similarly, the absence of safe, private sanitation facilities subjects women to a humiliating, stressful, and uncomfortable daily routine that can damage their health (UNMP 2005a, pp. 23–5). When designing water and sanitation facilities in camps for refugees and internally displaced persons, special attention should be given to prevent gender-based violence. For example, facilities should be provided in safe areas near dwellings (UNHCR 2005).

Second, water and sanitation should be *economically accessible*, including to those living in poverty. Poverty is associated with inequitable access to health services, safe water, and sanitation. If those living in poverty are not enjoying access to safe water and adequate sanitation, the State has a duty to take reasonable measures that ensure access to all.

Third, water and sanitation should be *accessible* to all *without discrimination* on any of the grounds prohibited under human rights law, such as sex, race, ethnicity, disability, and socioeconomic status.

Finally, reliable *information* about water and sanitation must be *accessible* to all so that they can make well-informed decisions.

Acceptable
The right to health requires that water and sanitation facilities be respectful of gender and life-cycle requirements and be culturally *acceptable*. For example, measures should ensure that sanitation facilities are mindful of the privacy of women, men, and children.

Quality
Both water services and sanitation facilities must be of good *quality*: This reduces susceptibility to anaemia, diarrhoea, and other conditions that cause maternal and infant mortality and morbidity (UNMP 2005a, p. 18). Water required for personal and domestic use should be safe and free from 'micro-organisms, chemical substances and radiological hazards which constitute a threat to a person's health' (UNCESCR 2003, para. 12(b)). States should establish water quality regulations and standards on the basis of the *WHO Guidelines for Drinking Water Quality* (WHO 2006c).

---

[17] Other Special Rapporteurs have documented violence and discrimination based on sexual orientation (UNCHR 2001, paras. 48–50; UNGA 2001, paras 17–25).

[18] For example, 'criminalization of homosexual activity . . . would appear to run counter to the implementation of effective education programmes in respect of HIV/AIDS prevention' (UNHRCttee 1994, para 8.5).

Similarly, each person should have affordable access to sanitation services, facilities, and installations adequate for the promotion and protection of their human health and dignity. Good health requires the protection of the environment from human waste; this can only be achieved if everyone has access to, and utilizes, adequate sanitation (UNCHR 2004, para. 44).

New tools and techniques

The 'Human rights' section introduced the idea, which is increasingly recognized, that one way of vindicating the right to the highest attainable standard of health is by way of the 'policy approach' i.e. the integration of the right to health in national and international policy-making approaches. For this approach to prosper, the traditional human rights techniques—taking test cases in the courts, 'naming and shaming', letter-writing campaigns, slogans, and so on—will not be sufficient. The 'policy approach' demands the development of new right-to-health skills and tools, such as budgetary analysis, indicators, benchmarks, and impact assessments. In recent years, the health and human rights community has made significant progress towards the development of these new methodologies. Here, by way of illustration, indicators, benchmarks, and impact assessments are briefly introduced in the context of the right to the highest attainable standard of health.

A human rights-based approach to health indicators

The international right to the highest attainable standard of health is subject to progressive realization. Inescapably, this means that what is expected of a State will vary over time. With a view to monitoring its progress, a State needs a device to measure this variable dimension of the right to health. The most appropriate device is the combined application of indicators and benchmarks. Thus, a State selects appropriate indicators that will help it monitor different dimensions of the right to health. These indicators might include, for example, maternal mortality ratios and child mortality rates. Most indicators will require disaggregation, such as on the grounds of sex, race, ethnicity, rural/urban, and socioeconomic status. Then the State sets appropriate national targets or benchmarks in relation to each disaggregated indicator.

In this way, indicators and benchmarks fulfil two important functions. *First*, they can help the State to monitor its progress over time, enabling the authorities to recognize when policy adjustments are required. *Second*, they can help to hold the State to account in relation to the discharge of its responsibilities arising from the right to health, although deteriorating indicators do not necessarily mean that the State is in breach of its international right to health obligations (UNCHR 2006, para. 35). Of course, indicators also have other important roles. For example, by highlighting issues such as disaggregation, participation, and accountability, indicators can enhance the effectiveness of policies and programmes.

Health professionals and policy makers constantly use a very large number of health indicators, such as the HIV prevalence rate. Is it possible to simply appropriate these health indicators and call them 'human rights indicators' or 'right to health indicators'? Or do indicators that are to be used for monitoring human rights and the right to health require some special features? If so, what are these special attributes?

The considered view is that some of these health indictors may be used to monitor aspects of the progressive realization of the right to health, provided the following conditions are met (UNGA 2004):

1. They correspond, with some precision, to a right to health norm.
2. They are disaggregated by at least sex, race, ethnicity, rural/urban, and socioeconomic status.
3. They are supplemented by additional indicators—rarely found among classic health indicators—that monitor five essential and inter-related features of the right to health:
   - A national strategy and plan of action that includes the right to health
   - The participation of individuals and groups, especially the most vulnerable and disadvantaged, in relation to the formulation of health policies and programmes
   - Access to health information, as well as confidentiality of personal health data
   - International assistance and cooperation of donors in relation to the enjoyment of the right to health in developing countries
   - Accessible and effective monitoring and accountability mechanisms

In this way, many existing health indicators, such as the maternal mortality ratio and HIV prevalence rate, have an important potential role to play in measuring and monitoring the progressive realization of the right to health, provided that they conform to these conditions.

Impact assessments and the right to the highest attainable standard of health

A further tool that can be employed to monitor the fulfilment of the right to health and hold duty-bearers to account is through impact assessments. They are an aid to equitable, inclusive, robust, and sustainable policy making, and have the objective of informing decision-makers and the people likely to be affected by a new policy, programme, or project so that the proposal can be improved to reduce potential negative effects and increase positive ones. They are one way of ensuring that the right to health—especially of marginalized groups, including the poor—is given due weight in all national and international policy-making processes. From the right to health perspective, an impact assessment methodology is a key feature of a health system and an essential means by which a government can gauge whether or not it is on target to realize progressively the right to health.

At least two distinct methodological approaches are available: To develop a self-standing methodology for human rights impact assessments such as has been done in other fields, such as environmental and social policy; or to integrate human rights into *existing* types of impact assessments. The second approach is consistent with the call on governments to mainstream human rights into all government processes and requires interdisciplinary collaboration (UNGA 2007, para. 39).

In order that an impact assessment uphold rights-based principles, it must: (1) Use an explicit human rights framework, (2) aim for progressive realization of human rights, (3) promote equality and non-discrimination in process and policy, (4) ensure meaningful participation by all stakeholders, (5) provide information and protect the right to freely express ideas, (6) establish mechanisms to hold the State accountable, and (7) recognize the interdependence of all human rights (Hunt and MacNaughton 2006, p. 32).

If the second approach above is adopted, there are six steps that should be followed to ensure that the right to health is integrated into existing impact assessments: (1) Perform a preliminary check on the proposed policy to determine whether or not a full-scale right-to-health impact assessment is necessary; (2) prepare an assessment plan and distribute information on the policy and the plan to all stakeholders; (3) collect information on potential right-to-health impacts of the proposed policy; (4) prepare a draft report comparing the potential impacts with the State's legal obligations arising from the right to health; (5) distribute the draft report and engage stakeholders in evaluating the options; and (6) prepare the final report detailing the final decision, the rationale for the choices made and a framework for implementation and evaluation.

Overall, the human rights framework for impact assessment adds value because human rights (1) are based on legal obligations to which governments have agreed to abide, (2) apply to all parts of the government encouraging coherence to policy-making and ensuring that policies reinforce each other; (3) require participation in policy making by the people affected, enhancing legitimacy and ownership of policy choices; (4) enhance effectiveness by demanding data disaggregation, participation and transparency; and (5) demand mechanisms through which policy makers can be held accountable.

Conclusion: Key features of a health system from a right to health perspective

The right to the highest attainable standard of health can be understood as a right to an effective and integrated health system, encompassing healthcare and the underlying determinants of health, which is responsive to national and local priorities, and accessible to all.

At the heart of this understanding of the right to health is a package of health services, facilities, and goods, extending to healthcare and the underlying determinants of health, such as access to safe water, adequate sanitation, and health-related information. This package must be available, accessible, and of good quality. Also, it must be sensitive to different cultures. While this package will have many features that are common to all countries, there will also be differences between one country and another, reflective of different disease burdens, cultural contexts, resource availability, and so on. This chapter has signalled some elements of this package in relation to neglected diseases, mental disability, sexual and reproductive health, and water and sanitation.

However, besides this essential package of health services, facilities, and goods, a health system must have some additional features if it is to reflect the right to the highest attainable standard of health. These additional features derive from international norms, including CESCR's General Comment 14 on the right to the highest attainable standard of health. While some of these additional features have been described in the preceding paragraphs, they include the following:

1. Formal legal recognition of the right to health in either a national Constitution, or bill of rights, or other statute.

2. An elaboration of what the right to health means, for both the public and private sectors, for example by way of regulations, guidelines and codes of conduct.

3. Research and development for national and local health priorities.

4. A comprehensive situational analysis identifying, inter alia, the health needs of the population, upon which (5) is based.

5. A comprehensive national health plan, including objectives, timeframes, who is responsible for what, reporting procedures, indicators and benchmarks (to measure progressive realization), and a detailed budget.

6. A health financing system that is equitable and evidence-informed.

7. An ex-ante right to health impact assessment methodology that permits the Government to foreshadow the likely impact of a draft law, policy, or programme on the enjoyment of the right to the highest attainable standard of health, thereby enabling it, when necessary, to revise the projected initiative.

8. As much 'bottom up' participation as possible, in relation to policy-making, implementation, and accountability.

9. Access to health-related information and data; data will have to be disaggregated so that the health situation of disadvantaged populations is properly understood, enabling the authorities to devise measures that address health inequities and disadvantage; at the same time, however, arrangements must be in place to ensure that personal medical data remains confidential.

10. As well as effective mechanisms for co-ordination within the health sector, there must also be effective mechanisms for inter-sectoral coordination in health, because the right to health extends beyond the health sector; moreover, where relevant, there must be effective coordination and referral with traditional health systems.

11. A sufficient number of domestically trained health workers enjoying good terms and conditions of employment; they should be reflective of the country's cultural diversity, including language, and strike a balance between men and women; health workers' training should include human rights.

12. An international dimension, for example, low-income countries should seek international assistance and cooperation in health and high-income countries should provide it.

13. Educational campaigns and other arrangements so that the public knows about its right to health entitlements and how to vindicate them.

14. Effective, transparent, and accessible monitoring and accountability mechanisms, including redress, for both the public and private health sectors.

States have a legal obligation to ensure that their health systems not only include an appropriate package of health services, facilities, and goods, but also the additional features briefly summarized in points 1–14.

Key points

◆ The right to the highest attainable standard of health is enshrined in several international treaties and numerous national constitutions.

◆ It gives rise to legally binding obligations on States.

◆ There is a complementary relationship between public health and the right to the highest attainable standard of health.

◆ The right to health analytical framework deepens understanding of contemporary public health issues and can help to identify appropriate responses to them.

◆ The right to the highest attainable standard of health can be understood as a right to an effective and integrated health system, encompassing healthcare and the underlying determinants of health, which is responsive to national and local priorities, and accessible to all.

References

ACHPR (African Commission on Human and Peoples' Rights) (2001). *Communication No. 155/96: The Social and Economic Rights Action Center for Economic and Social Rights v. Nigeria.* Fifteenth Annual Activity Report of ACHPR, 2001–2002, Annex V.

Annan, K. (2001). *Speech to the National Urban League Conference.* 30 July 2001, Washington DC.

Bartram, J. *et al.* (2005). Focusing on improved water for sanitation and health. *Lancet,* **365**, 810–12.

Beaglehole, R. (2002). Overview and framework. In *Oxford Textbook of Public Health* (ed. R. Detels), 4th edition. OUP, Oxford.

Chapman and Russel (eds.) (2002). *Core obligations: Building a framework for economic, social and cultural rights,* Intersentia, 2002.

CCSA (Constitutional Court of South Africa) (2002). *Minister of Health et al v. Treatment Action Campaign et al.* Case CCT 8/02, decided on 5 July 2002.

Cook, R., Dickens, B. *et al.* (2006). *International policy on sexual and reproductive health and rights.* Swedish International Development Cooperation Agency.

Coreil, J., Mayard, G., and Addiss, D. (2003). *Support groups for women with lymphatic filariasis in Haiti.* Report Series No. 2, Social, Economic and Behavioural Research, Special Programme for Research and Training in Tropical Diseases (TDR), 2003, p. 42.

Council of Europe (1950). *Convention for the protection of human rights and fundamental freedoms.* ETS No. 5.

DFID (Department for International Development) (2005). *How to reduce maternal deaths: Rights and responsibilities.* DFID, London.

ECSR (European Committee on Social Rights) (1998). *International Commission of Jurists v. Portugal.* Case No. 1/1998.

ECtHR (European Court of Human Rights) (1979). *Winterwerp v. The Netherlands, Judgement 24 October 1979.* Application No. 6301/73. Reported at 2 EHRR 387.

ECtHR (European Court of Human Rights) (1990). *E. v. Norway, Judgement of 29 August 1990.* Application No. 11701/85, Series A, No. 181–A.

ECtHR (European Court of Human Rights) (1994). *Lopez Ostra v. Spain, Judgement of December 9, 1994.* Case No. 41/1993/436/515.

Espino, F., Coops, V., and Manderson, L. (2004). *Community participation and tropical disease control in resource-poor settings.* UNICEF/UNDP/World Bank/WHO Special Programme for Research and Training in Tropical Diseases, Geneva.

Evans, B. *et al.* (2004). *Closing the sanitation gap: The case for better public funding of sanitation and hygiene behaviour change.* Organization for Economic Co-operation and Development (OECD) 13th Round Table on Sustainable Development. OECD, Paris.

Freedman, L. (2003). Human rights, constructive accountability and maternal mortality in the Dominican Republic: A Commentary. *International Journal of Gynecology and Obstetrics,* **82**.

Freedman, L. (2005). Achieving the MDGs: Health systems as core social institutions. *Development,* **48**(1).

Gostin, L.O. (2000). Human rights of persons with mental disabilities: The ECHR, *International Journal of Law and Psychiatry,* **23**.

Gostin, L.O. and Gable, L. (2004). The human rights of persons with mental disabilities: A global perspective on the application of human rights principles to mental health. *Maryland Law Review,* **63**.

Guthman, J. *et al.* (1997). Patients' associations and the control of leishmaniasis in Peru. *Bulletin of the World Health Organization,* **75**: 6–13. p.17.

Howard, G. and Bartram, J. (2002). *Domestic water quantity: Service level and health.* World Health Organization (WHO) 2002. WHO, Geneva.

Hunt, P. and MacNaughton, G. (2006). *Impact assessments, poverty and human rights: A case study using the right to the highest attainable standard of health.* UNESCO. http://www2.essex.ac.uk/human_rights_centre/rth/docs/Impact%20Assessments%209Dec06[1].doc

IACHR (Inter-American Commission on Human Rights) (1997). *Victor Rosario Congo v. Ecuador.* Case 11.427, Report No. 12/97, OEA/Ser.L/V/II.95 Doc. 7 rev at 257 (1997)

IACHR (Inter-American Commission on Human Rights) (2000). *Jorge Odir Miranda Cortez et al v. El Salvador.* Case 12.249, Report No. 29/01, OEA/Ser.L/V/II.111 Doc. 20 rev. at 282 (2000).

ICJ (International Court of Justice) (1996). *Advisory opinion: Legality of the threat or use of nuclear weapons,* ICJ Reports 1996. Vol. I. ICJ, The Hague.

Kinney, E. (2001). The international human right to health: What does this mean for our nation and world? *Indiana Law Review,* **34**.

Kinney, E. and Clark, B.A. (2004). Provisions for health and health care in the constitutions of the countries of the world, 37 *Cornell international law journal,* 285.

Lewis, O. (2002). Protecting the rights of people with mental disabilities: The ECHR. *European journal of health law,* **9**(4).

MDRI (Mental Disability Rights International) (2002). *Not on the agenda: Human rights of people with mental disabilities in Kosovo.* MDRI, Washington.

OAS (Organization of American States) (1948). *American declaration of the rights and duties of man.* OAS Res. XXX, adopted by the Ninth International Conference of American States (1948). OAS, Washington DC.

OAS (Organization of American States) (1969). *American convention on human rights.* OAS Treaty Series No. 36, 1144 U.N.T.S. 123. Adopted at the Inter-American Specialized Conference on Human Rights, San Jose, Costa Rica, 22 November 1969. OAS, Washington DC.

OAS (Organization of American States) (1994). *Inter-American convention on the prevention, punishment and eradication of violence against women, "Convention of Belém do Pará".* Adopted at the 24th Regular Session of the General Assembly, 9 June 1994. OAS, Washington.

Rosenthal, E. *et al.* (2000). Implementing the right to community integration for children with disabilities in Russia: A human rights framework for international action. *Health and Human Rights: An International Journal,* **4**.

Shiffman, J. and Garces del Valle, A. (2006). Political histories and disparities in safe motherhood between Guatemala and Honduras. *Population and Development Review,* **32**(1).

Skogly, S. (2006). *Beyond national borders: States' HR obligations in their international cooperation,* Intersentia.

UN (1945). *UN Charter,* adopted 26 June 1945, entered into force 24 October 1945, as amended by GA Res. 1991 (XVIII) 17 December 1963, entered into force 31 August 1966 (557 UNTS 143); 2101 of 20 December 1965, entered into force 12 June 1968 (638 UNTS 308); and 2847 (XXVI) of 20 December 1971, entered into force 24 September 1973 (892 UNTS 119). UN, New York.

UN (1948). *Universal declaration of human rights.* GA Resolution 217A (III), UN GAOR, Resolution 71, UN Document A/810. UN, New York.

UN (United Nations) (1965). *Convention on the elimination of all forms of racial discrimination,* (ICERD). UN GA Resolution 2106A (XX). UN, New York.

UN (1966a). *International Covenant on Civil and Political Rights*, (ICCPR). UN GA Resolution 2200A (XXI), 16 December 1966. UN, New York.

UN (1966b). *International Covenant on Economic, Social and Cultural Rights*, (ICESCR). UN GA Resolution 2200A (XXI), 16 December 1966. UN, New York.

UN (1979). *Convention on the elimination of all forms of discrimination against women* (CERD). GA Resolution 34/180, UN GAOR, 34th Session, Supplement No.46 at 193, UN Document A/34/46. UN, New York.

UN (1989). *Convention on the rights of the child*, (CRC). UN GA Resolution 44/25, 20 November 1989. UN, New York.

UN (1990). *International convention on the protection of the rights of all migrant workers and members of their families*, (ICRMW). GA Resolution 45/158, 18 December 1990. UN, New York.

UN (1991). *Principles for the protection of persons with mental illness and the improvement of mental health care*, GA Resolution 46/119, 17 December 1991. UN, New York.

UN (1993). United Nations General Assembly. *Vienna declaration and programme of action. World conference on human rights*, Vienna 14–25 June 1993, UN Document A/CONF.157/23. UN, New York.

UN (1994). *International conference on population and development.* 5–13 September 1994, Cairo, Egypt.

UN (1995). *Report of the fourth world conference on women.* Beijing, China 4–15 September 1995. UN Document A/CONF.177.20.

UN (2002). *Johannesburg plan for the implementation of the world summit on sustainable development.* 26 August–4 September 2002, Johannesburg, South Africa.

UN (2005). *Sub-Commission draft guidelines for the realisation of the right to drinking water and sanitation.* Adopted by the Sub-Commission in Resolution 2006/10. UN Document A/HRC/Sub.1/58/L11.

UNCEDAW (United Nations Committee on the Elimination of Discrimination Against Women) (1999a). *General Recommendation No. 24 on Women and Health*, EDAW/C/1999/1/WGII/WP2/Rev.1. UN, Geneva.

UNCEDAW (United Nations Committee on the Elimination of Discrimination Against Women) (1999b). *Concluding Observations on Colombia.* 5 February 1999. UN Document A/54/38, paras. 337–401. UN, Geneva. para. 393.

UNCESCR (United Nations Committee on Economic, Social and Cultural Rights) (1990). *General Comment No. 3 (Fifth Session). The nature of States parties obligations (Art.2, par.1).* UN Document E/1991/23. UN, Geneva.

UNCESCR (United Nations Committee on Economic, Social and Cultural Rights) (1994). *General Comment No. 5 (Eleventh Session). Persons with disabilities.* UN Document E/C.12/1194/13. UN, Geneva.

UNCESCR (United Nations Committee on Economic, Social and Cultural Rights) (2000). *General Comment No. 14 (Twenty Second Session). The right to the highest attainable standard of health.* UN Document E/C.12/2000/4. UN, Geneva.

UNCESCR (United Nations Committee on Economic, Social and Cultural Rights) (2003). *General Comment No. 15 (Twenty Ninth Session). The right to water.* UN Document E/C.12/2002/11. UN, Geneva.

UNCHR (United Nations Commission on Human Rights) (1991). *Second progress report of Mr Danilo Turk, special rapporteur on the realization of economic, social and cultural rights*, 18 July 1991, UN Document E/CN.4/Sub.2/1991/17. UN, Geneva. paras. 6–48.

UNCHR (United Nations Commission on Human Rights) (2001). *Civil and political rights, including the question of disappearances and summary executions: Report of the special rapporteur*, 11 January 2001, UN Document E/CN.4/2001/9). UN, Geneva.

UNCHR (United Nations Commission on Human Rights) (2002a). *Access to medication in the context of pandemics such as HIV/AIDS*, Resolution 2002/32, 22 April 2002. UN, Geneva.

UNCHR (United Nations Commission on Human Rights) (2002b). *Human rights of persons with disabilities*, Resolution 2002/61, 25 April 2002. UN, Geneva.

UNCHR (United Nations Commission on Human Rights) (2003a). *The right of everyone to the enjoyment of the highest attainable standard of physical and mental health, Report of the Special Rapporteur*, 13 February 2003, UN Document E/CN.4/2003/58). UN, Geneva.

UNCHR (United Nations Commission on Human Rights) (2003b). *The right of everyone to the enjoyment of the highest attainable standard of physical and mental health.* 22 April 2003, Resolution 2003/28. UN, Geneva. Preamble and para 6.

UNCHR (United Nations Commission on Human Rights) (2003). Extrajudicial, summary or arbitrary executions, *Report of the Special Rapporteur*, 11 January 2001, UN Document E/CN.4/2001/9). UN, Geneva. paras 48–50.

UNCHR (United Nations Commission on Human Rights) (2004). *Relationship between the enjoyment of economic, social and cultural rights and the promotion of the realization of the right to drinking water supply and sanitation: Final report of the UN sub-commission Special Rapporteur.* 14 July 2004. UN Document E/CN.4/Sub.2/2004/20. UN, Geneva, para 44.

UNCHR (United Nations Commission on Human Rights) (2006). *The right of everyone to the enjoyment of the highest attainable standard of physical and mental health, report of the Special Rapporteur*, 3 March 2006, UN Document E/CN.4/2006/48). UN, Geneva.

UNCRC (United Nations Committee on the Rights of the Child) (2003). *General Comment No. 4. Adolescent health and development in the context of the Convention on the Rights of the Child.* UN Document CRC/GC/2003/4. UN, Geneva. paras 9 and 19.

UNDP (United Nations Development Programme) (2006). *Human development report: Beyond scarcity: Power, poverty and the Global Water Crisis.* UN, Geneva.

UN ECOSOC (United Nations Economic and Social Council) (1985). *Siracusa principles on the limitation and derogation provisions in the international covenant on civil and political rights.* UN Document E/CN.4/1985/4, Annex.

UNGA (United Nations General Assembly) (1993). *Standard rules on the equalization of opportunities for persons with disabilities.* Adopted by Resolution 48/96, 20 December 1993. UN, New York.

UNGA (United Nations General Assembly) (2000). *United Nations Millennium Declaration.* Adopted by Resolution 55/2, 8 September 2000.

UNGA (United Nations General Assembly) (2001). *Question of torture and other cruel, inhuman or degrading treatment or punishment, Note by the Secretary-General.* 3 July 2001, UN Document A/56/156. paras 17–25.

UNGA (United Nations General Assembly) (2003). *Progress of efforts to ensure the full recognition and enjoyment of the human rights of persons with disabilities: Report of the Secretary General.* 24 July 2003, UN Document A/58/181. UN, New York. para 43.

UNGA (United Nations General Assembly) (2004). *Report of the Special Rapporteur on the right of everyone to the enjoyment of the highest attainable standard of physical and mental health*, 8 October 2004, UN Document A/59/422. UN, New York.

UNGA (United Nations General Assembly) (2007). *Report of the Special Rapporteur on the right of everyone to the enjoyment of the highest attainable standard of physical and mental health*, 8 August 2007, UN Document A/62/214. UN, New York.

UNHCR (United Nations High Commissioner for Refugees) (2005). *Access to water in refugee situations: Survival, health and dignity for refugees.* UNHCR, Geneva.

UNHRCttee (UN Human Rights Committee) (1994). *Toonen v. Australia*, 4 April 1994, UN Document CCPR/C/50/D/488/1992. UN, New York. para 8.5.

UNHRCttee (UN Human Rights Committee) (2003). *Karen Noelia Llantoy Huaman v. Peru* (*K.L. v. Peru*). UN Document CPR/C/85/D/1153/2003. UN, New York.

UNHRC (United Nations Human Rights Council) (2007). *Report of the Special Rapporteur on the right of everyone to the enjoyment of the highest attainable standard of physical and mental health,*

Paul Hunt, 17 January 2007, UN Document A/HRC/4/28. UN, New York.

UNMP (United Nations Millennium Project) (2005a). *Health, Dignity and Development: What Will it Take?* Report of the Task Force on Water and Sanitation. UN, New York. pp. 23–25.

UNMP (United Nations Millennium Project) (2005b). *Taking action: Achieving gender equality and empowering women.* Report of the Taskforce on Education and Gender Equality. Earthscan, London.

UNMP (United Nations Millennium Project) (2005c). *Who's got the power?* Report of the Task Force on Child Health and Maternal Health. UN, New York.

UNOHCHR (United Nations Office of the High Commissioner for Human Rights) (2006). *Frequently asked questions on a human rights based approach to development cooperation*, 2006, UN Document HR/PUB/06/8. UN, New York and Geneva.

UNOHCHR (United Nations Office of the High Commissioner for Human Rights) (2006). *Principles and guidelines for a human rights approach to poverty reduction strategies.* UN, Geneva. para 77.

WHO (World Health Organization) (1946). *Constitution of the World Health Organization*, adopted by the International Health Conference, New York, 19 June-22 July 1946, and signed on 22 July 1946. WHO, Geneva.

WHO (World Health Organization) (1978a). *Declaration of Alma-Ata: International conference on primary health care.* 6–12 September, USSR.

WHO (World Health Organization) (1978b). *A joint report by the Director-General of the WHO and the Executive Director of UNICEF presented at the international conference on primary health care*, 1978, Alma-Ata. WHO, Geneva.

WHO (World Health Organization) (2001). *A human rights approach to tuberculosis.* WHO, Geneva. p.12.

WHO (World Health Organization) (2001). *World Health Report 2001. Mental health: New understanding, new hope.* WHO, Geneva. pp. 112–15.

WHO (World Health Organization) (2002). *Global defence against the infectious disease threat.* WHO, Geneva.

WHO (World Health Organization) (2003). *Safe abortion: Technical and policy guidance for health dystems.* WHO, Geneva.

WHO (World Health Organization) (2004a).*Intensified control of neglected diseases: Report of an international workshop, Berlin, 10–12 December 2003.* WHO/CDS/CPE/CEE/2004.45. WHO, Geneva. p22.

WHO (World Health Organization) (2004b). *Water, sanitation and hygiene links to health: Facts and figures*, 2004. WHO, Geneva.

WHO (World Health Organization) (2004c). *Mental health policy, plans and programmes.* WHO, Geneva.

WHO (World Health Organization) (2005a). *Resource book on mental health, human rights and legislation.* WHO, Geneva.

WHO (World Health Organization) (2005b). *World Health Report 2005, make every mother and child count.* WHO, Geneva.

WHO (World Health Organization) (2006a). *World Health Report 2006, Working together for health.* WHO, Geneva.

WHO/UNICEF (World Health Organization/United Nations Children's Fund) (2006b). *Joint monitoring programme, meeting the MDG global water and sanitation target, the urban and rural challenge of the decade.* WHO, Geneva.

WHO (World Health Organization) (2006c). *Guidelines for drinking water quality.* WHO, Geneva.

WHO (World Health Organization) and TDR (Special Programme for Research and Training in Tropical Diseases) (2007). *Neglected diseases: A human rights analysis.* Document reference TDR/SDR/SEB/ST/07.2. WHO, Geneva.

4.2

Comparative national public health legislation

Robyn Martin and Alexandra Lo Dak Wai

Abstract

Law is an important tool in containment of communicable and non-communicable disease. International instruments require states to undertake measures which require legal underpinning. However, the meaning of 'law', and understandings of the extent to which the state can intervene in private life for the benefit of public health, differ across states. In some legal cultures, law is to be found in a form other than legislation, making difficult a comparison of state legislation. This chapter will examine limitations to a world comparison of public health legislation, and consider representative national laws from Western and Asian legal cultures in relation to three public health threats—communicable disease, tobacco harms, and obesity—to analyse ways in which law can play a part in global public health. The legislation discussed in the course of this chapter is that in force in December 2007.

Introduction

Early public health practice focused on poor sanitation and hygiene as sources of disease transmission. Law played an important role in underpinning public health interventions by providing surveillance duties together with powers of compulsory detention, quarantine, and in some instances, powers of compulsory vaccination or treatment. Improvements in scientific medicine throughout the twentieth century enabled the focus of public health to shift from sanitation to medical prevention and cure of disease. Non-medical interventions were considered less important, and by the mid-twentieth century, the role of law in public health had declined. Law came to be considered a redundant mechanism for disease control.

More recently, faced with new and re-emerging infectious diseases, we have been forced to recognize that science alone cannot contain threats posed by communicable disease. While science has made enormous strides in developing medical means of protection and containment, disease has consistently kept one step ahead of medicine. A legal framework for disease control measures is essential to public health disease containment strategy, and it is now also clear that a legal framework is equally important for effective containment of non-communicable diseases. Law is an essential tool in the armoury of contemporary public health, yet states the world over have looked to their public health legislation only to find that it is based on outdated science, and premised on outdated notions of the balance between public good and private right.

Since 2003 and the threat of SARS, many states have begun the process of rethinking and reforming their public health laws. This process has been made more urgent by the requirements of the revised WHO International Health Regulations (IHR) (Fidler & Gostin 2006). While some states have simply amended their laws to bring new disease threats within traditional legal disease frameworks, other states have taken the view that nineteenth-century legislative approaches are no longer valid, and have begun the process of designing entirely new laws to fit new public health environments. Much public health law across the world is in the process of reform, and the legislation discussed in this chapter is that in force in December 2007.

Comparing national public health legislation

The importance of political and social context to the content of public health law means that there is little to be gained in a simple comparison of legal rules or a compilation of state legislation. We must place any comparative analysis within its legal culture, the 'way in which values, practices, and concepts are integrated into the operation of legal institutions and the interpretation of legal texts' (Bell 1995). One way of going about this would be to locate legal systems in the context of world legal 'cultural families' (Van Hoecke & Warrington 1998). Any detailed comparison of laws across cultural families is of limited value as these cultures differ fundamentally in their approach to what constitutes law, and the role of law in society. We can, however, examine legal systems within a legal culture in order to identify the different ways in which public health laws are used to solve particular public health problems (Zweigert & Kötz 1998).

There is no universal understanding of the meaning of 'law' or 'regulation'. Some legal cultures recognize law only as the content of a written statutory act, code, or regulation, or the decision of a court. The WHO in the context of food law defines 'regulation' more widely to include 'any law, statute, guideline or code of practice issued by any level of government or self-regulatory organization' (WHO 1996). Other cultures have an even wider understanding of law which would include administrative orders, guidelines, local edicts and customary law. Legal pluralism, whereby traditional, religious, kinship, tribal, local, and community laws coexist alongside state laws, is common in many parts of the world. Public health is an issue which will in some states be governed not only by 'hard' law but also by 'soft' law which cannot be found in any formal document. It would be misleading then to assume that because a state has no public health legislation, then it has no public health laws. The requirement of compliance with the revised IHR, and the globalization of disease information and exchange, have prompted many states to formalize their primary public health laws, such that increasingly states are enshrining laws in publicly accessible legislation. However, it remains the case that in many states, particularly those not influenced by Western approaches to law, public health powers and duties fall within the domain of 'soft law', complicating any comparison of laws across states.

Much comparative law literature has been devoted to the identification of world legal cultures or families. Any such categorization will inevitably be simplistic and, if applied uncritically, potentially biased towards Western concepts of law because in Western legal philosophy the sources of law are more easily identifiable. Contemporary comparative legal theory has taken a social anthropological approach to defining legal systems which share fundamental characteristics, identifying four distinct legal cultures: Western, Asian, Islamic, and African (Van Hoecke & Warrington 1998). Grouping legal cultures in this way permits some macro-comparison of underlying concepts and underpinning theories, and enables us to take example states from legal families to make more manageable a world comparison. More importantly, some, even if superficial, understanding of the meaning and purpose of law in different legal cultures is essential to any examination or comparison of national laws in order to avoid drawing misleading conclusions about comparative public health legal regimes and in order to avoid examining national public health laws through a filter of Eurocentric legal theory.

The ideal approach in this chapter would have been to examine legislation in states from these four legal cultures. Such an ideal is, however, confounded by the fact that many states have no dedicated public health laws in the sense of published 'hard' law, although there may be conventional powers of quarantine, exclusion, or even compulsory treatment contained within traditional or 'soft' laws. This is particularly the case in states within Islamic or African legal cultures. Sources of public health law such as the WHO International Digest of Health Legislation focus primarily on states that have addressed public health by means of a parliamentary process and that have published laws in the Western tradition, and contain little information about public health laws and practices in states within Islamic and African legal cultures.

It is inevitable then that this comparison of public health legislation will focus on public health law within Western and Asian legal cultures, where states have chosen to enact dedicated public health legislation. This chapter will consider selected legal systems within these two legal families in order to compare approaches to public health law. It is important, however, not to forget that other legal cultures take different approaches to the use of law as a public health tool, and where possible reference will be made to approaches in other legal cultures.

The analysis will be undertaken on the premise that only laws which perform the same function are susceptible to comparison. This approach complies with the 'principle of functionality' (Mechlem 2000) whereby a comparative analysis should start with a legal question rather than with a legal norm. The discussion will focus on three public health questions: How can law support infectious disease control, how can law help to reduce the harms caused by tobacco, and the potential role of law in tackling obesity. In the course of comparison, issues of compliance of national laws with human rights and with the revised IHR will be addressed.

Defining public health law

What is public health law?

While communicable diseases still pose a catastrophic threat to health in many parts of the world, mortality and morbidity in the developed world are primarily the consequence of non-communicable diseases such as heart disease, stroke, and cancer, and their common risk factors such as diet, tobacco, and alcohol. This requires new public health strategies and new public health interventions. Defining public health law is not an easy task when it is realized that public health responsibility now extends to matters such as road traffic safety, domestic violence, lifestyle choice, media freedom, and taxation. The most commonly accepted definition is that by Gostin (2000):

Public health law is the study of the legal powers and duties of the state to assure the conditions for people to be healthy (e.g. to identify, prevent, and ameliorate risks to health in the populations) and the limitations on the powers of the state to constrain the autonomy, privacy, liberty, proprietary or other legally protected interests of individuals for the protection or promotion of community health.

This definition makes clear that public health law is about the relationship between the state and its populations rather than between health practitioners and patients. Public health law governs the organized efforts of the state for population health on the assumption that a state has responsibility for the health, and the conditions for health, of its citizens. Law may be needed to authorize interventions to address foreseeable risks of harm even where those interventions infringe the rights of individuals. At the same time, a public health end does not justify all possible means, and public health law will operate to set appropriate limits to infringement of individual rights and freedoms.

Law also has a wider role to play in the protection of public health. Laws might operate initially by means of direct provision of powers and duties, but will also serve to make a public statement of acceptability of behaviour which will indirectly alter public attitudes and actions. Laws against pollution or smoking in public places are effective only in part because of enforcement provisions. They are effective also because they have created minimum acceptable standards of protection. Laws, regardless of the legal system in which they operate, can change socio-cultural norms.

The absence of law also serves to send messages about acceptable behaviours. Where there is no law to regulate tobacco use, this implies that there is nothing socially unacceptable about cigarette advertising or smoking in proximity to others. Increasingly where individuals have little control over their living environments, even within Western individualistic societies, populations expect the state to intervene to reduce health risks and to set health standards.

Hence the content of public law has a value which is greater than the sum of its parts. Public health law reflects the importance that a government attributes to addressing threats to health, and reflects the standards that the state expects of its citizens in relation to health behaviours. Unreformed public health laws, based on outdated science and cultural values, create a dissonance between law and contemporary public health practice. Law reform must reflect social context, and it can prove counterproductive to transplant laws from another jurisdiction with a different social culture. Where law conflicts with contemporary understandings of the balance between individual right and public benefit, and where law fails to accommodate advancements in public health science, then law undermines the work of the state to protect its citizens from harm by eroding respect for public officials charged with implementing law.

Public health law in context

Gostin's definition presents a universal framework for the scope of public health law, but does not dictate the content of law. Public health law in each state will depend on the political and social context of that state. The recognition of health risk which might justify the application of law will vary according to understandings of medical science, public appreciation of risk, and public belief in the possibility of the control of risk. Where Western medical science is only one health belief system alongside others such as traditional medicine or religion, then law will play a different role in risk reduction. Public health operates within an ethical framework of communitarianism and utilitarianism, presupposing both that there are circumstances in which the greater good of the community justifies the overriding of autonomy of the individual, and that the intervention which results in the greatest health benefit for the greatest number is the most appropriate. However, the balance between communitarianism, utilitarianism, and autonomy is dependant on acceptance of state intervention in private life in pursuance of public health goals. The relationship between citizen and state, and the acceptability of intervention into individual rights for the public good, will be different, for example, in an authoritarian state than in a democracy. While Western health and legal systems prioritize autonomy as an underpinning health principle, other states, where the organization of society is based on religious or communitarian norms, may support more intrusive state activity to achieve public health goods.

Because of the importance of social and political context to the content of public health law, it will be useful, before examining legislation, to consider a brief overview of differing approaches to law within Western and Asian legal cultures.

Western legal culture

Western legal culture accommodates both common law and civil law states. Britain, Australia, Canada, New Zealand, and the United States, for example, have common law systems based on the English tradition in which law is embodied both in judicial decisions and in statutory form. So also do states and territories such as Cyprus, Malta, India, Hong Kong, Singapore, and Malaysia, although in these states the British system has been adapted to accommodate aspects of other cultures such as Asian or, in the case of Malaysia, Islamic legal culture. Former African colonies also apply English common law. Kenya has a basis of common law overlain with Islamic customary and tribal law, and the legal system of Nigeria is substantially common law combined with customary law.

France, Germany, Spain, Portugal, Italy, Turkey, along with South American and North African states with European colonial histories, have adopted the civil law tradition in which authoritative law has been codified, deriving from Justinian (Roman) law and developed by the French Code Civile or the German BGB. Other states such as the Philippines, South Africa, and Sri Lanka have legal systems containing both the common law and civil law traditions as a consequence of their history of colonialism, in each case overlain with values derived from Asian or African social traditions.

Legal systems within Western legal culture are secular, and independent of religion and morality. Law in a Western culture provides the main method of conflict resolution amongst individuals and between individuals and the state. One consequence of secularism is that of rationalism, whereby the legal system is organized according to principles and rules which must be justified by logic or reason rather than by religious or moral belief. A primary feature of Western legal culture is its presumption of autonomy of the individual. Western legal philosophy has given rise to an emphasis on human rights in both the civil and political, and social and economic spheres. While many of these human rights are universal and embedded in international treaties and conventions, the origin of much human rights doctrine in Western political philosophy has resulted in some distrust of human rights arguments in non-Western societies. In Western legal cultures, human rights focus on the relationship between the individual and the state and provide remedies for individuals in dispute with the state, and as such they constrain interference with private life even when that interference might be justified on the basis of a wider community or public benefit. Other legal cultures place more value on family and collective relationships, and hence individual human rights play a more significant role in Western legal culture than elsewhere.

Asian legal culture

The family of Asian legal systems includes China, Japan, the Republic of Korea, and Thailand. Other Asian states and territories such as Singapore, Malaysia, and Hong Kong, which inherited a common law system; Vietnam, which has a legal system based on Marxist–Leninist ideology; Macau, which inherited the Portuguese civil law legal system; and the Philippines, which has a mixed common law and civil law system, interpret law through a filter of Asian and/or Islamic values. In many respects, the legal systems of Asian states have little in common. Their political contexts vary widely and they have all introduced some Western law superimposed over traditional laws giving rise to pluralist systems. Nevertheless, there are aspects of Asian legal systems which contrast them from other legal cultures, most notably the influence of Confucianism and Buddhism which impose duties of loyalty to family and society. Additionally, most Asian governments are characterized by a strong bureaucracy and the absence of a doctrine of separation of powers.

Asian legal culture differs from Western culture in relation to the role of law in the regulation of private or social life. Whereas Western legal systems presuppose that the private life of citizens falls within the remit of objective state law, and that the limits of law are imposed by a philosophy of liberalism which guarantees personal freedoms, in Asian legal tradition it is not rational thought but rather an accepted natural order of things, derived from religious and moral belief, which underpins law. In this tradition, each individual has a status in the societal hierarchy. The duty of the individual is not to question, challenge, or debate, but rather to accept and obey the natural order. Individuals are characterized by duty rather than by autonomy. There is no consensus as to whether and to what extent modern Asian systems maintain this traditional approach, but there is nevertheless an accepted view that Asian legal culture shuns the adversarial style of Western dispute resolution in favour of a system of conciliation and compromise, whereby the end goal is not a vindication of rights but rather a result which restores harmony or creates the least disturbance to the natural order. This can still be seen in the reliance on mediation rather than litigation in the redress of rights in many Asian cultures.

The most significant consequence of respect for the natural order has been the approach to the balance between public good and private right. In Asian legal culture, rights are inseparable from duties (Diokno 2000), and there is in consequence a greater willingness on the part of individuals to suffer sacrifice for the benefit of the family or community. Government authority and some curtailment of rights are considered necessary to state welfare and social and political order. There has developed some resistance in Asia to Western approaches to human rights on the basis that human rights are values which derive from history and culture, giving rise to the claim for recognition of 'Asian values' (Bell 1996). Attempts to impose Western human rights on Asian legal systems have led to accusations of cultural imperialism (Svennson 2000). It has been argued that in developing Asian states, economic and social rights need to be constrained in pursuance of economic growth (Neary 2002), although some critics dispute that rights do in fact hamper economic growth (Sen 1997). Chinese scholars defend Asian interpretations of human rights (De Bary & Tu 2001), arguing that rights are communitarian and dependant on context. The view that Asian legal philosophy accepts wider government responsibility and greater intrusion into private life is still prevalent (Brems 2001). The Chairman of China's National People's Congress notes that Asian civilizations have developed through mutual influences based on a tradition that values harmony, and this should continue so as to allow Asian countries to develop their own cultural and foreign policies (South China Morning Post 2007).

Public health legislation in Western legal culture

Legislation supporting communicable disease control in Western legal culture

Public health legislation across much of Western legal culture has undergone little updating since the mid-twentieth century. Hence law is based on outdated science and fails to recognize human rights and ethics. Within Western legal culture, there is a range of approaches to legal public health powers and duties addressing communicable disease control. A study of legislation governing tuberculosis in 14 European states (Coker *et al.* 2007) demonstrates that approaches to public health law fall into four broad typologies, authoritarian (Russia, Estonia, Switzerland, and Norway), moderate (England, Germany, Israel, the Czech Republic, Hungary, Poland, and Finland), preventive (France and the Netherlands), and *laissez faire* (Spain). Differences of approach can be explained in part by the social and political histories of each state.

Nevertheless there are some common features to Western approaches to public health law. Most Western public health law focuses on protection of the healthy from sources of disease, including from human sources of disease, rather than on treatment and care of the ill. Most Western law provides penalties for persons who expose others to risk of disease by their health behaviours. It is now accepted in most Western states that human rights doctrine must provide limits to the power of the state to intervene for the public good, and human rights arguments have been used to challenge state public health powers. In *Enhorn v Sweden*, the European Court of Human Rights upheld a claim against the state of Sweden by an HIV-positive man detained under Swedish public health legislation, on the grounds that detention breached the claimant's right to liberty and to private and family life by being disproportionate to the public health risk (Martin 2006a).

Legislation supporting communicable disease control in England and Wales

The legal system in England and Wales is the English common law system. Authoritative law can be found both in the form of legislation (statutes and regulations) and of judicial decisions binding on lower courts by means of the doctrine of precedent. The main source of English public health law is in statutory form.

England led the world in developing legal powers and duties for population health. In the early nineteenth century, Britain faced environmental health threats from developing industrialization and urban populations well before other states. After the influenza and typhoid epidemics in 1837 and 1838, the lawyer Edwin Chadwick conducted an enquiry which concluded that much spread of disease resulted from living conditions. The first Public Health Act was passed in 1848 and the revised Public Health Acts became a model for legal regulation of public health across the world. British colonies from Hong Kong to Australia inherited British legislation, and states such as Japan, with very different legal systems, borrowed the British public health legal framework as a starting point for developing their own public health law (Tatara 2002).

The principles of public health law in England and Wales remain little changed since this early legislation. Disease control is governed by the Public Health (Control of Disease) Act 1984 and the Public Health (Infectious Disease) Regulations 1988. The other UK countries, Scotland and Northern Ireland, have similar legislation. Public health powers can only be invoked in relation to diseases classified as notifiable, as listed in the Act and in the Schedule to the Regulations. SARS and H5N1 influenza, for example, are currently not notifiable diseases and so there are no powers in relation to these diseases. The Act imposes a duty on medical practitioners to report notifiable diseases, and provides to the local authority powers of compulsory medical examination, powers of removal, and powers of detention in a hospital of persons with specified diseases. There are no powers of quarantine of persons exposed to disease, and no powers of isolation of persons with disease other than in a hospital. The Act imposes penalties on persons who expose others to risk of disease, although as the legislation is based on outdated science, some provisions provide penalties for behaviour that creates no public health risk. It is an offence, for example, for a person suffering from disease to return books to the library, although there is no known disease risk associated with library books (Atenstaedt 2006).

The 1984 Public Health Act is a consolidation of old public health laws, and powers were formulated at a time when it was accepted that private rights could be infringed for the benefit of a public good. There is concern that some powers provided by the Act may now be vulnerable to challenge under the Human Rights Act 1998 which brought into domestic law provisions of the European Convention for the Protection of Human Rights and Fundamental Freedoms. The decision of the European Court of Human Rights in *Enhorn v Sweden* (above) suggests that the exercise of public health powers which infringe liberty and private life can only be justified in circumstances where detention is proportional to the public health risk, and where detention is a last resort measure. As English public health legislation does not authorize measures less intrusive than hospital detention, some exercises of detention powers will not be a last resort (Martin 2006a). The absence of review and appeal procedures, and the fact that applications for detention can be made *ex parte* (such that the subject of the application cannot oppose it), make the legislation vulnerable to challenge under Article 6 of the European Convention which protects the right to a fair trial (Harris & Martin 2004).

Consistent with Western approaches to the public/private balance, only minor infringements of the rights to privacy and to private life will be tolerated even where the health of the population is threatened. English law does not, for example, authorize compulsory treatment or compulsory vaccination, whatever the public health risk, as consent to treatment is a fundamental principle of English jurisprudence.

English public health law is currently undergoing a process of amendment to ensure compliance with the revised IHR. There have long been calls for reform of the legal framework of public health (Coker & Martin 2006). In March 2007, a Consultation Paper was published (Department of Health 2007) proposing that revised legislation take an 'all hazards' approach rather than be based on notifiable diseases, and so cover new diseases as well as chemical or radiation contamination. The proposals recommend recognition within the legislation that powers be subject to principles of human rights. New powers of quarantine and compulsory counselling are proposed, powers of detention and medical examination are refined, and consistent with the principle of autonomy, powers of compulsory medical treatment are rejected. The paper argues against the requirement that subjects of public health powers be notified of applications to exercise powers so as to enable them to mount a defence, but does propose that there be opportunity for an order for exercise of compulsory powers to be reviewed. Statutory surveillance procedures are to be simplified and brought up to date in line with IHR requirements.

Legislation supporting communicable disease control in France

France is a republic with a centralist government structure. Despite the strong powers of central government, French philosophy favours individual over collective rights and there is reluctance in France to impinge on personal freedoms, what is known as the 'French paradox' (Morella 1996). The French legal system is a civil law system, in which authoritative law is codified. Law (*loi*) in the French legal system has a somewhat broader meaning than in English law, and covers the constitution, codes, statutes, *ordonnances* (which are time limited and lapse without later statutory ratification), regulations (*décrets* issued by the president or prime minister and *arrêtes* issued by a minister or mayor), orders, and circulars. There is no doctrine of precedent as in the English legal system, although court decisions are influential in the interpretation of law.

The *Code de la Santé Publique* recognizes the fundamental right to protection against health threats, guarantees equal access to the best possible health security, and protects the right to respect for dignity and freedom from discrimination.

The history of public health in France is very different from that in Britain. The association between hygiene, morality, and disease meant that the church for a long time played a role in public health initiatives. Indeed, there was suspicion around the involvement of the state in the private matter of health (Da Lomba & Martin 2004). Early public hygiene measures instituted by the church included detention, exclusion, and coercive treatment, but these measures were unsupported by legislation.

The first significant state intervention into public health came with the 1916 *Lois Bourgeois* and the 1919 *Honnorat* which created dispensaries for the purpose of detecting incidences of tuberculosis, and provided medicines to the poor and public sanitoriums. The 1994 *Loi relative á la santé publique et á la protection sociale* simplified the disease control framework. As a result, disease control in France relies primarily on notification of specified diseases and compulsory vaccination, including compulsory vaccination of both school children (vaccination is a precondition to public benefits such as schooling) and of persons working in specified activities (*Code de la Santé Publique*). There are also some powers of exclusion from activities (*Code de la Santé Publique*), but there are now no statutory powers of detention, quarantine, compulsory medical examination, or compulsory treatment, favouring instead voluntary and non-statutory measures and respect for the primacy of the patient/doctor relationship of trust. However, specific groups such as prisoners (*Code de Procédure Pénale* 1999) and foreigners (*Décret* no 46-1574 of 1946) may be subject to powers of compulsory medical examination and isolation in relation to diseases such as tuberculosis, and there are powers of containment of persons suffering from smallpox (*Décret* no 2003-313 of 2003). The Prefect of each *département* has the power to issue laws (*arrêtés*) in the short term in case of emergency, and central government has emergency powers, so law could provide powers in a public health emergency. Overall, however, France has few legislated public health powers compared to England or other Western states (Coker *et al.* 2007). France is considering the introduction of statutory powers of compulsory medical examination (where there is suspicion of disease), quarantine, and isolation in response to the SARS epidemic and in the light of the revised IHR (Sommade 2004).

Public health law reform for communicable disease in Western legal culture

The threat of SARS and pandemic influenza, and the requirement of compliance with the revised IHR, have provided an incentive to all states to revisit the role of law in public health. Public health legislation in Western legal culture has tended to be reactive, responding to existing public health concerns and consisting of precise duties and powers with little room for exercise of discretion (Martin 2006b). Law reform proposals tend to be more open-textured, more flexible, and more focused on rapid response to public health risk than traditional legislation.

Another feature of law reform proposals is an overt examination of the underpinning rights and values which provide the framework of public health activity, and in particular recognition that in Western jurisprudence, individual rights such as autonomy and privacy can only in exceptional circumstances be sacrificed to the public good. Whereas traditional public health legislation made no reference to the constraints of public health ethics or human rights, law reform proposals tend to make clear the balance between public good and private right in the context of the particular culture of the state.

An early example of law reform is the Australian Capital Territory's Public Health Act 1997. The ACT has a common law legal system. The Act introduced an approach to public health law driven by the notion of risk, with the objectives of providing tools for rapid response to public health risk and ensuring protection of individual liberty and privacy. The Health Minister may declare at any time a particular activity that might give rise to transmission of disease or that might otherwise affect the health of individuals, to be a public health risk activity. Any person carrying out a public health risk activity is obliged to comply with a code of practice, enforced by registration and licensing procedures. Duties of disease notification apply only where notification is necessary to protect public health, and powers of confinement of individuals apply only where confinement is necessary to avert an imminent and serious risk to public health.

Quebec, Canada, which has a civil law legal system, introduced its new Public Health Act in 2001. The legislation establishes a public health ethics committee with responsibility for overseeing public health surveillance so as to ensure ethics compliance, and notification is based on risk to public health. The Act allows for compulsory exclusion, isolation of both persons with disease and persons exposed to disease, medical examination, and, more unusually, for the compulsory medical treatment of persons with disease with the objective of reducing contagion. In a case of public health emergency, the Act provides compulsory vaccination powers. There is recognition of responsibility to sufferers of disease as well as to the healthy in the form of a general duty to see that all persons with disease are provided with access to medical care and treatment.

Scotland, which has a legal system based on Roman Dutch and common law, has published a consultation paper on public health law reform (Scottish Executive 2006). A focus of the paper is the determination of rights and values which are to provide a framework for public health practice in Scotland, suggesting that those primary values might be personal autonomy and privacy, along with care for others. Responsibility for the public's health lies with the individual as well as with the state. The Scottish proposals recognize that public health responsibilities and powers should reflect the objective of risk reduction. Proposed duties of notification are predicated on the requirement that the disease or condition pose an appreciable risk to the public's health. Duties of notification would consider moral and cultural sensitivities and comply with ethical and legal guidance. Powers of medical examination, exclusion, quarantine, or detention would need to be consistent with human rights principles of least restrictive alternative, proportionality, and individual rights. The Scottish proposals, like the English proposals, do not entertain the possibility of compulsory medical treatment in recognition of the primacy of the autonomy of the individual.

Legislation to address tobacco harms in Western legal culture

The use of law in the control of non-communicable disease is comparatively recent. Law is particularly important in this area because much non-communicable disease is a product of lifestyle choices and environmental influences on choices. Law has the power both directly and indirectly to change lifestyle environments, to ensure informed lifestyle choices, and to control commercial exploitation.

While the effectiveness of legal intervention into smoking behaviours is still subject to research, preliminary studies suggest that voluntary codes of behaviour do not work (Jones 1999), and that enforced smoking prohibitions serve both to improve the health environment of non-smokers, and to assist in discouraging smoking behaviours (Euromonitor International 2006a; Allwright 2005; Fichtenberg 2002). Within Europe, a number of states, including Ireland, the United Kingdom, Italy, Malta, Spain, the Netherlands, Norway, and France, have introduced laws restricting or prohibiting smoking in public places. Germany, the largest consumer of tobacco in Europe, is planning laws to ban smoking in restaurants, bars, and transport facilities. More widely in the Western world, laws have been introduced in Canada, the United States, New Zealand, and Australia providing smoke-free environments and regulating tobacco advertising, tobacco packaging and warnings, taxation on tobacco products, and restrictions on the sale of tobacco. Other laws such as occupational health and discrimination laws also provide protection from tobacco harms. In Australia, an asthmatic successfully sued a hotel under the Disability Discrimination Act 1992 because failure to provide a smoke-free environment prevented her, as a sufferer of asthma, from using hotel premises (*Francey and Meeuwissen v. Hilton Hotels of Australia* 2000).

The importance of law as a tool in the control of tobacco harms was recognized in the first ever global public health treaty, the WHO Framework Convention on Tobacco Control, adopted in 2003. In February 2005, the Convention became international law, and set international standards on tobacco price and tax increases, tobacco advertising and sponsorship, labelling, trade, and second hand smoke. The Convention requires signatory states to impose restrictions on tobacco sale, advertising, sponsorship and promotion, to regulate tobacco labelling, to protect indoor places from smoke polluted air, and to criminalize tobacco smuggling. Indeed legal interventions constitute the backbone of the Convention strategies.

Legislation to address tobacco harms in England and Wales

The United Kingdom ratified the Framework Convention on Tobacco Control in 2004, and subsequently individual UK countries produced legislation in compliance with the framework. The Health Act 2006 provides generally for designation of smoke-free areas, for possible exemptions from smoking prohibitions, and for signage to make clear where smoking is permitted. In England smoking prohibitions are contained in the Smoke Free (Premises and Enforcement) Regulations 2006 and the Smoke Free (Exemptions and Vehicles) Regulations 2007 has similar regulations. Any enclosed or substantially enclosed area or vehicle which is open to the public, or where people work, must now be smoke-free and must display signs making this clear. This includes restaurants, cafes, pubs, cinemas, clubs, public transport, company cars, offices, and factories. Exemptions from the prohibitions include prisons, adult residential care homes, residential mental healthcare centres, and designated hotel rooms. Significant warnings on tobacco packaging are required by the Tobacco Products Labelling (Safety) Regulations 1991 as updated, and the Tobacco Products (Manufacture, Presentation and Sale) Regulations 2002.

The 2005 European Union Tobacco Advertising Directive applies to tobacco advertising and sponsorship with a cross-border dimension but is limited to merchandizing and sports sponsorship. In England and Wales, the Tobacco Advertising and Promotion Act 2002 and regulations prohibit national advertising, promotion and sponsorship of tobacco products, including brandshare products (Tobacco Advertising and Promotion (Brandshare) Regulations 2004), with limited exceptions such as advertising near the till where cigarettes are to be sold in shops. The Children and Young Persons (Sale of Tobacco etc.) Order 2007 amends the Children and Young Persons (Protection from Tobacco) Act 1991 to raise the age at which young persons can be sold tobacco products from 16 to 18. Further laws are planned to prohibit the display of cigarettes in shops and supermarkets, requiring tobacco products to be kept under the counter. Similar laws are being considered in Scotland, Norway, New Zealand, and Scotland. The government also hopes to pass laws to prohibit vending machines in pubs, to fine persons who drop cigarette butts, and to restrict the sale of packs of 10 cigarettes as smaller packets are more attractive to children. Small packs of cigarettes are already prohibited in Australia, New Zealand, Canada, France, and some US states.

Legislation to address tobacco harms in France

Cigarette smoking has long been a feature of French café culture. France is also a producer of tobacco. Attempts to prohibit smoking in public places have been strongly resisted on both economic and cultural grounds. In 1991, France passed law to ban direct tobacco advertising, to require health warnings on tobacco packs, and to require all restaurants and bars to provide no-smoking areas. The restrictions on smoking in public places were in practice rarely enforced. In 1999, the French government issued a circular restricting smoking in healthcare establishments (Circular DGS/DH/SP 3 No 99-330 of 8 June 1999). France ratified the WHO Framework Convention on Tobacco Control in 2003 and in 2007 a smoking ban came into effect to include schools, shops, transport facilities, offices, public buildings, and other enclosed spaces. The smoking bans were not promulgated in legislative form but rather by government decree following a parliamentary committee recommendation (*Décret* no 2006-1386 of 15 November 2006). Smoking prohibitions in restaurants, bars, and nightclubs were delayed until 2008. Prohibition on tobacco advertising was introduced in France in 1993 (*Loi Evin*). These laws were amended to allow televised sports events from states where tobacco advertising is not prohibited. Sale of tobacco products to persons under 16 is prohibited by *Loi* no *2003-715 of 2003*, and the sale of cigarettes in packets of 10 is prohibited.

The potential role of law in tackling obesity in Western legal culture

WHO recognizes obesity to be one of the greatest public health challenges of the twenty-first century and a disease in its own right (WHO 2003). Law has long had a role in controlling toxic food content but until recently played no part in constraining and influencing lifestyle choices. Law has traditionally been predicated on the understanding that humans are rational actors, but theories of behaviouralism, which propose that external events and circumstances can bias the ability to make rational judgements, have paved the way for law's involvement in countering market manipulation of preferences (Harvard Law Review Note 2003). Research on the influence of advertising on food choices (Borzekowski *et al.* 2001) and on misleading food labelling has provided an evidence base for law. This 'new frontier of public health law' (Mello *et al.* 2006) has not been free of controversy. Legal intervention has prompted civil liberties arguments of freedom of choice and freedom of speech. Ethics literature has raised concerns of the 'nanny state' and of paternalism in relation to issues of personal responsibility (Holm 2007). While tobacco can be classified as a dangerous substance, much food at the centre of obesity arguments is not in itself dangerous, only becoming so as part of an overall unhealthy diet. One food manufacturer commented in relation to a chocolate bar, '. . . health warnings are for dangerous things. Whilst we recognise the

problem I do not think that a Curly Wurly is a dangerous thing' (House of Commons UK 2004). However, it is now accepted that some foods can be classified as healthy or unhealthy, and the food industry itself has begun to promote what it terms 'healthy eating' ranges of food.

The role of law in the relationship between food and public health has become more important in the changing dynamic of food systems (Lang 2006). Governments, concerned about the rising costs of obesity, are looking to law not only as a means of controlling market practices but also as a means of shaping consumers' knowledge and understanding of health risks, their purchasing patterns, and their eating habits.

The role of law in tackling obesity in England and Wales

Obesity is one of the most pressing public health concerns in Britain. Public health interventions to prevent increasing levels of obesity are a government priority (Department of Health 2004, 2006). The government has recognized the health problems posed by obesity in a series of papers which reflect changing approaches to the role of the state in obesity (Martin 2008). Obesity is categorized as a medical problem (National Audit office 2001), an economic problem (Wanless 2002, 2004), a societal problem (House of Commons 2004), and a public health problem (Department of Health 2004) in which the role of government is to:

> . . . support consumers, providing them with easier access to a wide range of healthier foods and, crucially, the information and knowledge needed to make informed choices about their diets. And this may mean targeting action to meet the needs of particular groups and tackle inequalities.

More recently obesity has been classed as a personal problem whereby 'Our problems are not, strictly speaking, public health questions at all. They are questions of individual lifestyle. . . . They are not epidemics in the epidemiological sense. They are the result of millions of individual decisions' (former prime minister Tony Blair 2006a). In this context, the government has on the whole favoured voluntary industry regulation.

However, industry has been slow to achieve the levels of protection demanded by the public health community, and gradually the government is turning to law to enforce food health standards. The Education (Nutrition Standards for School Lunches) (England) Regulations 2006 set minimum nutritional requirements in the provision of school lunches. The Food Labelling Regulations 1996 have been amended to require clearer labelling of food content, although labelling of the nutritional content of food is currently only required where the manufacturer makes particular nutritional claims for its product. The Food Standards Agency recommend a 'traffic lights' system of food labelling to allow easy identification of healthy foods, but some major supermarkets have rejected this approach in favour of a system based on percentage of guideline daily amount (GDA) of a nutrient, resulting in inconsistent labelling across the industry. In recognition of the relationship between breastfeeding and childhood obesity, the English government is considering the introduction of laws to protect breastfeeding in public along the lines of the Breastfeeding (Scotland) Act 2005.

The most contested area of legal intervention in obesity control is the proposal to prohibit the advertising of unhealthy foods targeted at children. The foods most commonly advertised to children in the United Kingdom (Hastings 2003), as elsewhere (Caraher 2006), are those which have high levels of fat, salt, and sugar. The House of Commons Health Committee acknowledges '... the food industry's relentless targeting of children through intense advertising and promotion campaigns, some of which explicitly aim to circumvent parental control by exploiting "pester power"' (House of Common Health Committee 2004). The Food Standard Agency accepts the '... causal link between promotional activity and children's food knowledge, preference and behaviours' (Food Standards Agency 2003).

In 2006, Ofcom, the independent regulator of television, radio, telecommunications, and wireless communications services in the United Kingdom, published a consultation document in which it concluded that self-regulation alone would not be sufficient to deal with the problem of advertising to children. Ofcom recommended that advertising of food and drink products be prohibited during programmes aimed at children or which will be of interest to children aged between 4 and 9 years, extended to cover programmes for children aged 4 to 15 in 2008 (Ofcom 2007). The public health community argued that these restrictions were insufficient to protect children and proposed that all food and drink advertising should be prohibited before 9 pm. As a result the 2007 Private Members Television (Food Advertising) Bill, proposed prohibiting advertising between 5 am and 9 pm of foods which fail to meet specified nutritional standards. It must be borne in mind that national legislation regulating television content in Europe is weakened by the European Television without Frontiers Directive which specifies that broadcasting is governed by the laws of the country in which it originates. This allows British viewers to access television programmes from other European states where there is no regulation of food advertising. The Directive on Audiovisual Media Services proposed in 2008–09 will attempt to limit advertising of food, tobacco, and alcohol products across Europe.

The role of law in tackling obesity elsewhere in Western legal culture

Obesity is a health concern across the Western world, and states are increasingly considering legal interventions. In Europe, in 2006, the WHO Ministerial Conference adopted a European Charter on Counteracting Obesity (WHO Regional Office for Europe 2006) which acknowledged that obesity posed a serious problem not only for health but also for economics and social development in Europe. The Charter recommends that governments and national parliaments ensure consistency and sustainability of approach to obesity through regulatory action, including legislation. A report by the International Association of Consumer Food Organizations for the World Health Organization consultation on a global strategy for diet and health has recommended international controls on food advertising including cross-border controls (IACFO 2003).

In Australia, obesity levels are particularly high. Laws in relation to health are devolved to state governments and so differ from state to state despite there being no real borders between states. Approaches in Australia to issues such as food content, food labelling, and the placement of food vending machines tend to favour voluntary industry regulation. Food labelling, for example, is governed by the Australian Food Standards Code which provides uniform food standards and outlines food labelling requirements. It is planned to amend the Code to introduce a 'traffic' light system

of food labelling along the lines of the proposed British system, but this will continue to be embodied in a code of practice rather than in law. Some Australian states have begun to introduce legislation in recognition that voluntary industry compliance has not been successful.

Elsewhere, Laws in Sweden and Norway prohibit advertising of junk food aimed at children under 12, but programmes for older children are often accompanied by advertisements for crisps and soft drinks (WHO 2006). Viewers have access to television programmes from other European states with no restrictions. In Canada, Quebec has legislated to restrict all marketing of food and beverage products to children under 13, but as with European legislation, protection is weakened by access to viewers in Quebec to programmes from other Canadian states and from the United States. New Zealand has introduced a food classification scheme which will restrict food advertising on terrestrial television in designated time bands. France now requires advertising of unhealthy food to carry a health warning. Spain has a Code of Self Regulation of the Advertising of Food Products Directed at Minors which requires that there be caution on advertisements aimed at children under 12, and prohibits use of celebrities in advertisement of unhealthy foods. Ireland has prohibited television advertising of fast foods and sweets, as well as the use of celebrities in the promotion of junk food to children.

Some states, Canada and the United States, for example, have legislated to require that the trans fat content of all pre-packaged foods be displayed on labels, and the New York City Health Code prohibits restaurants in New York from serving foods that contain more than 0.5 g of trans fat per serving (Gostin 2007). The Australia New Zealand Food Standards Code 2002 introduced mandatory nutrition labelling of packaged foods for Australia and New Zealand. Germany and Norway are planning on raising taxes on foods high in fats, sugars, and salt. School vending machines are prohibited in some jurisdictions, for example, in Latvia, California, and France, and are restricted in what they can sell in other places, such as Chicago. In New Zealand, the National Administration Guidelines were amended in 2007 to require schools to limit the sale of unhealthy food and drink in vending machines.

States across Western legal culture are actively exploring ways in which law might be used to control production, sale, advertising, and access to unhealthy foodstuffs. Objections by the food industry have carried little weight since voluntary industry codes have been unsuccessful, and food manufacturers are now changing approach. Many major food suppliers have introduced sugar-, salt-, and fat-reduced products, along with 'healthy' food ranges. Much food advertising now focuses on the health value of products, and many manufacturers have begun to improve food labelling, although not always in a manner consistent across the industry. Industry objections to television advertising have so far proved more successful based on freedom of speech arguments, but again the failure of voluntary codes has led many states to consider legislation. As the full health and economic consequences of obesity become more apparent, there is willingness across the Western world to use legislative tools to intervene in lifestyle choices, especially where children are at risk. Western consumers are generally in support of stronger controls. While protection of privacy and freedom of speech are fundamental Western rights, there is sufficient public concern about obesity to accept that laws are needed to ensure informed consumer choice in relation to diet and lifestyle.

Public health legislation in Asian legal culture

Legislation supporting communicable disease control in Asian legal culture

Legislation supporting communicable disease control in China

The revised IHR (2005) give member states new mandates and responsibilities to prevent, protect against, and control the international spread of disease. This development constituted the most far-reaching change in international public health regulation since the nineteenth century (Fidler 2005), and was the outcome of a shift from a 'Westphalian' (reliance on state sovereignty) to a 'post-Westphalian' (global health governance and international co-operation) regulatory model (Fidler 2004). China was at the epicentre of the 2003 SARS epidemic, and learned first hand the importance of law in support of public health. Since then China has enacted much needed public health legislation.

Public health programmes and interventions must be planned and delivered in the context of national health and political systems (Merson 2006). Under the Constitution of the People's Republic of China, the National People's Congress (NPC) is the highest organ of state power. The NPC and its Standing Committee are empowered with rights of legislation, decision, supervision, election, and removal. The State administration is collectively known as the Central People's Government and is responsible for carrying out the principles and policies of the Communist Party of China. In practice much of the detail of contemporary Chinese law has its origins in Japanese law, the civil law systems of Germany and France, and the common law of England and the United States. However, it remains the case that cultural influences have survived in the practice and enforcement of laws.

The primary legislation is the Communicable Diseases Law, promulgated at national level in 1989 and substantially revised in 2004. The Ministry of Health acknowledged in the promulgation notice that the law was amended in the light of experience gained from the SARS epidemic, and that its revision aimed to enhance the overall standard of disease prevention (zheng ti shui ping) and to achieve perfection (jian li, wan shan) of the public health system. Article 1 states the purpose of the law, to prevent, control, and eliminate the occurrence and spread of communicable diseases in order to protect the health of individuals and the public. Article 1 also clarifies the legislation's policy focus (zhi dao si xiang) on prevention (yu fang wei zhu), to include a combination of preventive and therapeutic measures (fang zhi jie he), and the adoption of 'diverse control measures' (fen lei guan li) based on scientific knowledge and the needs of the people. The infectious diseases (chuan ran bing) covered by the legislation fall into three categories. Type A includes plague and cholera, Type B includes SARS, avian influenza, anthrax, pulmonary tuberculosis, viral hepatitis, dysentery, typhoid, AIDS, syphilis, and measles, and Type C contains a long list of infectious diseases. Other diseases may be added to Types B and C on the decision of the national health authority attached to the State Council, as necessitated by outbreaks, the epidemiological situation or disease seriousness. SARS, anthrax, and avian influenza, which are highly pathogenic to humans and classified as Type B, may at times be subject to more rigorous preventive and control measures as if they were Type A diseases.

Article 8(1) entrenches the role of traditional medicine such as Chinese medicine (TCM) as a complementary partner to modern medicine in the prevention and treatment of communicable disease. While the role of TCM is protected by the Chinese Constitution, the reiteration here is a reflection of the belief that the use of TCM in China contributed significantly to the control and abatement of the spread of SARS, particular in the Guangdong region. The role of international co-operation is expressly encouraged (Article 8(2)). Individuals and units (dan wei) within the PRC are now required under Article 12 to comply with measures such as investigation, inspection, sample collection, isolation (ge li), and supply of accurate information as required by the health authorities, subject to the duty to respect privacy and the right of appeal. A new surveillance system (Article 17), warning system (Article 18), and pathogen databank (Article 26) are to be established. The 'diverse control measures' (fen lei guan li) focus on health promotion activities (Article 13), vaccination programmes with emphasis on free vaccination for children (Articles 14–16), enforcement through medical institutions (yi liao ji gou) (Article 21), laboratories (Article 22), blood collection, supply, and research institutions (Article 23), and agricultural ministries with responsibility for zoonosis (Article 25). Article 24 envisages that further regulations will be enacted with regard to AIDS, while provinces are expressly required to take more active steps to contain HIV/AIDS.

The Frontier Health and Quarantine Law 1986, Food Hygiene Law 1995, Law on Practising Doctors 1998, and Law on the Prevention and Treatment of Occupational Diseases 2001 are other examples of national law relevant to disease prevention. In 2003, Regulations on the Urgent Handling of Public Health Emergencies were promulgated by State Council. State Council also has the power to enact national administrative legislation under the Chinese Constitution, and through its ministries and bureaux, industry-specific administrative regulations. Such regulations must comply with national law to be valid. The Implementing Rules of the Frontier Law 1989 and the Regulations on the Handling of Major Animal Epidemic Emergencies 2005 are examples. At a further level, administrative bureaux such as the Ministry of Health and the State Administration of Quality Supervision, Inspection and Quarantine are vested with authority to enact measures such as the Measures for the Handling of Food Poisoning Incidents 2000, the Measures for the Administration of Information Reporting on Monitoring Public Health Emergencies and Epidemic Situation of Infectious Diseases 2003 and the Regulation on the Urgent Handling of the Entry-Exit Inspection and Quarantine of Frontier and Port Public Health Emergencies 2003.

Provincial national people's congresses and governments have legislative power to enact law governing their territories that are consistent with national law, which may further regulate activities in accordance with regional needs. Article 4 of the Communicable Diseases Law gives provincial governments the power to bring within the legislation locally prevalent diseases as Type B or C diseases without prior central government approval, though the notice of publication has to be filed with the central government. Article 10 of the Public Health Emergency Regulations empowers provincial governments to formulate regional plans for handling emergencies taking into consideration local circumstances, to supplement the national plan.

Border control issues are dealt with under the Frontier Law of 1986. Diseases are classified either as quarantinable (jian yi chuan ran bing) or monitored diseases (*jian ce chuan ran bing*). These provisions reflect the international obligations undertaken by China under the IHR 1969. The key obligation is set out in Article 7, which provides that all persons (*ren yuan*) and conveyances (*jiao tong gong ju*) are subject to quarantine inspection at the first frontier port of their arrival. Article 24 of the Frontier Law provides that where the provisions of the law differ from those of international treaties on health and quarantine to which China is a party, the provisions of such international treaties shall prevail with the exception of treaty clauses in relation to which the PRC has declared reservations.

An overview of Chinese public health law is not complete without reference to the stringent legal liability regime introduced by the Public Health Emergency Regulations in the wake of the SARS epidemic. Officials can be sanctioned, demoted, or removed from office if they fail to perform their reporting or other duties, or delay or cause false reports to be made directly or by enabling others to conceal information. Criminal sanctions may apply if such behaviour results in disease spread. While China was criticized for initially withholding information in relation to the SARS outbreak, China was quick to demonstrate that the delay was caused by decisions of recalcitrant officials who were subsequently removed from office, rather than state policy. Administrative or criminal sanctions will also apply to persons who propagate rumour, artificially push up prices, or defraud consumers during a public health emergency period (Articles 45–52).

Legislation supporting communicable disease control in Japan

Under the Japanese Constitution of 1947, the National Diet is the highest organ of state power. The Japanese legal system was modelled on the feudal Chinese legal system, but after the Meiji reformation, the legal system has largely followed the German model. As in China, laws are supplemented by administrative directions and suggestions (*gyôsei shidô*). Article 25 of the Constitution provides that all people shall have the right to maintain the minimum standards of wholesome and cultured living, and the State shall use its endeavours for the promotion and extension of social welfare and security, and of public health, in all spheres of life.

The main legislation on communicable diseases control in Japan is the 1999 Law Concerning the Prevention of Infectious Diseases and Medical Care for Patients of Infections, under which doctors are required to report 86 infectious diseases classified in 5 categories. In 1997 the epidemiology arm of The National Institute of Infectious Diseases was reformed as an independent Infectious Disease Surveillance Centre, with power to monitor and collect reports of infectious agents from prefectures, ordinance designated cities, and special wards (prefectures). The NIID also has power to conduct investigations in the event of an infectious disease outbreak and to exchange information with overseas agencies.

Pursuant to a requirement that the legislature review the law after 5 years, substantial amendments were introduced in 2004, with emphasis on tackling problems brought about by bioterrorism (anthrax and smallpox), the threat of terrorist attacks, and SARS. These amendments relate principally to strengthening the role of government in infectious disease control in an emergency, reviewing the control strategy of zoonosis, and reviewing the list of categorized diseases, especially Category IV. Article 15 empowers the national government to conduct epidemiological investigations in addition to those carried out by regional governments, and to provide suggestions for handling an outbreak. In a threatened breakout, the national government may require prefectures to establish concrete preparedness plans (Articles 9 and 10) and may issue directives to the local governors of the prefectures (Articles 51(2) and 63(2)).

Supplementary decisions made by the Diet provide that examination of patients with suspected SARS infection must take place only at specified hospitals. There is to be education at places of work and schools to ensure against discrimination and prejudice in relation to patients with infectious diseases and their families. Education is to be provided to ensure consideration of disease patients' human rights. Finally, international medical cooperation is to be promoted through WHO and through bilateral deliberations between countries.

The Quarantine Law was amended simultaneously to provide powers to expand the range of medical examinations and inspections at quarantine stations and to oblige persons suspected of suffering from an infectious disease to report their health conditions for a period after entry into Japan. In 2005, the Tuberculosis Control Law was revised with particular emphasis on medical screening in line with a further amendment to the Infectious Diseases Control Law in 2006, and the two laws are expected to improve control of infectious diseases.

Legislation supporting communicable disease control in Hong Kong

The Quarantine and Prevention of Disease Ordinance (Cap. 141) and the Prevention of the Spread of Infectious Diseases Regulations (Cap. 141B) constitute the legislative framework for the prevention and control of infectious diseases in Hong Kong. This legislation is based on early English public health laws. The primary legislation applies mainly to the 1969 IHR quarantinable diseases (cholera, plague, and yellow fever) and the regulations apply to other infectious diseases as listed in the First Schedule to the primary legislation. The legislation needs to be amended every time a new disease is added, and in 2003 there were delays in control measures in relation to SARS while the amendment procedures were undertaken (LegCo Select Committee Hong Kong 2004).

Under the regulations medical practitioners have a duty to report disease where they have reasonable grounds to suspect the existence of disease, and others such as police officers, relatives, occupiers, and hotel keepers have a duty to report when they have knowledge of disease. There is a presumption of knowledge such that the burden lies on the person with reporting responsibility to show that he had no knowledge. The regulations provide powers of entry onto premises, powers of forcible removal of persons from premises, powers of quarantine of persons exposed to disease, and powers of detention of a person with disease until he is no longer infectious. Statutory public health offences include exposure of others to risk of disease and failure to comply with a public health order. Certain extraordinary amendments were made during SARS. The Prevention of the Spread of Infectious Diseases (Amendment) Regulations 2003 inserted into the main legislation a new Part VIA with powers to restrict persons from leaving Hong Kong, to stop and detain, and to conduct medical examination of persons arriving in or leaving Hong Kong.

Hong Kong also has the Public Health and Municipal Services Ordinance (Cap. 132), which focuses on sanitary sources of disease, and the Emergency Regulations Ordinance (Cap. 241) which enables the Chief Executive in Council to make any regulations in a circumstance of public emergency and danger which he considers to be in the public interest. There are currently no regulations in pursuance of this Ordinance. The Hong Kong Bill of Rights Ordinance (Cap. 838) protects the right to life, liberty, freedom from torture, and rights to privacy, honour, and equality before the law. There are some exceptions to these rights on grounds such as public health, and measures may be taken in derogation of human rights in a situation of emergency.

In February 2007, proposals were introduced to the Panel on Health Services of Hong Kong's legislature to enable Hong Kong to comply with the revised IHR. The paper proposes amendments to strengthen the ability to respond to outbreaks and to provide for preventive and control measures by requiring travellers to produce proof of vaccination, prophylaxis, or declarations, to submit to medical examination, tests, and isolation measures. There will be powers to refuse entry or exit of travellers. It is also proposed to provide legal powers for combating and controlling the effect of public health emergencies and to ensure the territory's preparedness for public health emergencies. Proposed amendments include updating and expanding the list of notifiable diseases, requiring notification of any release of dangerous infectious agents, surrender or submission of specimens, requiring doctors to provide information, and placing sick persons under medical surveillance.

Legislation supporting communicable disease control in other Asian states

Asian states have high incidences of many infectious diseases and are particularly vulnerable to H5N1 strain influenza attributable in part to unhygienic poultry husbandry and lax biosecurity (Melville and Shortridge 2004). One of the common difficulties encountered in Asian states is that while the legal framework may be in place, resources and political will can be lacking.

Malaysia has a legal system based on English common law, but Islamic law also constitutes a significant source of law particularly in relation to private relationships. Malaysia has a large population of migrant workers from Vietnam, China, and Nepal suffering high incidences of tuberculosis, syphilis, and hepatitis B. All semi-skilled and unskilled foreign workers are screened before visas are issued and are required to undergo regular medical examination. Foreign travellers entering Malaysia from specified countries are required to show proof of vaccination against diseases such as yellow fever. The 1988 Prevention and Control of Infectious Diseases Act provides a wider range of duties and powers than equivalent legislation in Western cultures. As well as powers of isolation, medical examination, and quarantine, there are powers to enter into any vehicle arriving in Malaysia, to examine any person or property on board, and to take necessary samples. The Minister has the power to order any area of Malaysia to be designated an infected area, and in relation to an infected area there are powers to put persons under surveillance and powers of compulsory treatment and immunization. Malaysian legislation is currently undergoing reform to enhance surveillance capacity in compliance with the IHR 2005.

The legal system of the Philippines is a mixture of common and civil law. The 1987 Constitution of the Republic of the Philippines provides that the state shall protect and promote the right to health of the people and shall instil health consciousness. Principal law-making powers lie with the Congress of the Philippines, but there is considerable decentralized law-making power. Law may take the form of a presidential decree, a statute of the republic, an executive order, a local government ordinance, or a barangay (community) ordinance. Under Executive Order 102 of 1999, health services are devolved to local governments. The central Department of Health continues to provide services in relation to specific programmes such as tuberculosis and malaria eradication, to manage disease and surveillance systems, and to articulate national policy. The Local Government Code 1991 gives responsibility to local government for health promotion and prevention in relation to communicable and non-communicable diseases, and local health boards carry out this work. In case of widespread public health threats or epidemics, the Secretary of Health can be directed by the President of the Republic to take temporary control of health operations in a local government area for the duration of the emergency.

The prevalence of communicable diseases in the Philippines is high. Philippines has one of the highest incidences of TB in Asia, and non-completion of treatment is common. The Philippine Department of Health Web site attributes TB prevalence to the low priority given to anti-tuberculosis activities, poor availability of anti-TB drugs, insufficient laboratory networking, poor health infrastructures, and lack of trained personnel. These problems are now being addressed, and Directly Observed Therapy has been introduced to ensure completion of treatment. Childhood vaccination against diseases such as tuberculosis and hepatitis B is compulsory (Republic Act No. 7846 of 1994).

The Quarantine Act 2004 gives to the Bureau of Quarantine within the Department of Health powers of examination at ports of entry in relation to both domestic and international vessels, powers and duties of surveillance, and power to enforce rules and regulations necessary to prevent introduction, transmission or spread of 'public health emergencies of international concern'. The Director of the Bureau has power to exercise, in relation to port entry, intervention strategies such as health education, compulsory vaccination of persons entering the Philippines, medical examination of travellers, apprehension, detention, quarantine, and surveillance. Regulations under the Act enable, in an outbreak of a public health emergency, the Bureau Director to recommend to the Secretary for Health a range of disease control measures including apprehension, detention/isolation, and surveillance of suspect cases, surveillance of persons exposed to disease and the power to declare an area or community under quarantine.

Legislation to address tobacco harms in Asian legal culture

Legislation addressing tobacco harms in China

When China ratified the WHO Framework Convention on Tobacco Control in 2005, the Regional Director for the WHO Western Pacific Region stated in a press release that it was 'perhaps the clearest indication yet that the world is increasingly committed to addressing the global tobacco epidemic' (WHO 2005). Studies had predicted a significant increase in tobacco-related mortality in China (Liu 1998; Lam 2001). Current Ministry of Health figures suggest that in China there are 350 million smokers and 450 million passive smokers, and despite the fact that 100 000 die annually from passive smoking, only a third of the population is aware of the dangers of passive smoking (Reuters 2007a).

In 2000, at the National Conference on Policy Development on Tobacco Control in China in the twenty-first Century, participants from the Chinese Academy of Preventive Medicine, Ministry of Health, the WHO, and from other states proposed comprehensive legislation on tobacco control to include increases in tobacco tax, advertising, promotion and sponsorship bans, and package warnings, together with measures to reduce second-hand smoke and strengthen national mass-media campaigns (John Hopkins 2000). In ratifying the Framework Convention, the Chinese government declared that it was committed to strong tobacco control policy in order to fulfil its treaty obligations, and the Standing Committee of the National Peoples Congress took the opportunity to ban cigarette automatic vending machines (National People's Congress 2005). In 2007 eight ministries were established to co-ordinate treaty compliance operations. The 2007 China Tobacco Control Report was released in May 2007 to coincide with the Global Smoke Free Day (Ministry of Health China 2007).

Tobacco harms, particularly those to children, were already covered by the Law on the Protection of Minors 1991, the Law on the Prevention of Juvenile Crime 1999 which imposed duties on parents and teachers to educate minors not to smoke, Tentative Measures on the Administration of Tobacco Advertisements, the Implementing Measures on the Designation of Smoke Free Cities within China 2003, and the Measures on the Prohibition of Smoking in Public Transport and Waiting Rooms 1997. In 2006 substantial amendments were made to the Law on the Protection of Minors to introduce a ban on sale of cigarettes to persons under 18, and a complete ban on smoking in schools, nurseries, and youth activity centres. However, such policies were not implemented without dissent. It was reported (Reuters 2007b) that an official of the State Tobacco Monopoly Association told NPC delegates that while 'smoking harms people's health, restraining smoking threatens social stability', based on the estimate that the tobacco industry contributed 80 billion yuan per day in tax.

China continues to face tension between tobacco ownership interests and public health arguments. The 2007 Tobacco Control Report painted an alarming picture (Ministry of Health China 2007). For example, 180 million passive smokers in China are children under 15. It was recognized that '. . . our country is still considerably far from fulfilling the goals set down by the treaty'. The Report acknowledged that legislation prohibiting smoking in public places is an effective way of tobacco control, citing laws in other countries as well as survey results suggesting that the smoking bans would not be detrimental to businesses. Coupled with China's treaty obligation to prevent passive smoking under Article 8, the Report provides an incentive for the government to take tougher control measures. At the same time, China is the world's largest producer of tobacco with the Chinese government controlling monopoly interests in tobacco production (Peng 1997). Tobacco sales contribute significantly to tax revenues and the tobacco market in China is predicted to continue to expand (Euromonitor International 2006B).

China gave directions to health authorities, universities, and NGOs to promote the 20th Global Smoke Free Day on 31 May 2007, stating that China would be the first nation to host an Olympic games after the implementation of the Tobacco Framework. With international commitment and national pride in favour of tobacco control, China's policy to implement the Framework seems to have gained the upper hand. However, determination and concern for the health and well-being of its population are crucial if China is to counter economic objections and enforce laws in accordance with the requirements of the Tobacco Framework.

Legislation addressing tobacco harms in Japan

As recently as 2004, Japan was still home to over 31 million smokers, with high rates of smoking in young men and women (Omi 2004). Smoking prevalence among physicians and nurses was also high (WHO 2004). After ratifying the Tobacco Framework Convention in 2004, the Japanese government through the National Institute of Public Health began to strengthen its national programmes to control the use of tobacco. It was recognized that tobacco control might be a uniquely different issue in Japan because the Japanese tobacco industry was administered by the government. Indeed the Tobacco Industry Law of 1984 called for activities that promoted tobacco, and tobacco sales constituted a substantial source of revenue (Mochizuki-Kobayashi 2004). This is also reflected in the fact that the Ministry of Finance holds a nearly 50 per cent share in Japan Tobacco, and upon retirement from political life, officials of the Ministry often assume high positions in the company, so powerful individuals have an interest in maximizing tobacco profits (Mochizuki-Kobayashi 2004). The Ministry of Finance and the Ministry of Health, Labour and Welfare presented opposing views during the Framework deliberations. The Health Minister proposed a focus on ways to reduce tobacco consumption so as to promote health, but the Finance Minister argued that the role of government should be to provide information to enable individuals to decide for themselves and that no measures should be taken to reduce or ban tobacco use (Hanai 2003).

Much early tobacco legislation in Japan is contained in local ordinances. In 2001, a municipal ordinance in Aomori Prefecture prohibited the placement of vending machines for cigarettes. In 2002, Chiyoda Ward in Tokyo introduced an ordinance which prohibited smoking and discarding cigarette butts in designated areas. The first national legislation was the 2003 Health Promotion Law containing a provision on the responsibility of administrators for the prevention of passive smoking in public places, and so prompting large enterprises such as Japan Railway to adopt smoke-free policies in railway stations. Government buildings, schools, department stores, hospitals, cinemas, and theatres became smoke-free, but smoking in workplaces and other public places has yet to be prohibited. It remains to be seen what restrictions Japan will implement with regard to the obligation to undertake a comprehensive ban of all tobacco advertising, promotion, and sponsorship as required by the Framework Convention.

Legislation addressing tobacco control in Hong Kong

The Smoking (Public Health) (Amendment) Ordinance (Cap.371) was enacted in Hong Kong in 1982 providing prohibitions against smoking in areas such as banks and shopping malls, and stipulating that restaurants providing seating for over 200 people must designate not less than one-third of such area as smoke-free. However, the public was still subjected to considerable second-hand smoke. The bodies with responsibility for regulation are the Hong Kong Council on Smoking and Health established in 1987 under the Hong Kong Council on Smoking and Health Ordinance (Cap. 389) and the Tobacco Control Office within the Department of Health. To comply with the Framework Convention, the Smoking Ordinance was substantially revised in 2006. Changes pertained to expansion of statutory no smoking areas to cover most indoor areas in workplaces and public places, tightening of restrictions on advertisement, promotion and sponsorship of tobacco products, and requiring tobacco packages to bear health warnings with pictorial or graphic content. During the early days of application of the Ordinance there was confusion as to the meaning of terms such as 'indoor' areas, leading to a large number of exemptions being granted. Despite these unresolved issues, the amendments have resulted not only in cleaner air in indoor settings, but also a cultural shift whereby inconsiderate smokers are no longer condoned.

Legislation addressing smoking harms in other Asian states

Most Asian states are signatories to the Framework Convention on Tobacco Control including India, Pakistan, Republic of Korea, and People's Democratic Republic of Korea, Myanmar, Thailand, and Vietnam. Many states are introducing tobacco control legislation but as in Japan, smoking is an ingrained part of Asian culture and there is much resistance.

Singapore, a Convention signatory, began legislating against tobacco use in 1970. The Smoking (Prohibition in Certain Places) (Amendment) Notifications 1997 extended the ban so that it covered schools, universities, cinemas, air-conditioned restaurants, and air-conditioned shops. Further amendments in 2006 extended the smoking ban to cover outdoor food outlets, karaoke bars, and nightclubs. The 1998 amendments to the Smoking (Control of Advertising and Sale of Tobacco) (Licensing) Regulations regulate sale of tobacco to minors and tobacco advertising. Singapore now has one of the strongest anti-smoking regimes in the world.

Malaysia, also a signatory to the Convention, has one of the highest rates of smoking in the region. Malaysia passed the Control of Tobacco Products Regulation in 1993 but tobacco industry pressures resulted in limited prohibition (Assunta & Chapman 2004). Amendment regulations in 1997 prohibited the sale of tobacco products to persons under the age of 18 and increased the number of places where smoking is prohibited. Smoking is now prohibited in most public places including schools, government buildings, public waiting areas, air-conditioned restaurants, shopping malls, and sports complexes. However, indirect advertising of tobacco products still takes place and much needs to be done to comply with the Framework Convention.

Smoking incidence is high in the Philippines but appears to be declining among adolescents (CDC 2005). Tobacco is a major source of revenue for the Philippines. The 2003 Tobacco Regulation Act attempts a compromise between health and revenue, stating that it is the policy of the state both to protect the right to health, and to protect workers and other stakeholders in the tobacco industry. The result is that the emphasis of the tobacco control movement is on education and warnings of health risks. Smoking is prohibited in schools and recreational facilities for persons under 18, hospitals, and transport facilities. Other public areas such as covered areas open to the public, private workplaces and restaurants are required to provide designated smoking areas. No tobacco product can be sold within 100 m of a school. Tobacco advertising is allowed but must not be aimed at minors, must not feature celebrities, must not use cartoons, must not be placed in printed media where more

than 25 per cent of readers are under 18, and must not be placed on a billboard or mural near a school. Parallel to these measures are compensation measures for farmers who voluntarily cease to grow tobacco to support them in the change to other crops, and provisions to assist displaced cigarette factory workers.

The potential role of law in tackling obesity in Asian legal culture

Obesity may once have been primarily a Western problem, but no longer. One-fifth of the population in China is now overweight, and China has seen an alarming increase in childhood obesity (Wu 2006). The health risks associated with obesity tend to occur at lower body mass index (BMI) in Asian populations, and the Western Pacific Region of WHO have proposed new definitions of overweight and obesity based on lower levels of BMI for Asia (Regional Office for the Western Pacific 2000).

Obesity in Asia has been attributed to changing Asian diets and the adoption of Western food practices, together with low levels of exercise (Tee 2002). Asian culture has traditionally regarded excess weight as evidence of wealth and prosperity, and parents are proud of fat babies (Ip 1999). The result is that while obesity in the Western world is associated with poverty, in Asia it is associated with affluence (China Daily 2006). The opening up of Asian markets, particularly the enormous and lucrative Chinese market, to foreign foods and media advertising has resulted in the targeting of Asian populations by major food and drink manufacturers.

While there have been some restrictions on advertising in China, restrictions have tended to focus on cultural impact rather than on health (Ha 1996). However, evidence suggests that parents in China perceive that food advertising to children encourages poor quality, and expensive, eating habits and there is increasing pressure on government to regulate aggressive and deceptive advertising (Chan & McNeal 2003). Elsewhere in Asia, in 2007, South Korea announced restrictions on the advertising of 'fast' food from 2008, to be extended in 2010 to all foods containing high levels of sugar or fat. In June 2007, the government of Malaysia announced that fast-food companies were banned from sponsoring children's television programmes. In Thailand, all food advertisements must be approved by a national government body.

In South Korea, from 2007, the Korean Food and Drug Administration will require all foods to be labelled to make clear the levels of trans fat, and by 2010 no packaged food will be allowed to contain more than 1 per cent of trans fat. From 2007, in Malaysia, all fast-food chains will be required to label their food with cholesterol, fat, and sugar content. In Singapore, labelling of trans fats is voluntary but the largest supermarket chain, FairPrice, declares trans fats on its own brand labels and plans to reduce the number of its products containing trans fats. Thailand, the Philippines, Brunei Darussalam, Indonesia, and Singapore all restrict false advertising of the nutritional content of products (Tee 2002). The Philippine Food Fortification Act 2000 goes further and in recognition that the Filipino diet is deficient in nutrients, legislates for food fortification for locally processed products and food products for sale and distribution in the Philippines. For example, rice is to be fortified with iron; and wheat, sugar, and cooking oil, with vitamin A.

In South Korea, from 2007, no fast foods can be sold within 200 m of a school. Following a report by the Delhi Diabetics research centre, the Delhi government has proposed a ban on all junk food in schools.

China and Malaysia also regulate the content of school foods. Vietnam prohibits marketing of food and beverage products in schools.

Concern about the rapid increase in obesity and obesity-related health problems in Asian states has prompted consideration of government intervention in content, labelling, and marketing of processed foodstuffs. Because there is in general greater acceptance in Asian culture of state intervention in private life, particularly in states with some Islamic laws, civil liberties arguments have carried little weight. Concern has been more for economic consequences of restrictions, but unlike in the tobacco context where governments have a vested financial interest in tobacco production, these have not been sufficient to counter public health concerns for the health and economic consequence of obesity. Asian states are keen to learn from the problems faced by Western countries and to pre-empt the development of Western levels of obesity, and this has resulted in increasing regulation of food products with high levels of fat, salt, and sugar. Such measures are in accord with the concern of Asian states to protect cultural traditions, including traditional food practices, from Western influences, making food control laws more popular and less controversial than in Western states. However, WHO notes that most self-regulatory codes of practice on issues of food have developed in Europe, Australasia, and North America rather than in Asia, and that there has been relatively little activity to restrict marketing in low- to middle-income countries where promotional activities are growing faster and have the greatest impact (WHO 2006).

Conclusion

Increasingly states are resorting to law to provide a sound framework for non-medical interventions in public health. Increasingly also, international legal instruments are being developed to provide some coherence and consistency in approach to global public health problems.

In the context of communicable disease the revised IHR 2005 have the objective of achieving global public health security by strengthening national disease surveillance, prevention, control and response systems, and by strengthening WHO global alert and response systems. While the IHR 1969 focused on disease control at borders, the IHR 2005 address not only strengthening of border controls but also disease prevention and control at disease source, requiring states to introduce national measures to prevent the spread of disease. The IHR 1969 applied only to three diseases (cholera, plague, and yellow fever), but the IHR 2005 apply to all public health threats of international concern. The IHR also introduce into state and global disease responses respect for internationally recognized human rights. State parties to the Regulations are obliged to implement the core capacity requirements of the IHR by 2009. Law in statutory form, at least in a non-authoritarian state, must result from a parliamentary process which is inevitably slow. Hence many states are, at the time of writing, either in the process of reforming their public health legislation, or designing new legislation to strengthen 'soft' law public health powers.

In the context of tobacco control the 2003 WHO Framework Convention on Tobacco Control, developed in recognition of the global nature of the tobacco epidemic, requires signatory states to provide protection against tobacco smoke, regulation of tobacco product content, sale and traffic, regulation of tobacco labelling and warnings, regulation of tobacco advertising, promotion and

sponsorship, and health education and promotion. The greater part of these requirements requires legal underpinning because the requirements involve interference with commercial activity and constraint on individual lifestyle behaviours. Again many states have begun to frame law to implement the framework, requiring new legislation aimed specifically at the control of public health tobacco harms.

The WHO has not yet used its law-making powers for obesity, but has initiated a Global Strategy on Diet, Physical Activity and Health to support policies that promote accessibility to foods low in fat, salt, and sugar. In 2006 WHO published reports on Reducing Salt Intake in Populations, on The Extent, Nature and Effects of Food Promotion to Children: A Review of the Evidence, and on Marketing of Food and Non-alcoholic Beverages to Children, for the purpose of developing an evidence base on mechanisms for reducing obesity levels. The reports recognize that self- regulation has not proved sufficient, particularly in reducing the volume of food and drink marketing to children and in minimizing the effects of marketing. The reports recommend that self-regulation operate in a legal framework in which there are incentives for compliance (WHO 2006).

These global instruments provide a common framework of legislative public health tools, but the content of law in response to the IHR and the Framework Convention will differ widely across states. Unlike science, which purports to be neutral, objective, and universally applicable, law is the formalization of social contracts between the state and its citizens and will reflect the social relationships ingrained in the culture of the state. National history, politics, geography, and economics will have forged very different understandings of what law is, who has the power to exercise it, and how it operates. Cultural and political circumstances and public awareness will influence the nature of restrictions appropriate to particular health threats (WHO 2006).

Over time it may be that these differences in understanding will be eroded by the effects of globalization. Global media reports, global recognition of the need for intervention for the protection of public health, and global agreement to international health and human rights instruments may eventually lead to some harmonization, or at least convergence, of public health laws. We have not yet reached that point, and for now approaches to law as a tool for public health vary widely.

It has not therefore been possible to identify world themes of public health law. It has not even been possible to collate a representative sample of national public health legislation across the world, given that the term 'legislation' already imposes a Western approach to control of populations and population behaviour. Much public health intervention is operated, particularly in African and Islamic legal cultures, on the basis of customary law or authority of the state without the need for legislation. The agreement of such states to international instruments such as the IHR or the Framework Convention has prompted some legislative activity, and there has been some minimal commonality of content of national legislation across signatory states. But as can be seen by the response of Japan and the Philippines to the Framework Convention, local conditions and local culture have led to very different commitments to tobacco prohibition.

This chapter has focused on Western and Asian legal cultures because legislation plays a more significant role in the meaning of law in these cultures. Approaches to law in the Western states we have examined demonstrate that autonomy and private rights are fundamental to the framing of law, and only rarely does law in Western legal culture envisage measures such as treatment and vaccination without consent, even when it might be in the public interest to treat or vaccinate. Recognition of human rights documents also plays a significant role in the extent to which Western states are prepared to interfere with privacy and autonomy, particularly in relation to communicable disease where public health measures might call for infringement of physical liberties. However, Western states have generally been rigorous in legislating restrictions on tobacco use, even where restrictions impinge on commercial interests and constrain lifestyle choices. Similarly Western states have been ready to use law in relation to other 'lifestyle' diseases such as obesity, regulating food content, food advertising, and food labelling.

States which have elements of Asian legal culture, prioritizing community and state interests over individual interests, have been prepared to adopt more stringent legal measures for communicable disease control than Western states. Hence Asian states are more likely to legislate for powers that potentially infringe autonomy such as compulsory treatment and vaccination. This is not because Asian states are prepared to override human rights, but rather because recognition of Asian values results in different interpretations of the meaning of rights. At the same time, Asian states have been less prepared to interfere with cultural lifestyle choices where to do so would impinge on state commercial interests, public revenue, employment rights of workers in the tobacco industry, and cultural smoking behaviours. Tobacco laws in Asian states have emphasized health education and health warnings over interference with smoking practices. There are signs, however, that Asian states are prepared to intervene in dietary choices, particularly in relation to imported Western food practices which threaten not only health of populations and the economy of the state but are also harmful to cultural food practices and traditions.

Globalization inevitably leads to some measure of cultural imperialism, and over time the predominance of Western approaches to regulation, rights, and legislative expression of law is filtering into approaches in other legal cultures. The significant presence of persons from Western cultures in international organizations, and their representation in the framing of international instruments, has meant that Western approaches to public health and to rights have influenced the content of international public health frameworks. International frameworks presuppose that national laws are formalized, with the result that all states will over time enshrine their public health laws in statutory form.

We are a long way from a common international stance on the use of law as a public health tool, but the renewed willingness of the WHO to use its treaty and law-making powers in the interests of global health will slowly lead to some convergence of national public health legislation. Only when all states choose to use statutory powers, published in legislative form and publicly available, to endorse public health interventions, will we able to undertake a comprehensive worldwide analysis of national public health legislation.

Key points

- Law is an important tool for containment of both communicable and non-communicable disease.

- Law is not a neutral instrument, and the meaning and process of 'law' differ widely across legal cultures.

- Any comparison of national public health legislation is made difficult by absence of legislation addressing public health in many states. States within Western and Asian legal cultures are more likely to enshrine law in legislative form.

- Many states within Western and Asian legal cultures have legislated to control communicable disease and to control tobacco harms, and are beginning to consider legislation to address obesity.

- International legal instruments such as the revised International Health Regulations and the Framework Convention for Tobacco Control will require many more states to consider legislation to comply with international requirements.

References

Allwright, S., Paul, G., and Bernie, J. (2005). Legislation for smoke-free workplaces and health of bar work before and after study. *British Medical Journal*, **331**, 1117–26.

Assunta, M. and Chapman, S. (2004). Industry sponsored youth smoking prevention programme in Malaysia: A case study in duplicity. *Tobacco Control*, **13**, ii37–42.

Atenstaedt, R. (2006). Does danger lurk in the library? *Public Health*, **120**(8), 776–7.

Bell, D. (1996). The East Asian challenge to human rights: Reflections on an East West dialogue. *Human Rights Quarterly*, **18.3**, 641–67.

Bell, J. (1995). Comparative law and legal theory. In *Prescriptive formality and normative rationality in modern legal systems* (eds. W. Krawietz, N. MacCormick, and G. von Wright). Duncker and Humblot, Berlin.

Borzekowski, D. and Robinson, T. (2001). The 30-second effect: An experiment revealing the impact of television commercials on food preferences of preschoolers. *Journal of the American Diet Association*, **101**, 42–6.

Brems, E. (2001). *Human rights: Universality and diversity*. Martinus Nijhoff, The Hague.

Caraher, M. (2006). Television advertising and children: Lessons from policy development. *Public Health Nutrition*, **9**(5), 596–605.

CDC (2005). Tobacco use among students aged 13 to 15 years – Philippines, 2001 and 2003. *MMWR*, February 4, 2005.

Chadwick, E. (1842). *Report on the sanitary conditions of the labouring population of Great Britain*, London.

Chan, K. and McNeal, J. (2003). Parental concern about television viewing and children's advertising in China. *International Journal for Public Opinion Research*, **15**(2), 151–66.

China Daily (2006). Hong Kong parents must take lead in obesity battle. *China Daily*, 3 October 2006.

Coker, R. and Martin, R. (2006). Introduction: The importance of law for public health policy and practice. *Public Health*, **120**(Suppl.) 2–8.

Coker, R., Mounier-Jack, S., and Martin, R. (2007). Public health law and tuberculosis control in Europe. *Public Health*, **121**(4), 266–73.

Dalacoura, K. (2003). *Islam, liberalism and human rights*. L.B.Tauris, London.

Da Lomba, S. and Martin, R. (2004). Public health powers in relation to infectious tuberculosis in England and France: A comparison of approaches. *Medical Law International*, **6**, 117–47.

De Bary, Tu. (2001). *Confucianism and human rights*. Columbia University Press, Columbia.

Department of Health (2004). *Choosing health: Making healthy choices easier*. Department of Health White Paper, 16 Nov 2004.

Department of Health Western Australia (2005). *A new public health Act for WA*. Department of Health, Perth.

Department of Health (2006). *Forecasting obesity to 2010*. Department of Health July 2006.

Department of Health (2007). Review of Parts II, V and VI of the Public Health (Control of Disease) Act 1984: a Consultation. Department of Health, London.

Diokno, M. (2000). Once again, the Asian values debate: The case of the Philippines. In *Human rights and Asian values* (eds. M. Jacobsen and O. Bruun). Curzon Press, Richmond.

Durand de Bousingen, D. (2001). French court enforces Formula 1 tobacco advertising ban. *Lancet*, **9273**, 2036.

Enhorn v Sweden [2005] E.C.H.R. 56529/00.

Euromonitor International (2006a). *NRT smoking cessation aids in Ireland*.

Euromonitor International (2006b). *Tobacco in China*. December 2006.

Fidler, D. (2004). SARS, governance and the globalization of disease. Palgrave, McMillan, UK.

Fidler, D. (2005). From international sanitary conventions to global health security: The new international health regulations. *Chinese Journal of International Law*, **4**(2), 325–92.

Fidler, D. and Gostin, L. (2006). The new international health regulations: An historic development for international law and public health. *Journal of Law and Medical Ethics*, 85–94.

Fichtenberg, C. and Glantz, S. (2002). Effect of smoke-free workplaces on smoking behaviour: systematic review. *British Medical Journal*, **325**, 188–94.

Food Standards Agency (2003). Academic panel examines food promotion and children reviews. 26 November 2003.

Francey and Meeuwissen v Hilton Hotels of Australia H 97/50, 10 March 2000.

Gostin, L. (2000). *Public Health Law: Power, duty, restraint*, p. 4. University of California Press, Berkeley.

Gostin, L. (2007). Law as a tool to facilitate healthier lifestyles and prevent obesity. *JAMA*, **298**, 87–90.

Hanai (2003). Reported in Mochizuki-Kobayashi Y *et al.* (2004). Tobacco Free*Japan. Recommendations for Tobacco Control. Tobacco Free*Japan, Tokyo and Institute for Global Tobacco Control, Department of Epidemiology, Johns Hopkins Bloomberg School of Public Health, at 268.

Ha, L. (1996). Concerns about advertising practices in a developing country: An examination of China's new advertising regulations. *International Journal of Advertising*, **15**, 91–102.

Harris, A. and Martin, R. (2004). The exercise of public health powers in an era of human rights: The particular problem of tuberculosis. *Public Health*, **118**(5), 312–22.

Harvard Law Review Note (2003). The elephant in the room: Evolution, behaviouralism and counteradvertising in the coming war against obesity. *Harvard Law Review*, **116**(4), 1161–84.

Hastings, G. *et al.* (2003). *Review of the research on the effects of food promotion to children*. Centre for Social Marketing, Glasgow.

Holm, S. (2007). Obesity interventions and ethics. *Obesity Reviews*, **8**(1), 207–10.

House of Commons UK (2004). *Response to consultation by the select committee on health, Third Report*. House of Commons, London.

House of Commons Health Committee (2004). Press Notice, 'Obesity Report Published'. 26 May 2004.

IAFCO (2003). *Broadcasting bad health*. July 2003.

Ip, H. (1999). Comment by Dr Henrietta Ip, Chair, Hong Kong Child Health Foundation, to the BBC. May 23 1999.

Jacobsen, M. and Bruun, O. (eds.) (2000). *Human rights and Asian values*. Curzon Press, Richmond.

Johns Hopkins (2000). *National conference on policy development on tobacco control in China in the 21st century*, reported at http://www.jhsph.edu./global_tobacco/policy_development/china_national_plan/.

Jones, K., Wakefield, M., and Turnbull, D. (1999). Attitudes and experiences of restaurateurs regarding smoking bans in Adelaide, South Australia. *Tobacco Control*, **8**, 62–6.

Lam, T., Ho, S., Mak, K. *et al.* (2000) Mortality and smoking in Hong Kong: Case-control study of all adult deaths in 1998. *British Medical Journal*, **323**, 361.

Lang, T. (2006). 'Food, the law and public health'. *Public Health*, Special edition edited by Coker, R. and Martin, R., **120**, 30–41.

LegCo Select Committee Hong Kong (2004). *Report of the Select Committee to inquire into the handling of the severe acute respiratory syndrome outbreak by the government and the hospital authority*. Legislative Council, Hong Kong.

Liu, B-Q., Peto, R., Chen, Z-M. *et al.* (1998). Emerging tobacco hazards in China: 1. Retrospective proportional mortality study of one million deaths. *British Medical Journal*, **317**, 1311–1422.

Maffeis, C. and Tatò, L. (2001). Long term effects of childhood obesity on morbidity and mortality. *Hormone Research*, **55**(1), 42–5.

Martin, R. (2006a). The exercise of public health powers in cases of infectious disease: Human rights implications. *Medical Law Review*, **14**(1), 132–43.

Martin, R. (2006b). The limits of law in the protection of public health and the role of public health ethics. *Public Health*, Special edition edited by Coker, R. and Martin, R., **120**, 71–80.

Martin, R. (2008). The role of law in the control of obesity in England: looking at the contribution of law to a healthy food culture. *Australia and New Zealand Health Policy*. In press.

Mbeke, T. (2000). *HIV=AIDS controversy: What's all this then?* Thabo Mbeke's letter to world leaders on AIDS in Africa.

Mechlem, K. (2000). Legal reform in developing countries: The use of comparative law and law and economics. In *Governance, decentralization and reform in China, India and Russia* (ed. J. Dethier). Kluwer Academic Press, Dordrecht/London/Boston.

Mello, M., Studdert, D., and Brennan, T. (2006). Obesity—the new frontier of public health law. *New England Journal of Medicine*, **354**(24), 2601–10.

Melville, D. and Shortridge, K. (2004). Influenza: Time to come to grips with the avian dimension. *Lancet Infectious Diseases*, **4**(5), 261–2.

Merson, M., Black, R., and Mills, A. (2006). *International public health: Diseases, programs, systems, and policies*. Jones and Bartlett, Sudbury, Mass.

Mill, J. (1869). *On Liberty*. Longman, Roberts and Green, London.

Ministry of Health China (2007). *China tobacco control report 2007*. Office of the Team of Leaders for Conforming to the FCTC, Ministry of Health, Beijing, May 2007 (Chinese only).

Ministry of Health New Zealand (2002). *Public health legislation: Promoting public health, preventing ill health, and managing communicable diseases*. Ministry of Health, Wellington.

Mochizuki-Kobayashi, Y. *et al.* (2004). *Tobacco Free * Japan. Recommendations for Tobacco Control*. Tobacco Free*Japan, Tokyo and Institute for Global Tobacco Control, Department of Epidemiology, Johns Hopkins Bloomberg School of Public Health.

Morella, A. (1996). *La Défaite de la Santé Publique*, pp. 266–9. Flammarion, France.

National Audit Office (2001). *Tackling obesity in England*. National Audit Office, 15 February 2001.

National People's Congress (2005). Decision of the standing committee of the tenth national people's congress about ratifying the framework convention on Tobacco Control promulgated on 28 August 2005, reported at http://www.lawinfochina.com.

Neary, I. (2002). *Human rights in Japan, South Korea and Taiwan*. Routledge, London.

Ofcom (2006). *Television advertising of food and drink to children: Options for new restrictions*. 28 March 2006.

Ofcom (2007). *Television advertising of food and drink to children: Final statement*. 22 February 2007.

Omi, S. (2004). *Message for tobacco free Japan. Forward to recommendations for tobacco control policy*. WHO Western Pacific Region Office.

Parliament of South Australia (2007). *Fast food and obesity inquiry*. Adelaide, 27 March 2007.

Peng, Y. (1997). *Smoke and power: The political economy of Chinese tobacco*, University of Oregon PhD thesis, referenced in de Bayer, J. *et al.* (2004), *Research on tobacco in China*, Health, Nutrition and Population Discussion Paper, World Bank.

Pickett, K., Kelly, S., Brunner, E. *et al.* (2005). Wider income gaps, wider waistbands? An ecological study of obesity and income inequality. *Journal of Epidemiology and Community Health*, **59**, 670–4.

Prime Minister Tony Blair (2006a). Healthy living. July 2006.

Prime Minister Tony Blair (2006b). How do we lead healthier lives? 26 July 2006.

Regional Office for the Western Pacific (2000). *The Asia-Pacific perspective: Redefining obesity and its treatment.* WHO, February 2000.

Reuters (2007a). '100,000 Chinese die annually from passive smoking'. 29 May 2007.

Reuters (2007Bb). 'Smoking curb could "upset China stability"'. 7 March 2007.

Scottish Executive (2006). *Public health legislation in Scotland.* Scottish Executive, Edinburgh.

Sen, A. (1997). Human rights and Asian values: What Lee Kuan Yew and Le Peng don't understand about Asia. *The New Republic*, July 14.

Sommade, C., Haut Comité Français pour la Défense Civile (2004). Quarantine Conference, Wilton Park, 22 January 2004.

South China Morning Post (2007). The debate on Asian values gets a revival. April 23. Hong Kong.

Stanton, R., Mehta, A., Morton, H. *et al.* (2005). Food advertising and broadcasting legislation – a case of system failure? *Nutrition and Dietetics*, **62**(1), 26–32.

Svennson, M. (2000). The Chinese debate on Asian values and human rights: Some reflections on relativism, nationalism and orientalism. In *Human rights and Asian values* (eds. M. Jacobsen and O. Bruun). Curzon Press, Richmond.

Tan Poh-ling (1997). *Asian legal systems.* Butterworths, Australia.

Tatara, K. (2002). Philosophy of public health: Lessons from its history in England. *Journal of Public Health Medicine*, **24**(1), 11–15.

Tee, E-S. (2002). Nutritional labelling and claims: Concerns and challenges; experiences from the Asia Pacific Region. *Asia Pacific Journal of Clinical Nutrition*, **11**, S215–S223.

Van Hoecke, M. and Warrington, M. (1998). Legal cultures, legal paradigms and legal doctrine: Towards a new model for comparative law. *International and Comparative Law Quarterly*, **47**, 495–536.

Wanless, D. (2002). *Securing our future health: Taking a long-term view.* HM Treasury, London.

Wanless, D. (2004). *Securing good health for the whole population.* HM Treasury, London.

WHO (2000). WHO Western Pacific region tobacco-free initiative country specific database, quoted in *Tobacco Free * Japan. Recommendations for Tobacco Control.* Tobacco Free*Japan, Tokyo and Institute for Global Tobacco Control, Department of Epidemiology, Johns Hopkins Bloomberg School of Public Health, at 270.

WHO (2003). Factsheet: *Obesity and overweight,* http://www.who.int/hpr/NPH/docs/gs_obesity.pdf.

WHO (2005). *'China joins the global war on smoking'*. Press release 30 August 2005.

WHO (2006). *Marketing of food and non-alcoholic beverages to children.* WHO, Geneva.

WHO Regional Office for Europe (2006*). European charter on counteracting obesity.* Istanbul 16 November 2006.

Wu, Y. (2006). Overweight and obesity in China. *British Medical Journal*, **333**, 362–3.

Zweigert, K. and Kötz, H. (1998). *Introduction to comparative law.* Clarendon Press, Oxford.

4.3

International public health instruments

Douglas Bettcher[1], Katherine DeLand[1], Jorgen Schlundt[1], Fernando González-Martín[1], Jennifer Bishop, Summer Hamide, and Annette Lin

Abstract

Norms, standards, agreements, and regulations have been used, since the nineteenth-century International Sanitary Conferences, as governance tools in public health diplomacy. With globalization attaining an unprecedented level at the end of the twentieth century, it appeared that some public goods were increasingly difficult to provide efficiently at the state level. The reason for this is that as states increased their interconnectedness, the interrelation between domestic public goods common to the interacting states also increased. Correlatively, the singular nature of some of what were once solely domestic public goods progressively declined and the creation and maintenance of those public goods became shared enterprises. This led to the emergence of the concept of the global public good (GPG). This chapter examines the ideas of health as a GPG and international law in general, and international health instruments in particular, as intermediate GPGs utilized to protect and promote health. As intermediate GPGs for health, international legal instruments take on an additional layer of importance in global health governance. In providing a robust framework for improving and occasionally even creating health, these instruments are important not only for what they are already doing, but for the potential new instruments that may be developed. Through the presentation of case studies examining three international instruments that the World Health Organization (WHO) has been involved in developing, the chapter focuses on the evolution and implementation of emerging, salient international health-specific legal agreements. As WHO continues to grow into its normative role, it is likely that additional opportunities to exercise its constitutional quasi-legislative powers will present themselves. The three examples of intermediate GPGs examined in this chapter have laid a solid foundation on which WHO and its Member States may build, to continue working toward achieving the GPG of health.

Notwithstanding over 150 years of the use of regulatory approaches to public health protection and promotion, their
relevance is still intensely debated. In today's world characterized by the phenomenon of globalization, what is the relevance of norms, standards, agreements, and regulations in multilateral disease control initiatives? In what ways could the usefulness and utility of regulatory and normative mechanisms be enhanced to diminish the morbidity and mortality burdens of communicable and non-communicable diseases on vulnerable groups in developing countries? Can normative and regulatory mechanisms play any meaningful role in financing global health, and the distribution of health dividends as GPGs in a sharply divided world?

This chapter will first present the economic concept of GPGs and examine the idea of health as a GPG and international health instruments as intermediate GPGs utilized to protect and promote health (Kaul *et al.* 1999; Taylor & Bettcher 2000; Fidler 2003). Next, through the presentation of case studies examining three international instruments that the WHO has been involved in developing, the chapter will focus on the evolution and implementation of emerging, salient international health-specific legal agreements. Finally, the chapter will provide a brief discussion of the 'soft law' and 'hard law' international legal paradigms, and WHO's role in creating these instruments.

As the WHO Constitution provides, health is not merely the absence of disease or infirmity, but is also 'a state of complete physical, mental, and social well being' (WHO 2007a). Because of the broad nature of health, concerted multinational action on all levels is required to provide health. This chapter aims to provide some insight and overview into the relationship between international law and the improvement of public health using the concept of GPGs.

---

[1] The author is a staff member of the World Health Organization. The author alone is responsible for the views expressed in this publication, and they do not necessarily represent the decisions or the stated policy of the World Health Organization.

Section I: Global public goods—health and international health instruments

Health as a global public good

The concept of public goods form a core economic tool used since the eighteenth century to think about and analyse national governance. A public good is a good that has two characteristics: (1) It is non-rival in consumption; that is, its consumption by an individual does not impede someone else from consuming it, and (2) it is non-excludable, which means that one cannot prevent someone from consuming it. For instance, a public park can be considered a public good. The fact that someone is spending some time in a public park does not, under normal circumstances, impede someone else from coming into the park. Furthermore, in a normal situation, a public park is open to anyone and no one is allowed to prevent someone else from accessing it. It should be noted, however, that public goods do not necessarily have to be tangible. For instance, security or education can also be considered public goods. Since public goods tend to be underprovided in the absence of government intervention, due to the 'free-rider problem' (i.e. taking advantage of a public good without providing for its existence or maintenance), governments often focus on activities dedicated to providing public goods.

With globalization attaining an unprecedented level at the end of the twentieth century, it appeared that some public goods were increasingly difficult to provide efficiently at the state level. The reason for this is that as states increased their interconnectedness, the interrelation between domestic public goods common to the interacting states also increased. Correlatively, the singular nature of some of what were once solely domestic public goods progressively declined and the creation and maintenance of those public goods became shared enterprises. This led to the emergence of the concept of the GPG. Kaul *et al.* (1999) define GPG as a public good having three characteristics:

1. It covers more than one group of countries.

2. Its benefits [...] reach [...] a broad spectrum of the global population (which means that access to them must not be limited to certain economic classes, gender, religious groups, or any other discrete community).

3. It meets the needs of present generations without jeopardizing those of future generations.

Based on these criteria, health is arguably a GPG. As a public good, health is a positive sum: One person's good health does not detract from another's. Indeed, better individual health usually has positive effects on entire populations—for example, through reduced disease transmission. As health is not only an end in itself, but is also inseparable from social and economic welfare, health is also a key element for economic and social growth. An improvement in individual health can improve the community-level economy and social fabric.

Furthermore, although the onus of providing health remains primarily on national governments, globalization means that the determinants of health, as well as the requisite means to deliver health, are increasingly global (Jamison *et al.* 1998). Countries are more and more interdependent with regard to health issues. This is clearly true for those matters related to communicable disease, as illustrated by the 2002 SARS outbreak, which required concerted, multilateral action to contain. Though less obvious, this is no less true for non-communicable diseases (Beaglehole & Yach 2003). In fact, a range of non-infectious transnational health threats have emerged in recent years, including *inter alia* the marketing of tobacco, environmental degradation, alcohol and illicit drug use, anti-microbial resistance, hunger and food insecurity, and diet and obesity, all of which now constitute globalized threats to health and human security. As these threats demonstrate, globalization is not limited to the movement of people and goods across borders, but also can affect individual and collective behavioural patterns which can, in turn, have dramatic impact on health.

Two forces are moving health progressively toward the centre of the stage in the discussion of GPGs. First, as already noted, enhanced international linkages in trade, migration, and information flows have accelerated the cross-border transmission of disease and the international transfer of behavioural health risks. Second, intensified pressure on common-pool global resources, such as air and water, has generated shared, transnational environmental threats. The result is that diseases, and other threats harmful to health, present enormous international (and often global) challenges that are beyond the governance capabilities of individual nation states. Accordingly, efficiently addressing these issues requires coordination and action at a supranational level.

It should be noted, however, that the notion of health as a GPG is not uncontested. It has been argued that an individual's health—or even an entire county's health status—primarily benefits only the individual or country and that the resources necessary to provide better health are indeed 'predominantly rival and exclusive' (Woodward & Smith 2003). This school agrees that some aspects of health may be GPGs, including control of globally threatening communicable disease, like HIV/AIDS and tuberculosis, but there is some concern that 'relaxing' the interpretation of GPG to include health may dilute the usefulness of GPGs as means to secure funding (Smith & Woodward 2003). Perhaps most importantly, if health as a GPG is limited to very prescribed circumstances, like control of certain infectious disease, then it loses its capacity as an organizing principal for global health priorities (Smith *et al.* 2004).

Nonetheless, even among those who maintain that health is not a GPG, there is a strong sense that collective action and coordination, as the core notion of GPGs, can be used to great and measurable effect to promote and improve global health. While this chapter argues that heath is, in and of itself, a GPG, it does so in the same spirit as those who contest this first, basic notion. Namely, the idea of health as a GPG is a useful tool, both to an intellectual examination of global health status, progress and possibilities, and to the development of practical, applicable health interventions. Insofar as this chapter focuses on international instruments, developed via collective global action, its premise finds the common ground between the health as a GPG camp and the opposing view.

As well as being the means to a GPG end (in this case, health), the coordination and actions themselves could also be considered GPGs, insofar as they provide a shared platform for the process of improving social and economic welfare. The agreements to coordinate and to act in concert, while critical for reaching a GPG, are part of the process rather than an outcome in and of themselves. This conceptualization allows us to introduce a typology that distinguishes two different types of GPGs—final GPGs and intermediate GPGs:

1. Final GPGs are outcomes rather than 'goods' in the standard sense. They may be tangible (such as the environment or the

common heritage of mankind) or intangible (such as peace or financial stability).

2. Intermediate GPGs, such as international regimes, contribute towards the provision of final GPGs (Kaul *et al.* 1999).

The WHO Framework Convention on Tobacco Control (WHO FCTC) provides an example of an intermediate GPG. As an intermediate GPG, the WHO FCTC establishes a rubric of coordinated action among states, which will bring about a significant health improvement not otherwise efficiently obtainable by states acting on their own (Taylor *et al.* 2003).

Health-related international instruments as intermediate GPGs

The evolution of normative and regulatory approaches to the transnational spread of disease dates back to the European-led International Sanitary Conferences in the mid-nineteenth century. The European cholera epidemics of 1830 and 1847 catalysed the earliest regulatory and normative approaches to cross-border disease control. From 1851 to the end of the nineteenth century, ten International Sanitary Conferences were convened, and eight sanitary conventions were negotiated on the cross-border spread of cholera, plague, and yellow fever in Europe.

Insofar as these instruments were negotiated long before any of the European countries had experienced an epidemiologic transition from infectious to chronic disease burdens (Omran 1971), these normative, regulatory frameworks were narrowly focused on infectious disease control, the primary threat to health and a substantial cross-border concern. The agreements were a prominent feature of the European-led international sanitary conferences and the emphasis on infectious disease was mirrored in the disease surveillance-oriented mandates of pioneer multilateral health organizations, including the Pan American Sanitary Bureau, Office International d'Hygiene Publique, Health Office of the League of Nations, and Office International des Epizooties.

The globalization of public health provides a context in which the continued development and implementation of public health-related global norms and standards is becoming increasingly relevant. As there is no supranational authority that can ensure the provision of GPGs, the implications of globalization include the need for increased transnational cooperation and partnerships, as well as greater intersectoral action. Intermediate GPGs, like international norms, agreements, and regulations, play an important role in this dynamic (Kaul *et al.* 2003; Taylor *et al.* 2003; Fidler 2002). The globalization of public health has catalysed global health governance, involving states, international organizations, and non-state actors in the process of designing multinational health interventions and agreements (Kickbusch 2003; Dodgson *et al.* 2002; Taylor & Bettcher 2000).

Although WHO has made limited use of its constitutional powers to adopt agreements under Article 19, regulations under Article 21 and recommendations under Article 23, during the 1990s, the Organization launched two initiatives suggesting that international law may be seen as a more important instrument of global public health policy in the future. The first involved the revision of the International Health Regulations (IHR) to make them more relevant to the global problems caused by emerging and re-emerging infectious diseases. The second was the decision to develop the WHO FCTC. Additionally, although not exclusively about health, many

multilateral instruments negotiated by states, intergovernmental organizations (IGOs), and non-governmental organizations (NGOs) in areas like international environmental law, international trade law, international human rights law, international humanitarian law, international law on arms control, international law on narcotic drugs and international labour law have included the protection of human health as an embedded objective (Taylor *et al.* 2002).

Using the intermediate GPG international law to achieve the GPG for health

The use of international law in the production of health as a GPG comprises four essential aspects. First, states use international law to establish formal institutions empowered to work on global public health problems. The modern classic example of this is, of course, the WHO, but it is reasonable also to see certain others, including the United Nations Environment Program (UNEP) and the International Labor Organization (ILO), that also, if somewhat indirectly, promote and foster health.

Second, states use international law to establish procedures through which states and non-state actors can tackle specific global public health problems. For example, in order to effectively address the transnationalization of health risks and diseases, instruments like the WHO FCTC and the International Health Regulations (IHR) provide frameworks for efficient multilateral information and surveillance systems. Implementation and ongoing evolution and improvement of these systems are critical and the complexity inherent in this kind of information gathering is exemplified by WHO's strengthening global monitoring and alert systems, which link together, *inter alia*, specialized laboratories, disease surveillance systems, sources of relevant expertise, and state governments via electronic and printed media.

Third, states use international law to craft substantive duties in connection with particular global public health challenges. The IHR, for example, obligates WHO Member States to notify the Organization of specific public health events. The WHO FCTC requires Parties to implement specific obligations, like adhering to a discrete tobacco product labeling and warning regime, as well as to incorporate the general obligations and objectives of the Convention into their approaches to providing health.

Fourth, states use international law to create mechanisms to enforce substantive legal duties undertaken by states that have agreed to be bound by international instruments. Enforcement mechanisms come in many forms, from states self-reporting on progress made in connection with certain goals articulated in a treaty, as is common in multilateral environmental agreements like the Basel Convention (1992), to formal adjudication of state-to-state disputes by an international tribunal, as seen in the WTO's dispute-settlement mechanism.

While various instruments can be intermediate GPGs for health, international legal agreements are among the most important. International legal agreements provide a foundation for many other intermediate products with global public benefits, including institutionalized forums for global cooperation, research, surveillance, technical assistance programmes, and information clearinghouses. Global agreements like the WHO FCTC, the IHR, and the Codex Alimentarius are negotiated to secure global cooperation and that cooperation, in turn, leads to the sustained creation and promotion of health and related GPGs.

Section II: Case studies

The intermediate GPGs that comprise health-related international normative agreements, strategies, and instruments, will improve public health, reduce the burden of disease, and lead to reductions in poverty and increases in economic development. Globalization has been a cardinal factor triggering the expansion of international health law, which is recognized as inextricably interrelated to other areas of international normative concern, including international environmental law, labour law, and arms control. The WHO FCTC signalled a turning point in WHO's approach to international health lawmaking, and its entry into force heralded a new era in international health cooperation. As demonstrated by the WHO FCTC and the revision of the IHR, the forces of globalization at work in international health are compelling the international community to think creatively and to develop new models of cooperation, including the expanded use of international health law, to protect and promote the health of populations worldwide.

The three case studies that follow illustrate the relevance of norms, standards, agreements, and regulations in transnational disease control and discuss the impact of such instruments now and in the future. First we will examine the WHO FCTC, the first global health treaty negotiated under the auspices of WHO. The Convention is an evidence-based treaty that represents a paradigm shift in developing a regulatory strategy to address addictive substances; in contrast to previous drug control treaties, the WHO FCTC asserts the importance of demand reduction strategies as well as supply reduction issues. Second, we will present the IHR, WHO's legally binding regulations designed to address the spread of general and specific infectious disease. States Parties to the IHR are required to develop, strengthen, and maintain core surveillance and response capacities to detect, assess, notify, and report public health events to WHO and respond to public health risks and public health emergencies. Third, we will discuss the International Food Safety Authorities Network (INFOSAN) and the Codex Alimentarius, which has become the global reference point for consumers, food producers and processors, national food control agencies, and the international food trade as the benchmark against which national food measures and regulations are evaluated within the legal parameters of the WTO Agreements.

Case study: The WHO Framework Convention on Tobacco Control

The WHO FCTC is a carefully balanced legal instrument, adopted following vigorous negotiations, which took into account scientific, economic, social, and political considerations. The launch of WHO's first treaty negotiation was catalysed by a unique convergence of a number of factors:

- The accumulation of solid scientific evidence over a 50-year period, demonstrating the causal links between tobacco use and more than 20 major categories of disease (Doll 1998), and evidence pointing to the global toll of tobacco-related diseases;
- The strengthening of the evidence pointing to the adverse economic implications of the tobacco epidemic (World Bank 1999)
- The strengthening of the evidence that cost-effective tobacco control measures exist (World Bank 1999)
- The release as a result of litigation in the United States of over 35 million pages of previously secret tobacco industry documents, which provided a unique opportunity to better understand the strategies and tactics of the tobacco industry and, in doing so, to advance the public health agenda (Yach & Bettcher 2000)
- The establishment of a WHO cabinet project, the Tobacco Free Initiative, to focus international attention, resources, and action on the global tobacco epidemic
- The examples of different countries with successful tobacco control experiences
- The support of civil society in the form of public pressure on governments for strengthened tobacco regulations as the public became more aware of the dangers of tobacco (Da Costa e Silva & Nikogosian 2003)

The WHO FCTC focuses on the global implementation of evidence-based strategies to decrease demand rather than focusing solely on the supply side of the equation (Yach & Bettcher 2000). It is designed to act as a global complement to, not a replacement for, national and local tobacco control programmes and activities.

This case study explores the economic and public health evidence that provides the foundation for the WHO FCTC, demonstrates how the provisions of the Convention promote evidence-based interventions that have been proven to effectively reduce the demand for tobacco, and finally discusses how the WHO FCTC is an intermediate GPG for health.

The globalization of the tobacco epidemic

The WHO FCTC was developed in response to the ongoing globalization of the tobacco epidemic, which was amplified by a variety of complex factors with cross-border effects, including trade liberalization, foreign direct investment, global marketing, transnational tobacco advertising, promotion and sponsorship, and the international movement of contraband and counterfeit cigarettes. To strengthen and coordinate global responses to the tobacco epidemic, the World Health Assembly adopted, on 24 May 1999, a resolution to pave the way for accelerated multilateral negotiations on a framework convention on tobacco control and possible related protocols. This represented the first time that WHO Member States had exercised their treaty-making powers under Article 19 of the WHO Constitution (WHO 2007a).

Tobacco use is the second leading cause of death worldwide (WHO 2002c). Annually, 5.4 million people die prematurely from tobacco-related disease and it is expected that the developing countries' share of total tobacco-related deaths will reach 84 per cent in 2030 (Mathers & Loncar 2006). Indeed, while the number of tobacco consumers in developed countries is now quite stable (and even decreasing in a few countries), it has been rapidly increasing in developing countries. As a result, 84 per cent of tobacco users are in developing countries and this share is expected to reach 88 per cent by 2025, even if we assume a decrease of 1 per cent in prevalence annually (Guindon & Boisclair 2003). The consequences will be dramatic: By 2030, the number of deaths per year attributable to tobacco globally will be 8.3 million (Mathers & Loncar 2006).

Besides the harm that tobacco causes its users, it is now well established that second-hand smoke also considerably increases the risk of contracting tobacco-related illnesses, both for adults and children. The health consequences for them can be dramatic and immediate. Finally, a well-known impact of tobacco use on others is the effects it can have on unborn babies, particularly when mothers smoke or are exposed to second-hand smoke.

Economic consequences of the tobacco epidemic

In recent years, the adverse impact of tobacco consumption on economic development has been confirmed by an increasing number of studies. The European Commission has stated that it 'clearly recognizes the importance of tobacco control as a development issue' (European Commission 2003).

There are a number of ways in which tobacco consumption can have negative economic impact. National revenue is directly reduced because tobacco kills about a quarter of its consumers in their middle age, depriving families of essential financial resources. This in turn reduces the level of education and health which are 'critical input[s] into poverty reduction, economic growth, and long-term economic development at the scale of whole societies' (WHO 2001). The fact that purchasing tobacco products requires a greater proportion of income the poorer a consumer is also detracts from the basic needs of families with tobacco users. For instance, it is estimated that, in Bangladesh, 'over 350 young children per day could be saved from death by malnutrition, if their parents redirected some of their tobacco money to food' (Efroymson *et al.* 2001).

The healthcare costs attributable to smoking are particularly high in developed countries and are increasing in developing countries. When these costs are borne by the government, they decrease the ability of the government to provide other services and the kinds of infrastructure that are essential for economic growth. When borne by individuals, these costs represent a heavy financial burden on the smokers and their families.

Another crucial economic issue related to tobacco use is the effect that it can have on employment. The tobacco industry has abundantly used the argument that tobacco growing and manufacturing provide jobs in communities and are therefore important for many economies. However, this argument is misleading. First, in high-income countries, tobacco manufacturing is highly capital intensive and provides for only a very few jobs (World Bank 1999). In these countries, if tobacco consumption were to decrease, the money previously spent on tobacco products would shift to other, probably more labour intensive goods, thereby creating more jobs. In low- and middle-income countries, while the tobacco industry employs a large number of people, these jobs often represent a 'poverty trap' for an important proportion of those employed. The *bidi* factories in India and Bangladesh, for example, employ mostly women and children, many of whom work 11–16 h per day, without enough pay to cover their basic needs (Blanchet 2002; Raghavan 2002). The employment of children by the tobacco industry prevents them from receiving a proper education, as well as putting them at risk for the severe health problems associated with tobacco cultivation, including 'green tobacco sickness' and pesticide exposure (Blanchet 2002; Raghavan 2002). Additionally, imported raw tobacco, heavy dependence on government subsidies, trade barriers, and prohibitive loans that reinforce the global tobacco oligopsony all make tobacco farming unprofitable for farmers and governments (World Bank 1999).

Finally, international tobacco smuggling presents both serious public health and economic problems. As documented in the World Bank Report *Curbing the Epidemic*, it is estimated that some 30 per cent of internationally traded cigarettes, which amounts to about 355 billion pieces, are lost to smuggling each year (World Bank 1999). Tobacco smuggling undermines the legal tobacco market, thereby needlessly causing governments to lose substantial tax revenue. Moreover, young people, who are most sensitive to the prices of tobacco products (World Bank 1999), are most at risk from smuggled cigarettes, which often are sold more cheaply than legal cigarettes and often do not contain the legally mandated product warnings and information that legal cigarettes do.

Demand-side measures: Evidence-based interventions to reduce tobacco use

It has been clearly demonstrated that cost-effective demand reduction interventions for tobacco use can be useful in reducing tobacco consumption in both developing and developed country settings (World Bank 1999; WHO 2002). The WHO FCTC incorporates evidence-based provisions that reaffirm the right of all people to the highest standard of health. The Convention's objective provides a solid foundation for the treaty to reduce the public health and economic damage inflicted on individuals, communities, and countries by tobacco use.

This section maps out the evidence-based interventions that have been proven to reduce tobacco consumption and outlines the main provision of the WHO FCTC that correspond to these interventions; the WHO FCTC provides a global roadmap for comprehensive tobacco control.

Price measures

Price and tax measures are an important and effective means of reducing tobacco consumption, especially among young people (World Bank 1999)—a fact specifically recognized in the WHO FCTC in Article 6. Many countries have experienced important reductions in tobacco consumption after having increased their tax level. South Africa increased its taxes on tobacco, making the price of cigarettes go up by nearly 85 per cent between 1993 and 1999 and its estimated smoking prevalence decreased by 14.4 per cent (Van Walbeek 2002). Generally, it is estimated that a 10 per cent increase in the price of cigarettes will reduce consumption by approximately 4 per cent in a high-income country and by approximately 8 per cent in a low- or middle-income country (World Bank 1999). Furthermore, it has been shown that tax increases have a stronger impact on young people, which is particularly important, as the risk of lung cancer increases exponentially with the duration of smoking. Lastly, increases in tobacco taxes increase government revenue.

Non-price measures

Protection from exposure to tobacco smoke. Article 8 of the WHO FCTC requires Parties to provide 'for protection from exposure to tobacco smoke in indoor workplaces, public transport, indoor public places and, as appropriate, other places' (WHO 2003c). Where a Party lacks legal jurisdiction to do this at the national level, it is to 'actively promote' equivalent measures at the subnational level. For the United States, where the workplace is covered by this provision, it is estimated that consumption was reduced 4 to 10 per cent when these kinds of restrictions were implemented (World Bank 1999). Recognizing the importance of protection from tobacco smoke, the second session of the Conference of the Parties to the WHO FCTC (the governing body for the Convention) adopted guidelines for the implementation of Article 8 that include a ban on smoking in public and work places.

Packaging and labeling of tobacco products. When warning labels contain large, graphic, thought provoking, and factual information, they are effective in deterring tobacco use. This is recognized in Article 11 of the WHO FCTC, which contains obligations for Parties to appropriately label packages of tobacco products.

Tobacco product label warnings are unique in prevention because the consumer receives the warning at the time of use. When new and graphic cigarette labels were introduced in Canada in 2000, 41.2 per cent of those surveyed in one study had intentions to quit smoking within 6 months (Hammond 2003). In Poland, new warning labels occupying 30 per cent of the largest sides of cigarette packs greatly influenced smokers' decisions to halt or reduce their smoking (World Bank 1999).

Communication, media, and dissemination of scientific information. In the area of education, communication, training, and public awareness, addressed in Article 12 of the WHO FCTC, Parties are required to adopt legislative, executive, administrative, or other measures that promote public awareness and access to information on the dangers of tobacco.

As more people become educated regarding the effects of tobacco, fewer choose to use it. In the United States, tobacco consumption declined 30 per cent from the 1930s to the end of the 1970s (World Bank 1999), a period during which there were three tobacco information shocks, including the groundbreaking tobacco control report issued by the Surgeon General in 1964 (United States 1964). In areas where funds are limited, including developing countries, an inexpensive method that has been used to achieve similar information shocks is to record smoking behaviour on individuals' death certificates and then publicly disseminate the resulting data.

The use of counter-advertising in various media has channeled negative images of smoking to the public. A study conducted between 1954 and 1981 in Switzerland revealed that counter-advertising in the media dramatically reduced smoking by 11 per cent (World Bank 1999). Finland and Turkey have had similar success with anti-smoking campaigns.

Tobacco advertising, promotion, and sponsorship. Bans on cigarette promotion can also reduce smoking. A comparison of 100 countries, some with complete bans on advertising and others with no such bans, showed that countries that banned advertisements had a significant decrease in consumption (World Bank 1999).

Article 13 of the WHO FCTC requires each Party to undertake comprehensive bans of all tobacco advertising, promotion, and sponsorship, as far as constitutionally possible for each Party. This is a centrepiece of an evidence-based approach for reducing the demand for tobacco products. Parties whose constitution or constitutional principles do not allow them to undertake a comprehensive ban must apply a series of restrictions on all advertising, promotion, and sponsorship of tobacco products.

Cessation interventions

Cessation interventions include individual training, hospital treatment, counselling, and numerous pharmacological products known as nicotine replacement therapy (NRT) that have the benefit of being self-administered. Patches, gums, sprays, and inhalators are types of NRT that deliver small doses of nicotine free of harmful tobacco smoke. They are considered safe and effective and have been shown to help double the success rate of other cessation efforts (World Bank 1999). Models based on data from the United States suggest that if NRT were made available over the counter, rather than just by prescription, significantly more people would quit smoking (World Bank 1999). Furthermore, there is evidence that smokers want this type of help: In the United States, sales of NRT products increased by 150 per cent between 1996 and 1998

(World Bank 1999). The roles of policy-makers, health professionals, researchers, and the international community are important in the cessation movement (WHO 2003a).

In the area of cessation, Article 14 of the WHO FCTC requires Parties to endeavour to:

- Create cessation programmes, not only in healthcare facilities, but also in workplaces, educational institutions, and other settings
- Include diagnosis and treatment of nicotine dependence in national health programmes
- Establish programmes for diagnosis, counselling, and treatment in healthcare facilities and rehabilitation centres
- Collaborate with other Parties to the Convention to increase the availability of cessation therapies, including pharmaceutical products

Supply side measures: Elimination of illicit trade in tobacco products

The World Bank has concluded that the only supply side measure that leads to effective demand reduction is the elimination of illicit trade (World Bank 1999). The causes of illicit trade in tobacco products are multi-factorial, requiring concerted multilateral action by all countries. Contrary to assertions by tobacco companies that price differentials between countries are the only significant cause of illicit trade, World Bank research has also identified corruption as an equally important cause of illicit trade in tobacco (World Bank 1999).

The WHO FCTC in Article 15 recognizes that the elimination of smuggling and all forms of illicit trade in tobacco products is an essential component of tobacco control. Moreover, the WHO FCTC includes a detailed provision on the illicit trade in tobacco products which incorporates provisions on tracking and tracing of such products. At the second session of the Conference of the Parties to the WHO FCTC, the Parties recognized that the elimination of smuggling and counterfeiting is an essential component of global tobacco control and, as such, it established a subsidiary body to negotiate the Convention's first protocol, which will address illicit trade in tobacco products.

Comprehensive multisectoral intervention

The best results in the reduction of tobacco use within a country are achieved when several interventions are combined. India experienced success with this approach, as noted by the tobacco industry and reflected in a report in the Tobacco Journal International, a tobacco industry publication. The report states that India's tobacco industry suffered a 4 per cent decline during the 1999–2000 period, due to excise duty on cigarettes, smoke-free workplaces, bans on tobacco sales at railway stations, and cigarette advertising bans (Tobacco Journal International 2000). In this regard, the WHO FCTC in one of its core guiding principles acknowledges that 'comprehensive multisectoral measures and responses to reduce consumption of all tobacco products at the national, regional and international levels are essential' (WHO 2003c).

Impact of WHO FCTC

All of the WHO FCTC's methods have already proven their impact over time. The most obvious of these impacts have been in the economic and public health areas, but ground has been gained on the political and multisectoral fronts as well.

Empirically, increasing the price of tobacco products is the primary method of curbing consumption. The potency of this measure is clear in economic terms: A 33 per cent increase in the price of tobacco would yield a cost-effectiveness ratio of US$3 to US$42 for every disability adjusted life year (DALY) averted in low- and middle-income countries, and US$85 to US$1773 for every DALY averted in high-income countries (Jamison *et al.* 2006). Levels of taxation currently avert about 15 million DALYs annually; further increases can avert even more DALYs (Shibuya *et al.* 2003). An averted DALY has sizable financial implications, with less public and private expenditure on healthcare for tobacco-attributed illnesses. And contrary to critics' fears, taxation on tobacco products actually raises government revenues because consumption usually falls at a slower rate than price increases (Frank *et al.* 2000).

These financial gains are linked with public health and broader economic gains. A healthy and long-living workforce, with incentives to invest in human capital, has positive implications for long-term development. Increasing tobacco prices by 70 per cent could avert 10–26 per cent of all smoking-related deaths globally, an outcome that would particularly affect low- and middle-income countries, young people, and men (Jamison *et al.* 2006). But tax increases can be more effective if implemented with other measures—in developed countries, the demand is price-inelastic, and additional methods, such as comprehensive bans on tobacco advertising, bans of smoking in public and work places, and strong counter-marketing measures must be utilized (Shibuya *et al.* 2003). Non-price methods, such as nicotine replacement therapies, can be more expensive than raising cigarette prices, but are still cost effective, if also 'extremely sensitive to context'—where public health messages are readily absorbed, such costs could be low (Jamison *et al.* 2006). Promoting cessation among current smokers will have its impact during the next 50 years, and prevention efforts will have their impact afterwards (Jamison *et al.* 2006).

Less apparent than the economic and health impact of the WHO FCTC's methods is its political and multisectoral impact. Cooperation and political resolve have become essential as more sectors become involved with the battle against the tobacco epidemic. There is a growing awareness of the effectiveness of the multisectoral approach's synergistic core; as Dr Margaret Chan, Director-General of WHO, stated: 'multiple sectors influence health, and should pay attention to the health impact of their policies' (Chan 2007). Each of the WHO FCTC's measures enhances the efficacy of the others—thus the whole of the WHO FCTC is greater than the sum of its parts.

The WHO FCTC provides the context for a substantial scale up of WHO's efforts at country-level to reduce the non-communicable burden of disease by implementing a core package of cost-effective, demand reduction measures. The treaty itself has catalysed Organizational and national programmatic movement to address the effects of non-communicable disease and its determinants.

The WHO FCTC as an intermediate global public good for health

The WHO FCTC and the process of negotiating the WHO FCTC both have important intermediate GPG characteristics. The Convention and its negotiation are intermediate GPGs in that both have facilitated the development of tobacco control policies globally (Taylor *et al.* 2003). Having entered into force, the WHO

FCTC provides a mechanism to respond to the GPG aspects of tobacco control. The WHO FCTC will facilitate the flow of information about tobacco control and serve as a mechanism to coordinate various transnational aspects of tobacco control, including smuggling, advertising, packaging, and labelling. It will enhance global surveillance, information exchange, and international technical, legal, and financial cooperation in support of the GPGs of tobacco control. Even now, the WHO FCTC process continues to provide a global instrument for public health professionals to distribute their evidence to governments and to get this evidence incorporated into binding agreements (Wipfli *et al.* 2002), including future protocols to the Convention.

Conclusion

The strength of the WHO FCTC resides primarily in three elements. First, it is an evidence-based treaty. All the tobacco control measures required by the WHO FCTC have been proven to be effective and are based on numerous experiences and facts. Second, it is a comprehensive tool that addresses all the effective tobacco control policies that can be implemented to reduce tobacco consumption; its effect will exceed the sum of the results of each measure taken separately because some measures increase the effectiveness of others. Third, the global aspect of the convention will enhance its effectiveness far beyond action implemented at the national or even regional level. The burden of disease induced by the tobacco epidemic is huge and increasing. The number of smokers in the world is estimated to be about 1.3 billion and it is expected that, if the current trend continues, this number will increase to 1.7 billion in 2025 (WHO 2003a; Guindon & Boisclair 2003). Half of these people will eventually die from tobacco-related illnesses.

It has been estimated that reduction of consumption and initiation of tobacco use by 50 per cent by 2050 has the potential to avert up to 200 000 000 deaths from tobacco use (Peto & Lopez 2000). As a powerful intermediate GPG designed to reduce tobacco consumption, the WHO FCTC will significantly decrease this burden, which will in turn lead to improved overall health and economic conditions.

Case study: The international health regulations

While the WHO FCTC was the WHO Member States' first exercise of the WHO Constitutional powers to adopt conventions or agreements within the purview of the Organization's mandate, the power to adopt regulations found in Article 21 of the WHO Constitution was tapped into decades ago, in response to the threat of infectious disease. The result was the International Health Regulations (IHR), legally binding regulations adopted by most countries to contain the threats from diseases that may rapidly spread from one country to another (WHO 2007b). The current IHR are designed to address not only emerging infectious diseases like SARS, but also those cross-border threats that arise as a result of public health risks and emergencies like chemical spills or waste that has been dumped.

The version of the IHR that was in place through the end of the twentieth century, the 1969 IHR, included only three diseases: Cholera, plague, and yellow fever. The measures were oriented to border control and the notification and control measures were relatively passive, reflecting a strong sense of independent, domestically oriented disease control. When the WHO Member States called for a revision of the 1969 IHR, it was based on the need for stronger, more collaborative measures to adequately respond to the globalized nature of infectious disease. Its revision in 2005 demonstrates a global commitment to contain public health risks and emergencies at the source, not only at national borders. The revised IHR, the 2005 IHR, was adopted by the World Health Assembly in May 2005, and came into force, generally, on 15 June 2007.

The compelling question of whether or not the IHR constitutes an intermediate GPG for health was addressed by Giesecke prior to the 2005 adoption by the World Health Assembly of the 2005 IHR (Giesecke 2003). Giesecke accurately projected what a revised IHR would need to contain to be considered an intermediate GPG for health. Indeed, his vision of the revised IHR as an intermediate GPG for epidemic control mirrors, to a great extent, what was ultimately adopted by the 192 WHO Member States at the close of the decade-long process of revising the 1969 IHR.

This case study describes the relevant new provisions in the Regulations and seeks, in part, to illustrate how the 2005 IHR, or aspects thereof, may be considered an intermediate GPG for health.

Strengthening of the IHR through increased roles and responsibilities for WHO and Parties

The 2005 IHR increased the rights and obligations of WHO and Parties both substantially and substantively. This expansion of roles is analysed below in the context of the Regulations as an intermediate GPG for health.

New mandates for WHO

Five key changes to the 1969 IHR found a place in the final text of the 2005 IHR. These changes strengthen WHO's role and contribute to establishing the Regulations as an effective tool to attain the ultimate GPG for epidemic control. These include (1) use of other information sources by WHO; (2) informal and confidential notification to WHO; (3) a wider remit (scope); (4) guaranteed assistance by WHO to control outbreaks; and (5) a rapid, transparent decision mechanism to make recommendations on any necessary health measures.

The use of information from sources other than official governmental notifications or consultations and provisional confidentiality of notified information. For the past decade, WHO's alert and response operations team has been using information from non-official sources to detect public health events of international importance and to conduct timely risk assessment with countries. With the advent of the 2005 IHR this mechanism has been further refined and formalized. Article 9.1 of the 2005 IHR firmly establishes WHO's mandate to 'take into account reports from sources other than notifications and consultations' with the proviso that these reports must be assessed on the basis of sound epidemiological principles and communicated to the country where the event is occurring (WHO 2005). Before taking action on these reports, WHO is required to seek verification thereof from the Party in which the event is allegedly occurring (WHO 2005).

Consultation. WHO is no stranger to consultations with its Member States' public health officials and has engaged in countless discussions on public health events of national and potentially international concern with key personnel in ministries of health. Article 8 of the 2005 IHR provides a legal framework for this consultation process, including consultation under circumstances where the information available may be insufficient to perform the assessment required for notification to the Organization. Critically, the information communicated to WHO under this provision is subject to the provisional restrictions placed on its dissemination to other Parties as set out in Article 11 of the 2005 IHR. According to the text of Article 11, WHO must, as a general matter, consult with the Party in whose territory the event is occurring as to its intent to make this information available to other States.

A broader purpose and scope. As has been discussed earlier, the purpose and scope of the 2005 IHR are far broader than those of the 1969 IHR, which was limited to Parties being required to notify WHO only when one of three diseases (cholera, plague, and yellow fever) became apparent in their jurisdictions. By contrast, one of the cornerstones of the 2005 IHR is notification to WHO of public health events on the basis of contextual criteria without restriction to a limited list of diseases. While not intended to detract from this broad language, for a number of political and policy reasons, WHO Member States were in favour of including a short list of diseases for mandatory notification, although the value of including a list of notifiable diseases in the Regulations is debatable.

WHO support to States Parties in their response to public health risks and emergencies of international concern. The Organization has been supporting countries in their response to national and international public health emergencies for many years, including through the Global Outbreak Alert and Response Network, managed by the WHO alert and response operations group. The 2005 IHR further institutionalizes and harmonizes these processes for both Parties and WHO. Articles 10 (Verification) and 13 (Public health response) of the 2005 IHR carve out a specific role for WHO in terms of when and how the Organization is required to support Parties. The verification procedure established in Article 10 requires that WHO, when it receives information of an event that may constitute a public health emergency of international concern (PHEIC), offers to collaborate with the Party concerned to assess the potential for international disease spread, possible interference with international traffic, and the adequacy of control measures. Although a Party is not necessarily obliged to accept such an offer, a refusal on its part does not prevent WHO from sharing available public health information with other Parties should this be warranted by the 'magnitude of the public health risk' involved, while taking into account the views of the Party (World Health Organization 2005). With regard to public health response, in Article 13 WHO is required generally to collaborate with Parties 'in the response to public health risks and other events by providing technical guidance and assistance and by assessing the effectiveness of the control measures in place, including the mobilization of international teams of experts for on-site assistance, when necessary' (World Health Organization 2005).

A transparent decision-making process within WHO. A number of countries raised concerns regarding the decision-making procedure at WHO during the 2003 SARS crisis, which in turn had a profound impact on the IHR negotiations in 2004 and 2005. Indeed, World Health Assembly resolution WHA56.28 expressly requested the Director-General of WHO 'to take into account evidence, experiences, knowledge and lessons acquired during the SARS response when revising the International Health Regulations' (WHO 2003b). This request was accommodated in the 2005 IHR, which, for example, establishes a specific procedure for the *determination* of a PHEIC by the Director-General and the issuance of any corresponding health measures (WHO 2005). Although it remains the duty of the Director-General to determine whether a particular public health event constitutes a PHEIC, s/he is required to first seek the view of an Emergency Committee of relevant independent experts before informing other countries of his/her decision, unless the affected Party agrees with the determination. With regard to the adoption of specific control measures following such a determination, the Director-General must invariably take into account the views of the Committee. It should be noted that the views of the Committee are not binding on the Director-General, who may decide to reject them.

New rights and obligations for States Parties

With regard to Parties' obligations, the need to strengthen national surveillance was central to creating a successful IHR. From the perspective of promoting a GPG for health, epidemiology training and capacity building, including improved communications and laboratory facilities, are prerequisite to the successful control of epidemics. Annex 1A of the 2005 IHR establishes a set of minimum core public health capacities for surveillance and response that all Parties to the Regulations must meet within a pre-defined time period set out in Articles 5 (Surveillance) and 13 (Public health response). These new provisions stipulate that each Party 'shall develop, strengthen and maintain, as soon as possible, but no later than five years from the entry into force of these Regulations, the capacity:

(1) To detect, assess, notify and report events

(2) To respond promptly and effectively to public health risks and public health emergencies of international concern

It should be noted that this 5-year period may be extended 'on the basis of a justified need and an implementation plan' for an additional 2-year period. Finally, on an exceptional basis, the Director-General may grant a Party an additional 2-year extension to meet its obligations under Articles 5 and 13 of the 2005 IHR. The Director-General's decision, however, is contingent on first consulting the Review Committee.

The 2005 IHR as an intermediate global public good for health

The concept of public goods and what make them global have been defined and discussed elsewhere in this chapter and will, therefore, be dealt with only briefly here. Relevant to the examination of the IHR, disease control at the national level through the adoption of regulatory measures can be seen as a public good for health. That is, such a public good is non-excludable because it benefits those who are not even aware that there is a risk (of disease) and non-rivalrous due to the fact that one person benefiting from disease control does not prevent another from also benefiting. With regard to the global nature of the public good of infectious disease control it is clearly the intent of the 2005 IHR to be a transboundary, globally inclusive instrument. Article 3 (Principles) of the 2005 IHR provides that the implementation of the new rules 'shall be guided by the goal of their universal application for the protection of all people of the world from the international spread of disease' (WHO 2005).

In terms of the IHR as an intermediate GPG for health, the freedom from epidemics (or epidemic control) is a final GPG for health, while the surveillance and control mechanisms required to attain this goal are an intermediate GPG for health. A functioning IHR provide the set of rules that establish administrative and legislative structures in support of these intermediate GPGs for health. Therefore, inasmuch as they deal with epidemic control, the 2005 IHR may constitute an intermediate GPG for health. The conditional is employed here because, as the Regulations entered into force only on 7 August 2007 for all WHO Member States that adopted them in May 2005, it is too early to tell what the level of compliance with the new rules will be and whether the 2005 IHR are being successfully implemented. Indeed, for the fate of the 2005 IHR to be different than that of the 1969 Regulations, which had become largely ineffective, full implementation and respect for its provisions are pre-requisite to play this enabling role as an intermediate GPG for health. The ineffectiveness of the 1969 IHR resulted, in part, from their scope being limited to three diseases; the failure by WHO Member States to notify WHO of outbreaks in a timely fashion, in accordance with the Regulations; and the application by Member States of excessive measures affecting traffic and trade.

Although it is premature to assess the extent to which the 2005 IHR will be an effective tool to curb epidemics, it is clear that its purpose and scope make it a firm candidate as an intermediate GPG for health. This is shown by the broad scope of the IHR as set out in Article 2 of the Regulations which provides that:

> The purpose and scope of these Regulations are to prevent, protect against, control and provide a public health response to the international spread of disease in ways that are commensurate with and restricted to public health risks, and which avoid unnecessary interference with international traffic and trade. (emphasis added) (WHO 2005)

The scope is further delineated through the definitions of key terms such as PHEIC, disease, international traffic, and public health risk. Given the far-reaching scope of the 2005 IHR and, with 194 Parties and its quasi-universal geographical coverage, it could easily be argued that the 2005 IHR has the potential to become an intermediate GPG for health, as described above. Although the scope of the proposed revised Regulations was somewhat controversial during the revision negotiations in 2004 and 2005 (Plotkin *et al.* 2007), and the text itself is not explicit on this point, the coverage of the 2005 IHR is considered broad enough to encompass relevant public health risks involving biological, chemical, or radiological agents (WHO 2007), including those that are naturally occurring, accidental, or intentional in nature (Fidler & Gostin 2006). It is also important to highlight that, as was the case with the 1969 version of the Regulations, the 2005 IHR is designed to contain the international spread of disease while at the same time ensuring that the international movement of people and goods is not unnecessarily restricted. This nexus between public health and international traffic, as well as between the law of infectious disease and trade law, is an important and defining aspect of the Regulations, both today and historically.

Conclusion

The 2005 IHR clearly has the potential to become an intermediate GPG for health, as discussed in this case study. Their purpose of preventing and protecting against the international spread of disease, including epidemic control, while avoiding unnecessary interference with world traffic, falls squarely within the definition of a public good. Moreover, the global nature of this public good is clear, given the Regulations' textual intent of universal application. Whether or not the 2005 IHR actually plays this enabling role as an intermediate GPG for health, however, will largely depend on its effective implementation. The most important challenge is, therefore, to create incentives for States Parties to comply with the 2005 IHR (Aginam 2005) and rally support for their implementation. This will require substantial human and financial resources and a strong commitment from a broad array of partners and stakeholders, including the donor community. Without this, the 2005 IHR role as an intermediate GPG for health will remain purely aspirational. Every effort must be made to ensure that governments and international organizations, including WHO, prioritize their effective implementation.

Case study: Food safety—the Codex Alimentarius Commission (CAC) and the International Food Safety Authorities Network (INFOSAN)

Food safety and food control have been recognized as important issues in many countries for decades. Many major initiatives both in safe food production and in control philosophy have contributed to systems perceived by many to be efficient in the prevention of foodborne disease in most developed countries. The recent outbreaks of foodborne disease have, however, shaken the consumers' trust in these food safety systems. BSE, dioxin, *Escherichia coli* O157, *Salmonella*—all foodborne hazards that were virtually unknown 10–15 years ago are now household names in most families.

Many countries now realize that foodborne disease continues to be a major public health issue. Foodborne diseases are some of the most widespread health problems in the world and they have implications on both the health of individuals and the development of societies. Deeply concerned by this, the Fifty-third World Health Assembly adopted a resolution in May 2000 calling upon WHO and its Member States to recognize food safety as an essential public health function (WHO 2000). The resolution also called for the development of systems to enable a reduction of the burden of foodborne disease.

One of the primary multilateral responses to the need for food safety management is the Codex Alimentarius Commission (CAC), an intergovernmental body operated under the auspices of the Food and Agriculture Organization of the United Nations (FAO) and WHO. The objective of the CAC is to protect the health of consumers and to ensure fair practices in the food trade, while promoting coordination of all food standards work undertaken by intergovernmental and non-governmental organizations (FAO and WHO 2007). The international food standards and related texts adopted by CAC constitute the *Codex Alimentarius*. All food standards and related texts in the Codex Alimentarius are of voluntary nature and may become binding only when they are converted into national legislation or regulation. The membership of CAC is open to all member nations and associate member nations of FAO and WHO, and currently covers more than 99 per cent of the world population. To complement the CAC standard setting, and in response to two World Health Assembly resolutions and a CAC request (CAC 2004), WHO established a list of primary official contact points in each of its Member States for the exchange of information in food safety emergency situations. This network, the International Food Safety Authorities Network (INFOSAN), also provides tools and support to increase Member State capacity to develop their national food safety systems and respond to health emergencies posed by natural, accidental, and intentional contamination of food.

This case study examines the global burden of foodborne disease and provides overviews of CAC and INFOSAN, the most salient international responses to food safety concerns. As part of the review of these mechanisms, the question of CAC and INFOSAN providing intermediate GPGs for health is considered.

Foodborne disease burden

It is estimated that up to 2 million people die each year from diarrhoeal diseases, mostly attributed to contaminated food and drinking water. Studies estimate that each year in the United States, foodborne diseases result in 76 million illnesses, 325 000 hospitalizations, and 5000 deaths (Mead *et al.* 1999). It is estimated that foodborne diseases in the United States caused by *Campylobacter*, *Salmonella*, *E. coli* O157, and *Listeria monocytogenes* cost almost US$7 billion annually.

Extrapolations such as this one from the United States, are scarce at the global level. In addition, data collected through surveillance systems for foodborne disease do not provide the real incidence of such diseases. Available data often pertain mostly to outbreaks, which are only the tip of the iceberg. Data on sporadic diarrhoeal illness (of which most are caused by food) is largely obtained through passive surveillance systems whose quality varies greatly between countries and diseases. For example, underreporting of *Salmonella* diarrhoea, including both sporadic and outbreak cases, differs from country to country and has recently been estimated at from 3.2 to 3.9 per cent in the United Kingdom (Adak *et al.* 2002; Wheeler *et al.* 1999) to 38 per cent in the United States (Mead *et al.* 1999). No information on under notification of diarrhoea is presently available for developing countries, but it could be assumed the underreporting is even more prevalent and therefore more important in areas with poorer general health coverage.

The additional contribution of foodborne disease to the vicious circle of malnutrition and diarrhoea should not be forgotten. The FAO estimates that malnutrition affects about 800 million people. Malnutrition increases host susceptibility to foodborne infections through a number of mechanisms. Diarrhoea caused by *E. coli*, which is probably the most important cause of children's diarrhoea in developing countries, has a longer duration and a greater potential for long-term nutritional consequences in malnourished children. In general malnutrition can result in a 30-fold increase in the risk for diarrhoea-associated death (Morris & Potter 1997).

It is important to reiterate that diarrhoeal diseases only constitute a fraction of disease caused by food. Microorganisms transmitted through food can cause many other types of disease, including very serious long-term infections. Even more important, the disease burden caused by chemical hazards in food is largely unknown, with estimation of a very serious fraction of all cancers caused by such hazards. Therefore, it is generally recognized that determinations of the impact of foodborne disease have always relied heavily on estimates and assumptions. We do not have the full picture yet.

Foodborne diseases not only significantly affect people's health and well-being; they also have economic consequences for individuals, families, communities, businesses and countries. These diseases impose a substantial burden on healthcare systems and markedly reduce economic productivity. The loss of income due to foodborne disease perpetuates the cycle of poverty. Estimating direct as well as indirect costs of foodborne disease is difficult. An estimate in the United States places the medical costs and productivity losses in a population of approximately 250 million in the range of US$6.6–37.1 billion (Butzby & Roberts 1997).

Global food trade is increasing with feed, food ingredients, partially processed food, and final food products being bought and sold around the world. Food is also sent abroad for processing and then returned to the country of origin for sale. According to FAO trade statistics, the value of trade in agricultural products was estimated at US$552 billion in 2005. International travel also represents a significant source of foodborne disease for some countries. For example, in 2005, Sweden reported that 80.2 per cent and The Netherlands reported 87 per cent of their salmonellosis cases acquired their infection while overseas (EFSA 2007).

Thus, it has become imperative to address the matters related to food safety at the international level—to complement and assist in the actions taken by national governments that carry the primary responsibility to ensure food safety for their population.

The Codex Alimentarius Commission (CAC)
Legal basis and organizational structure
The CAC was established as a joint commission on the basis of Article VI.1 of the FAO Constitution (FAO 1961) and under Article 18 of the WHO Constitution (WHO 1963), as the executive organ of the Joint FAO/WHO Food Standards Programme. CAC enjoys certain autonomy on procedural and programmatic matters, whereas the strategic direction of the Joint Programme is laid out by the Member States in the respective governing bodies of the two parent organizations. The highest governing body of Codex Alimentarius is the CAC. It meets annually in Rome and in Geneva on an alternate basis. The CAC is assisted by an Executive Committee. The Secretary of the CAC is jointly appointed by the Directors-General of FAO and WHO from the staffs of these organizations.

The preparatory work of the Codex Alimentarius (i.e. development of draft international standards and related texts), is undertaken by the subsidiary bodies of CAC—Codex committees and task forces. They are classified into two categories. The general subject committees address horizontal aspects of food standards (additives, contaminants, labelling, methods of analysis, and sampling, etc.); the commodity committees address specific groups of commodities (fish and fishery products, milk and milk products, etc.).

The provision of scientific advice, based on risk analysis principles, by FAO and WHO to Codex and to member states, occurs through expert committees, such as: Joint FAO/WHO Expert Committee on Food Additives (JECFA), Joint FAO/WHO Meetings on Pesticide Residues (JMPR), and Joint FAO/WHO Expert Meetings on Microbiological Risk Assessment (JEMRA).

Operations and procedure
The operation of the CAC system is guided by the Rules of Procedure, adopted by CAC and endorsed by the Directors-General of FAO and WHO. The process of elaboration and adoption of international standards and related texts follows a procedure consisting of eight steps:

Step 1: A proposal for new work is reviewed and a decision on whether or not to undertake new work is taken by the Commission.

Steps 2–4: A draft text is prepared and circulated to governments and all interested parties for comment, followed by review by the relevant Committee.

Step 5: The Commission reviews the progress made and agrees that the draft should go to finalization.

Steps 6 and 7: The approved draft is sent again to governments and interested parties for comment and is finalized by the relevant Committee.

Step 8: Following a final round of comments, the Commission adopts the draft as a formal Codex text.

An accelerated procedure whereby the elaboration of a text is concluded by adoption at Step 5 can be used, thereby skipping steps six through eight.

International importance
The Codex Alimentarius has become the global reference point for consumers, food producers and processors, national food control agencies, and the international food trade. The status of Codex Alimentarius standards recognized in the World Trade Organization's (WTO) Agreement on the Application of Sanitary and Phytosanitary Measures (WTO/SPS Agreement) and the Agreement on Technical Barriers to Trade (WTO/TBT Agreement) both encourage the international harmonization of food standards. As a result, Codex Alimentarius standards have become the benchmarks against which national food measures and regulations are evaluated within the legal parameters of the WTO Agreements.

In particular, the SPS Agreement specifically designates Codex Alimentarius standards, guidelines, and recommendations as the international standards in food safety, with which WTO members are encouraged to harmonize their sanitary measures. The SPS Agreement acknowledges that governments have the right to take sanitary measures necessary for the protection of human health. WTO members applying measures that are more stringent than Codex standards are allowed to do so but are required to provide scientific justification for those measures.

The International Food Safety Authorities Network (INFOSAN)
In collaboration with FAO, WHO initiated INFOSAN in 2004. The mandate to establish INFOSAN lies in two World Health Assembly Resolutions. World Health Assembly Resolution 53.15, adopted in 2000, called for improved communication among WHO and its Member States on matters of food safety (WHO 2000). World Health Assembly Resolution 55.16, adopted in 2002, expressed serious concern about natural, accidental, and intentional contamination of food that can lead to health emergencies (WHO 2002a). Member States requested that WHO provide tools and support to increase their capacity to respond to such emergencies. The INFOSAN mandate was also based on recommendations from a series of international conferences which called for a coordinated approach for the effective management of public health emergencies, including those caused by contaminated food. In 2004, the CAC requested that WHO establish a list of primary official contact points in each of its Member States for the exchange of information in food safety emergency situations.

Based on these mandates, and recognizing the continuous increase in global food trade and travel, INFOSAN was developed to share food safety information and experience, as well as to promote collaboration between food safety authorities at national and international levels. An integral part of the INFOSAN network is the rapid exchange of emergency information between such authorities relative to food safety events or emergencies. This is known as INFOSAN Emergency.

As of February 2009, INFOSAN has 172 member countries and is advised on its strategic functions by an external advisory group. To facilitate the sharing of food safety experience, INFOSAN Information Notes, describing the latest food safety knowledge, are developed 6–12 times per year. Multilateral communication is also encouraged as a means of countries learning from each others' experiences.

INFOSAN Emergency operates within the International Health Regulations (2005) (WHO 2005) and oversees all food safety related events, inclusive of food contamination and foodborne disease. On average, 200 food safety events per month are investigated to determine their public health impact, including events of unusual or unexpected natures, distribution, and possible trade restrictions. The network actively shares information about 1 or 2 such events per month deemed of international public health significance. For example, when two shigellosis outbreaks occurred in two countries both implicating baby corn from a third country, INFOSAN Emergency sought information from the exporting country. Through this process it was determined that a further three countries were at risk since they had imported the affected baby corn. INFOSAN Emergency alerted all three countries, enabling a process where these countries could determine the risk for their population and implement their own appropriate risk management options. In the baby milk powder event in China, involving the export of different products contaminated with melamine, the Chinese authorities actively used INFOSAN to communicate information on needed recalls to a number of other countries.

Membership in INFOSAN is voluntary. However, the legal obligation with regard to INFOSAN Emergency is a mix of both hard and soft law: The 2005 IHR (hard law) and the instruction to WHO to maintain a list of primary contacts from the CAC (soft law). Codex Alimentarius encourages the rapid notification of food safety events or emergencies associated with imported foods to international bodies and to the exporting country.

CAC and INFOSAN as intermediate GPGs for health

Both CAC and INFOSAN have proven capacity to improve health and health systems, the predicate for an intermediate GPG for health. The success of the CAC as the multilateral framework for global food safety is the result of the global scale and scope of over 180 commodity standards, 1112 food additives provisions, covering 292 food additives and 2930 Maximum limits for pesticide residues, covering 218 pesticides (FAO and WHO 2006). In addition, many consider Codex Alimentarius and CAC a successful United Nations initiative because of a high level of transparency ensured by the participation of a number of governmental and non-governmental observer organizations in the 8-step rule-based standards-setting process.

Contributing to the success of the Codex Alimentarius is the Codex Trust fund. The trust fund was established to provide financial support to developing countries, so that their officials can participate directly in CAC meetings. The Codex Alimentarius contributes significantly to a general public health improvement in many countries, where the expertise and food safety system necessary to obtain the most recent scientific information and knowledge of food safety advice and regulation is not available. As developing nations and regions move to comply with WTO trade and SPS obligations and monitor the impact of agri-food industry globalization and global food trade liberalization on food safety, the work of the CAC in establishing a basis for standards harmonization continues to grow in importance.

INFOSAN has demonstrated its function as an intermediate GPG for health, strengthening international as well as national food safety systems and providing a platform for the development of the GPG of health, itself. The provision of INFOSAN Information Notes provides technical support for national food regulators when considering the impact and management of evolving food safety issues. INFOSAN Emergency activities enable rapid alerts to countries about food safety events or emergencies that may impact both the health and the economy of these countries. INFOSAN also assists national governments with the necessary public health response as required.

Conclusion

The ability of national governments to regulate food safety as they simultaneously move to increase food security presents many challenges. The necessary changes in food production systems should be matched with the food safety lessons learned throughout the developments in the industrialized food producing countries. There is no need to repeat the food safety mistakes in these countries in other parts of the world. At the present time, national governments are forced to acknowledge the inability of nations to unilaterally regulate domestic food systems. When confronted with growing levels of international food trade, cross-border competition, increasing corporate and supplier power, and rapid consolidation of global agri-food markets and industries, governments increasingly engage in collective policy action at the multilateral level to protect citizens and to achieve the collective good.

The high level of foodborne disease, together with the globalization of the food trade and international travel, signify that foodborne disease is an issue of international public health concern. In recognition of this, WHO has developed, in collaboration with other United Nation and international agencies, the Codex and INFOSAN–both strong examples of intermediate GPGs for health.

Section III: International legal paradigms, enforcement, and intermediate global public goods for health

As noted earlier in this chapter, the production of GPGs for health is most effective when states create international legal instruments that contain four essential aspects:

1. The establishment of formal institutions empowered to work on global public health problems

2. The establishment of procedures through which states and non-state actors can tackle specific global public health problems

3. The enumeration of substantive duties in connection with particular global public health challenges

4. The creation of mechanisms to enforce substantive legal duties undertaken by states that have agreed to be bound by international instruments

The WHO FCTC and the 2005 IHR both integrate all four aspects, as they address institutional, procedural, substantive, and enforcement aspects of the regulation of tobacco products and disease spread, respectively. As binding instruments, these instruments are often called 'hard law'. However, as demonstrated by the non-binding Codex Alimentarius and the voluntary INFOSAN, it is not only binding multilateral legal instruments that make up the landscape of intermediate GPGs for health. Those agreements and arrangements that are non-binding, and sometimes identified as 'soft law', can play a critical role in establishing the foundations required to produce the ultimate GPG—in this case, health.

This section provides a brief review of health as a GPG in the context of international law and the spectrum of agreements between nations. The contrasts and similarities between hard and soft international law are presented and the institutional capacity, responsibility, and role of WHO in the creation of intermediate GPGs for health is examined.

Law and non-law: Binding and non-binding international instruments and GPGs for health

The ideas and characteristics of soft law and hard law, and their relationship and usefulness, are common themes among international legal scholars and practitioners. With regard to the GPG of health, a very cogent and useful set of articles on this area was presented in the Bulletin of the WHO in December 2002, a special edition focusing on international law and public health (WHO 2002b).

As exemplified by the case studies in this chapter, public health concerns are becoming increasingly complex as globalization progresses; so, too then, must and have the international responses been. In overcoming the Westphalian notion of single nation solutions, 'the complex network of global health governance structures that are emerging . . . indicates the need for an inclusive approach to engagement with new global health actors', including civil society, private actors, and public organizations (Taylor & Bettcher 2002; Taylor 2002). It is perhaps reasonable, then, to assert that the first step to producing the GPG of health is to examine the entire spectrum of stakeholders and create processes that are inclusive, to ensure that the intermediate GPG international legal instruments are as effective and efficient as possible.

Among the intermediate GPG legal instruments, traditional legal instruments—namely, treaties—provide the strongest, most effective tools for improving health (Taylor 2002), though they are commensurately difficult to negotiate because they bind parties to discrete, identifiable obligations. Although treaties have variable success in being implemented and enforced, the gestalt created by a negotiation, adoption, and entry into force can be tremendous (Taylor 2002). This certainly was the case for the WHO FCTC process, during which 'the power of the process' was often noted as one of the key ingredients to its success. In this way, not only the instrument, but also the attendant process and investment by interested entities, becomes an intermediate GPG for health.

Perhaps because of the substantial challenges inherent in successfully negotiating a treaty on a topic as multifaceted as health, non-binding instruments have become increasingly utilized as nations seek to reach agreement and move a number of multilateral agendas forward (Chopra *et al.* 2002). The force behind this is likely that non-binding agreements provide the kind of flexibility that allows nations to act cooperatively and in concert without limiting their own autonomy (Chopra *et al.* 2002). In their article, Taylor and Bettcher note, however, that the position and essential nature of non-binding instruments like resolutions and codes, sometimes called soft law and sometimes called 'non-law', remain unsettled in the rubric of international law (Taylor & Bettcher 2002). In terms of intermediate GPGs for health, non-binding arrangements like the Codex and INFOSAN certainly have demonstrated their usefulness, even in the face of not having the more robust implementation and enforcement opportunities that come with traditional international legal instruments.

Global health and global health governance is a dynamic, exciting arena with an increasingly complex landscape being painted with each new transboundary health challenge that emerges or is identified. The relationship between hard and soft law has and will continue to adapt to best respond to the needs of global communities, which will in turn look to the WHO FCTC, 2005 IHR and the Codex as models of intermediate GPGs on which to build.

WHO and institutional roles and responsibilities in the creation of intermediate GPGs for health

In a review of the nature and usefulness of international instruments for health, it would be remiss not to consider the role of WHO, as the United Nations specialized agency for health, in the creation of these intermediate GPGs for health. As the institutional umbrella home of all the instruments considered in this chapter, it plays a key and central role in fostering and providing a forum for its Member States to create agreements. Notwithstanding this, though, the question of what it can do and what it should do remain topics worth considering.

According to its Constitution, WHO is not simply an institutional home for multilateral health programmes and technical expertise; WHO is vested with substantial normative functions as well, including the Articles 19 and 21 powers to adopt conventions and regulations on matters within its competence (WHO 2007a). Though, with the exception of regulations, these powers are only 'quasi-legislative' in that Member States are not automatically bound to provisions of a given negotiated text, this is nonetheless one of the Organization's most important functions (Burci & Vignes 2004). As Taylor notes, 'WHO's leadership in coordinating codification and implementation efforts among the diverse global actors actively engaged in health lawmaking could, in theory, foster the development of a more effective, integrated and rational legal regime and, consequently, better collective management of global health concerns' (Taylor 2002). The Organization has, essentially, a bully pulpit and, if exercised with care, political acumen, and vision, there is tremendous opportunity to promote international law as a primary tool for the GPG of health.

By design of its founding Member States, WHO does not, and perhaps should not, have full legislative capacity (Burci & Vignes 2004). It does have substantial comparative advantage, though, in being the agent for actualizing international agreements on health. The Organization has the capacity to coordinate its Member States, promote dialogue, and set the global health agenda and provide a platform for negotiations (Taylor 2002), provided it maintains adequate supporting political will and consensus among its constituency (Burci & Vignes 2004; Taylor 2002). WHO is one of, if not *the*, most potent sources of intermediate GPGs for health.

Conclusion

As intermediate GPGs for health, international legal instruments take on an additional layer of importance in global health governance.

In providing a robust framework for improving and occasionally even creating health, these instruments are important not only for what they are already doing, but for the potential good new instruments might be able to deliver. As WHO continues to grow into its normative role, it is likely that additional opportunities to exercise its Constitutional quasi-legislative powers will present themselves. The three examples of intermediate GPGs examined in this chapter, the WHO FCTC, the 2005 IHR, and the Codex and INFOSAN, have laid a solid foundation on which WHO and its Member States may build to continue to work toward achieving the GPG of health.

Acknowledgement

The authors would like to acknowledge Obijiofor Aginam and Kazuaki Miyagishima for their contributions towards this chapter.

Key points

◆ Health is arguably a GPG: One person's good health does not detract from another's and an improvement in individual health can improve the community-level economy and social fabric. Furthermore, although the onus of providing health remains primarily on national governments, globalization means that the determinants of health, as well as the requisite means to deliver health, are increasingly global.

◆ Insofar as international health instruments provide an infrastructure critical for reaching GPGs, but are part of the process rather than an outcome in and of themselves, they can be considered intermediate GPGs.

◆ The WHO Framework Convention on Tobacco Control (WHO FCTC), with its foundations in economic and public health, promotes evidence-based interventions that have been shown to improve health by effectively reducing the demand for tobacco, is an intermediate GPG for health.

◆ Intended to prevent and protect against the international spread of disease, including epidemic control, while avoiding unnecessary interference with world traffic the 2005 International Health Regulations (IHR) clearly have the potential to become an intermediate GPG for health, if effectively implemented.

◆ Insofar as both the Codex Alimentarius and INFOSAN strengthen international as well as national food safety systems and provide a platform for the development of the GPG of health, they are also both intermediate GPGs for health.

◆ WHO is one of, if not *the*, most potent sources of intermediate GPGs for health; the Organization has the capacity to coordinate its Member States, promote dialogue and set the global health agenda and provide a platform for negotiations, provided it maintains adequate supporting political will and consensus among its constituency.

References

Aginam, O. (2005). *Global health governance: International law and public health in a divided world*, p. 82. University of Toronto Press, Toronto.

Adak, G.K., Long, S.M., and O'Brien, S.J. (2002). Trends in indigenous foodborne disease and deaths, England and Wales: 1992 to 2000. *Gut*, **51**, 832–41.

Beaglehole, R. and Yach, D. (2003). Globalization and the prevention and control of noncommunicable disease: The neglected chronic diseases of adults. *The Lancet*, **362**, 903–8.

Blanchet, T. (2002). Child work in the bidi industry – Bangladesh. In *Tobacco and poverty: Observations from India and Bangladesh* (ed. D. Efroymson), pp. 37–43. PATH Canada, Dhaka.

Burci, G.L. and Vignes, C-H (2004). Normative functions. In *World Health Organization*, pp.124–53. Kluwer Law International, The Hague.

Butzby, J.C. and Roberts, T. (1997). Guillain-Barré syndrome increases foodborne diseases costs. *Food Review*, **20**, 36–42.

CAC (2004) Principles and guidelines for the exchange of information in food safety emergency situations. CAC/GL 19-1995, Rev.1-2004. www.codexalimentarius.net/download/standards/36/CXG_019e.pdf

Chan, M. (2007). Speech to interns. 24 August 2007, World Health Organization, Geneva.

Da Costa e Silva, V.L. and Nikogosian, H. (2003). Convenio marco de la OMS para el control del tabaco: la globalizacion de la salud publica.[WHO Framework Convention on Tobacco Control: the globalization of public health.] *Prevencion del Tabaquismo* [Prevention of tobacco addiction], **5**, 71–5.

Dodgson, R., Lee, K., and Drager, N. (2002). Global health governance: A conceptual review *Key Issues in Global Health Governance Discussion Paper No. 1* Centre on Global Change & Health and World Health Organization, Geneva. Available from: http://whqlibdoc.who.int/publications/2002/a85727_eng.pdf

Doll, R. (1998). Uncovering the effects of smoking: historical perspective. *Statistical Methods in Medical Research*, **7**, 87–117.

Efroymson, D., Saifuddin, A., Townsend, J. *et al.* (2001). Hungry for tobacco: An analysis of the economic impact of tobacco consumption on the poor in Bangladesh. *Tobacco Control*, **10**, 212–17.

European Commission (2003). *Tobacco control in EC development policy: A background paper for the high level round table on tobacco control and development policy*, p. 2. European Commission, Brussels.

European Food Safety Authority (EFSA) (2007). *The Community Summary Report on trends and sources of zoonoses, zoonotic agents, antimicrobial resistance and foodborne outbreaks in the European Union in 2005.* EFSA, Brussels.

FAO/WHO (2006) Understanding the Codex Alimentarius. Third Edition. Rome. ftp://ftp.fao.org/codex/Publications/understanding/Understanding_EN.pdf

FAO/WHO (2007) Codex Alimentarius Commission. Procedural Manual. Seventeenth Edition, Rome. ftp://ftp.fao.org/codex/Publications/ProcManuals/Manual_17e.pdf

Fidler, D. (2002). *Global health governance: Overview of the role of international law in protecting and promoting global public health* (*Key issues in Global Health Governance Discussion Paper 3*). World Health Organization and London School of Hygiene and Tropical Medicine. Available from: http://www.lshtm.ac.uk/cgch/ghg3.pdf

Fidler, D. and Gostin, L. (2006). The new International Health Regulations: An historic development for international law and public health. *Journal of Law, Medicine and Ethics*, **34**, 85–94.

The Food and Agriculture Organization (FAO) (1961). 11th FAO Conference Resolution No. 12/61, FAO, Rome.

Frank, J., Chaloupka, F.J., Hu, T. *et al.* (2000). The taxation of tobacco products. In *Tobacco control in developing countries* (eds. P. Jha and F. Chaloupka), pp. 237–72. Oxford University Press, Oxford.

Giesecke, J. (2003). International health regulations and epidemic control. In *Global public goods for health*: *Health economic and public health perspectives* (eds. R. Smith, R. Beaglehole, D. Woodward and N. Drager), pp. 196–211. Oxford University Press, Oxford.

Guindon, G.E. and Boisclair, D. (2003). Past, current and future trends in tobacco use *HNP Discussion Paper No.6, Economics of Tobacco Control Paper No. 6*. The World Bank, Washington, DC.

Hammond, D., Fong, G.T., McDonald, P.W. *et al.* (2003). Impact of the graphic Canadian warning labels on adult smoking behaviour. *Tobacco Control*, **12**, 391–5.

Jamison, D.T., Frenk, J., and Knaul, F.I. (1998). International collective action in health: Objectives, functions, and rationale. *The Lancet*, **351**, 514–7.

Jamison, D.T., Breman, J.G., Measham, A.R. *et al.* (2006) Cost-effective strategies for noncommunicable diseases, risk factors, and behaviors. *Priorities in health*, pp. 97–128. Oxford University Press, New York.

Kaul, I., Grunberg, I., and Stern, M.A. (1999). Defining global public goods. In *Global public goods, international cooperation in the 21st century* (eds. I. Kaul, I. Grunberg, and M.A. Stern), pp. 2–19. Oxford University Press, Oxford.

Kickbush, I (2003). Global health governance: Some theoretical considerations on the new political space. In *Health impacts of globalisation: Towards global governance* (ed. K.), pp. 192–203. Palgrave, Macmillan, London.

Mathers, C. and Loncar, D. (2006). Projections of global mortality and burden of disease from 2002 to 2030. *PLoS Medicine*, **3**, 2011–30.

Mead, P.S., Slutsker, L., Dietz, V. *et al.* (1999). Food-related illness and death in the United States. *Emerging Infectious Disease*, **5**, 607–25.

Morris, J.G. Jr. and Potter, M. (1997). Emergence of new pathogens as a function of changes in host susceptibility. *Emerging Infectious Diseases*, **3**, 435–41.

Omran, A. (1971). The epidemiologic transition: A theory of the epidemiology of population change. *Milbank Quarterly*, **49**, 509–38.

Plotkin, B., Hardiman, M., González-Martin, F. *et al.* (2007). Infectious diseases surveillance and the international health regulations. In *International Disease Surveillance* (eds. N.M. M'Ikanatha, R. Lynfield, C.A. Van Beneden, and de Valk, eds.), pp. 18–31. Blackwell Publishing, Oxford.

Raghavan, P. (2002). Bidi workers in Ahmedabad, India: Monotonous work, low pay. In *Tobacco and poverty: Observations from India and Bangladesh* (ed. D. Efroymson), pp. 31–6. PATH Canada, Dhaka.

Report of the Commission on Macroeconomics and Health (2001). *Macroeconomics and health: Investing in health for economic development*, chaired by Jeffrey D. Sachs, World Health Organization, p.21.

Shelton, D. (2000). Law, non-law and the problem of "soft law" In *Commitment and compliance: The role of non-binding norms in the international system* (ed. D. Shelton), pp. 1–20. Oxford University Press, Oxford.

Shibuya, K., Ciecierski, C., Guindon, E. *et al.* (2003). WHO framework convention on tobacco control: Development of an evidence based global public health treaty. *British Medical Journal*, **327**, 154–7.

Smith, R.D. and Woodward, D. (2003). Global public goods for health: Use and limitations. In *Global public goods for health: A reading companion*. World Health Organization, Geneva. Available at http://www.who.int/trade/distance_learning/gpgh/gpgh9/en/index.html

Smith, R., Woodward, D., Acharya, A. *et al.* (2004) Communicable disease control: A 'Global Public Good' perspective. *Health Policy and Planning*, **19**, 271–8.

Taylor, A.L. (2002). International health law and the WHO. *Bulletin of the World Health Organization*, **80**, 975–80.

Taylor, A.L., Bettcher, D.W., and Peck, R. (2003). International law and the international legislative process: The WHO Framework Convention on Tobacco Control. In *Global public goods for health: Health economic and public health perspectives* (eds. R. Smith, R. Beaglehole, D. Woodward, and N. Drager), pp. 212–32. Oxford University Press, Oxford.

Taylor, A.L. and Bettcher, D.W. (2002). WHO framework convention on tobacco control: A global 'good' for public health. *Bulletin of the World Health Organization*, **78**, 920–9.

Taylor, A.L., Bettcher, D.W., Fluss, S.S. *et al.* (2002). International health instruments: An overview. In *Oxford Textbook of Public Health: The scope of public health* (eds. R. Detels, J. McEwen, R. Beaglehole, and H. Tanaka), pp. 359–86. Oxford University Press, Oxford.

United States (1964). Smoking and health: Report of the advisory committee to the Surgeon General of the public health service. *Public Health Service Publication No. 1103* Public Health Service, Office of the Surgeon General.

Van Walbeek, C. (2002). Recent trends in smoking prevalence in South Africa: Some evidence from AMPS data. *South African Medical Journal*, **92**, 468–72.

World Bank (1999). *Curbing the epidemic: Governments and the economics of tobacco control*. World Bank, Washington, DC.

World Health Organization (WHO) (1963). Article 18 of the WHO Constitution, the 16th World Health Assembly Resolution WHA16.42, WHO, Geneva, Switzerland.

WHO (1983) *International Health Regulations, 3rd annotated edition*. WHO Press, Geneva.

WHO (2000). Food Safety. *World Health Assembly Resolution WHA53.15*. Available from http://ftp.who.int/gb/archive/pdf_files/WHA53/ResWHA53/15.pdf.

WHO (2002a). Global public health response to natural occurrence, accidental release or deliberate use of biological and chemical agents or radionuclear material that affect health. *World Health Assembly resolution WHA55.16*. Available from: http://www.who.int/gb/ebwha/pdf_files/WHA55/ewha5516.pdf.

WHO (2002b). Special theme issue: Global public health and international law. *Bulletin of the World Health Organization*, **80**, 923–1000.

WHO (2002c). *The World Health Report 2002: Reducing risk, promoting health life*, p. 8. WHO Press, Geneva.

WHO (2003a). *Policy recommendations for smoking cessation and treatment of tobacco dependence*. WHO Press, Geneva.

WHO (2003b). *Revision of the International Health Regulations*. World Health Assembly resolution WHA56.28. Available from: http://www.who.int/gb/ebwha/pdf_files/WHA56/ea56r28.pdf.

WHO (2003c). *WHO framework convention on tobacco control*. WHO Press, Geneva.

WHO (2005). *Revision of the International Health Regulations*. World Health Assembly resolution WHA58.3. Available from: http://www.who.int/gb/ebwha/pdf_files/WHA58/WHA58_3-en.pdf.

WHO (2007a). *Basic Documents*, 46th edition, pp.1–18. WHO Press, Geneva.

WHO (2007b). *The World Health Report 2007: A safer future: Global public health security in the 21st century*, p. 5. WHO Press, Geneva.

Wheeler, J.G., Sethi, D., Cowden, J.M. *et al.* on behalf of the Infectious Intestinal Disease Study Executive (1999). Study of infectious intestinal disease in England: Rates in the community, presenting to general practice, and reported to national surveillance *British Medical Journal*, **318**, 1046–50.

Wipfli, H., Bettcher, D., Subramaniam, C. *et al.* (2001). Confronting the global tobacco epidemic: Emerging mechanisms of global governance. In *International co-operation in health* (eds. M. McKee, P. Garner, and R. Stott), pp. 189–231. Oxford University Press, Oxford.

Woodward, D. and Smith, R.D. (2003). Global public goods and health: Concepts and issues. In *Global public goods for health: A reading companion*. World Health Organization, Geneva. Available at http://www.who.int/trade/distance_learning/gpgh/gpgh1/en/index.html

Yach, D. and Bettcher, D. (2000). Globalisation of tobacco industry influence and new global responses. *Tobacco Control*, **9**, 206–16.

Tobacco Journal International (2000). Taxation structure hits Indian cigarette market: Country Special, India. *Tobacco Journal International*.

4.4

Ethical principles and ethical issues in public health[1]

Nancy Kass

Abstract

Public health ethics examine and consider the moral dimensions of public health practice and public health research. While the field of medical ethics dates back hundreds of years, and writings on bioethics began to emerge in the 1960s and 1970s, the field of 'public health ethics', articulated as such by name, did not appear significantly in the literature for several more decades. More recently, there has been an explosion of interest in defining public health ethics, examining how it resembles or differs from medical ethics or bioethics, laying out frameworks and codes, and trying to provide both conceptual and practical guidance on how ethics plays a role in public health practice and research. This chapter will describe briefly the history of medical ethics and bioethics; work in bioethics with direct relevance for public health; the principles, codes, and frameworks recently articulated to provide guidance on public health ethics; and discuss the recent and growing literature on ethics and public health *research*, including whether and how public health research ethics might differ from the ethical guidance and regulations that have been created to more broadly oversee the ethics of research with human participants.

History of medical ethics and bioethics

Medical ethics has a long and important history. While some cite the Hippocratic Oath as the first articulation of the moral duties of physicians, and others cite nineteenth century writers such as John Gregory and Thomas Percival as giving birth to medical ethics, clear codes and teachings about the moral duties of the physician as a professional and as a caretaker have existed for hundreds, if not thousands, of years (Percival 1985; McCullough 1998). The depth of this work has grown: It is the focus of significant scholarship both in philosophy and other disciplines, the American Medical Association has longstanding professional codes of medical ethics,

and instruction on medical professionalism is currently required by 99 per cent of US and Canadian medical schools (Kao *et al.* 2003). The American Association of Medical Colleges insists that principles related to medical ethics should be taught as part of the Graduate Medical Education (GME) Core Curriculum (Allen 2007). Medical history, understandably, remains focused predominantly on the individual interactions between a physician and his or her patient.

Bioethics, in contrast, emerged within the last 50 years, bringing with it an explicitly broader focus. Emerging out of questions of resource allocation, moral questions raised by new reproductive and genetic technologies, a growing patients' rights movement, and a lack of oversight in human subject research, bioethics focused significantly on the societal and public policy implications of healthcare, research, and new medical and/or scientific discovery. The name 'bioethics' began to appear in the 1960s and 1970s. Early issues animating this new field of bioethics included whether social 'worth' should be relevant in allocating early kidney dialysis, whether Karen Ann Quinlan, a young woman in a persistent vegetative state, ought to be removed from a respirator when she had no meaningful cognition, and how to respond to a series of US-government-funded research studies viewed as potentially exploitive and inappropriate. Important scholarship grew in all of these areas and, in the early 1970s, a national commission was convened at the request of the US Congress to examine questions of ethics and human research. The National Commission drafted the *Belmont Report* (National Commission for the Protection of Human Subjects of Biomedical and Behavioral Research 1979) that delineated three ethics principles to be followed in conducting human research—beneficence, respect for persons, and justice.

Bioethics as a field took off. Centres were created, journals were started, meetings were convened, and professionals from a variety of disciplines began to call themselves 'bioethicists'. The three 'Belmont principles' became the foundation for one of the preeminent texts in bioethics (Beauchamp & Childress 1979) and, while some suggested alternative approaches to navigate through tough situations of bioethics, they remain widely cited both by scholars and as a practical framework through which to reason moral problems in healthcare and research (Clouser 1995; Jonsen 1995; Pellegrino 1995).

The early framers of these three principles suggested that no principle, a priori, ought to have moral superiority over any other. Nonetheless, the issues that animated bioethics in the early

[1] The first half of this chapter (until the section heading Public Health Research) is drawn significantly from two previously published articles by the author: 1. Kass, N., Public health ethics: From foundations and frameworks to justice and global public health, *The Journal of Law, Medicine, and Ethics*, 2004, **32**(2), 232–42; 2. Kass, N. An ethics framework for public health, *American Journal of Public Health*, 2001, **91**(11), 1776–82.

years—the need to tell patients and research subjects the truth and the right to refuse medical care or research participation—were ones where the principle of respect for autonomy, perhaps given too little moral attention previously, was now given pre-eminent moral status (Callahan 1984; Pellegrino & Thomasma 1988; Steinbock 1996). Informed consent, a practical application of the autonomy principle, became a hallmark of the new bioethics. Codes of ethics for clinical practice, which had focused for a century on not harming patients and upholding professional decorum, now added clauses requiring physicians to 'best protect the dignity of man in patients or research subjects' (Ramsey 1973).

The sub-field of *public health ethics*, articulated as such, did not appear significantly in the literature until approximately 10 years ago. An important exception, however, was a chapter, 'Ethics and Public Health', in the 1986 edition of the Maxcy-Rosenau text *Public Health and Preventive Medicine* (Lappe 1986).[2] This chapter outlined some of the core challenges in public health ethics: Fair distribution of resources, rights of individuals vs. those of groups, and promoting efficiency while recognizing the 'special standing of those in greatest need of health protection and services'. Moreover, Lappe compared medical ethics to public health ethics. Medical ethics is more concerned with individual autonomy and the duties of single health professionals, whereas public health ethics focuses more on equity and efficiency in the distribution of health resources as well as on the community in having its health protected. Lappe suggested that individual rights can be compromised for the sake of community interests, but only when there is proportionality. That is, the benefit must be larger than the sacrifice, and the absolute level of infringement on individual rights must be minimal. Related, since many public health programmes do not grant individuals the right of refusal, there must be evidence that the programmes will provide the good on which they are premised. At least as much as community good vs. individual rights being at stake, he suggested, there is an inevitable tension between utilitarianism and justice or, stated differently, between efficiency and equity. An ethic of public health captures the urgency for efficiency, while recognizing the special standing of those in greatest need of health protection and health services.

An additional exception worth noting is the work of Dan E. Beauchamp. Beauchamp suggested that social justice and communitarian traditions are and ought to be the driving forces behind public health practice and that these might define a somewhat separate 'ethic' (Beauchamp 1976). While public health practitioners had recognized, importantly, for more than a century, the relationship between social conditions and health (Fee 1977),[3] Beauchamp's work was striking in laying out as a new idea *within bioethics* that exclusive attention to individual interests, particularly

through a notion of market justice, 'plague attempts to protect the public's health … This new ethical paradigm will require thinking about and reacting to the problems of disability and premature death as primarily collective problems of the entire society' (Beauchamp 1976).

Furthermore, Beauchamp challenged bioethics to realize that much of the work of public health is to further the interests of community. Community, Beauchamp asserted, does not mean simply that the government ensures that individuals' interests are not offended by the actions of others. Rather, community means that we have shared commitments to one another, and that through collective actions related to health and safety, for example, we share a commitment to the common life, 'a central practice by which the body politic defines itself and affirms its values' (Beauchamp 1985). While Beauchamp did not literally use the words 'public health ethics', his work is foundational in describing how public health has its own set of moral priorities, and that these are critical to the functioning of a civil society.

Similarly, some of the issues that animated bioethics discourse in the 1960s and 1970s produced a literature that now, arguably, would be categorized as centrally relevant to questions of public health ethics despite not using the language, 'public health ethics'. In the next section, three of these ethics issues will be described: Ethics and health promotion, resource allocation, and the civil liberties vs. public health questions precipitated by the HIV/AIDS epidemic.

Ethics and health promotion

The degree to which governments should become involved in regulating personal behaviour became a matter of heated debate, and several scholars began to address the ethics issues inherent to health promotion, government involvement, and public health. At the core of the debates was whether it was acceptable to intervene only when behaviour change was relevant to protecting the health of others, as traditionally had been the norm in public health, or whether, now, paternalistic justifications, allowing intervention to improve the health of the person who would be the object of an intervention, also would be considered morally acceptable. Daniel Wikler, an important scholar for this body of literature, further suggested that promoting certain lifestyles or modes of behaviour itself conveyed a certain set of moral values about what constitutes right behaviour: 'It is not self-evident that this vision of a safe society, with its lack of immoderation, stress, and risk-taking, is to be favoured over others whose constitutive elements have incidental adverse effects upon health' (Wikler 1978).

Edmund Pellegrino, considered as one of the 'fathers of bioethics', wrote about an ethics of prevention (Pellegrino 1981). Preventive interventions, he suggested, ranged in how voluntary the intervention was, citing approaches like health education, opinion manipulation through mass media, tax and insurance incentives and disincentives, legal prohibitions. Pellegrino reminded us that health education and promotion include at the very least persuasion and, at times, coercion in the name of what some consider to be 'the good life'. And yet, he rightly explains, there 'is unlikely to be universal consensus on these matters in a democratic society that promises a maximal degree of personal choice'. Nonetheless, as a society, we inevitably are forced to make decisions about what constraints we will accept to further the common good.

---

[2] Note that the 11th edition of the same text book (1980) had a chapter entitled 'Legal and Ethical Issues in Public Health' by Sidney Shindell. The bulk of this chapter is devoted to legal issues in public health, however, rather than ethics issues, and thus is not discussed here.

[3] Note that this article describes the work of Edward Chadwick in England in the early 1800s demonstrating that differences in social conditions led to a more than twofold difference in life expectancy between upper and lower classes. Also in the 1800s, governments began conducting investigations of housing conditions and garbage heaps and mapping them in relation to outbreaks of disease, and by the end of the nineteenth century, state and local boards of health were being created to enforce sanitary regulations.

Faden and Faden, similarly, described a spectrum of interventions from facilitation to persuasion to manipulation to coercion, and argued that the acceptability of such approaches ultimately rests on how rational they are, and how resistible they are (Faden & Faden 1978). Described here, to be cited frequently throughout future public health ethics writings, was the concept of *proportionality*: The burden posed by interventions (particularly non-voluntary interventions) should be low and the benefit high. As such, incentives should be favoured over disincentives, true education should be favoured over manipulative messages, and government intervention ought not occur unless there is considerable evidence about the effectiveness of the proposed intervention.

Scholars of this period agree that voluntary approaches are ethically preferable to compulsory ones. The Society of Public Health Educators' code of professional ethics goes further, however, calling voluntariness as the *only* acceptable approach. According to the Code, health educators must 'support change by choice, not by coercion' (Society for Public Health Education 1976).

Purely voluntary interventions do not always work, however (Glanz *et al.* 1997; Roter *et al.* 1998). The operative question for ethics scholars, then, became whether or under what conditions more directive or controlling interventions could be implemented. Furthermore, since it would be governments implementing stricter measures, how could one ensure that the agenda was related to public health rather than to politics (Faden 1987)? Involuntary measures also assume 'a benign, wise, and responsive government, something history finds singularly rare' (Pellegrino 1981).

Shifting in focus from what governments can impose on individuals was Dan Beauchamp. Beauchamp suggested that the legal authority of public health should be used to regulate the behaviour of those who market and distribute harmful products rather than regulating the behaviour of individuals (Beauchamp 1976). If outside influences allow an individual unknowingly to alter his or her preferences, this diminishes the autonomy with which those choices are made (Wikler 1978). Coercive measures may be needed to control the facilitation, persuasion, and manipulation of messages that run counter to the interests of public health.

Resource allocation (Faden & Kass 1991)

In the 1970s and 1980s, a significant body of literature emerged regarding the fair distribution of healthcare resources. Articles examined access to healthcare and whether there was a moral 'right' to healthcare (Fried 1975; Fried 1976; Beauchamp & Faden 1979; Daniels 1981; Menzel 1983; Engelhardt 1986). The President's Commission for the Study of Ethical Problems in Medicine and Biomedical and Behavioral Research commissioned papers on this topic (President's Commission for the Study of Ethical Problems in Medicine and Biomedical and Behavioral Research 1983), and other scholars built on this work.

Since many political figures and advocates were calling for a right to healthcare, philosophical examinations of rights theory emerged during this period. A right to healthcare differs from healthcare being a privilege, or being provided out of charity (Beauchamp & Faden 1979). Given that there is no legal right to healthcare in this country, scholars have examined whether morally there is the obligation to provide citizens with healthcare. During this period, contrasting views of justice were put forward (Brody 1981; Gibbard 1982; Green 1983; Walzer 1983; Buchanan 1984; Daniels 1985),

yet all scholars agreed that healthcare access must be improved. Furthermore, despite differences about how to achieve it, there was agreement that individuals should be guaranteed some minimum of healthcare services.

Inevitably, questions of increasing access to healthcare led to questions of how to most fairly allocate limited resources (Winslow 1986; Churchill 1987; Blank 1988; Callahan 1988; Pellegrino 1988). There were calls to recognize both the implicit rationing inherent in the American healthcare system and the need for a morally acceptable and explicit rationing policy. One of the more controversial proposals was to ration by age. Both Daniel Callahan and Norman Daniels wrote books suggesting it is morally defensible to use age in resource allocation decisions (Callahan 1988; Daniels 1992). Pellegrino and Thomasma, in contrast, stated that most of the hard rationing decisions could be avoided if we shifted spending from less valuable goods, such as the US$65 billion spent on cosmetics or the US$30 billion spent on alcohol (Pellegrino & Thomasma 1988).

While the allocation and rationing literature of this period did not explicitly discuss public health or invoke the language of public health ethics, scholars ultimately argued that preventive and primary care services should be privileged in resource allocation decisions. Mainstays of public healthcare delivery—prenatal care and immunizations—often were cited as among the least controversial services to be included in a basic, minimum package of services (President's Commission for the Study of Ethical Problems in Medicine and Biomedical Behavioral Research 1983; Churchill 1987).

HIV and bioethics

Few public health challenges have forced the examination of ethics issues as often as HIV/AIDS. Essentially all of the classic public health ethics tensions emerged, from societal rights vs. individual liberties to justice and healthcare access, and issues emerged in range of core functions of public health: Surveillance, disease reporting, containment, and resource allocation. As policy makers contended with tough decisions, a large body of bioethics literature emerged, much in what might now be called public health ethics. Indeed, arguably, it was the HIV epidemic that introduced much of the bioethics world to the world of public health, its priorities, tools, and responses.

In 1983, the Public Health Service recommended that gay men be discouraged from donating blood (CDC 1983). Ronald Bayer, among the founders of public health ethics, responded with one of the earliest pieces on ethics and HIV (Bayer 1983). Two major US public policy documents, *Confronting AIDS* from the quasi-public Institute of Medicine (IOM 1986) and the *Report of the Presidential Commission on the Human Immunodeficiency Virus Epidemic* (Presidential Commission on the Human Immunodeficiency Virus Epidemic 1988) included significant sections on the ethical issues raised by the epidemic. Fear and uncertainty precipitated calls for restrictive proposals, from tattooing infected persons to full quarantine. While there was almost uniform rejection from the bioethics and legal communities of isolation of this sort (Gostin & Curran 1986; Koop 1986; Macklin 1986; Musto 1986; Porter 1986), policy proposals continued that advocated for the exclusion of HIV-infected persons from specific opportunities, such as employment, housing, insurance, and school. The bathhouses of San Francisco and the case of Ryan White—a child with haemophilia and HIV barred from his school—became symbols of the fear and discrimination that prompted questions about how to respond to the new public health crisis. Bioethics could not help but jump into the fray to help articulate an appropriate public health response.

Bridging clinical and public health ethics were examinations of the moral responsibilities of physicians to the wives of bisexual men, particularly HIV-infected bisexual men. Public health traditionally has protected unknowing contacts from risks of infection, while clinical medicine has enforced a tradition of patient confidentiality. Could bioethics help navigate the right response when these duties conflicted? Arguably, the area in which bioethics most engaged with the HIV epidemic and traditional public health was in debates about how best to design HIV screening programmes. Screening is a mainstay of public health. Back in the 1920s, criteria were established that needed to be satisfied before screening programmes could be implemented (Wilson & Jungner 1968; Cochrane & Holand 1971; Whitby 1974). In response to HIV, bioethicists, for the first time, put forward ethical requirements that must be in place before a public health screening programme can be imposed (Bayer 1989; Bayer *et al.* 1986; Gostin & Curran 1987; Gostin *et al.* 1987; Hunter 1987; Childress 1987). What types of screening programmes should be implemented was particularly vexing in the mid 1980s, a time when the screening tool had been licensed, but no treatments were yet available. Thus, those screened would not be helped, and they would be subject to discrimination. HIV screening was put forward so that infected persons might learn their status and, theoretically, would take precautions to prevent the spread to unknowing others. Little empirical evidence was available to demonstrate whether this assumption was true, however. Indeed, the limited research available provided somewhat contradictory findings (Doll *et al.* 1987; Coates *et al.* 1988; McCusker *et al.* 1988; Van Griesven *et al.* 1988). One study found that, while HIV-infected persons decrease their risky sexual practices once learning their status, uninfected persons engage in riskier behaviour once they are told they are uninfected (Fox *et al.* 1987). Such findings have tremendous implications given that, even in the highest prevalence communities, screening is likely to identify more uninfected persons than infected ones.

HIV also renewed interest in the ethics of other traditional tools of public health. Calls were made for mandatory reporting of HIV, contact tracing, and partner notification. Advocates of reporting suggested that more accurate understanding of the disease could be achieved with mandatory reporting and that education and potential treatments could be targeted to those found to be infected. Critics argued that education and potential treatments can be provided with or without reporting, while reporting was an unjustified invasion of privacy, particularly when strong antidiscrimination laws did not exist. As a result, they feared, at risk individuals would be driven from testing out of fear of the consequences. Not surprising, the momentum for mandatory reporting increased when treatments became available.

HIV also prompted ethics analysis regarding health education, duty to treat, resource allocation, access to care, and healthcare financing. Indeed, HIV stimulated public policy debate in almost every existing area of public health. As HIV gripped the United States, so did it grip the community of bioethicists, who became introduced to public health, why it exists, and how it operates. Through this more intimate knowledge of public health, bioethics

began to ponder when, ethically, public health should use particular response tools, and what criteria must be satisfied before the more invasive tools of public health can be dispatched. The phrase 'public health ethics', again, was not yet used, but the foundation of the field had been laid.

Public health ethics

After the important work of Beauchamp and Lappe, there was somewhat of a hiatus in thinking about public health ethics, formally, for another 15 years. Much more recently, however, there was a ground swell within bioethics recognizing that the ethics issues that emerged through public health were somewhat different in nature from ethics issues raised through medicine or other areas of bioethics and/or that similar ethics challenges emerged, but deserved to be *resolved* differently when encountered through public health. Several commentators offered frameworks, definitions, and analyses of public health ethics, claiming public health ethics to be its own subfield of bioethics, with its own priorities and approaches. In 2001 and 2002, four articles were published that defined public health ethics, its territory, and/or offered tools to use in its analysis (Kass 2001; Callahan & Jennings 2002; Childress *et al.* 2002; Roberts & Reich 2002), and in 2002, for the first time, the American Public Health Association, an organization that had existed since 1832, published its first code of ethics (APHA Code of Ethics 2002).

One article called for a framework of analysis for public health ethics that might differ from the existing frames for medical and research ethics (Kass 2001). Such a framework would give priority to certain public health interests while keeping in moral check the legally sanctioned police powers of public health. Another article sought to 'map the terrain' of public health ethics and identified particular ethics considerations that arise predictably in public health, from maximizing utility to preventing harm to distributing benefits fairly (Childress *et al.* 2002). Both of these contributions provide frameworks for analysis that include identifying programme goals, determining effectiveness, minimizing burdens, proportionality, and procedural justice.

Callahan and Jennings pointed out that public health has been concerned with social and economic inequality since nineteenth century, while bioethics, in its first decades, was more visibly concerned with the good of the individual. They identified four areas of public health that typically raise ethics issues: Health promotion, risk reduction, epidemiologic research, and interventions to reduce structural and economic disparities (Roberts & Reich 2002). Notably, they call for bioethics as a community to become more aware of the ethics issues that arise in public health.

Not coincidentally, all three of these articles also devote attention to social justice. Social justice is highly correlated with better health outcomes, and social justice is a recurring theme of public health (Powers & Faden 2006). Indeed, as will be described subsequently, public health practitioners rarely go far in examining epidemiologic correlations without finding important associations between poor health outcomes and social class and/or social position. An important question for public health ethics, then, is to what extent do public health professionals have an affirmative obligation to better *social* rather than, narrowly, health-related, conditions, in the name of public health? Such 'positive duties' remain more controversial than do the 'negative duties' of ensuring that citizens' health, rights, and opportunities are not interfered with by others, and yet there is growing literature within public health and public health ethics that such affirmative duties, at least to ensure the conditions under which individuals can be healthy, is indeed an obligation of public health.

Public health research

Literature related to ethics and public health research fall into two categories. First, there are articles that try to examine how public health research can be distinguished, both conceptually and operationally, from public health practice (CDC 1999; Casarett *et al.* 2000; Bellin & Dubler 2001; Amoroso & Middaugh 2003). This body of literature tries to lay out criteria defining when an activity is 'simply' quality assurance or evaluation vs. when it crosses the line to become research with humans. At stake in such a distinction is not simply intellectual precision; activities deemed to be research with humans cannot be conducted until they have been approved by an Institutional Review Committee, in accordance with the Code of Federal Regulations pertaining to human research, and individuals cannot be asked to participate or contribute their data until they have provided written consent or until those in charge obtain a waiver.

Second, there is a body of literature related to public health research and ethics that focuses more specifically on activities that unquestionably are research, but that ask whether public health research is different, again, from clinical research. As such, ought it to be exempt from certain types of review or requirements, and, in addition, do different ethics challenges emerge when one targets populations rather than individuals to be the subject of research intervention and inquiry. Both of these bodies of literature will be summarized briefly here.

Distinguishing public health research from non-research activities of public health

An early and widely cited document that sought to distinguish public health research from non-research was put forward by the Centers for Disease Control and Prevention (CDC) in 1999 (CDC 1999). This document built on an earlier published report from two CDC staff members (Snider & Stroup 1997). The CDC guidelines were written in response to queries from outsiders that certain activities conducted by CDC in the name of public health practice perhaps ought to have been categorized as research (Burris, Buehler & Lazzarini 2003). While the CDC guidelines were written primarily for CDC employees to help guide them in their own work, the distinctions raised are relevant to others in public health as well. The document acknowledges that federal regulations, when drafted, did not address whether or how they would apply to the mandatory data collection requirements of health departments. Specifically, all health departments have statutory authority to collect systematic data from individuals, using methods similar to those used in formal research investigations. And while federal regulations provide a definition of human research, the definition does not adequately distinguish public health research from 'non-research'. The 1999 CDC guidelines outline three public health activities—surveillance, emergency response, and evaluation—that are particularly susceptible to the quandary over whether the activity is research or non-research (CDC 1999). According to the CDC document, distinctions rest on what was the primary intent of the activity. If, primarily, the activity is designed to help a public health department do its job furthering the health interests of a particular community, even if it *also* produces data of more generalizable interest, the activity can and should be called non-research. Research, in contrast, always is intended to produce generalizable data, and the activity is designed from the beginning to have relevance beyond the population or programme from which data were collected. Surveillance activities, for example, are likely to be considered non-research when they are in response to 'lawful state disease reporting or monitoring' activities. When they are collected to learn information more broadly about similar populations or settings or more broadly about a given health condition, then activities are more likely to be considered as research. Sometimes, a state health department could be engaged in both. That is, they may be collecting data for purposes of statutorily authorized surveillance and reporting. However, they may also be collecting additional data on etiological causes of disease that would be of broader interest. This latter component may then be considered a research activity, but the data collected more narrowly for surveillance purposes would retain its categorization as a non-research activity. Conducting an evaluation is viewed by the CDC guidelines similarly. If the evaluation is conducted to examine how well a particular programme achieved its own objectives within a given setting or population, it likely would be considered non-research. If, instead, the evaluation were conducted to see if programmes *of this sort* generally worked with populations *of this sort*, then the activity likely would be considered research. Moreover, to the extent that environments are manipulated (e.g. one group receives a programme and the other does not, and outcomes are compared), activities are more likely to be considered research.

The CDC states that outbreak investigations and other emergency responses are and must be considered non-research. Indeed, state and local health departments arguably could not conduct their state-mandated functions if they were not classified in this way.

Academic scholars also have taken on this question of when an activity is research vs. non-research. Casarett *et al.* proposed two criteria for distinguishing quality improvement from research activities. While not focusing on the public health context *per se,* these authors set forward criteria that are quite different from those urged by the CDC. Rather than focusing on the purpose or intent of the activity, these authors are perhaps more consequentialist. Activities should be regulated as research, they say, if (1) the majority of patients involved are not expected to benefit directly from the knowledge to be gained and (2) additional risks and burdens exist as a result of wanting findings to be generalizable. That is, rather than asking if the activity is designed to gather generalizable knowledge, they ask, does creating generalizable knowledge change the risk/benefit ratio. They further suggest that their approach is more practical, contending that it may be difficult to determine intent and also that the results of most QI activities are generalizable to some degree. When lines are blurry, they say, it is appropriate to consider risk. This recommendation is corroborated, to some extent, by the recommendations from a CDC workshop on the topic of practice vs. research (MacQueen 2004). MacQueen and Buehler describe participants at this workshop debating two particular cases and recommending that the need for research oversight be determined on level of risk, while also stressing the need to ensure ethical and professional conduct, rather than making distinctions based on primary intent.

Bellin and Dubler, in contrast, say that an activity can be considered QI (rather than research) if there is a commitment, in advance of data collection, 'to a corrective action plan given any one of a number of possible outcomes. The sponsor of this review must have both clinical supervisory responsibility and the authority to impose change' (Bellin & Dubler 2001). That is, an activity should be considered quality improvement if there is a direct and clear commitment from someone with the power to make changes that evaluation results will lead to modifications, as necessary, in how the programme is structured or run. Otherwise, they say, the activity must be considered research. Amoroso and Middaugh continue the theme, suggesting that practice refers to interventions designed solely to enhance the well being of *specific* individuals, whereas research creates generalizable results (Amoroso & Middaugh 2003). They acknowledge, however, that in actual cases, categorizing particular activities can be challenging and they emphasize that such decisions should be made in advance and not left to journals to decide whether submitted manuscripts need to have had their work reviewed by an IRB.

Burris *et al.*, however, take on a more conceptual question. They contend that, while many of the tools and activities of public health practice resemble the tools and activities of research, a fundamental moral difference exists between public health departments performing these activities and others doing so. Public health departments are government agencies, 'carrying out a statutory mission to protect and promote collective health'. As such, when *they* collect data, they are doing so as a means of fulfilling their government-mandated *practice functions*. Burris, then, believes that the work of public health departments systematically should be exempt from the federal regulations and posits that those who suggest otherwise simply do not understand what public health agencies do. Under such a view, even those activities conducted by public health departments that others would put in the 'research' category—activities designed to gather generalizable knowledge— would be exempt from oversight by the Common Rule, expressly *because* they are conducted by public health departments. Importantly, however, an alternative, internal system would need be created to ensure that the 'human beings who become involved in activities that increase our knowledge (whether defined as research or not) should be protected'. Having internal review rather than using the preexisting Common Rule system is suggested not only out of efficiency (so that critical public health data collection activities can occur in a timely manner), it also is suggested because of a view that the usual balancing IRBs are asked to perform when they review research is misplaced if applied to public health departments. That is, most human research reviewed by IRBs ultimately is discretionary while the research of public health departments, in these authors' view, is less so since it is conducted as a means of fulfilling their public mandate. They propose that systems be put in place to ensure that data collection activities are conducted in the least harmful, least restrictive, and most respectful way possible, but should be judged less on whether or not they should be conducted (Burris *et al.* 2003).

The National Bioethics Advisory Commission (NBAC) suggested that, just as the physician performs clinical activities on behalf of the individual patient, public health professionals act on behalf of the population as a whole (National Bioethics Advisory Commission 2001). Furthermore, public health practice professionals are bound by a variety of laws that provide comparable ethics protections to the safeguards offered by IRBs. Specifically, public health laws 'address the requirements for informed consent, protections for privacy and confidentiality, procedures for collecting and handling information . . . and penalties for public health professionals when they do not comply with legal requirements' (National Bioethics Advisory Commission 2001). NBAC, however, takes a different position from Burris and, echoing CDC guidelines, suggests that projects *intended* to produce generalizable knowledge must be subject to the oversight provided by the Common Rule.

Perhaps the strongest voices in the literature for continued and ongoing oversight of public health data collection activities come from Fairchild and Bayer. Their view is that *all* data collection activities conducted by federal or state governments should be subject to ethical review, whether classified as practice or research. While not suggesting that IRBs necessarily perform this review, they advocate for universal review of these activities. Indeed, they argue, it is expressly because of the statutory requirement for data collection in public health that someone must ensure that public health does not overstep its reach: 'The invocation to act, especially when the individual rights of privacy and liberty may be impinged, must be subject to limits' (Fairchild & Bayer 2004). They provide as a hypothetical example that public health might try to link HIV registries with school registries, a proposal that might be denied if reviewed by an ethical board. Ethical review, they suggest, would help to keep public health authorities' power to collect identifiable data in check.

Ethical issues raised by public health research

The second body of literature summarized here examines activities clearly labelled as research. At stake, however, is whether ethics issues in *public health research* might differ somewhat from those of clinical research. Related, this literature asks whether the review considerations of IRBs should change to some degree when evaluating investigations labelled as public health research.

A series of papers, drafted mostly by epidemiologists, began to appear in the literature in the 1970s that suggested the need for certain types of epidemiological studies to maintain identifiers and, importantly, to waive the usual requirement for individual informed consent (Gordis *et al.* 1977; Kelsey 1981; Waters 1985). Gordis *et al.* contended that epidemiologists have important responsibilities in maintaining confidentiality, but also maintained that requiring patients' consent for researchers accessing patients' medical records would make retrospective record review studies essentially impossible to conduct (Gordis *et al.* 1977). They provide dozens of examples, from identifying the link between cigarette smoking and lung cancer, to the link between high concentrations of oxygen for premature infants and blindness, to the link between oral contraceptives and stroke, illustrating that epidemiologic record review studies have contributed enormously to our clinical and public health knowledge. Kelsey went further and suggested that, in some cases, written consent also should be waived for interview studies conducted in person, suggesting that the spirit of consent is important, but the act of signing may discourage some individuals from enrolment and simply may not be necessary for lower risk research

(Kelsey 1981). As a whole, these papers point out that epidemiologic research is less likely than clinical research to include patients and associated drug risks and more likely to be analysing records with associated privacy risks. Thus, they begin to suggest that there might be ways in which public health research is 'different' from clinical research. More specifically, they suggest that risks generally are low in epidemiologic research, leading them to make procedural recommendations for research review and oversight.

More recently, a conceptual literature has begun to explore whether and how population-based research and/or prevention research differ in ethically relevant ways from clinical research. Taylor and Johnson suggest that the research ethics literature generally has focused on the important ethics challenges from clinical research (generally with individuals) but has given little attention to issues raised by population-based research (Taylor & Johnson 2007). For example, population-based research may not allow individual participants the opportunity to refuse participation, something generally considered fundamental to ethical research with humans. Providing interventions at the level of the community rather than the level of the individual, by definition, means that everyone in that community automatically is exposed to the intervention. Studies, for example, have evaluated community-wide interventions, such as measuring the effect of fortifying flour or cereals in some but not all communities' rations, or determining the impact of health promotion media campaigns provided in some communities and not in others. When individuals cannot refuse their participation in a study, IRBs must determine that the level of risk for individuals is minimal and that the public health benefit resulting from the research outweighs the compromise to autonomy imposed by individuals' inability to refuse. Almost always in such cases, data are collected at the population level and without any individual identifiers. In some cases, there are mechanisms to inform the population as a whole that the research is being conducted, allowing for some level of disclosure or 'informing' to occur, even absent the ability to individually agree or decline participation.

Another ethics risk that may be more likely to exist in population-based research is social stigma or stereotyping of identifiable groups. Population-based research sometimes will target specific geographic, religious, or ethnic communities, or may target groups defined by a risk behaviour such as injection drug use or sexual orientation. As such, it has the potential to create social harms seen less often in clinical research that targets individuals. Specifically, not only might individuals enrolled in studies that target particular groups be at social risk by virtue of being associated with the study; moreover, the research study's results may be used to label or stereotype the population as a whole. Thus, even if researchers rigorously follow usual measures to safeguard confidentiality of individual identities, population-based research carries the risk that outsiders might think differently about an entire social group due to the research having been conducted. Consequently, it is from population-based research that community advisory boards (Strauss et al. 2001; Morin et al. 2003; Quinn 2004) and community-based participatory methods (Israel et al. 1998; Macaulay et al. 1999) have emerged as a means to get community input into planned designs as well as into how findings will be disseminated and described afterward. When communities potentially are put at risk by research, it is important, ethically, to get the views of groups best able to represent community-wide interests, just as individuals

must provide input for clinical research. Communities can give voice to, and respond to how rights and interests of communities will be protected in proposed research and how benefits that might offset any existing risks will be realized.

Finally, in the same way that traditional clinical trials have faced the question of whether successful interventions needed to be provided to research subjects—or at least to those who had been in the placebo group—after the trial is over, population-based trials increasingly are needing to consider what, if anything, will be made available to study communities when the research is completed. Particularly for research conducted in resource-poor communities, this new question has become quite contentious and has been the subject of significant bioethics attention. This has been the focus of some literature on Community Based Participatory Research. Also, guidelines of the Council for International Organization of Medical Sciences (CIOMS), drafted to advise researchers on ethical conduct for research in resource-poor settings, delineate that successful research interventions should be made 'reasonably available for the benefit of that population or community', although this is qualified in the CIOMS commentary by saying that decisions about what should be provided and in what manner must be decided on a case-by-case basis (CIOMS 2002). The World Health Organization's guide for developing countries on creating research ethics committees similarly says that 'a description of the availability and affordability of any successful study product to the concerned communities following the research' is a reasonable piece of ethics committee review but does not suggest that research should be approved only when future access can be guaranteed (WHO 2000). The National Bioethics Advisory Commission went further, suggesting that 'prior agreements'—that is, 'arrangements made before a trial begins that address the post-trial availability of effective interventions to the host community and/or country after the study has been completed'—should be made among 'producers, sponsors, and users' of research products; such agreements likely would lay out what will be available, to whom, for how long, and who will pay (National Bioethics Advisory Commission 2001). While clearly an attractive idea in principle, some have criticized this recommendation, saying that many policy commitments from donors and/or governments for translating important research findings into public health practice never could have been secured until the dramatic study results were in hand. Requiring agreements in advance, they say, would stifle important research from going forward. An empirical study with a variety of stakeholders, however, showed that 83 per cent of participants, 29 per cent of IRB chairs, and 42 per cent of researchers thought that an HIV-related intervention, if shown to be effective in a study, should be made available to all HIV-infected persons globally either for free or at a level they could personally afford (Pace et al. 2006). Another study showed that 37 per cent of US investigators working on intervention studies in developing countries believed it was 'true or sometimes true' that 'the intervention being tested is unlikely to be available to most citizens of the developing country in the foreseeable future' (Kass et al. 2003).

Finally, important in the evolution of thinking about public health research and ethics was a controversial legal case of 2001 related to a lead abatement trial conducted in the 1990s in Baltimore (Ericka Grimes vs. Kennedy Krieger Institute, Inc. 2001). This trial targeted low income housing units in old neighbourhoods that had both significant lead paint in units and where units often were in disrepair; that is, where children would be at risk of lead poisoning due to the existing poor conditions (Farfel & Chisolm 1990; Farfel & Chisolm 1991; Farfel & Chisolm 1994; Pollak 2002). Despite evidence for decades of the danger of lead paint, particularly to children, and despite continued high rates of lead poisoning among children in Baltimore, no laws existed requiring that houses be safe or abated before they could be rented to families. Thus, in the trial, households were randomized to one of several different lead abatement strategies in order to see the effect on both household lead dust and children's own blood lead levels of the varying abatement strategies. Two families later brought lawsuits, charging that researchers failed to warn them in a timely manner of children's continued risk of exposure and that families had not been fully informed of the risks of the research. The judge's ruling in the case garnered significant public attention for many reasons, including that he stated that this research was analogous to the Tuskegee syphilis study of 1932–1972 where poor, African-American men were deliberately denied penicillin for their syphilis. The judge further stated that families were 'enticed . . . into living in potentially lead-tainted housing', while researchers claimed that families benefited from having houses at least partially abated, given that public policy otherwise allowed landlords to rent completely unabated housing units to low-income families in these neighbourhoods.

This case was paradigmatic of certain types of public health research, in that it targeted a particular community, it dealt with prevention of a major public health problem and, significantly, it was designed to respond to a series of baseline conditions that were harmful to public health. Thus, debate ensued focused on what research ethics requires when public health research interventions are being evaluated in *settings of neglect*. Are public health researchers responsible for eliminating all of the neglect in order to be able to work in such environments? Or can public health researchers test interventions meant to ameliorate the harmful effects of such environments? Related, a panel was convened by the National Academy of Sciences to investigate ethics and prevention research in response to the issues raised by this case (Lo and O'Connell 2005).

To date, there continues to be no consensus regarding whether research is exploitive when situated in settings of neglect and when testing interventions that may improve conditions, but will not improve them as much as other, existing, currently unavailable interventions. Scholars have raised whether conducting research on 'partial solutions' condones the idea that partial solutions are adequate for the disadvantaged (Spriggs 2004; Farmer and Campos 2004; Buchanan and Miller 2006; Kass [under review]).

A few key ethics questions arise with this type of research. First, do the preexisting, risky background conditions (in this case, of lead paint poisoning) count as a risk of the study, or the condition being studied (Spriggs 2005)? Second, how likely, actually, is it that the partial solutions being tested through the research will have a better chance of being translated into practice, if shown to be effective, than 'full solutions' had been previously? That is, what justifies conducting research on partial abatement, or short course AZT for pregnant HIV-infected women in poor countries, or a number of other 'partial solutions' is that they might be simpler, more affordable, or otherwise generally more realistic as a policy option for governments, health departments, and individuals to consider using on a widespread basis. Presumably, studies of this sort only are considered where the 'full solution', existing interventions

(like full lead abatement, or longer courses of AZT for pregnant women) simply are not required or not otherwise being provided to communities at risk.

Miller and Buchanan suggest that rejecting all research on partial solutions out of a 'presumption that a particular conception of justice will eventually prevail'—that is, that the disadvantaged eventually will get access to existing, better interventions they have previously been unable to access—sacrifices the welfare of 'literally millions' of (in this case) children who could benefit from the results of the partial solutions tested through public health prevention research. Related, they assert that it is inappropriate to blame researchers for 'the lack of social consensus' on the right to better social conditions and that doing so is 'misplaced indignation' (Buchanan & Miller 2006).

Others, however, suggest that even the perception of exploitation raised through this case is harmful for the research enterprise and suggests a need for 'true partnership in the research enterprise, particularly when proposed research involves vulnerable communities' (Mastroianni & Kahn 2002).

Conclusion

Public health has only recently been given significant attention in the bioethics literature, both in terms of public health practice and public health research. However, the population focus of public health means that its duties are to safeguard the wellbeing of communities and populations as a whole rather than, primarily, the rights and well being of individuals. As such, public health practice must balance furthering the health of communities through education, surveillance, interventions, and regulations with needing to restrict the freedoms or privacy of individuals affected to the minimum degree possible. Public health is granted statutory authority to protect the public's health and, indeed extraordinary public health improvement has been achieved through sanitary measures, restaurant inspections, immunizations, and health education. At the same time, it is expressly because of this authority that ethics has such a critical role to play. Clear frameworks of ethics that lay out a need for data, minimizing of harms, and fair procedures, and clear principles to follow, including transparency, reciprocity, and equity, can help public health to do its duty to improve health on behalf of all of us, while allowing individuals who comprise 'the public' to feel confident that any restrictions are appropriate and fairly defined. Public health research requires some new considerations for research ethics. Research ethics will continue to require prior review by ethics committees—or IRBs—and will continue to require that benefits and risks be balanced and study populations be chosen fairly. Within public health research, however, new considerations will allow IRBs to be more mindful of the implications of research for populations as a whole, for finding creative ways to seek community-wide input, and to begin to consider how to ensure that communities, as well as individuals, realize research benefit.

References

Allen, R. (2007) Fostering professionalism during medical school and residency training. CME Report 3-A-01. *Report of the Council on Medical Education*. American Medical Association, Chicago.

American Public Health Association (2002). *APHA Code of Ethics*. Washington, DC.

Amoroso, P. and Middaugh, J. (2003). Research vs. public health practice: when does a study require IRB review? *Preventive Medicine*, **36**, 250–3.

Bayer, R. (1983). Gays and the stigma of bad blood. *Hastings Center Report*, **13**, 5–7.

Bayer, R. (1989). Ethical and social policy issues raised by HIV screening: the epidemic evolves and so do the challenges. *AIDS*, **3**, 119–24.

Bayer, R., Levine, C., Wolf, S.M. (1986). HIV antibody screening: an ethical framework for evaluating proposed programs. *Journal of the American Medical Association*, **256**, 1768–74.

Beauchamp, D.E. (1976). Alcoholism as blaming the alcoholic. *International Journal of Addiction*, **11**, 41–52.

Beauchamp, D.E. (1985). Community: the neglected tradition of public health. *The Hastings Center Report*, **15**, 28–36.

Beauchamp, D.E. (1985). Public health as social justice. *Inquiry*, **13**, 1–14.

Beauchamp, T.L. and Childress, J.L. (1979). *Principles of Biomedical Ethics.* Oxford University Press, Oxford.

Beauchamp, T.L. and Faden, R.R. (1979). The Right to Health and the Right to Health Care. *Journal of Medicine and Philosophy*, **4**, 118–131.

Bellin, E. and Dubler, N.N. (2001). The Quality Improvement-Research Divide and the Need for External Oversight. *American Journal of Public Health*, **91**, 1512–1517.

Blank, R.H. (1988). *Rationing Medicine*. Columbia University Press, New York.

Brody, B. (1981). Health Care for the haves and have nots. Toward a just basis of distribution. Shelp E.E., ed. In *Justice and Health Care*. Reidel, Boston, 151–159.

Buchanan, A.E.(1984). The right to a decent minimum of health care. *Philosophy and Public Affairs*, **13**, 55–78.

Buchanan, D.R. and Miller, F.G. (2006). Justice and Fairness in the Kennedy Krieger Institute Lead Paint Study: the Ethics of Public Health Research on Less Expensive, Less Effective Interventions. *American Journal of Public Health*, **96**, 781–787.

Burris, S, Buehler, J, Lazzarini, Z (2003). Applying the Common Rule to Public Health Agencies: Questions and Tentative Answers about a Separate Regulatory Regime. *J Law Med Ethics*, **31**, 638–653.

Callahan, D. (1984). Autonomy: A Moral Good, Not a Moral Obsession. *The Hastings Center Report*, **14**, 40–42.

Callahan, D. (1988). Meeting Needs and Rationing Care. *Law, Medicine and Health Care*, **16**, 261–66.

Callahan, D. (1988). *Setting Limits: Medical Goals in an Aging Society.* Touchstone Books, New York.

Callahan, D. and Jennings, B. (2002). Ethics and Public Health: Forging a Strong Relationship. *American Journal of Public Health*, **92**, 169–176.

Casarett, D., Karlawish, J.H.T., Sugarman, J. (2000). Determining When Quality Improvement Initiatives Should Be Considered Research: Proposed Criteria and Potential Implications. *Journal of the American Medical Association*, **283**, 2275–2280.

Centers for Disease Control (1983). Current Trends Prevention of Acquired Immune Deficiency Syndrome: Report of Inter-Agency Recommendations. *Morbidity and Mortality Weekly Report*, **32**, 101–3.

Centers for Disease Control (1999). *Guidelines for Defining Public Health Research and Public Health Non-Research*. Atlanta.

Childress, J.F. (1987). An Ethical Framework for Assessing Policies to Screen for Antibodies for HIV. *AIDS Public Policy Journal*, **2**, 28–31.

Childress, J.F. *et al.* (2002). Public Health Ethics: Mapping the Terrain. *Journal of Law, Medicine, and Ethics*, **30**, 170–178.

Churchill, L. (1987). *Rationing Health Care in America*. University of Notre Dame Press, Notre Dame.

Clouser, K.D. (1995). Common Morality as an Alternative to Principlism. *Kennedy Institute of Ethics Journal*, **5**, 219–236.

Coates, T.J., Stall, R.D., Kegeles, S.M., Lo, B., Morin, S.F., McKusic, L (1988). AIDS antibody testing. *American Psychology*, **43**, 859–64.

Cochrane, A.L. and Holland, W.W. (1971). Validation of Screening Procedures. *British Medical Bulletin*, **27**, 3–8.

Council for International Organizations of Medical Sciences (2002). *International Ethical Guidelines for Biomedical Research Involving Human Subjects*, World Health Organization, Geneva.

Daniels, N. (1981). Health-care needs and distributive justice. *Philosophy and Public Affairs*, **10**, 146–79.

Daniels, N. (1985). *Just Health Care*. Cambridge, New York. 245.

Daniels, N. (1992). *Am I My Parent's Keeper? An Essay on Justice Between the Young and Old*. Oxford University Press, New York.

Doll, L.S., Darrow, W., O'Malley, P., Bodecker, T., Jaffe, H. (1987). *Self-reported Behavioral Change in Homosexual Men in the San Francisco City Clinic Cohort*. Presented at 3rd International AIDS Conference, Washington, DC.

Engelhardt, H.T. (1986). Rights to Health Care, Social Justice, and Fairness in Healthcare Allocations. In *Foundation of Bioethics*. Oxford University Press, New York.

Ericka Grimes, v. Kennedy Krieger Institute, Inc. (2001). West's Atl Report. 2001, **782**, 807–62. Baltimore, MD.

Faden, R.R. (1987). Ethical issues in government sponsored public health campaigns. *Health Education Quarterly*, **14**, 27–37.

Faden, R.R. and Faden, A.I. (1978). the ethics of health education as public policy. *Health Education Monographs*, **6**, 180–197.

Faden, R.R. and Kass, N.E. (1991). Bioethics and public health in the 1980s: resource allocation and AIDS. *Annual Reviews of Public Health*, **12**, 335–360.

Fairchild, A.L., Bayer, R. (2004). Public health: ethics and the conduct of public health surveillance. *Science*, **303**, 631–632.

Farfel, M.R. and Chisolm, J.J. (1990). Health and environmental outcomes of traditional and modified practices for abatement of residential lead-based paint. *American Journal of Public Health*, **80**, 1240–1245.

Farfel, M.R. and Chisolm, J.J. (1991). An evaluation of experimental practices for abatement of residential lead-based paint: report on a pilot project. *Environmental Research*, **55**, 199–212.

Farfel, M.R. and Chisolm, J.J. (1994). The longer-term effectiveness of residential lead paint abatement. *Environmental Research,* **66**, 217–221.

Farmer, P. and Campos, N.G. (2004). New malaise: bioethics and human rights in the global era. *Journal of Law and Medical Ethics,* **32**, 243–251.

Fee, E. (1977). History and development of public health. In *Principles of Public Health Practice* (Scutchfield F.D., Keck C.W., eds.). Delmar Publishers, Boston, 10–30.

Fox, R., Odaka, N.J., Brookmeyer, R., and Polk, B.F. (1987). Effect of HIV antibody disclosure on subsequent sexual activity in homosexual men. *AIDS*, **1**, 241–46.

Fried, C. (1975). Rights in health care—beyond equity and efficiency. *New England Journal of Medicine*, **293**, 241–245.

Fried, C. (1976). Equality and rights in medical care. *Hastings Center Report*, **6**, 29–34.

Gibbard, A. (1982). The prospective Pareto principle and equity of access to health care. *Milbank Memorial Fund Quarterly*, **60**, 399–428.

Glanz, K., Lewis, F.M., and Rimer, B.K. (1997) *Health Behavior and Health Education: Theory, Research and Practice (2nd Ed.)* Jossey-Bass, San Francisco.

Gordis, L., Gold, E., and Seltser, R. (1977). Privacy protection in epidemiologic and medical research: a challenge and a responsibility. *American Journal of Epidemiology*, **105**, 163–168.

Gostin, L. and Curran, W.J. (1986). The limit of compulsion on controlling AIDS. *Hastings Center Report*, **16**, 24–29.

Gostin, L. and Curran, W.J. (1987). Legal control measures for AIDS: reporting requirements, surveillance, quarantine, and regulation of public meeting places. *American Journal of Public Health*, **77**, 214–218.

Gostin, L., Curran, W.J., and Clark, M.E. (1987). The case against compulsory casefinding in controlling AIDS—testing, screening and reporting. *American Journal of Law and Medicine*, **12**, 7–53.

Green, R.M. (1983). The priority of health care. *Journal of Medical Philosophy*, **8**, 373–380.

Hunter, N.D. (1987). AIDS prevention and civil liberties: the false security of mandatory testing. *AIDS Public Policy Journal*, **2**, 1–10.

Institute of Medicine (1986). *Confronting AIDS: Directions for Public Health, Health Care, and Research*. National Academies Press, Washington, DC.

Israel, B.A., Schulz, A.J., Parker, E.A., Becker, A.B. (1998). Review of community-based research: assessing partnership approaches to improve public health. *Annu Rev Public Health*, **19**, 173–202.

Jonsen, A.R. (1995). Casuistry: an alternative or complement to principles? *Kennedy Institute of Ethics Journal*, **5**, 237–251.

Kao, A., Lim, M., Spevick, J., Barzansky, B. (2003). Teaching and evaluating students' professionalism in US Medical Schools, 2002–2003. *JAMA*, **290**, 1151–1152.

Kass, N.E. Just research in an unjust world [manuscript under review].

Kass, N.E. (2001). An Ethics Framework for Public Health. *American Journal of Public Health*, **91**, 1776–1782.

Kass, N., Dawson, L., Loyo-Berrios, N.I. (2003). Ethical oversight of research in developing countries. *IRB Ethics & Human Research*, **25**, 1–10.

Kelsey, J.L. (1981). Privacy and confidentiality in epidemiological research involving patients. *IRB*, **3**, 1–4.

Koop, C.E. (1986). Surgeon generals report on acquired immune deficiency syndrome. *Journal of the American Medical Association*, **256**, 278–89.

Lappe, M. (1986). Ethics and public health. In *Maxcy-Rosenau Public Health and Preventive Medicine, Twelfth Edition* (Last J.M., ed.), Appleton-Century-Crofts, Norwalk, Connecticut, 1867–77.

Lo, B. and O'Connell, M.E. (2005). Ethical considerations for research on housing-related health hazards involving children. *Committee on Ethical Issues in Housing-Related Health Hazard Research Involving Children, Youth and Families*, National Academies Press, Washington DC.

Macaulay, A.C. *et al.* (1999). Participatory research maximizes community and lay involvement. *British Medical Journal*, **319**, 774–778.

Macklin, R. (1986). Predicting dangerousness and public health response to AIDS. *Hastings Center Report*, **16**, 16–23.

MacQueen, K.M. and Buehler, J.W. (2004). Ethics, practice, and research in public health. *American Journal of Public Health*, **94**, 928–931.

Mastroianni, A.C. and Kahn, J.P. (2002). Risk and responsibility: ethics, Grimes v Kennedy Krieger, and public health research involving children. *American Journal of Public Health*, **92**, 1073–1076.

McCullough, L.B., ed. (1998). *John Gregory's Writings on Medical Ethics & Philosophy of Medicine*, Kluwer Academic Publishers, Dordrecht.

McCusker, J, Stoddard, A.M., Mayer, K.H., Zapka, J, Morrison, C, Salzman, S.P. (1988). Effects of HIV antibody test knowledge on subsequent sexual behaviors in a cohort of homosexually active men. *American Journal of Public Health*, **78**, 462–67.

Menzel, P.T. (1983). *Medical Costs, Moral Choices: A Philosophy of Health Care Economics in America*. Yale University Press, New Haven.

Morin, S.F., Maiorana, A., Koester, K.A., Sheon, N.M., Richards, T.A. (2003). Community consultation in HIV prevention research: a study of community advisory boards at 6 research sites. *JAIDS*, **33**, 513–520.

Musto, D.F. (1986). Quarantine and the problem of AIDS. *Milbank Memorial Fund Quarterly*, **64**, 113.

National Bioethics Advisory Commission (2001). *Ethical and Policy Issues in Research Involving Human Participants: Volume I: Report and Recommendations of the National Bioethics Advisory Commission*. Bethesda, MD.

National Commission for the Protection of Human Subjects of Biomedical and Behavioral Research (1979). *The Belmont Report: Ethical Principles and Guidelines for the Protection of Human Subjects of Research*.

Pace, C. *et al.* (2006). Post-trial access to tested interventions: the views of IRB/REC chair, investigators, and research participants in a multinational HIV/AIDS study. *AIDS Research and Human Retroviruses*, **22**, 837–841.

Pellegrino, E.D. (1981). Health promotion as public policy: the need for moral groundings. *Preventive Medicine*, **10**, 371–378.

Pellegrino, E.D. (1988). Rationing health care: the ethics of medical gatekeeping. In *Medical Ethics: A Guide for Health Professionals* (Monagle J.F., Thomasma D.C., eds), Aspen, Rockville, MD, 261–70.

Pellegrino, E.D. (1995). Toward a virtue-based normative ethics for health professions. *Kennedy Institute of Ethics Journal*, **5**, 253–277.

Pellegrino, E. and Thomasma, D.C. (1988). *For the Patient's Good: The Restoration of Beneficence in Health Care*. Oxford University Press, New York.

Percival, T. (1985). Medical Ethics; or a Code of Institutes and Precepts, adapted to the Professional Conduct of Physicians and Surgeons . . . together with an Introduction by Edmund D. Pellegrino. Classics of Medicine Library, Birmingham.

Pollak, J. (2002). The lead-based paint abatement repair and maintenance study in Baltimore: historic framework and study design. *Journal of Health Care Law and Policy*, **6**, 89–108.

Porter, R. (1986). History says no to the policeman's response to AIDS. *British Medical Journal*, **293**, 1589–90.

Powers, M. and Faden, R. (2006). *Social Justice: The Moral Foundations of Public Health and Health Policy*. Oxford University Press, New York.

Presidential Commission on the Human Immunodeficiency Virus Epidemic (1988). *Final Report*. Government Printing Office, Washington DC.

President's Commission for the Study of Ethical Problems in Medicine and Biomedical and Behavioral Research (1983). *Securing Access to Health Care: The Ethical Implications of Differences in the Availability of Health Services*. Volume One: Report, 1983. Government Printing Office, Washington DC, 201.

Quinn, S.C. (2004). Ethics in public health research: protecting human subjects: the role of Community Advisory Boards. *American Journal of Public Health*, **94**, 918–22.

Ramsey, P. (1973). The nature of medical ethics. In Veatch R.M., Gaylin W., Morgan, eds, *National Conference on the Teaching of Medical Ethics*, pp. 14–28. New York: Hastings Center.

Roberts, M.J. and Reich, M.R. (2002). Ethical analysis in public health. *The Lancet*, **359**, 1055–9.

Roter, D.L., Hall, J.A., Merisca, R., Ruehle, B., Cretin, D., Svarstad, B. (1998). Effectiveness of interventions to improve patient compliance: a meta-analysis. *Medical Care*, **36**, 1138–61.

Snider, D.E. and Stroup, D.F. (1997). Defining research when it comes to public health. *Public Health Reports*, **112**, 29–112.

Society for Public Health Education (1992). *Code of Ethics for the Health Education Profession*. Section 4. http://www.sophe.org/ Accessed 11/4/03.

Spriggs, M. (2004). Canaries in the mines: children, risk, non-therapeutic research, and justice. *Journal of Medical Ethics*, **30**, 176–81.

Steinbock, B. (1996). Liberty, responsibility, and the common good. *The Hastings Center Report*, **26**, 45–47.

Strauss, R.P. *et al.* (2001). The role of Community Advisory Boards: involving communities in the informed consent process. *American Journal of Public Health*, **91**, 1938–43.

Taylor, H.A. and Johnson, S. (2007). Ethics of population-based research. *Journal of Law, Medicine & Ethics*, **35**, 295–9.

Van Griesven, G.J.P. *et al.* (1988). Impact of HIV antibody testing on changes in sexual behavior among homosexual men in the Netherlands. *American Journal of Public Health*, **79**, 1575–77.

Walzer, M. (1983). *Spheres of Justice*. Basic Books, New York.

Waters, W.E. (1985). Ethics and epidemiological research. *International Journal of Epidemiology*, **14**, 48–51.

Wikler, D.I. (1978). Coercive measures in health promotion: can they be justified? *Health Education Monographs*, **6**, 223–41.

Wikler, D.I. (1978). Persuasion and coercion for health. *Milbank Memorial Fund Quarterly/Health and Society*, **56**, 303–33.

Whitby, L.G. (1974). Screening for disease: definitions and criteria. *Lancet*, **819**.

Wilson, J.M.G. and Jungner, F. (1968). *Principles and Practice of Screening for Disease*. Public Health Papers, No 34. World Health Organization, Geneva.

Winslow, G.R. (1986). Rationing and publicity. In *The Price of Health* (eds Agich, G.J. and Begley, C.E.) Reidel, Boston, 199–215.

World Health Organization (2000). *Operational Guidelines for Ethics Committees That Review Biomedical Research*. WHO, Geneva.

Index

Page numbers in **bold** refer to major sections of the text.

Since the major subject of this title is public health, entries under this keyword have been kept to a minimum, and readers are advised to seek more specific references.

Indexing style
Alphabetical order. This index is in letter-by-letter order, whereby hyphens, en-rules and spaces within index headings are ignored in the alphabetization. Terms in brackets are excluded from initial alphabetization.

Main abbreviations used
AIDS acquired immunodeficiency syndrome
ANOVA analysis of variance
BMI body mass index
CJD Creutzfeldt-Jakob disease
COPD chronic obstructive pulmonary disease
HIV human immunodeficiency virus
SARS sudden acute respiratory syndrome
STIs sexually transmitted infections

Other abbreviations are defined in the index

M

McGill Pain questionnaire 417
Machupo virus 1398
macroeconomic policy 107
macroergonomics 920
macro errors 466
magnetic resonance imaging 842
Mahler, Halfdan 318
malaria 58, **1231**
　anopheline mosquito vectors 1235
　　capacity and entomological inoculation
　　　rate 1236
　　geographical patterns of
　　　transmission 1236
　antimalarial drug resistance 1241
　　epidemiology 1242
　antimalarial drugs 1241
　cerebral 1238
　control 48, 1244
　　adult vector control 1244
　　breeding site and larva 1244
　　insecticide-impregnated-treated
　　　bednets 1245
　　vector control 1244
　DALYs *858*
　diagnosis 1240
　diversity of disease 1238
　endemicity 1232
　epidemiology 1238
　　human activities and 1239
　forced migrants 1522
　and gender 1430
　global disease burden 1603
　history 1231
　and HIV 1239
　mortality 263, *858*
　　children 262
　parasites 1233, *1233*
　　biological differences 1234
　　life cycle 1233–4
　　molecular biology 1235
　　sporogonic development 1233
　pathogenesis 1236
　　disease and malaria species 1237
　　genetic factors 1237
　　host response 1237
　　infection and disease 1236
　　undernutrition and micronutrient
　　　deficiencies 1237
　in pregnancy 1239
　　maternal mortality ratio 1240
　public health importance 1232
　treatment
　　at home 1245
　　intermittent preventive 1245
　　passive case finding 1245
　　prophylaxis 1245
　　vaccines 1245
　　see also antimalarial drugs
　under-fives 1443
　urban 1389
　vaccines 1243, *1243*
Malaria Eradication Programme 701
malathion 1612
Malawi, mortality by age 737
Malaysia
　legislation
　　communicable disease control 362
　　obesity 363
　　tobacco 363

Maldives, natural disasters *1699*
male condoms 1199
Mali, disability prevalence *1484*
malnutrition 178, 194, *827*
　adolescents 1458
　case management 1444
　causes 178
　children
　　mortality 262
　　rickets 138
　　and skilled birth attendance 114–16
　　under-fives 1444
　forced migrants 1523
　and malaria 1237
　micronutrients 181, *181*
　prevention 1444
　see also micronutrient deficiencies
management 318, *319*, 783, **788**
　challenges 793
　　disease spectrum and health
　　　emergencies 793
　　health-care reform and financing 794
　　health workforce 793
　　technology and infrastructure 793
　definition 788
　nonprofit organizations 791
　in public health 792
　skills 791
　theory 790
management information systems 398
man-made disasters 1698
Mantel-Haenszel test 515, 518, 602
manual handling 919
　nursing 919
maple syrup urine disease *146*
marasmus 179
Marburg virus 1265, 1398
Marfan syndrome *143*
markers 139
　elimination 885
　of exposure 874
marriage 1414
　age of 1416
　gay 1417
Marx, Karl 108
masks 1406
mass-action principle 669, 677
mass miniature radiography 1623
mass vaccination 682
　impact of 688–9
　reduction of disease incidence 691
matched-pair design 544
　analysis 549, 551
matching, case-control studies 612
material circumstances 105, 109
material progress 295
maternal age 1416
maternal and child health care 42
maternal mortality 302, 1421, 1714
　human rights approach 343
mathematical models *see* modelling
maximum likelihood 598
mean 645
　comparison of 658, *658, 665*
　sampling distribution of 652
　standard error of 653
measles *671*, 1604
　age-dependent mortality 691
　case notifications 678, 690
　duration of infection *686*

epidemiology *685*
forced migrants 1522
island communities *680*
mortality *864*
quarantine 1614
vaccine 50–1, 1607
measure of association 619
measure of effect 619
　derivation 632, *633*
measurement validity 599–600, 607
mebendazole *217*, 1609
mechanically recovered meat 1165
media, violence depicted in 1355
median 645
mediation 756
medical examinations 907
medical examiner reports 708
Medical Expenditure Panel Survey 402
Medical Outcome Study Short Forms 52
medical sociology 719
　areas of investigation 725
　　chronic illness 725
　　sociology and place 726
　consensual theories 720
　qualitative research 722
　　data analysis 724
　　data collection 723
　　research designs 722
　　study numbers and sampling 723
　　synthesis 725
　　validity 724
　quantitative research 721
　　assumptions and procedures 721, *722*
　　data collection 722
　social action theories 721
　structural theories 720
　structure and agency 721
medium chain acyl CoA dehydrogenase
　deficiency *146*
MEDLINE 428, 435, 626, 634
MedlinePlus 428
mefloquine 1241, 1265
megacities 1377
meiosis 139
melanoma 847, 1011
melioidosis 1371, *1397*
men
　drinking habits 1428
　life expectancy *1420*
　mortality 1420, *1420–1*
　see also gender
Mendelian inheritance 139–40
Mendelian randomization 963
meningitis 206
　aetiology 206, *207*
　bacterial *671*
　medical treatment 207
　presentation and diagnosis 207, *207*
　prevention 208
meningococcal meningitis
　in forced migrants 1523
　mortality *864*
mental health 1081, **1098**
　definition 1081
　determinants of 1093
　　social 1093, *1095*
　forced migrants 1524
　and gender 1429
　and global health 1098
　ideology 1087

needs assessment (*continued*)
  rapid assessment procedures 1557
  severe obesity 1559
  stages of 1552
  stakeholder advisory group 1551–2
  strengths and weaknesses *1558*
  timing 1550
  undertaking 1551
  value of 1557
needs-based formulas 1541–2
needs and wants 1537
negative externalities 802
neglected diseases, human rights
      approach 340
negotiation 790
Neisseria
  *N. gonorrhoeae 671,*859, *1174,* 1604, 1610
    chemoprophylaxis 1609
    control 1605
  N. meningitidis 207, 1268
neo-liberalism 87, 800
neonatal care 1417, 1439, *1440,* 1441
neonatal screening 145, *146,* 1634, *1634*
  cystic fibrosis *146*
  phenylketonuria 145, *146*
  sickle cell disease *146,* 1631
    outcome *1632*
neonatal sepsis 204, *204*
  aetiology 204
  bacterial causes *205*
  diagnostic criteria *204*
  epidemiology 204
  evidence-based interventions 204
  medical treatment 204, *205*
  prevention 206
neoplasms *see* cancer
Nepal
  community health workers *1690*
  life expectancy *1420*
  mortality, under-fives *1421*
  sanitation 44
nerve entrapment syndromes 922
Netherlands
  age-standardized mortality *301*
  asthma prevalence *1031*
  CJD
    case numbers *1164*
      mortality 1162
  health inequaliy *1568*
  height differences *1569*
  mental health disorders *1083*
  mortality 972, *1564*
  resource allocation 1675
  socioeconomic health inequality 1575
  trade in pharmaceuticals *89*
Net Reproduction Rate 741
networking 831
networks 397
neural tube defects
  genetic associations *141*
  prevention 1594
neurofibromatosis *143*
neurologic diseases **1132**
  dementia 1141
  epilepsy 1138
  headache 1133, *1133*
  multiple sclerosis 1150
  parkinsonism 1148
  peripheral neuropathy 1146
  traumatic brain injury 1136

neuropathy
  diabetic 1074, 1147
  peripheral 1146
    carpal tunnel syndrome 1147
    clinical overview 1146
    infection-related 1148
    nutritional 1147
neutraceuticals 194
New Caledonia, measles persistence *680*
new drugs 1673
New Hebrides, measles persistence *680*
new public health 720, 752
new public management 812
New Zealand
  age-standardized mortality *301*
  asthma prevalence *1031*
  mortality 972
NHANES 401, 472, 881, 936, 1643
  sampling methods 478
nickel *1004*
nico test 966
nicotine dependence 1284
nicotine replacement therapy 373, 1292
NIDA Clinical Trial Network 1310
Niger
  life expectancy *1420*
  mortality, under-fives *1421*
Nigeria
  mental health disorders *1083*
  overweight population *96*
Nipah virus 232, 491, 1266, 1371
Niue, measles persistence *680*
noise *827*
noise-induced hearing loss 897
non-alcoholic fatty liver disease 1258
  diagnosis 1259
  and metabolic syndrome 1259
  natural history 1260
  prevalence 1259
non-alcoholic steatohepatitis 1258
  diagnosis 1259
  and metabolic syndrome 1259
  natural history 1260
  prevalence 1259
non-communicable chronic diseases 3, 5–7, 93,
      263, 725, **1592**
  adaptation 726
  biographical disruption 725
  causation 1595
  causes 12
  DALYs 1594
  and diet 186
  environmental risk factors 1597
  future of 1599
  genetic and molecular epidemiology 1597
  global burden 54, 1592–3
  infectious causes 859, *859*
  mortality 1592–3
  prevention 192, 1593
    health care 1596
    health promotion 1595
    integrated approach 1598
    life-course approach 1597
    screening 1594, *1595*
  projections 268
  risk factors 1715
  self-management 726
  social determinants of health 1596
  suffering and loss of self 726
  see also individual diseases

Non-communicable Disease Prevention
    Program (CINDI) 558
non-differential errors 601
non-discrimination 340
non-financial incentives 1686
non-governmental organizations (NGOs) 44,
      370
  mitigation of consequences of war 1374
non-inferiority 528
non-ionizing radiation, and cancer 1003
non-marital childbearing 1415–16
non-probability sample 643
nonprofit organizations, management 791
non-refoulement 1519
non-response 476
  adjusting for 478
  biological samples 477
  improving 477
  item non-response 478
non-State actors 335
normal distribution 647, 649–51
  standard 650
    working with 650
norms, societal 1672
norovirus *210*
North America
  fertility 735
  Internet usage *428*
  iodine deficiency *183*
  life expectancy 735
  mortality, adolescents *1455*
  obesity/overweight *1054*
    children *1055*
  older population 1498
  typhoid fever *214*
North Karelia Project **557**
  results 562
Norway
  age-standardized mortality *301*
  e height differences *1569*
  health inequaliy *1568*
  mortality *1564*
notification systems 706
Nottingham Health Profile 417
nuclear weapons 1369
  treaties 1373
nucleotide 139
nuisance 26
null bias 601
number needed to screen 965, *966*
number needed to treat 632, 965
nutrigenomics 151
nutrition 20, **177**, 1715
  and chronic disease 186
  and disease prevention 194
  under-fives 1437
  see also diet
nutritional neuropathies 1147
nutritional status 179
nutrition transition 93, 194, 1051, 1053, *1054*

O
obesity 93, 95, *96,* 122, 190, *190,* 194, 292, 802,
      1046, 1429
  abdominal 1048, *1048*
  adolescents 1458
  and asthma risk 1035
  biological and societal maintenance 1059,
      1060
  BMI *see* body mass index